Paediatric
Handbook

Paediatric Handbook

NINTH EDITION

Edited by

Amanda Gwee

General Paediatrician & Infectious Diseases Physician
Department of General Medicine
Honorary Fellow
Murdoch Childrens Research Institute
Victoria, Australia

Romi Rimer

General Paediatrician
Department of General Medicine
Victoria, Australia

Michael Marks

General Paediatrician
Department of General Medicine
Associate Professor
Department of Paediatrics
University of Melbourne
Honorary Fellow
Murdoch Childrens Research Institute
Victoria, Australia

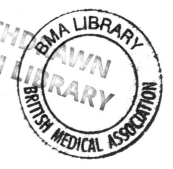

WILEY Blackwell

This edition first published in 2015 © 2015 by John Wiley & Sons Ltd

Registered office: John Wiley & Sons, Ltd, The Atrium, Southern Gate, Chichester, West Sussex, PO19 8SQ, UK

Editorial offices: 9600 Garsington Road, Oxford, OX4 2DQ, UK
    The Atrium, Southern Gate, Chichester, West Sussex, PO19 8SQ, UK ·
    1606 Golden Aspen Drive, Suites 103 and 104, Ames, Iowa 50010, USA

For details of our global editorial offices, for customer services and for information about how to apply for permission to reuse the copyright material in this book please see our website at www.wiley.com/wiley-blackwell

Library of Congress Cataloging-in-Publication Data

Paediatric handbook (Royal Children's Hospital)
    Paediatric handbook / edited by Amanda Gwee, Romi Rimer, Michael Marks. – Ninth edition.
      p. ; cm.
    "From Royal Children's Hospital in Melbourne."
    Includes bibliographical references and index.
    ISBN 978-1-118-77748-0 (pbk.)
    I. Gwee, Amanda, editor.   II. Rimer, Romi, editor.   III. Marks, Michael (Michael Kenneth), editor.   IV. Royal Children's Hospital, issuing body.   V. Title.
    [DNLM: 1. Pediatrics–Handbooks.   WS 39]
    RJ48
    618.92–dc23

                                                                                2015004077

A catalogue record for this book is available from the British Library.

Wiley also publishes its books in a variety of electronic formats. Some content that appears in print may not be available in electronic books.

Cover photo and design: The Royal Children's Hospital Educational Resource Centre

Set in 7.5/9.5pt Frutiger Light by Aptara Inc., New Delhi, India
Printed and bound in Malaysia by Vivar Printing Sdn Bhd

1   2015

Contents

Contents

Contributors

George Alex, MBBS, FRACP, MMed, MRCP, PhD
Paediatric Gastroenterologist
Department of Gastroenterology
Royal Children's Hospital
Victoria, Australia

Roger Allen, MBBS, FRACP
Paediatric Rheumatologist
Department of General Medicine
Royal Children's Hospital
Victoria, Australia

David Amor, MBBS, PhD, FRACP, FFSc(RCPA)
Clinical Geneticist and Medical Director
Victorian Clinical Genetics Services
Murdoch Childrens Research Institute
Victoria, Australia

Peter Barnett, MBBS, FRACP, MSc, FACEM, MSpMed
Deputy Director
Emergency Department
Royal Children's Hospital
Clinical Associate Professor, University of Melbourne
Victoria, Australia

Antun Bogovic, BPharm, MSHP
Deputy Director
Pharmacy Department
Royal Children's Hospital
Victoria, Australia

Fergus Cameron, BMedSci, MBBS, DipRACOG, FRACP, MD
Head, Diabetes Services and Deputy Director
Department of Endocrinology and Diabetes and
    Centre for Hormone Research
Royal Children's Hospital and Murdoch Childrens
    Research Institute
Victoria, Australia

George Chalkiadis, MBBS, DA(Lon), FANZCA,
FFPMANZCA
Staff Anaesthetist
Head, Children's Pain Management Service
Royal Children's Hospital and Murdoch Childrens
    Research Institute
Clinical Associate Professor, Department of
    Paediatrics, University of Melbourne
Victoria, Australia

Michael Cheung, Bsc (Hons), MBChB, MRCP, MD, FRACP
Director, Department of Cardiology, Royal Children's
    Hospital
Heart Research Group Leader, Murdoch Childrens
    Research Institute
Principal Fellow, University of Melbourne
Victoria, Australia

Tom Clarnette, MBBS, MD, FRACS (Paeds)
Consultant Paediatrician Surgeon
Royal Children's Hospital
Victoria, Australia

Michael Clifford, MMBS (Hons), FCICM, FANZCA,
PGDipCU
Resuscitation Officer
Department(s) of Paediatric Intensive Care and
    Anaesthesia and Pain Management
Royal Children's Hospital
Victoria, Australia

Tom Connell, BMedSci, MRCPI, FRACP, PhD
Paediatrician, Infectious Diseases Physician
Department of General Medicine
Royal Children's Hospital
Victoria, Australia

Noel Cranswick, MBBS, BMedSci, FRACP
Director, Clinical Pharmacology
Director, Australian Paediatric Pharmacology
    Research Unit
Royal Children's Hospital and Murdoch Childrens
    Research Institute
Associate Professor, University of Melbourne
Victoria, Australia

Nigel Crawford, MBBS, MPH, PhD, FRACP
General Paediatrician
Medical Head, Immunisation Services, Department of
    General Medicine, Royal Children's Hospital
Deputy Director, SAEFVIC, Murdoch Childrens
    Research Institute
Senior Fellow, Department of Paediatrics, University
    of Melbourne
Victoria, Australia

List of Contributors

Nigel Curtis, BArts, MArts, MBBS, DipTropMed and Hygiene, FRCPCH, PhD
Head of Paediatric Infectious Diseases Unit, Department of General Medicine
Royal Children's Hospital and Murdoch Childrens Research Institute
Chair of Infectious Diseases, Department of Paediatrics, University of Melbourne
Victoria, Australia

Margot Davey, MBBS, FRACP
Associate Professor
Director, Melbourne Children's Sleep Centre
Monash Children's Hospital
Victoria, Australia

Leo Donnan, MBBS, FRACS
Orthopaedic Surgeon
Royal Children's Hospital
Associate Professor, University of Melbourne
Victoria, Australia

Trevor Duke, MD, FRACP
Intensive Care Specialist
Director, Centre for International Child Health
Royal Children's Hospital
Associate Professor, Department of Paediatrics, University of Melbourne
Victoria, Australia

Daryl Efron, MBBS, FRACP, MD
Consultant Paediatrician, Department of General Medicine
Co-ordinator of Clinical Services, Centre for Community Child Health
Royal Children's Hospital
Victoria, Australia

James Elder, MBBS, FRANZCO, FRACS
Department of Ophthalmology
Royal Children's Hospital
Associate Professor, Department of Paediatrics, University of Melbourne
Victoria, Australia

Susan Gibb, MBBS, FRACP
Paediatrician
Department of General Medicine
Royal Children's Hospital
Victoria, Australia

Anthea Greenway, MBBS (Hons), FRACP, FRCPA
Paediatric Haematologist, Department of Clinical Haematology and Laboratory services
Royal Children's Hospital
Honorary Fellow, Murdoch Childrens Research Institute
Victoria, Australia

Sonia Grover, MBBS, FRANZCOG, MD
Director, Department of Gynaecology
Royal Children's Hospital
Research Fellow, Murdoch Childrens Research Institute
Clinical Professor, Department of Paediatrics, University of Melbourne
Victoria, Australia

Kerrod Hallett, BDSc (Hons), MDSc, MPH, FRACDS, FICD
Paediatric Dentist
Director, Department of Dentistry
Royal Children's Hospital
Research Fellow, Clinical Sciences, Murdoch Childrens Research Institute
Clinical Associate Professor, University of Melbourne
Victoria, Australia

Diane Hanna
Paediatric haematology/oncology fellow
Children's cancer centre
Royal Children's Hospital
Victoria, Australia

Winita Hardikar, MBBS, FRACP, PhD
Head of Liver and Intestinal Transplantation
Department of Gastroenterology
Royal Children's Hospital
Victoria, Australia

Ralf Heine, MD FRACP
Paediatric Gastroenterologist/Allergist
Department of Gastroenterology & Clinical Nutrition
Department of Allergy & Immunology
Royal Children's Hospital and Murdoch Childrens Research Institute
University of Melbourne
Victoria, Australia

Yves Heloury, MD
Urology department
Professor of Paediatic Surgery
Royal Children's Hospital
Victoria, Australia

Rod Hunt, BMBS, MRCP(UK), FRACP, MMed, PhD
Director, Neonatal Medicine
Royal Children's Hospital
Senior Research Fellow, Murdoch Childrens Research
    Institute
Associate Professor, University of Melbourne
Victoria, Australia

John Hutson, MD, MB, DSc, FRACS, FAAP
Urology and General Surgery Departments
Royal Children's Hospital
Chair of Paediatric Surgery, Department of
    Paediatrics, University of Melbourne
Victoria, Australia

Jenny Hynson, MBBS, FRACP
Consultant Paediatrician
Victorian Paediatric Palliative Care Program
Royal Children's Hospital
Victoria, Australia

Bryn Jones, MBBS, FRACP, FCSANZ
Deputy Director, Department of Cardiology
Royal Children's Hospital
Clinical Senior Fellow, Department of Paediatrics,
    University of Melbourne
Victoria, Australia

Julian Kelly, MBBS, FRACP
Paediatrician, Department of General Medicine
Royal Children's Hospital
Senior Lecturer, University of Melbourne
Victoria, Australia

Andrew Kornberg, MBBS (HONS), FRACP
Director of Neurology
Department of Neurology
Royal Children's Hospital
Victoria, Australia

Joy Lee, MD, FRACP
Consultant Metabolic Physician
Department of Metabolic Medicine
Royal Children's Hospital
Victoria, Australia

Lionel Lubitz, MBChB (UCT), DCH, MRCP, FRACP
Consultant Paediatrician, Department of General
    Medicine
Royal Children's Hospital
Associate Professor (Clinical), Department of
    Paediatrics, University of Melbourne
Victoria, Australia

Mark Mackay, MBBS, FRACP
Paediatric Neurologist
Department of Neurology
Royal Children's Hospital
Research Affiliate, Murdoch Childrens Research
    Institute
Victoria, Australia

Wirginia Maixner, MBBS, FRACS
Director, Department of Neurosurgery
Royal Children's Hospital
Victoria, Australia

Catherine Marraffa, MBBS, FRACP, FRCPCH
Deputy Director Developmental Medicine
Royal Children's Hospital
Honorary Fellow, Murdoch Childrens Research
    Institute
Victoria, Australia

John Massie, FRACP, PhD
Respiratory Physician
Department of Respiratory Medicine
Royal Children's Hospital
Clinical Associate Professor, University of Melbourne
Victoria, Australia

Zoë McCallum, MBBS, FRACP
Paediatrician
Department of General Medicine
Department of Clinical Nutrition
Royal Children's Hospital
Senior Lecturer, Department of Paediatrics, University
    of Melbourne
Victoria, Australia

Sarah McNab, MBBS, FRACP
Paediatrician
Department of General Medicine
Royal Children's Hospital
Victoria, Australia

Francoise Mechinaud, MD, FRACP
Director, Children Cancer Centre
Royal Children's Hospital
Victoria, Australia

Michele Meehan, RN, RMDipCHN, DipHlthEd
Clinical Nurse, Consultant
Maternal and Child Health
Royal Children's Hospital
Victoria, Australia

List of Contributors

Jane Munro, MBBS, FRACP, MPH
Paediatric Rheumatologist
Head of Rheumatology Unit
Royal Children's Hospital
Group Leader, Rheumatology, Murdoch Childrens
  Research Institute
Victoria, Australia

Michael Nightingale, FRACS
Paediatric Surgeon
Department of Paediatric and Neonatal Surgery
Royal Children's Hospital
Victoria, Australia

Michele O'Connell, MRCPI, FRACP, MD
Staff Specialist
Department of Endocrinology & Diabetes
Royal Children's Hospital
Melbourne and Centre for Hormone Research,
  Murdoch Childrens Research Institute
Victoria, Australia

Ed Oakley, MBBS, FACEM
Director
Department of Emergency Medicine
Royal Children's Hospital
Clinical Associate Professor, Department of
  Paediatrics, University of Melbourne
Victoria, Australia

Mike O'Brien, PhD, FRCSI (Paed), FRACS (Paed)
Consultant Paediatric Urologist
Director of Urology
Chief of Surgery
Royal Children's Hospital
Victoria, Australia

David Orchard, MBBS, FACD
Dermatologist
Department of Dermatology
Royal Children's Hospital
Victoria, Australia

Greta Palmer, MBBS, FANZCA, FFPMANZCA
Specialist Anaesthetist and Pain Management
  Consultant
Royal Children's Hospital and Murdoch Childrens
  Research Institute
Clinical Associate Professor, University of Melbourne
Victoria, Australia

Georgia Paxton, MBBS, BMedSci, MPH, FRACP
Head Immigrant Health, Consultant Paediatrician
Department of General Medicine
Royal Children's Hospital
Victoria, Australia

Rod Phillips, MBBS, FRACP, PhD
Consultant in Paediatric Skin Disease
Department of General Medicine
Royal Children's Hospital and Murdoch Childrens
  Research Institute
Associate Professor, Monash University
Victoria, Australia

Chidambaram Prakash, MBBS, DPM, FRANZCP, Cert
Child Psychiatry (RANZCP)
Authorised Psychiatrist
Principal, Hospital Psychiatrist Mental Health
Royal Children's Hospital
Victoria, Australia

Sarath Ranganathan, MBChB, MRCP, FRCPCH,
FRACP, PhD
Director Respiratory Physician
Department of Respiratory Medicine
Royal Children's Hospital
Victoria, Australia

Dinah Reddihough, MD, BSc, FRACP, FAFRM
Paediatrician, Developmental Medicine
Royal Children's Hospital
Group Leader, Developmental Disability and
  Rehabilitation Research, Murdoch Childrens
  Research Institute
Honorary Professorial Fellow, University of
  Melbourne
Victoria, Australia

Sheena Reilly, BAppSc, PhD, MRCSLT, MSpAA
Director, Department of Speech Pathology
Royal Children's Hospital
Director, Healthy Development Theme, Murdoch
  Childrens Research Institute
Professor of Paediatric Speech Pathology,
  Department of Paediatrics, University of
  Melbourne
Victoria, Australia

Liz Rogers, BAppSci, MND, APD
Clinical Specialist Dietitian
Nutrition and Food Services
Royal Children's Hospital
Victoria, Australia

Elizabeth Rose, MBBS, FRACS
Otolaryngologist
Department of Paediatric Otolaryngology Head and
  Neck Surgery
Royal Children's Hospital
Victoria, Australia

Kathy Rowe, MBBS, MD, FRACP, MPH, Dip Ed (Lond), Grad
Dip Int Health
Consultant Paediatrician
Department of General Medicine
Royal Children's Hospital
Research Fellow, Murdoch Childrens Research
  Institute
Victoria, Australia

Matthew Sabin, MRCPCH (UK), PhD
Consultant Paediatric Endocrinologist, Department
  of Endocrinology and Diabetes
Royal Children's Hospital and Murdoch Childrens
  Research Institute
University of Melbourne
Victoria, Australia

Susan Sawyer, MBBS, MD, FRACP
Director, Centre for Adolescent Health
Royal Children's Hospital
Chair of Adolescent Health, Department of
  Paediatrics, University of Melbourne
Victoria, Australia

Joanne Smart, Bsc, MBBS, PhD, FRACP
Paediatric Allergist and Immunologist
Department of Allergy and Clinical Immunology
Royal Children's Hospital
Victoria, Australia

Anne Smith, MBBS, FRACP, MForensMed, FFCFM (RCPA)
Medical Director
Victorian Forensic Paediatric Medical Service
Royal Children's Hospital
Victoria, Australia

Mike Starr, MBBS, FRACP
Paediatrician, Infectious Diseases Physician,
  Consultant in Emergency Medicine
Director of Paediatric Education
Royal Children's Hospital
Victoria, Australia

Russell G. Taylor, FRACS
Consultant Paediatric Surgeon
Department of Paediatric and Neonatal Surgery
Royal Children's Hospital
Victoria, Australia

Michelle Telfer, MBBS (Hons), FRACP
Paediatrician and Clinical Lead
Adolescent Medicine, Centre for Adolescent Health
Royal Children's Hospital
Victoria, Australia

Dean Tey, MBBS, FRACP
Paediatric Allergist and Immunologist
Department of Allergy and Immunology
Royal Children's Hospital
Victoria, Australia

James Tibballs, BMedSc (Hons), MBBS, MEd, MBA, MD,
MHlth&MedLaw, DALF, FANZCA, FJFICM, FACLM
Intensive Care Physician and Resuscitation Officer
Principal Fellow, Australian Venom Research Unit
Department of Pharmacology
Principal Fellow, Department of Paediatrics,
  University of Melbourne
Victoria, Australia

Amanda M. Walker
Director, Department of Nephrology
Royal Children's Hospital
Honorary Fellow Manager, Murdoch Childrens
  Research Institute
Honorary Clinical Associated Professor, Department
  of Paediatrics, University of Melbourne
Victoria, Australia

George Werther, MD, FRACP, MSc (Oxon)
Director, Department of Endocrinology and Diabetes
  and Centre for Hormone Research
Royal Children's Hospital and Murdoch Childrens
  Research Institute
Professor, Department of Paediatrics, University of
  Melbourne
Victoria, Australia

Margaret Zacharin, DMed Sci, BS, FRACP
Endocrinologist
Department of Endocrinology and Diabetes
Royal Children's Hospital
Professor, Department of Paediatrics, University of
  Melbourne
Victoria, Australia

Acknowledgements

We greatly appreciate and acknowledge the contribution of the following people:

Editorial team of the ninth edition: Daryl Efron, Jane Munro, Michael Nightingale, Chris Sanderson, Mike Starr, Kate Thomson

Previous authors and other contributors:

Ruth Armstrong
Rob Berkowitz
Julie Bines
Avihu Boneh
Paul Brookes
Jim Buttery
Kay Gibbons
Kerr Graham

Michael Harari
Simon Harvey
John Heath
Colin Jones
Nicky Kilpatrick
Maria McCarthy
Peter McDougall
Mary O'Toole

Dan Penny
Heidi Peters
Damien Phillips
Andrew Rechtman
Jenny Royal
Mimi Tang
Garry Warne
Joshua Wolf

Foreword

Since it was first published in January 1964, the *Royal Children's Hospital Handbook* has provided invaluable guidance to clinicians managing health problems in children. Although this primary purpose has not changed since the first edition, the Handbook itself has changed greatly. The 1964 edition consisted of only 100 pages in a ring binder, so individual sections could be updated from year to year. It was called the *Resident Medical Officers' Handbook* and it slipped easily into the pocket of a white coat for, in 1964, Junior Medical Staff, as they were called, actually wore white coats and resided at the Hospital.

It may have been a convenient size, but the first edition made no mention of upper or lower respiratory tract infections, fever, asthma or convulsions, and cardiac disease was covered in two pages that were mainly about digoxin. Subsequent editions were more systematic; they provided practical guidance about the management of the common illnesses of children, including paediatric emergencies and the common causes of admission to hospital. From the 1989 edition onwards, there was an index so that information was easier to find, and sources of more detailed material were suggested. The eighth edition of 640 pages was published in 2009, by which time the Handbook had become so useful that it was widely used, not just at the Royal Children's Hospital, but throughout the world.

To make this ninth edition even more useful in clinical practice, it has been redesigned for easier navigation and updated with many more links to practice guidelines. The Handbook is now 50 years old, and it has matured into an extraordinarily useful resource. We are lucky to have it – and so are the children.

Frank Shann, AM, MBBS, MD, FRACP, FCICM
Staff Specialist in Intensive Care, Royal Children's Hospital
Professor of Critical Care Medicine, University of Melbourne
Victoria, Australia

RCH Handbook List

1st edition (1964). *Resident Medical Officers' Handbook*, Lawson JS, ed. (Foreword: Sloan LEG). 100 p. Snap-lock ring binder.

2nd edition (1975–1976). *Residents Handbook*, Roy N, Vance J, eds. (Foreword: Sloan LEG). 203 p. Snap-lock ring binder.

2nd edition, revised (1982–1983). *Residents Handbook*, Roy N, Vance J, eds. (Foreword: Westwood G). 228 p. Snap-lock ring binder.

3rd edition (1989). *Paediatric Handbook*, Smith LJ, ed. (Preface: Phelan PD). xiv, 287 p. Paperback. ISBN 0-7316-2463-7.

3rd edition (1990). *Paediatric Handbook Supplement*, 1989 Edition. 12 p. Paperback. ISBN 0-9590-6187-8.

4th edition (1992). *Paediatric Handbook*, Marks MK, ed. (Preface: Phelan PD). xiv, 234 p. Paperback. ISBN 0-86793-217-1.

5th edition (1995). *Paediatric Handbook*, Efron D, Nolan T, eds. (Foreword: Phelan PD). xv, 520 p. Paperback. ISBN 0-86793-337-2.

6th edition (2000). *Paediatric Handbook*, Smart J, Nolan T, eds. (Foreword: Smith PJ). xviii, 630 p. Paperback. ISBN 0-86793-011-X.

7th edition (2003). *Paediatric Handbook*, Paxton G, Munro J, Marks M, eds. (Foreword: Bowes G). xviii, 709 p. Paperback. ISBN 0-86793-431-X.

8th edition (2009). *Paediatric Handbook*, Thomson K, Tey D, Marks M, eds. (Foreword: Bines J). xv, 640 p. Paperback. ISBN 978-1-4051-7400-8.

Preface

We are very excited and proud to present the ninth edition of the Royal Children's Hospital *Paediatric Handbook*. The Royal Children's Hospital moved to an outstanding new building in November 2011. This edition is the first to be published since the move, with the front cover displaying some of the artistic beauty that lies within the "Main Street". Just as our new campus has been given a fresh look, so too this edition has taken a fresh approach on an already popular resource for medical students, general practitioners, paediatricians and other health professionals alike.

There are many improvements and updates in the latest edition. First, the Handbook is ordered with chapters according to systems. This will make it easier and more intuitive for clinicians to readily access the information they require about a given problem. In addition, the Handbook is now more closely aligned with the *Royal Children's Hospital Clinical Practice Guidelines*, which remains the most popular paediatric website in the Southern Hemisphere.

Some of the other new features include:
- Evidence-based information with revisions in all chapters of this Handbook
- The addition of a genetics chapter
- Completely new renal chapter
- Completely new oncology chapter
- Updated drug doses
- Electronic version of the Handbook

This Handbook was written collectively by a multitude of staff from the Royal Children's Hospital in Melbourne, including doctors, nurses and allied health. The authors are greatly respected clinicians in their fields and we are grateful for their time, effort and expertise, which has resulted in this world-class paediatric aid. We also sincerely appreciate the efforts of previous authors who laid the foundations for such a key resource. Special thanks to Professor Frank Shann for permitting us to utilise his drug doses book. The PDA version of this reference will be available in its entirety at www.drugdoses.net

Lastly, to the enthusiastic and dedicated editorial committee, thank you so much for your mammoth efforts in putting together this Handbook. Your support and assistance are greatly appreciated.

One of the great things about paediatrics, and indeed medicine in general, is that it is ever changing. So, whilst the information in this Handbook is up to date at the time of printing, we encourage our readers to continue to read the literature and check drug doses before administration.

Thank you, the readers, for your support of this paediatric handbook. We trust that you will find this a very important and useful tool when looking after the children of the world.

Amanda Gwee
Romi Rimer
Michael Marks

CHAPTER 1
Medical emergencies

Michael Clifford
Ed Oakley
James Tibballs

Cardiorespiratory arrest

Cardiorespiratory arrest may occur in a wide variety of conditions that cause hypoxaemia or hypotension, or both.

The initial cardiac rhythm discovered during early resuscitation is often severe bradycardia or asystole. Although the spontaneous onset of ventricular fibrillation in children is approximately 10%, it may occur more frequently with congenital heart conditions or secondary to poisoning with cardioactive drugs. In hospital, respiratory arrest alone is more common than cardiorespiratory arrest.

Diagnosis and initial management

- Cardiorespiratory arrest may be suspected when the patient becomes unresponsive or unconscious, is not moving or breathing normally or appears pale or cyanosed. Call for help immediately.
- Assess airway and respiration by observing movement of the chest, as well as listening and feeling for expired breath while positioning the head and neck to open and maintain an airway. Movement of the chest without expiration indicates a blocked airway.
- DO NOT delay resuscitation while feeling for a pulse. Start compressions in the presence of bradycardia before the pulseless state or if other signs of circulation (adequate ventilation, movement, consciousness) are absent.
- Whenever possible, manage in a treatment room. Carry the patient there if necessary. If this is not possible, get the resuscitation trolley brought to the patient.
- Cardiopulmonary resuscitation (CPR) must commence with basic techniques and be continued using advanced techniques (Fig. 1.1).

Airway maintenance and ventilation

- If airway obstruction is present, quickly inspect the pharynx. Clear secretions or vomitus by brief suction using a Yankauer sucker.
- Maintain the airway with backward head tilt, chin lift or forward jaw thrust.
- If adequate spontaneous ventilation does not resume, ventilate the lungs mechanically with a self-inflating resuscitator (e.g., Laerdal, Ambu, Air-viva) with added oxygen 8–10 L/min. If ventilation cannot be achieved with the resuscitator, use a mouth-to-mask technique. Give two initial breaths.
  Note: Self-inflating bags (e.g., Laerdal) will provide no gas flow to the patient unless they are compressed cyclically.
- **Whatever technique is used, ensure that ventilation expands the chest adequately.**
- Intubate the trachea via the mouth if possible, but do not cause hypoxaemia by prolonged unsuccessful attempts. Select the tube and insert it at a depth appropriate to the patient's age in years.

Endotracheal tube size and position

- Uncuffed tube size (internal diameter) = (age/4) + 4 mm (for patients over 1 year of age)
- Cuffed tube size (internal diameter) = (age/4) + 3.5 mm (for patients over 1 year of age)
- Depth of insertion is approximately (age/2) + 12 cm from the lower lip
  Neonates: see Neonatal Conditions (Table 21.1).

Paediatric Handbook, Ninth Edition. Edited by Amanda Gwee, Romi Rimer and Michael Marks.
© 2015 John Wiley & Sons, Ltd. Published 2015 by John Wiley & Sons, Ltd.

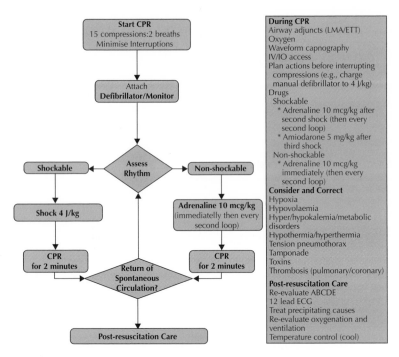

Fig. 1.1 Management of cardiorespiratory arrest. Adapted from guidelines at www.nzrc.org.nz/guidelines.

Secure the tube with cotton tape around the neck or affix it firmly to the face with adhesive tape to avoid endobronchial intubation or accidental extubation. Confirm placement by detecting end-tidal CO_2.

External cardiac compression
Start external cardiac compression (ECC) over the lower sternum if

- A pulse is not palpable within 10 seconds
- A pulse is less than
  - 60 beats/min (for infants)
  - 40 beats/min (for older children)
- Other signs of circulation (adequate ventilation, movement, consciousness) are absent

Place the patient on a firm surface and depress the lower sternum one-third the depth of the chest whilst avoiding pressure over the ribs and abdominal viscera:

- Newborn infant or an infant (<1 year) – two-thumb technique in which the hands encircle the chest
- Small child (1–8 years) – the heel of one hand
- Larger child (>8 years) and adult – the two-handed technique

Compression–ventilation rates and ratios
The rates and ratios recommended for health-care rescuers by the Australian Resuscitation Council (www.resus.org.au) are shown in Table 1.1. Use a ratio of 30:2 if a sole rescuer or 15:2 when two rescuers are present.

Table 1.1 Compression–ventilation ratios

	Give two initial breaths, then	
	One rescuer (expired air resuscitation) Compression:breaths	Two rescuers (bag–mask ventilation) Compression:breaths
Newborn infants	3:1	3:1
Infants (<1 year old)	30:2	15:2
Small children (1–8 year old)	30:2	15:2
Larger children (>8 year old)	30:2	15:2
Adults	30:2	30:2

Source: From the Australian Resuscitation Council. Adapted from guidelines at www.resus.org.au/policy/guidelines.

When using bag-to-mask ventilation or mouth-to-mask ventilation, the rescuer giving compressions should count aloud to allow the rescuer giving ventilation to deliver effective breaths during pauses between compressions with minimal interruption in compressions. Compression may be commenced at the end of inspiration. If the patient is intubated, DO NOT interrupt compressions. The *rate* of compressions should be 100/min.

If ventilation is given by bag and ETT, ECC may be continued during ventilation, provided lung expansion can be achieved. In this circumstance, restrict the number of ventilations to about 10/min. Aim for an end-tidal CO_2 of >15 mmHg.

Management of cardiac dysrhythmias
Determine the cardiac rhythm with defibrillator paddles or pads or chest leads.
- Give a single 4 J/kg DC shock if ventricular fibrillation or pulseless ventricular tachycardia is present. See Table 1.1 and Fig. 1.1.
- Give adrenaline if any other pulseless rhythm is present (see Fig. 1.1). The dose is
  - IV and intraosseous: 10 mcg/kg (0.01 mL of 1:1000 solution).
  - Endotracheal tube (ETT): 100 mcg/kg (0.1 mL of 1:1000 solution).
- Insert an IV cannula. Although this is the preferred access to the circulation, do not waste time (>90 seconds) with repeated unsuccessful attempts, as access can be achieved with the alternative techniques of
  - *Intraosseus administration* (see Chapter 4, *Procedures*, p. 36): all IV drugs and resuscitation fluids can be given via this route.
  - *ETT administration*: only adrenaline, atropine and lignocaine (lidocaine) can be given this way; this is the least effective method.
- A quick reference guide to drug doses and fluid volume is provided in Table 1.2.

Other drugs
Amiodarone
This is the only antidysrhythmic shown to be of benefit for VT/VF. The dose is 5 mg/kg given as a bolus. It can cause hypotension.

Calcium
This is a useful inotropic and vasopressor agent but has no place in the management of a dysrhythmia, unless it is caused by hypocalcaemia, hyperkalaemia or calcium channel blocker toxicity. It is not useful and probably harmful for asystole, ventricular fibrillation or electromechanical dissociation. The IV dose is 10% calcium chloride (0.2 mL/kg) or 10% calcium gluconate (0.7 mL/kg). Do not administer calcium via ETT and do not mix it with bicarbonate.

Adenosine
This is the preferred drug treatment (200 mcg/kg IV) for supraventricular tachycardia (SVT). See management of SVT in Chapter 6, *Cardiac conditions*, p. 64.

Table 1.2 Table of drugs, fluid volume, endotracheal tubes and direct current shock for paediatric resuscitation

Age	0	2 months	5 months	1 year	2 years	3 years	4 years	5 years	6 years	7 years	8 years	9 years	10 years	11 years	12 years	13 years	14 years
Bodyweight (kg)[a]	3.5	5	7	10	12	14	16	18	20	22	25	28	32	36	40	46	50
Height (cm)[a]	50	58	65	75	85	94	102	109	115	121	127	132	138	144	151	157	162
Adrenaline 1:1000 (mL)																	
10 mcg/kg	0.035	0.05	0.07	0.10	0.12	0.14	0.16	0.18	0.2	0.22	0.25	0.28	0.32	0.36	0.4	0.46	0.5
100 mcg/kg	0.35	0.5	0.7	1	1.2	1.4	1.6	1.8	2	2.2	2.5	2.8	3.2	3.6	4	4.6	5
Adrenaline 1:10,000 (mL)																	
10 mcg/kg	0.35	0.5	0.7	1	1.2	1.4	1.6	1.8	2	2.2	2.5	2.8	3.2	3.6	4	4.6	5
100 mcg/kg	3.5	5.0	7.0	10	12	14	16	18	20	22	25	28	32	36	40	46	50
Lignocaine (lidocaine) 1% (mL)																	
1 mg/kg	0.3	0.5	0.7	1.0	1.2	1.4	1.6	1.8	2.0	2.2	2.5	2.8	3.2	3.6	4.0	4.6	5.0
Sodium bicarbonate 8.4% (mL)																	
1 mmol/kg	3.5	5	7	10	12	14	16	18	20	22	25	28	32	36	40	46	50
Fluid volume (mL)																	
20 mL/kg	70	100	140	200	240	280	320	360	400	440	500	560	640	720	800	920	1000
Endotracheal tube																	
Size (mm) Age/4 + 4	3	3.5	3.5	4	4.5	4.5	5	5	5.5	5.5	6	6	6.5	6.5	7	7	7.5
Oral length (cm) Age/2 + 12	9.5	11	11.5	12	13	13.5	14	14.5	15	15.5	16	16.5	17	17.5	18	18.5	19
Direct current shock (J) unsynchronised																	
VF, VT 2 J/kg	7	10	20	20	20	30	30	30	50	50	50	50	70	70	70	100	100
VF, VT 4 J/kg	10	20	30	50	50	50	70	70	70	100	100	100	150	150	150	200	200
Direct current shock (J) synchronised																	
SVT 1 J/kg	3	5	7	10	10	10	20	20	20	20	30	30	30	30	50	50	50

Source: Oakley, P., Phillips B, Molyneaux E, & Mackway-Jones K. (1993) Paediatric resuscitation. Updated standard reference chart. British Medical Journal 1993;306(6892):1613. (Oakley 1993. Reproduced with permission by BMJ.)
[a]50th percentiles.

Extracorporeal cardiopulmonary resuscitation – extracorporeal life support

Centres with the capacity to provide paediatric cardiopulmonary bypass should consider the role of extracorporeal life support. ECLS for refractory cardiac arrest has been associated with increased survival. At RCH this is usually reserved for in-hospital arrests.

Post-resuscitation care
- Ensure adequate ventilation and normocarbia.
- Maintain adequate blood pressure with infusion of fluids and inotropic support as needed.
- Do not actively rewarm. If the child remains unconscious after resuscitation, institute therapeutic hypothermia to 33–34°C within 6 hours for 2–3 days.

Anaphylaxis

See also Chapter 19, *Allergy and immunology*.

The life-threatening clinical manifestations are
- Hypotension secondary to vasodilatation and loss of plasma volume due to increased capillary permeability
- Bronchospasm
- Upper airways obstruction due to laryngeal or pharyngeal oedema

Immediate treatment
- Vasopressor and bronchodilator therapy: give adrenaline 10 mcg/kg (0.01 mg/kg) at 0.01 mL/kg of 1:1000 solution by **intramuscular (IM)** injection or 0.01 mg/kg (i.e. 0.1 mL/kg of 1:10,000 solution) by slow IV injection (over 10 minutes). A continuous infusion (0.1–1.0 mcg/kg/min) may be required if manifestations are prolonged. *Note*: Do *not* use subcutaneous adrenaline as absorption is less reliable.
- Oxygen by mask: mechanical ventilation may be required.
- IV volume expander: give 0.9% saline at 20 mL/kg. Give repeat boluses of 10–20 mL/kg until the blood pressure is restored.
- Bronchodilator therapy with salbutamol: continuous nebulised (0.5%) or IV 5 mcg/kg/min for 1 hour, then 1 mcg/kg/min thereafter. Secondary therapy with a steroid, aminophylline and an antihistamine may be helpful for prolonged bronchospasm and capillary leak.
- Relief of upper airway obstruction: mild to moderate oedema may respond to inhalation of nebulised 1% adrenaline (1 mL per dose diluted to 4 mL) or 5 mL of nebulised 1:1000 solution, but intubation of the trachea may be required.
- Anaphylaxis can be biphasic and the patient may deteriorate again over the next few hours.
- All patients with anaphylaxis should be observed carefully for at least 12 hours, followed up for allergen testing, provided with self-injectable adrenaline and a Medi-alert bracelet.
- Refractory anaphylaxis has been shown to respond to both noradrenaline and vasopressin infusions. These will require central venous access.
- If drug-mediated anaphylaxis is suspected, a mast cell tryptase (serum tube) should be taken ideally between 1 and 4 hours after the reaction (earlier if hymenoptera (bee) sting suspected).
- See http://www.allergy.org.au

Septicaemic shock

Hypotension is due to vasodilatation, (early) leakage of fluid from capillary beds and depression of myocardial contractility.
- Collect blood for culture, but do not delay administration of an **antibiotic** if a blood sample cannot be collected.
  - Unknown pathogen: give flucloxacillin 50 mg/kg (max 2 g) IV 4 hourly and cefotaxime 50 mg/kg (max 2 g) IV 6 hourly.
  - Meningococcaemia: give cefotaxime 50 mg/kg (max 2 g) IV 6 hourly. Give benzylpenicillin 60 mg/kg (max 3 g) IV/IM 4 hourly if cefotaxime is not available.
  - For particular circumstances, consult the Appendix 3, *Antimicrobial Guidelines*.
- Treat shock with **0.9% saline solution**, 20 mL/kg initially (further boluses of 10–20 mL/kg may be needed).
- Give **oxygen** and monitor blood gases. Mechanical ventilation may be required.

- Commence infusion of an **inotropic agent**. Administration via a central vein is preferred but it may be given via a peripheral vein as a dilute solution (e.g. dobutamine 15 mg/kg in 500 mL at 10–40 mL/h = 5–20 mcg/kg/min). Dobutamine (5–20 mcg/kg/min) may be administered into a peripheral vein and is preferred initially. If still hypotensive, noradrenaline can be added when central access is obtained (0.15 mg/kg in 50 mL 5% hep/dex at 1–10 mL/h = 0.05–0.5 mcg/kg/min).
- Defer lumbar puncture if indicated, until the child has been stabilised.

Drowning

There is a global hypoxic–ischaemic injury often associated with lung damage from aspiration of water and gastric contents. The differences between freshwater and saltwater drowning are not usually clinically important. Poor prognostic signs include

- Immersion time >10 minutes
- Rectal temperature <30°C
- Absence of any initial resuscitative efforts
- Arrival in hospital with CPR in progress or in coma
- Requirement of CPR
- Initial serum pH <7.0

Management

- Adequate oxygenation and ventilation are of paramount importance. Mechanical ventilation is required for severe lung involvement, circulatory arrest or loss of consciousness. Lung hypoxic–ischaemic injury is compounded by pulmonary oedema or aspiration of water or gastric contents.
- Decompress the stomach, which is usually distended with air and water.
- Support the circulation:
  ○ IV infusion of colloid (e.g. 4% albumin) or 0.9% saline solution.
  ○ Commence infusion of an **inotropic agent**. Administration via a central vein is preferred but it may be given via a peripheral vein as a dilute solution (e.g. 15 mg/kg in 500 mL at 10–40 mL/h = 5–20 mcg/kg/min). Dobutamine (5–20 mcg/kg/min) may be administered into a peripheral vein and is preferred initially. If still hypotensive, noradrenaline can be added when central access is obtained (0.15 mg/kg in 50 mL 5% hep/dex at 1–10 mL/h = 0.05–0.5 mcg/kg/min).
- If signs of cerebral oedema are present (i.e. a depressed conscious state), administer mannitol 0.25–0.5 g/kg IV once.
- Correct electrolyte disturbances. Hypokalaemia in particular is common.
- Administer benzylpenicillin 60 mg/kg (max 3 g) IV 6 hourly if ventilation is required (to prevent the complication of pneumococcal pneumonia).
- If CPR is required, prevent hyperthermia and induce controlled hypothermia (33–34°C) for 72 hours for cerebral protection.
- Place a cervical collar if a diving injury is suspected. Early MRI will be required.

Acute upper airway obstruction

The most common cause is laryngotracheobronchitis (croup). Occasional causes include epiglottitis (see Chapter 7, *Respiratory conditions*), an inhaled foreign body, allergic oedema and trauma. The hallmark of obstruction is stridor, which when accompanied by a barking cough suggests croup, or when accompanied by dysphagia/drooling suggests epiglottitis. Severe obstruction stimulates forceful diaphragmatic contraction that results in a retraction of the rib cage, tracheal tug and abdominal protrusion on inspiration. Cyanosis and irregular respiratory effort are terminal signs.

Management

- Allow the child to settle quietly on their parent's lap in the position the child feels most comfortable.
- Observe closely with minimal interference.
- Treat specific cause – refer to **Croup**, **Anaphylaxis** and **Foreign Body in the Airway** clinical practice guidelines.
- Call **PICU** if worsening or severe obstruction occurs.

- Oxygen may be given while awaiting definitive treatment. This can be falsely reassuring because a child with quite severe obstruction may look pink in oxygen.
- Intravenous access should be deferred – upsetting the child can cause increasing obstruction.

Note: Lateral cervical soft tissue x-rays do not assist in management. In severe airways obstruction, x-rays cause undue delay in definitive treatment and may be dangerous (positioning may precipitate respiratory arrest).

Behavioural emergencies

Behavioural emergencies in late childhood and adolescence are uncommon, frightening, complicated and fraught with risk. The aetiology is multifactorial with variable contributions from

- Psychiatric and neurodevelopmental disorders (autistic spectrum disorder, intellectual disability)
- Personality and behavioural factors (poor impulse control or coping strategies, maladaptive responses learned at home, emerging personality disorders)
- Medical conditions (head injury, seizure, hypoglycaemia, brain tumours, meningitis, brain abscess and strokes)
- Substance intoxication or withdrawal
- Environmentally derived issues (fear, frustration, anxiety)

Evaluation

This occurs in tandem with stabilisation. Clinical aggression, active self-harm and absconding are dynamic events where simultaneous (and sometimes competing) priorities often require rapid changes in approach. The clinician needs to balance requirements around

- Duty of care
- Patient safety
- Respect for autonomy
- Mental Health law, in regards to competence
- Occupational health and safety
- Zero tolerance policy

Clinical features

Clinical aggression may be verbal or non-verbal. Typically aggression follows a well-defined pattern where escalating psychomotor agitation (pacing, gesticulating, angry facial expression, dilated pupils, sweatiness) is accompanied by increasingly aggressive verbal signals. The aggression peaks with a violent outburst, which is followed by a rapid return to calm, even remorse.

Assessment

It is useful for physical and mental health assessments to occur in tandem, with both the treating physician and mental health professional.

Assessment aims to define the origins of the behaviour in three broad terms: organic, behavioural and psychiatric. Key historical features include

- Antecedents and triggers of the behaviour
- Pre-existing conditions
- Development and personality
- Past history of similar behaviour
- Access to and use of substances

Interview with family members may be the only source of information. Mental state examination is crucial. Evidence of major psychiatric disease (psychosis, depression) should be sought. An organic aetiology is suggested by history of neurological disease or injury, infection or substance use.

Physical examination should focus on evidence of

- Inattention
- Clouding of consciousness (delirium)
- Fever (CNS infection, delirium)
- Head injury
- Neurological signs (space occupying lesion, encephalitis)
- Toxidrome, as well as
- Assessing and treating any injury arising from unstable behaviour

Investigations

There is no set of routine investigations. The history or examination might give rise to specifically indicated investigations, for example, a paracetamol level in a polypharmacy overdose or a CT brain when external signs of head injury are found. Urine drug screen has no role in guiding emergency treatment decisions.

Treatment

Prevention is the first step.

Clinicians should **not** place themselves in dangerous situations:
- Maintain a safe distance from agitated patients.
- See a patient in an area which is well observed and has an escape route.
- Make sure they are searched for weapons and other dangerous objects.

On initial approach
- Adopt an open posture with neutral or facilitative body language. Use calm, quiet, slow, simple language and recognise the problem from the viewpoint of the patient.
- Attempt to give the patient some control with simple, low-risk decisions.
- Rephrase the problem simply to show you understand.
- Set clear goals and expectations, and outline positive consequences, rather than issue threats.
- Meet the patient's needs. Offer food, drink, a toilet stop.
- Recognise substance withdrawal, in particular, nicotine craving.

With open engagement and skilful verbal de-escalation, many potentially risky situations can be brought under control.

Behavioural resuscitation

Physical, mechanical or chemical restraint are indicated when behaviour is due to medical, behavioural or psychiatric factors for which the patient needs treatment, when the risk to the patient is imminent and high and all other methods have failed (or will fail).

Restraint and apprehension for criminal activity, acting out or detainment for child protection concerns should be done by the police rather than health-care workers.

Restraint should be performed by a trained team of at least five people although the mere appearance of a five-person team can rapidly de-escalate the situation. The team should be aware of the hazards of biting and spitting, and use standard precautions. The aim is to terminate the aggressive behaviour through safe and calm but assertive physical intervention, with sheer numbers rather than individual strength of any one team member.

If physical restraint is needed, generally sedation should follow. The patient may accept oral diazepam or sublingual olanzapine; however, if refused, parenteral sedation should be used. Midazolam and either haloperidol or olanzapine can be used in combination for combined rapid onset/short duration and slower onset/longer duration. If insufficient clinical effect is seen after 10 minutes, a titrated repeat dose may be required. This combination will take effect within 5 minutes and last 1–2 hours, by which time the behavioural crisis may have resolved and more detailed assessment will have taken place.

USEFUL RESOURCES
- *www.resus.org.au* – Australian Resuscitation Council.
- *www.rch.org.au* – Royal Children's Hospital Clinical Practice Guidelines.
- *www.allergy.org.au* – Anaphylaxis information and action plans.
- *www.rch.org.au/clinicalguide/guideline_index/Septic_Shock* – Septic shock guidelines.

CHAPTER 2

Surgical emergencies

Russell Taylor
John Hutson
Tom Clarnette
Ed Oakley
Michael Nightingale

Neonatal surgical emergencies
Important warning signs
- Excessive drooling of frothy secretions from the mouth may suggest oesophageal atresia.
- Bile-stained or green vomiting is always abnormal (malrotation may be present and requires urgent treatment).
- Delayed passage of meconium (beyond 24 hours) is abnormal and may indicate Hirschsprung disease.
- Inguinoscrotal hernias need urgent attention to avoid strangulation.

All the conditions below require urgent paediatric surgical consultation and transfer to a tertiary centre.

Oesophageal atresia
- Excessive drooling of frothy, mucousy secretions from the mouth in a newborn suggests an inability to swallow.
- The test for oesophageal atresia is to pass a 10-French gauge catheter (which will not curl up) gently through the mouth. In the baby with oesophageal atresia, the catheter stops at 10 cm from the gums. In a normal baby, it passes to 20–25 cm and returns acid on litmus testing.
- First aid includes: Nil orally, IV fluids, frequent oropharyngeal suction (every 10–15 minutes) to prevent aspiration.
- Urgent transfer is required for surgical management.

Diaphragmatic hernia
- Respiratory distress in a newborn with a scaphoid abdomen suggests diaphragmatic hernia.
- Clinical cardiac displacement and a chest radiograph showing bowel loops in the chest (left side more commonly) confirm the diagnosis.
- If mechanical ventilation is required, only provide this via tracheal intubation; bag and mask ventilation may exacerbate respiratory distress by distending the stomach bowel.

Exomphalos/gastroschisis
- These anterior abdominal wall defects place the child at risk of heat and water loss from the exposed surface of the sac (exomphalos) or bowel (gastroschisis).
- The baby should be placed in a humidicrib and the entire torso covered in Glad Wrap. Great care must be taken to ensure any exposed bowel is not twisted and its blood supply is not compromised.
- Gastrointestinal decompression with a nasogastric tube and IV fluid management should commence whilst transfer to a tertiary surgical centre is undertaken.

Sacrococcygeal teratoma
- Any lump over the coccyx of a baby should be assumed to be a teratoma until proven otherwise. This needs immediate referral at birth.

Paediatric Handbook, Ninth Edition. Edited by Amanda Gwee, Romi Rimer and Michael Marks.
© 2015 John Wiley & Sons, Ltd. Published 2015 by John Wiley & Sons, Ltd.

Malrotation and volvulus

- A green vomit without an obvious septic cause is an indication for urgent surgical consultation.
- Malrotation occurs when the duodenojejunal flexure and the ileocaecal junction are adjacent to each other and results in a very short base to the small bowel mesentery. This predisposes to volvulus of the mesentery. If the mesentery twists through one full rotation, there is venous and lymphatic engorgement with bile-stained vomiting. Surgery at this point is likely to have a good outcome. Further rotation of the gut increases the risk of intestinal ischaemia and infarction.
- Initially, there may not be any clinical signs of abdominal disease. Abdominal distension is not usually seen in the early stages of presentation.
- The diagnosis is by an upper GI contrast study showing loss of the normal C-shaped loop of the duodenum. Volvulus may be seen by the cork screw passage of contrast through the twisting proximal small bowel.
- In regional settings, consider doing an urgent contrast study first if surgical review is not immediately available.
- Urgent surgical referral is necessary and an urgent laparotomy is performed if volvulus cannot be excluded.

Ambiguous genitalis

Genitalia that are frankly ambiguous need urgent consultation with an experienced paediatric endocrinologist or surgeon on the first day of life (see Chapter 13, *The endocrine system*). An enlarged clitoris in an apparent female is also abnormal and needs immediate referral. Hypospadias may overlap with ambiguous genitalia. This needs a careful initial assessment; if the diagnosis of hypospadias has been made, someone has already assumed the gender is male. If one or both testes are undescended, or the scrotum is bifid, or both, the baby should be treated as having ambiguous genitalia until proven otherwise with immediate referral for further investigation.

Childhood surgical emergencies

Major trauma

Rather than a thorough plan for managing all major trauma, this section is an overview of the issues and problems that need consideration.

Major trauma is an infrequent life-threatening problem encountered in children. A large proportion of severely injured children have significant head injuries. It ideally requires management by a team experienced in resuscitation, and the procedures that might be required for managing trauma.

A trauma team may consist of the following:

- Team leader (a clinician experienced in resuscitation)
- Airway doctor and nurse (consider an anaesthetist, intensivist or emergency physician confident with managing a child's airway)
- Procedure doctor and nurse
- Surgeon (ideally paediatric surgeon) to facilitate theatre when needed and as an expert in some procedures
- Social worker or nurse to manage the relatives and psychological needs of the child

Access to, or advice from, a neurosurgeon and orthopaedic surgeon is desirable.

Major trauma is ideally initially managed at a trauma centre, but if managed at another site early discussion with and appropriate transfer to the trauma centre are indicated.

- Resuscitation should follow the principles of resuscitations outlined in Chapter 1 (Medical emergencies chapter) and should concurrently manage Airway, Breathing, Circulation, and assessment of disability.
- Ensuring adequate oxygenation and blood pressure to perfuse the injured brain is of particular importance.
- Fluid resuscitation should begin with 0.9% NaCl or Hartmann's solution. If more than 40 mL/kg is needed, or there is obvious massive blood loss, blood should be immediately administered (initially O-negative, then crossmatched blood once available).
- Monitoring should at a minimum include continuous heart rate, pulse oximetry, frequent intermittent non-invasive BP, and intermittent measurement of temperature.

Throughout resuscitation a staff member should remain with the relatives and explain management and the patient's condition. Family should be allowed to witness the resuscitation (at least in part) if they so desire. Once possible the family should be given an opportunity to see, talk to and touch the injured child.

Life-threatening problems should be rapidly identified and corrected. These include

- Obstructed or inadequate airway
- Inadequate breathing

- Evidence of blood loss (tachycardia, poor perfusion, hypotension)
- Evidence of other complications such as pneumothorax/tension pneumothorax; haemothorax; pericardial tamponade; open wounds with active bleeding

Other management should follow the same plans and path of non-trauma resuscitation; however, vigilant and repeated examination should be undertaken to determine the presence and extent of any internal haemorrhage. Full but modest **exposure** of all parts of the body is necessary to ensure no injuries are missed.

Adequate analgesia is an important and often overlooked part of trauma resuscitation. Control of pain and anxiety will assist with assessment and management of the child. Morphine in 0.1 or 0.05 mg/kg aliquots is recommended.

All trauma patients must be considered to have injury to the spinal column until this can be assessed and cleared. Therefore, spinal alignment and *neck immobilisation in a cervical collar* is necessary until full assessment can be performed.

Procedures that might be needed in trauma resuscitation include

- Management of a damaged or bleeding airway
- Needle thoracostomy (for tension pneumothorax)
- Chest tube insertion (for pneumothorax or haemothorax)
- Large bore venous or intraosseous access for fluid resuscitation (with the possible need for multiple lines)
- Rapid fluid resuscitation and massive transfusion
- Urinary catheterisation
- Splinting of injured limbs

Investigations that may be needed

Blood tests

- Crossmatch of blood (mandatory for all major trauma)
- Blood gas analysis to assist with assessment of ventilation (maintenance of a normal PCO2 in a head-injured patient)
- Electrolytes
- Coagulation tests (in prolonged resuscitation or massive transfusion)

Imaging tests

- CXR should be performed in all major trauma.
- Lateral c-spine x-ray provides information on significant abnormalities.
- Pelvic x-ray should be performed in patients at risk of pelvic injury.
- FAST ultrasound scanning to identify intra-abdominal bleeding, pericardial effusion, and haemothorax or pneumothorax may be useful.
- CT scan (of brain, chest, abdomen, pelvis or spine may be indicated).

Rarely in children haemorrhage continues after initial resuscitation and ongoing resuscitation is required. If more than 40 mL/kg of blood is required in the first hour of arrival in hospital, consideration of urgent transfer to the operating theatre should be made for surgical management of the bleeding.

Issues to specifically consider in trauma:

- Immobilisation of the spine including a cervical collar.
- Persistent inadequate circulation due to fluid loss is blood loss and should be replaced with blood.
- Injuries to the head, neck, chest and abdomen may require urgent procedural intervention.
- Children rapidly become cold and hypothermia impairs coagulation.
- Transfer to a trauma centre should be arranged early.

Aspirated foreign body

First aid

- Give first aid (back slaps, chest thrusts) if obstruction occurs, otherwise allow the child to cough.
- Do not instrument the airways if the child is coping, but contact an anaesthetist and ENT surgeon.
- Give oxygen.

If partial obstruction occurs

- Place child upright in the position they feel most comfortable and arrange for urgent removal of foreign body in the operating theatre.

If complete obstruction occurs

- Open the airway and under direct vision (preferably using a laryngoscope) check in the mouth for a foreign body – if present remove it with Magill forceps.
- Place child prone with the head down.
- Apply five blows with the open hand to the interscapular area.
- Turn child face up.
- Apply five chest thrusts using the same technique as for chest compression during CPR.
- Check in the mouth to see if foreign body has appeared.
- Apply five lateral chest thrusts.
- If unsuccessful, repeat interscapular blows, central chest compressions and lateral chest thrusts.
- If this is unsuccessful, perform cricothyrotomy or tracheostomy.
- If respiratory failure is due to a foreign body lodged in the lower trachea or bronchi, attempt ventilation via an endotracheal tube while organising endoscopic removal.

Surgical management of an obstructed upper airway

- Several cricothyrotomy kits are now available in paediatric sizes. They are based on a Seldinger (catheter over wire) technique – know your own equipment.
- Adequate oxygenation (but not normal ventilation) can be obtained by inserting a 14-gauge IV cannula percutaneously into the trachea via the cricothyroid membrane (which lies between the thyroid and cricoid cartilage).
  - The patient should be lying straight, with the cannula in the midline and angled towards the feet.
  - Remove the needle of the IV cannula.
  - Connect the cannula to a resuscitator or a bagging circuit using a connector from a 3.0 mm endotracheal tube.
  - Oxygenate with sustained 100% oxygen inspirations.
  - Alternatively, connect the cannula to the compressed wall oxygen supply via a three-way IV tap (to allow expiration) and a length of plastic tubing.
  - A length of plastic tubing that has a side hole cut may also be used to allow expiration. Aid intermittent expiration by lateral chest compression.
- Alternatively, perform cricothyrotomy.
  - Identify and maintain stabilisation of the thyroid–cricoid region with one hand.
  - Incise the skin over the cricothyroid membrane.
  - Bluntly dissect into the trachea with forceps in the midline or incise vertically with scalpel.
  - Insert a small tracheostomy or endotracheal tube.
- Alternatively, perform percutaneous mini-tracheostomy.

Acute scrotum

- An acute scrotum is red, painful and tender. Any child with an acute scrotum should be seen by a surgeon as a matter of urgency.
- There are several causes of an acute scrotum but without surgical exploration, it is usually impossible to exclude testicular torsion.
- Other causes of an acute scrotum include torsion of the appendix testis, epididymo-orchitis and idiopathic scrotal oedema.

Testicular torsion

- Torsion of the testicle causes ischaemic infarction and must be urgently surgically corrected.
- Torsion of the testis can occur at any age, but is most common in infants and adolescents.
- In older children it is characterised by severe pain and vomiting. A testis lying horizontally in the scrotum indicates an anatomical predisposition to torsion and may cause intermittent testicular pain. When torted the testis is high riding, hard and exquisitely tender.
- Ultrasound is unreliable in distinguishing between torsion of the testis and torsion of the testicular appendage and often delays critical operative treatment.

Burns

The treatment of a burn aims to

- Prevent and treat shock
- Provide adequate analgesia
- Prevent infection
- Obtain early skin cover
- Prevent hypertrophic scar formation
- Restore function and correct cosmetic defect
- Prevent recurrence of injury and promote accident prevention

Assess the following

- Age – the younger the child, the more likely shock will occur for a given extent of burn.
- Estimating the body surface area burned (BSA).
  - The usual adult formula (rule of nines) is not applicable to children.
  - In infancy, the head is relatively large and contributes proportionately more to the total surface area. As the child grows, the lower limbs contribute more to the total surface area.
  - The burned areas should be plotted accurately on the body chart and the area calculated with the aid of the Lund–Browder chart. The extent of the burn is commonly overestimated, leading to excessive fluid administration.
- Assessment of the depth of burn – in most burns, there are varying grades of injury (see Table 2.1).

Management

First aid

- Remove clothing or smother the flame immediately.
- In minor burns, apply cold water from a bowl or by compressing for up to 30 minutes.
- In major burns, bathe for 20 minutes whilst awaiting transportation to hospital. Never use ice or ice slush.
- Cover to guard against hypothermia or cold injury with special foam transport dressing (if available) or plastic cling wrap, with a blanket for warmth. Give IV fluid, oxygen and morphine.
- Chemical and eye burns should be irrigated with copious volumes of cold water.
- Check tetanus immunisation status and boost with tetanus toxoid ± tetanus immunoglobulin as appropriate (see RCH *Tetanus-prone wounds* clinical practice guideline *http://www.rch.org.au/clinicalguide/guideline_index/Management_of_tetanusprone_wounds/*).

Pain relief

- Paracetamol (oral) 20–30 mg/kg.
- Codeine (oral) 0.5–1 mg/kg.
- Morphine (IV) 0.1 mg/kg given in titrated boluses.
- Morphine (IM) 0.2 mg/kg (useful if only a single dose is anticipated).

Table 2.1 Assessment of burn depth

Depth	Cause	Surface/colour	Pain	Treatment
Superficial (partial loss of skin)	Sun, flash, minor scald	Dry, minor blisters, erythema	Painful	Expose Non-adherent dressing
Superficial partial	Scald	Moist, reddened with broken blisters	Painful	Nanocrystalline silver dressing, e.g. Acticoat
Deep partial	Scald, minor flame, contact	Moist, white slough, red mottled	Painless	Nanocrystalline silver dressing, e.g. Acticoat
Deep (complete loss of skin)	Flame, severe scald, or contact	Dry, white, charred	Painless	Nanocrystalline silver dressing, e.g. Acticoat or SSD cream until split skin graft

Minor burns

Superficial burns <5% of the BSA are suitable for outpatient treatment, unless they occur on the face, neck, hands, feet or perineum. Infants <12 months are more likely to require admission.

Initial management

- Blisters should be left intact.
- Gently cleanse and remove loose skin.
- If burns are definitely superficial, dress with tulle gras and an absorbent dressing (e.g. gauze). Do not use Hypafix-type dressing directly on the burn.
- Immobilise with a crepe bandage, plaster slab or sling, if indicated.
- In partial thickness burns of indeterminate depth, the use of nanocrystalline dressing is recommended, for example Acticoat. These dressings should be left in place for 3 or 7 days depending on the product used.

Subsequent management

- Leave the initial dressing for 5–8 days. If the dressing is soaked by exudate, redress without disturbing the adherent tulle.
- If the healing process is not complete by the end of the second week, grafting may be required. Deep, second-degree burns not healing by 10 days should be referred to a burns unit.
- Pain, fever and soiled or offensive dressings indicate that the dressing should be changed and the child assessed and treated for infection if necessary.

Major burns

Superficial burns >5% of the BSA and deep burns may require admission to hospital.

For any child with burns >10% of the BSA, consider transfer to a specialist paediatric burns centre. Older children with more extensive superficial burns, such as sunburn, may be managed as outpatients.

General

- Document the time, causative agent, circumstances of the burn, therapy initiated and the child's general health. If the history is inconsistent with the injury, consider child abuse.
- Carefully chart the extent and depth of the burn.
- Weigh the patient if possible.
- In burns >10% of BSA, insert an IV line. If a central venous line is needed, a specialist burn centre should be involved. Plan IV therapy and commence treatment with Hartmann's solution.
- Draw blood for baseline laboratory studies, including haemoglobin, haematocrit and serum electrolytes. In severe burns include blood group and a crossmatch.
- In burns >15% of BSA, insert a silastic urethral catheter for hourly urine volume.
  Analgesia or sedation should be administered as necessary (see Chapter 3, *Pain management*).
- Prevent infection. Care should be taken in ward management to guard against cross-infection. Antibiotics should not be prescribed routinely.
- Observations of general condition, pulse, respiration rate, temperature, BP and fluid balance (including hourly urine output estimations) are necessary.
- A nasogastric tube should be placed if the burn is >15% of BSA.

Respiratory management

- With severe burns to the face, consider early endotracheal intubation. As the face swells, airway obstruction may occur, making intubation difficult.
- Smoke inhalation may lead to acute respiratory distress syndrome (ARDS) where ventilation perfusion defects result in hypoxemia, alveolar collapse, shunting and decreased lung compliance.
- Carboxyhaemoglobin (COHb) and cyanide concentration should be measured in all burn/smoke inhalation patients. Symptoms of hypoxemia manifest at levels >30% COHb. Treatment is oxygen therapy, as CO binding to Hb is reversible.

Fluid management

Fluid Resuscitation

- Fluid volume = 3 mL/kg body weight/% BSA in the first 24 hours.
- In less severe burns, fluid volume = 2 mL/kg body weight/% BSA may be sufficient.

- Type of fluid = 4% normal serum albumin solution (NSAS) and Hartmann's solution (use 50% of each solution concurrently).

Fluid maintenance
- 5% dextrose with 0.9% saline (to calculate maintenance fluid rate see Chapter 9, *Fluids and nutrition*, p. 107).

Rate of infusion (first 24 hours)
- First 8 hours: 1/2 resuscitation fluid plus 1/3 maintenance fluid.
- Second 8 hours: 1/4 resuscitation fluid plus 1/3 maintenance fluid.
- Third 8 hours: 1/4 resuscitation fluid plus 1/3 maintenance fluid.

For example, in a 16-kg child with 5% BSA burns
- Total resuscitation fluid = 3 × 16 kg × 5% = 240 mL (use 120 mL NSAS + 120 mL Hartmann's).
- Total maintenance fluid = 1300 mL.
  - First 8 hours = 120 mL (1/2 total resus fluid) + 433 mL (1/3 total maintenance fluid) = 553 mL (69 mL/h).
  - Second 8 hours = 60 mL (1/4 total resus fluid) + 433 mL (1/3 total maintenance fluid) = 493 mL (62 mL/h).
  - Third 8 hours = 60 mL (1/4 total resus fluid) + 433 mL (1/3 total maintenance fluid) = 493 mL (62 mL/h).

The 24-hour period commences from the time of burning, not from the time of admission.

Adjustments are made according to the hourly urine output, which is the best guide to the adequacy of fluid replacement. Expected flow is 0.75 mL/kg/h in children; in infants and toddlers, a urine output of up to 1 mL/kg/h is required. Record the urine specific gravity, serum and urine osmolality if renal function is poor.

Continue monitoring haemoglobin, haematocrit and electrolytes more frequently in severe injury. Restlessness may indicate inadequate fluid replacement (see Table 2.2).

Rate of infusion (second 24 hours and onwards)
After the initial 24 hours of fluid replacement, the type of fluid replacement will depend on urinary output, serum electrolytes and haemoglobin.
- The volume of burn resuscitation fluid is approximately 1/2 of that given for the first 24 hours.
- Total volume is given at an even rate over 24 hours.
- The volume and type of fluid given are adjusted according to urine flow and electrolyte estimations, and then decreased as the shock diminishes over the succeeding days. Diuresis occurs 2–3 days post-burn.

Oral fluids
Most children will tolerate small amounts of feeds (30–60 mL/h) after 4–8 hours. If this is tolerated, increase the quantity to 4 hourly. In minor burns, oral fluids may be commenced earlier. If vomiting secondary to gastric dilatation occurs, a nasogastric tube should be inserted.

After 48 hours, most fluid intake is usually oral. Children who refuse to drink, or who have burns to the face and mouth, may require nasogastric feeding.

Blood
Whole blood is not required initially except in severe, deep burns, and then usually only 24 hours post-burn, when the haemoglobin concentration is falling.

Local wound care
Minimal debridement of loose skin is done initially and management continued by exposed or closed methods.

Table 2.2 Fluid management for first 24 hours

	First 24 hours (volume)	First 8 hours (volume)	Second 8 hours (volume)	Third 8 hours (volume)
Resuscitation 50% of each of • 4% normal serum albumin solution (NSAS) • Hartmann's solution	3 × kg × % = — mL	1/2 of 24-hour volume	1/4 of 24-hour volume	1/4 of 24-hour volume
Maintenance	As per IV fluid protocol	1/3 of 24-hour volume	1/3 of 24-hour volume	1/3 of 24-hour volume
Total				

- Escharotomies should be considered if the peripheral circulation to a limb is jeopardised. Before commencing this procedure contact a paediatric burns unit.
- Respiratory difficulties require particular attention; intensive care or escharotomy to the trunk may be required.

Exposed
- Indications: for burns on the face, perineum, or one surface of the trunk.
- Treatment: apply paraffin gauze if superficial; nanocrystalline silver (Acticoat) dressing or topical silver sulfa-diazine (SSD) cream can be used depending on the extent of the burn.

Closed
- Indications: for small children and burns on extremities. Except for burns to the face or perineum, nearly all children are ultimately nursed with closed dressings.
- Treatment: an antiseptic tulle gras and gauze for superficial burns, or Acticoat dressing for deep burns. Fingers and toes are separated and wrapped together (not separately). Acticoat dressings can be left intact for either 3 or 7 days, per manufactures instructions for the dressing chosen.

Fever in patients with burns and antibiotic choice
- On admission, swabs should be taken of the burn area, nose, throat and rectum. In major burns, multiple 3-mL punch biopsy specimens are the most reliable method of detecting infection.
- Antibiotics are usually only given for proven infection and on the basis of sensitivity tests.
- If septicaemia is suspected clinically, blood culture should be performed and empiric antibiotics commenced. First-line antibiotics are flucloxacillin and gentamicin. Antibiotics to cover *Pseudomonas* sp. should be considered if there is no clinical improvement.

Nutrition
- All children with burns should receive a high-calorie diet containing adequate protein, vitamin and iron supplements.
- In severe burns there is a marked increase in metabolic rate and gastric tube feeding with a complete fluid diet (e.g. Isocal or Ensure) should be instituted early and adjusted to maintain or increase body weight. The involvement of a dietician is recommended.

Room temperature
- It is desirable that this is in the range of 22–26°C. If a child is partly exposed and nursed in a cool environment, metabolic requirements will increase.

Special therapy
- Physiotherapy and occupational therapy should be commenced early and continued throughout the course of burn care. Splints and pressure dressings are necessary to control hypertrophic scar formation. The play therapist also has an important role.
- Social rehabilitation is important, as many burned children come from disadvantaged homes. Maltreated children constitute approximately 6% of admissions to the burns unit. Psychological and psychiatric consultation is often required. The hospital teacher should also liaise with the child's schoolteachers.

Follow-up
- Healed burns and grafts are kept soft with emollient (e.g. Sorbolene cream).
- Pressure therapy and supervision of splints should be continued by a physiotherapist and occupational therapist.
- Parents and children need continuing support.
- Further operations are sometimes necessary to correct contractures and relieve cosmetic defects.

CHAPTER 3

Pain management

Jane Munro
George Chalkiadis

Numerous misconceptions contribute to under-treatment of paediatric pain, including
- Neonates and children do not experience pain or remember painful events.
- Children tolerate pain better than adults as their nervous systems are immature.
- All children are 'sensitive' to analgesics.
- Opioids are addictive or too dangerous to use in children.

These myths lead to poor pain prevention and management in neonates, children and adolescents. If unrelieved or inadequately treated, pain has negative physiological, psychological and emotional consequences.

Assessment of acute pain
Pain scores are important! They are the fifth vital sign on patients' observation charts. Pain assessment includes a combination of the following:

History
- Including site, onset, duration, quality, radiation, triggers and relievers, impact on functioning (including sleep disturbance and other activities), treatments tried and their effectiveness.
- In developmentally normal children, ask the child directly about their pain using appropriate tools.
- In neonates, pre-verbal children and cognitively impaired children, parents and regular caregivers are often best equipped to interpret the child's pain reliably.

Examination
- Behavioural observation (e.g. vocalisation, facial grimacing, posturing, movement).
- Physiological parameters (e.g. heart rate, respiratory rate, blood pressure) and physical signs (e.g. muscle spasm).
- Functional effects: for example, the ability to move (e.g. sitting up after laparotomy) and the tolerance of touch of the painful area usually signify adequate analgesia, whereas a child lying still and withdrawn may be in severe pain.

Use of pain-rating scales
Observe trends of change in an individual's pain score or function (e.g. ability to turn in bed comfortably, ability to walk to the toilet) rather than the 'raw' pain score.
- Verbal children
  - FACES scales for children >4 years, for example, Wong–Baker FACES Pain Rating Scale (Fig. 3.1) or Bieri revised
  - Visual analogue scale (e.g. 100-mm ruler)
  - Verbal numerical rating scale (e.g. 'out of 10 where 0 is no pain and 10 is the worst pain imaginable … ')
- Non-verbal children including neonates and cognitively impaired are particularly vulnerable (see Pain in children and adolescents with disabilities, p. 28)
  - FLACC: Face, Legs, Activity, Cry and Consolability
  - PATS (for neonates): Pain Assessment Tool Score

Paediatric Handbook, Ninth Edition. Edited by Amanda Gwee, Romi Rimer and Michael Marks.
© 2015 John Wiley & Sons, Ltd. Published 2015 by John Wiley & Sons, Ltd.

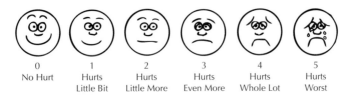

0	1	2	3	4	5
No Hurt	Hurts Little Bit	Hurts Little More	Hurts Even More	Hurts Whole Lot	Hurts Worst

Fig. 3.1 Wong–Baker **FACES** pain rating scale. Reproduced with permission from Hockenberry MJ, Wilson D, Winkelstein ML. *Wong's Essentials of Pediatric Nursing*, 7th ed., St. Louis, 2005, p. 1259. © Mosby. (Hockenberry 2005. Reproduced with permission of Elsevier.)

Analgesics for acute pain

Multimodal analgesia (MMA) involves the use of more than one drug and/or method of controlling pain to obtain additive beneficial effects, reduce side effects, or both.

MMA use is ideal for acute pain management including pain due to surgery, trauma or cancer, as it allows analgesia to be optimised and directed according to the multiple sources of pain (somatic, visceral and/or neuropathic).

Drug options include paracetamol, NSAIDs, COX-2 inhibitors, muscle relaxants (e.g. Buscopan for smooth and diazepam for skeletal muscle spasm), tramadol and neuropathic analgesics (such as gabapentin, pregabalin, amitriptyline, clonidine and ketamine).

Drugs can be administered by various routes. Specialised infusions (e.g. local anaesthetics, ketamine and opioids) can be via bolus and/or continuous infusion.

Use an analgesic ladder approach to manage acute pain (see Table 3.1). The progress up or down the steps varies according to

- the intensity of pain experienced;
- its anticipated duration; and
- the expected recovery period.

Each step up employs all the analgesics listed in the steps below. Once pain is controlled, wean back to the previous step. This varies with the speed of resolution of the painful condition and the number of breakthrough or rescue agents that are required in the higher category. If pain is poorly responsive to these measures, get consultant assistance. See Table 3.2 for dosing.

Table 3.1 Analgesic ladder approach

Degree of pain and setting	Analgesic 'steps'
Severe pain	
Inpatient	Add specialised infusion, for example ketamine, epidural local anaesthetic Add parenteral opioid by infusion (nurse or patient controlled)
Outpatient or emergency presentation	Add parenteral opioid by bolus or regular oral opioid (consider controlled release when long duration) Consider parenteral tramadol, NSAID, paracetamol Address sleep impairment and anxiety if present

Moderate pain	Add one (or combination) of:
	  Strong opioid, for example oral morphine, oxycodone
	  'Non-opioid': tramadol
	  Mild opioid: codeine
	Address environmental/psychosocial contributors

Mild pain	Begin with paracetamol and/or NSAIDs

Table 3.2 Analgesic medication

Drug	Dose	Route(s)	Indications	Side effects	Special notes/contraindications
Paracetamol	*Oral, rectal:* 15 mg/kg per dose 4 hourly *prn* rounded to appropriate suppository strength for rectal administration. Total daily maximum 60 mg/kg/day *IV:* 15 mg/kg qid	Oral: syrup or tablets Oral is preferred to rectal administration as absorption is more reliable and has an earlier peak concentration (oral 30–60 minutes vs. rectal 2–3 hours) IV (onset 15 minutes)	Effective for mild-to-moderate pain Also has antipyretic effects but physical measures are better	Hepatotoxicity Otherwise well tolerated	Hepatotoxicity has been reported in children. Use with caution in patients with severe liver disease, jaundice, malnutrition, glutathione depletion, dehydration and long-term ingestion Significant opioid sparing effects Adjust dosing to lean body mass in obese children
Opioid					
Oxycodone	0.1–0.2 mg/kg 4 hourly	Oral tablet (onset 30–60 minutes) Also available in slow release (SR) form	Stronger opioid	Nausea and vomiting, constipation Less itch than morphine or codeine	Cost is only slightly greater than codeine and no metabolism issues Avoids morphine stigma
Morphine	0.25–0.5 mg/kg 4 hourly orally 0.1 mg/kg 4 hourly iv	Oral (onset 40–60 minutes) Also available in controlled release (CR) form	Stronger opioid	As above	Stigma

(continued)

Table 3.2 (Continued)

Drug	Dose	Route(s)	Indications	Side effects	Special notes/contraindications
Tramadol	1–2 mg/kg 6 hourly	Oral; 50 mg or 100 mg capsules, IR (onset ~30–60 minutes) Also available in: SR tablet IV form (onset same as IV morphine)	For moderate-to-severe pain	Nausea and vomiting, dizziness, sedation Not as constipating and less itch and respiratory depression than opioids	Off-license use in <12-year olds requires anaesthetist-only prescription or Drug Usage Committee approval at RCH Avoid if history of seizures Mechanism of action via serotonin, noradrenaline reuptake and opioid receptors-dont prescribe with antidepressants (risk of serotonin syndrome) Opioid effect by metabolite M1 (requires CYP2D6 for conversion)
Fentanyl	1.5 mcg/kg (half into each nostril)	Intranasal (initial studies have used a specially designed atomiser)	Short-term analgesia		Initial emergency department studies have used 300 mcg/mL concentrations. Studies validating the use of 100 mcg/2 mL are pending.
NSAIDS					
Ibuprofen	5–10 mg/kg t.i.d–q.i.d	Oral: syrup 100 mg/5 mL 200 mg tablets (large)	For mild-to-moderate pain Particularly for muscular, bony or visceral pain	Gastrointestinal Renal Platelet inhibition (bleeding)	Caution in low volume status, poor urine output, renal failure, bleeding and asthma Avoid in severe asthma with nasal disease (because of NSAID/aspirin-exacerbated respiratory disease (ERD)) Can be used in mild asthma Generally NSAIDs are avoided in infants <6 months in Australia and <12 months in USA

Drug	Dose	Formulation	Uses	Cautions	Comments
Diclofenac	1 mg/kg b.i.d–t.i.d	Oral and rectal 25 and 50 mg tablet Rectal suppositories available at RCH			
Piroxicam	0.2–0.4 mg/kg (adult 10–20 mg) daily	Oral tablet			
Indomethacin	0.5–1.0 mg/kg per dose (adult 25–50 mg) 8 hourly (max 6 hourly)	Oral tablet			
Ketorolac	0.2 mg/kg IV (not IM)	IV available for anaesthetists to use at RCH			Off-license use <16 years
COX-2 inhibitor					
Celecoxib	2–4 mg/kg b.i.d	Oral capsule		No platelet inhibition	COX-2 s are OK in NSAID–ERD Off-license use <18 years
Local anaesthetics					
Lignocaine (lidocaine) 1–2% (1 mL of 1% = 10 mg)	Maximum doses: lignocaine (lidocaine) with adrenaline: 7 mg/kg Without adrenaline: 3 mg/kg	Injectable	Wound infiltration Nerve blocks/infusion	Neurological Cardiac	Do not inject adrenaline into 'end organs' such as fingers, toes, penis, nose or ears due to the risk of ischaemia
Bupivacaine 0.25–0.5%	Maximum dose 2–2.5 mg/kg e.g. <0.5 ml/kg of 0.5%				
Levobupivacaine 0.25–0.5%	Maximum dose 2–3 mg/kg, e.g. 0.4–0.6 ml/kg of 0.5%				

COX, cyclooxygenase; CR, controlled release; ERD, exacerbated respiratory disease; IR, immediate release; NSAIDs, non-steroidal anti-inflammatory drugs; SR, slow release.

Examples of patients with severe pain and suggested management
Femoral fracture
- Single-shot local anaesthetic femoral nerve block.
- Diazepam.
- Place in back slab or traction.
- Give other agents according to need.

Bowel obstruction requiring laparotomy
The patient will be nil orally and will universally require parenteral analgesia for severe pain. The following are suggested options. It is important that analgesia be commenced even if the child is to be transferred to a larger centre.
- Regular parenteral NSAID and paracetamol **and**
- Postoperative epidural local anaesthetic infusion **or**
- Opioid via patient-controlled analgesia (PCA) and ketamine infusion.

Metastatic cancer with bony metastases and large intra-abdominal mass
- Will benefit from regular dosing with a long-acting opioid such as MSContin or fentanyl patch (applied every 3 days).
- Manage breakthrough pain with immediate release morphine, fentanyl lozenges, sufentanil nasal/buccal spray or ketamine lozenges.

Procedural pain management
See Chapter 4, *Procedures*, p. 30.

Everyday events such as blood collection, cannula insertion, port cannulation, lumbar puncture and suturing are often a source of fear and anxiety for children. The aims of treating procedure-related pain are to prevent or minimise pain and distress.

Children with illnesses that require multiple painful procedures should be treated with care and sensitivity from the outset to avoid the development unnecessary psychological trauma.

Anticipation by staff and preparation of patients and their parents are of key importance. Consider
- The patient: age, previous experiences, emotional and physical condition of the child.
- The procedure: is it needed and how urgently, the level of expected pain and duration.
- The proceduralist: availability of appropriately skilled staff.

Always combine pharmacological and non-pharmacological techniques.
- Behavioural strategies (e.g. calico dolls, play therapy) can be used before all painful procedures. Use of appropriate distraction and breathing techniques are very helpful.
- Analgesic and sedative drugs are added when required.
- Remember that sedatives alone are not analgesics.
- It is difficult to assess pain and the effects of analgesia and sedation in neonates and children with cognitive impairments.

Before the procedure
General principles – preparation is the key
- Prepare yourself and the other staff involved.
- Ensure parents and the child understand what the procedure involves. Ideally, prepare the child <6 years immediately before the procedure and >6 years 1 week before.
- Avoid medical jargon; explain what is going to happen and in what order.
- Obtain consent from the parents (verbal or written as required).
- Set up your equipment before the child enters the procedure room.
- Encourage the parents to play an active role during the procedure by involving them in distraction techniques and comfort strategies. Avoid asking them to restrain their child.
- Children may be assisted to develop their own personal procedure routine, comfort or distraction strategies.
- An explanatory video may be helpful in preparing the child and their parent for the procedure.
- If considering procedural sedation, ensure adequate staffing and resources are available.

Pharmacological
- Topical anaesthetics (e.g. AnGel, EMLA for intact skin; Laceraine for wounds).
- Oral paracetamol, and/or NSAIDs and/or opioids, for example oxycodone.

During the procedure
General principles
- Give the child some feeling of control (e.g. choice of hand for IV, sitting up or lying down).
- Prompt the child to use the previously planned coping methods.
- Monitor the pain and effectiveness of pain management techniques during a procedure.
- If the child is not coping well, consider changing pain control measures or aborting the procedure.
- Consider sedation, depending on the procedure involved and the child's previous experience.

Comfort techniques
- Position for comfort (i.e. infants on parents' lap with physical/eye contact with parent).
- Have parents comfort child with gentle massage/touch or holding hands.
- Calm breathing.
- Swaddling for infants (<6 months).

Distraction techniques
- Choosing and playing an interactive iPad game, music CD or watching a favourite movie.
- Playing with developmentally appropriate toys.
- Counting objects in the room or looking at posters on the wall or ceiling.
- Reading interactive storybooks.
- Visual imagery (e.g. ask the child to imagine a place where they would like to be and to tell you about it).

Pharmacological techniques
- *Sucrose:* for infants (2 mL of 33% sucrose). Give 0.25 mL 2 minutes before the start of a procedure onto the infant's tongue. Offer a dummy if it is part of the infant's care. Give the remainder of the sucrose slowly during the procedure.
- *Topical local anaesthetic* (e.g. EMLA or AnGel)
  - IV cannulation, lumbar punctures and blood sampling are all potentially distressing for children.
  - Apply local anaesthetic cream 60–90 minutes before soft tissue needling procedures (this ensures skin analgesia a few millimetres deep).
  - Creams remain effective for up to 4 hours after application.
  - EMLA is a mixture of prilocaine 2.5% and lignocaine (lidocaine) 2.5%, and often vasoconstricts the area under application (onset 60–90 minutes).
  - AnGel (amethocaine 1%) has a faster onset than EMLA (60 minutes). If amethocaine is left on for >1 hour, erythema and itch can occur.
- For specific procedures: a *peripheral nerve block or IV regional anaesthesia* (e.g. Bier's block).
- *Local anaesthetic infiltration* (lignocaine (lidocaine), ropivacaine, bupivacaine or levobupivacaine)
  - The skin and subcutaneous tissues can be effectively infiltrated with local anaesthetic solutions.
  - Lignocaine (lidocaine) stings as it is injected. Stinging may be reduced by adding 1 mL of 8.4% sodium bicarbonate to 9 mL of lignocaine (lidocaine) solution.
  - The addition of adrenaline 1:200,000 or 1:400,000 (or 5–10 mcg/mL) may increase the duration of action, slows systemic absorption by up to 50% and reduces bleeding, **but adrenaline should not be used in 'end organs' such as fingers, toes, penis, nose or ears because of the risk of ischaemia.**
- *Nitrous oxide*
  - Useful inhalational analgesic agent which provides potent short-term analgesia for painful procedures such as wound dressings and the removal of catheters.
  - Rapid onset and offset.
  - Side effects may include sedation, nausea and vomiting. Bone marrow depression can occur with prolonged exposure (>12 hours) – consider in the child requiring daily repeat procedures.
  - Do not use in patients with head injuries, pneumothorax, cardiac disease and those who are obtunded.
  - The person administering nitrous oxide should have adequate airway management skills.

   ○ Fast patient before administration (2 hours for solids and liquids, or longer as clinically appropriate for more complex patients).
   ○ Methods of delivery include
     ▪ Entonox (a mixture of 50% nitrous oxide and 50% oxygen).
     ▪ Quantiflex (variable demand delivery system of nitrous oxide and oxygen).
● *Intranasal fentanyl*
   ○ Has been used in Australian emergency departments in the initial pain management of long-bone fractures.
   ○ A more concentrated solution of 300 mcg/mL was initially used, administered via an atomiser at a dose of 1.5 mcg/kg, given into one nostril only (where the child is >50 kg or if the less-concentrated solution is used, give half the dose into each nostril).
   ○ This has been administered prior to cannulation for subsequent opioid analgesia to be given intravenously.
   ○ *Note*: The role of this agent via this route as the neat standardly available solution (100 mcg/2 mL) in procedural sedation requires further delineation.

Anxiolytics and sedatives

Procedural sedation should only be undertaken by accredited staff members, with appropriate monitoring and equipment and line-of-sight nursing until return to baseline sedation score. Oral midazolam 0.5 mg/kg (usual max 15 mg) 20-30 minutes before treatment is routinely recommended. Intranasal delivery stings and is now avoided at RCH.

    Sedation is not analgesia! Sedation alone is useful for non-painful procedures, for example diagnostic ultra-sound. For painful procedures, analgesia is also necessary.

Cautions

● Observe the child in department or ward (line-of-sight nursing) until return to baseline sedation score.
● Usually recovery occurs by 60 minutes after oral/intranasal administration and 30 minutes after IV administration.
● Midazolam potentiates the sedative effects of other drugs, for example, opioids.
● Be prepared for a paradoxical reaction (agitation secondary to benzodiazepines).
● Midazolam should not be given to children with pre-existing respiratory insufficiency or neuromuscular disease (such as muscular dystrophy).

After the procedure

● Encourage the parent to remain with their child.
● Provide ongoing analgesia as needed.
● Document pain management techniques used and perceived success in minimising pain.
● Depending on the procedure, the child may need the opportunity to debrief. For example, staff and parents should focus on the helpful things the child did during the procedure. Staff may also like to suggest alternative techniques for any further procedures that may be planned.

Chronic or persistent pain management

Acute and chronic pain are distinct entities that require vastly different diagnostic and management skills; see Table 3.3.

Assessment

General principles

● Integrated multidisciplinary assessment and management is ideal.
● Assess the physical and psychosocial causes for the child's presentation.
● The factors maintaining persistent pain will determine specific treatment.
● An integrated approach with good communication between the involved healthcare providers is ideal.

History

● Is the pain
   ○ Nociceptive (arising from peripheral or visceral nociceptors)?
   ○ Neurogenic (arising at any point from the primary afferent neurone to higher centres in the brain)?
   ○ Psychogenic (occurs in the absence of any identifiable noxious stimulus or injurious process)?

Table 3.3 Comparison of the qualities and clinical course of acute versus chronic or persistent pain

Acute pain	Chronic or persistent pain
Tangible and understandable by the patient, family, friends and the treating doctor	Often nothing to see and minimal evidence of tissue damage
Usually brief, evoked by a recognised noxious stimulus and associated with an adaptive biological significance (e.g. protection of injured part to encourage healing)	Often present for prolonged duration
Usually improves rapidly and is associated with functional improvement and pain score reduction on a daily basis	May be evoked by minor trauma
Usually related to the nature and extent of tissue damage	Generally improves slowly over time with an undulating course
Responds to pharmacological intervention	Improvement and deterioration may be linked to life stresses
	Not necessarily related directly to the nature and extent of tissue damage
	Does not always respond to pharmacological intervention
	Often associated with secondary gains (e.g. school, sport or chore avoidance)

- Fixed factors (age, cognitive level, previous pain experience, witnessed examples of how other family members react to pain).
- Situational factors (social and academic functioning at schools, learned pain triggers, independent pain-reducing strategies).
- Suffering (fear, anxiety, anger, frustration, depression).
- Pain behaviour (overt distress, secondary gain, consultation with multiple health professionals factors, moaning, splinting, complaining of pain). Pain behaviour is exacerbated where the following factors are present:
  - Pain is central to communication (e.g. to receive a diagnosis or treatment).
  - Similarly, there is an absence of reinforcement for non-pain communication.
  - The child is fearful of increased pain (e.g. with movement).
  - The meaning of pain is fear-inducing.
  - The child and their parents may hold unhelpful beliefs and inadvertently maintain suffering, disability and dependency. The parents or child may obtain significant secondary gain from the child's maintained pain.
- Assess for
  - Unhelpful belief systems of child and/or family (e.g. if pain were cured the other problems would not exist).
  - Unrealistic expectations (e.g. it is others' responsibility to fix the problem).
  - Functional disability (e.g. inability to play sport, socialise with peers, attend school). Impaired sleep often occurs.

Examine the painful site

- What is causing the pain?
- Are there signs of complex regional pain syndrome (CRPS)? (see p. 27).
- Is there secondary deconditioning (e.g. muscle wasting, joint stiffening, tendon shortening)?
  - These can occur rapidly, especially when fear of touch or movement exists.

Management

The goals are to eliminate pain, restore function and reduce pain behaviour. It is desirable to identify the cause of pain, treat and eliminate it; however, this is not always possible. Therefore management aims to achieve a more active and fulfilling lifestyle, less constrained by pain with improved coping.

Coordinate outpatient appointments to facilitate achieving these goals and minimising school absenteeism, time off work for parents and discouraging adoption of the sick role.

When to refer to a multidisciplinary pain clinic

A multidisciplinary team should ideally include a pain medicine specialist, physiotherapist, clinical psychologist, occupational therapist and child psychiatrist. The team should have access to an orthopaedic surgeon, neurosurgeon, paediatrician, paediatric rheumatologist and a rehabilitation specialist.

Refer when
- Pain is more intense or persists longer than anticipated (e.g. after an injury).
- Character of pain is different to that expected.
- Pain responds poorly to medication.
- Loss of function results in secondary deconditioning (e.g. muscle wasting).
- Pain interferes with sleep, socialising with peers, school attendance and leisure activities.
- Pain behaviour manifests.
- CRPS is present.
- Pain is neuropathic.

Non-pharmacological techniques in chronic pain management

- Pain education
  - Help the patient understand that stress, anxiety and anger may contribute to pain. Identifying these stressors (often school or family) and managing these feelings more effectively may reduce or eliminate pain.
  - Help the patient understand that pain does not always mean damage, and that pain is not a hindrance to return to function.
  - Provide illness information (if one has been identified) outlining implications for the future. This can minimise anxiety.
- Cognitive behavioural techniques address the (often unhelpful) thoughts that maintain pain and disability.
  - Thought stopping or challenging techniques.
  - Mindfulness
  - Behaviour modification techniques: based on modifying the consequences of the child's pain experience and pain behaviour by rewarding positive behaviour.
- Pain coping strategies include
  - Relaxation techniques: muscle relaxation via body awareness techniques, meditation, self-hypnosis or biofeedback.
  - Distraction techniques: art, play or music therapy.
- Physiotherapy reconditioning programs
  - Involve gradual return to function.
  - Utilise: muscle stretches, postural exercises, reconditioning programs and stress loading (e.g. 'scrub and carry' techniques for the upper limbs, weight bearing for lower limbs).
  - Ultrasound treatment.
  - Heat/cold treatment.
  - Transcutaneous electrical nerve stimulation (TENS): activates large, myelinated primary afferent fibres (A fibres) that act through inhibitory circuits within the dorsal horn to reduce nociceptive transmission through small unmyelinated fibres (C fibres). TENS is more likely to be effective if pain responds to heat or cold.
- Pacing activity with reasonable goals.
- Management of setbacks.
- Sleep management.
- Family therapy
  - Addresses how family dynamics may maintain pain.
  - Addresses how pain affects the rest of the family (e.g. lack of attention for well siblings).
- Parental counselling
  - Parents may inadvertently support illness and ignore non-pain activities.
  - Addresses parental feelings of helplessness and loss of control.
  - Equips parents with strategies to manage pain behaviour.
- Assertiveness training.

- School liaison
  - Address bullying.
  - Modifications to allow return to school despite disability.
  - Equip teachers with strategies to deal with pain behaviour.
  - Graded return-to-school programs with involvement and education of teachers.
- Vocational counselling.
- Hydrotherapy.
- Acupuncture.

Pharmacological techniques in chronic pain management

Paracetamol

Limit the dose for long-term administration to 60 mg/kg per day.

Steroids

- Triamcinolone used for joint injections, trigger point injections, tendon sheaths and neuralgias.
- Dexamethasone administered by iontophoresis for soft tissue injuries.
- Epidural or root sleeve steroid administration for localised nerve root irritation due to disc herniation without motor weakness.

Non-steroidal anti-inflammatory drugs

- Topical gels (diclofenac, piroxicam, ibuprofen)
- Oral and rectal preparations (described in Table 3.2)

Anti-neuropathic medications

Tricyclic antidepressants (TCADs)/newer noradrenergic and serotonergic reuptake inhibitors (SSRIs)

Improve pain even if depression is not present by suppressing pathological neural discharges. Provides more effective analgesia, usually within days, once appropriate dose reached.

Indications

- Severe unremitting pain, especially if neuropathic
- CRPS
- Associated depression
- Poor sleep

Amitriptyline is the most commonly used TCAD, starting at 0.2 mg/kg per day increasing over 2 weeks to 2 mg/kg per day. Administer as a single dose before bed to take advantage of sedative properties. Increase dosage until the desired treatment goal is achieved or side effects become unacceptable, for example dry mouth, morning somnolence.

Anticonvulsants (e.g. gabapentin, pregabalin or carbamazepine)

Indicated for neuropathic pain and CRPS

Dosage should be in the therapeutic anticonvulsant range, although there is no evidence of any relationship between analgesic effect and the plasma level. Some recommend increasing the dosage to the point of side effects or analgesia. Gabapentin is not licensed for use in pain and incurs an out-of-pocket cost.

Opioids

- Only partially modulate central sensitisation.
- Usually ineffective in controlling neuropathic pain or pain secondary to CRPS.
- Indicated in cancer pain and nociceptive pain.
- Tramadol may be useful.

Other techniques can include ketamine, baclofen, clonidine, sympathetic and peripheral nerve blocks. Surgical techniques are rarely used in paediatrics.

Complex regional pain syndrome (CRPS), types I and II

This condition is of unknown aetiology and is more common in paediatrics than is generally realised. The diagnosis is clinical and treatment is easier when the condition is recognised early.

- **Type I** was formerly known as reflex sympathetic dystrophy (RSD). It often occurs after a noxious stimulus to the affected limb (e.g. minor trauma or surgery). Symptoms are disproportionate to the inciting event.
- **Type II** was formerly referred to as causalgia. It differs from type I because it occurs after peripheral nerve injury.

Clinical manifestations

The affected area, usually a limb, manifests autonomic, sensory and motor symptoms consisting of

- Pain
  - ○ Regional non-dermatomal distribution
  - ○ Hyperaesthesia (diffuse pain exacerbated by touch)
  - ○ Allodynia (pain elicited by a stimulus that is not usually painful)
- Temperature change (affected limb often colder)
- Changes in skin blood flow – often red/purple colour change
- Abnormal sweating
- Oedema
- Loss of function/reduced range of motion
- Motor dysfunction – weakness, tremor, dystonia
- Abnormal hair growth, skin and/or nail atrophy

Investigations

- Acute phase markers – normal
- Bone scan often abnormal – increased or decreased uptake
- Plain radiograph – osteopenia in prolonged cases
- MRI – diffuse marrow infiltration is sometimes present

Management

- Management requires early identification, skilful physical therapy, avoidance of immobilisation and multidisciplinary pain team input.
- Consider psychiatric assessment, pharmacological and interventional techniques.

Neuropathic pain

- Typified by continuous burning with an intermittent electric shock, stabbing or shooting-type discomfort.
- May be paroxysmal or spontaneous.
- Pain in an area of sensory loss.
- Pain in the absence of ongoing tissue damage.
- Associated with dysaesthesia (unpleasant, abnormal sensation; e.g. ants crawling on skin), allodynia and hyperalgesia (increased pain in response to noxious stimuli).
- Increased sympathetic activity may be present.
- Causes include CRPS type II, tumour, spinal cord injury, nerve damage (e.g. neuropraxia or avulsion, neuroma).
- Usually poor response to opioid medication.
- Consider the use of anti-neuropathic medications and early referral to a pain specialist and/or multidisciplinary pain management team if prolonged or refractory.

Pain in children and adolescents with disabilities

See also Chapter 23, *Child development*, p. 357.

Pain assessment in individuals with cerebral palsy, cognitive impairment and/or communication difficulties can prove challenging.

- No simple pain assessment tool exists.
- Caregivers are best placed to distinguish pain from 'normal' behaviour in the individual.
- Pain may manifest as crying, screaming, frequent waking, grimacing, arching, muscle spasm or self-injurious behaviour, but some individuals with cerebral palsy or intellectual disability may exhibit these behaviours without experiencing pain.
- Differential diagnosis includes seizures, muscle spasm, anxiety, depression and anger.
- A thorough search for the cause of pain will guide treatment options.

Sleep disturbance
- Occurs frequently and has implications for the functioning of the whole family.
- Address poor sleep hygeine.
- Address underlying worries and concerns.
- TCAD, via their analgesic and sedative effects, may be useful in reducing the frequency of waking.
- Melatonin may also be useful.

> **USEFUL RESOURCES**
> - *www.rch.org.au/anaes/pain_management/Acute_Pain_Management_CPMS/* – RCH Acute Pain Management Service Clinical Practice Guidelines. Links to many topics including: morphine by intermittent bolus guideline; opioid by infusion and patient controlled analgesia (PCA).
> - *www.rch.org.au/clinicalguide/guideline_index/Analgesia_and_Sedation/* [Analgesia & Sedation] – RCH Clinical Practice Guidelines including links to Nitrous Oxide and Ketamine Guidelines.
> - *www.pediatric-pain.ca* – Pediatric Pain Research Lab. Site created by a Canadian research group, devoted to the topic. Contains useful downloadable pamphlets and protocols.

CHAPTER 4

Procedures

Ed Oakley

Procedures can be pain- and anxiety-free with good planning and procedural pain management. It is easier to perform any procedure with a calm child and family. Ideally, procedures should be carried out in a designated procedure room, with equipment ready before the child enters the room. Procedural pain management includes both non-pharmacological techniques such as distraction, presence of a parent, and pharmacological techniques with analgesia and sedation as required. Agents that provide sedation may not provide pain relief. Suggested analgesia is included for procedures in this chapter, further details are included in Chapter 3, *Pain management*, p. 17. Universal precautions should be taken during any procedure. Gloves and protective eyewear should be worn and a hard plastic container should be within easy reach for the disposal of sharps. Procedures should be documented in the medical record.

For some simple ways of communicating procedures to parents and patients see RCH *communicating procedures to families* clinical practice guideline *http://www.rch.org.au/clinicalguide/guideline_index/Communicating_procedures_to_families/*

Venepuncture
Sites
- Cubital fossa
- Dorsum of the hand
- Others, as dictated by availability or necessity

Suggested analgesia
- Topical local anaesthetic, for example amethocaine or EMLA (lignocaine (lidocaine), prilocaine), can be used for any age except preterm neonates.
- Sucrose in infants <3 months (max 2 mL, 0.5 mL in infants <1500 g).
- Consider nitrous oxide in children >2 years.
- Consider sedation, for example midazolam oral 0.5 mg/kg (max 15 mg) intranasal/buccal 0.3 mg/kg (max 10 mg).

Equipment
Needle (straight or butterfly), syringe, alcohol wipe, tourniquet, cotton ball, band-aid/tape, blood collection tubes.

Technique
- In adolescents and older children, blood can be collected with a needle and syringe, as in adults. In infants and small children, a 23-gauge butterfly needle offers more stability.
- Wash the site with an alcohol preparation and allow to dry. Using a tourniquet around the limb, insert the needle into a vein and aspirate gently; once enough blood is collected, release tourniquet and apply local pressure with a cotton ball on the puncture site.
- Some visible veins are too small to be used to take blood. A palpable vein is more likely to be successful than a visible but non-palpable vein.
- With small children, an assistant can hold the limb still and provide a tourniquet at the same time.
- An alternative technique is to insert a 21- or 23-gauge needle into a vein and allow the blood to drip out directly into collection tubes. Several millilitres can be collected this way.

Paediatric Handbook, Ninth Edition. Edited by Amanda Gwee, Romi Rimer and Michael Marks.
© 2015 John Wiley & Sons, Ltd. Published 2015 by John Wiley & Sons, Ltd.

Blood culture collection
- Strict asepsis is required.
- Use alcoholic chlorhexidine or 70% alcohol-based preparations for skin preparation and wait at least 1 minute before taking blood. Do not touch the venepuncture site after skin preparation.
- Most paediatric blood culture bottles require 1–4 mL of blood; take as close to 4 mL as possible for optimal sensitivity.
- Consider anaerobic blood cultures (as well as aerobic) in: neonates where there has been prolonged rupture of membranes or maternal chorioamnionitis, poor dentition, severe mucositis, sinusitis, abdominal sepsis, perianal infections, bite wounds or in immunosuppressed patients.
- In patients with central venous access devices take paired peripheral and central line cultures.
- There is no need to change needles between venepuncture and injecting the blood culture bottles. Inject blood culture bottles first (before dividing blood into other specimen tubes).

Intravenous cannula insertion
Sites
- Dorsum of the non-dominant hand is preferred.
- Alternative sites include the anatomical snuffbox, volar aspect of the forearm, dorsum of the foot, great saphenous vein or cubital fossa.
- The site usually requires splinting and this should be taken into consideration (e.g. foot in a mobile child is less desirable).
- Scalp veins should only be used when there are no other possibilities.

Suggested analgesia
- As for venepuncture above.
- Consider injectable local anaesthetic in older children, for example lignocaine (lidocaine) 1%, applied intradermally.

Equipment
Dressing pack, antiseptic solution, IV cannula, blood collection tubes and syringe if needed, 0.9% saline flush, three-way tap/connection tubing (primed with 0.9% saline), tourniquet, splint, tapes, bandage.

Technique
- Be patient and look carefully for the best option. Ensure the child is warm and there is adequate light.
- If using the back of the hand in infants, grasp the wrist between the index and middle fingers with the thumb over the patient's fingers, flexing the wrist. This achieves both immobilisation and tourniquet (see Fig. 4.1).
- Insert the cannula just distal to and along the line of the vein at an angle of 10–15°. When a large vein is entered, a 'flash' of blood will enter the hub of the needle.

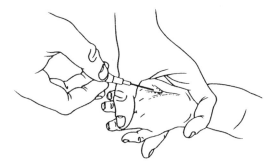

Fig. 4.1 Intravenous cannula insertion

- Advance the cannula a further 1–2 mm along the line of the vein, then remove the needle while advancing the cannula along the vein. If the cannula is in the vein, blood will flow back out along the cannula.
- Safety IV cannulae have a clip or mechanism which covers the needle tip when the needle is retracted fully from the cannula. It may be necessary to insert the cannula (with needle *in situ*) slightly further into the vein initially, as the safety mechanism often produces a backward movement as it retracts and may dislodge the cannula.
  - When trying to cannulate a small vein, there may not be a flashback of blood. Insert the cannula and when it is likely to be in the vein, partially remove the needle and watch for blood moving slowly back along the cannula. Advance the cannula along the vein gently. With safety cannulae it is not possible to remove the needle and reinsert.
- Take required blood samples at this stage. In neonates and young infants, blood can be collected by allowing it to drip directly into collection tubes (without a syringe).
- Connect a primed three-way tap/connector and tape the cannula. Place tape over the cannula, then a clear plastic dressing and further tape over the top.
- Flush the cannula with 0.9% saline to confirm IV placement. Connect the IV tubing and splint the arm to an appropriately sized board. Wrap the entire length of the board in a bandage.

Accessing central venous catheters
Types
- Catheter devices, for example Hickman or Broviac catheters, are central venous access devices that are tunnelled subcutaneously before they enter a central vein. They may be either single or double lumen. The external part of the line has a clamp and a connector which is accessed.
- Infusaports are central venous access devices that have a small chamber attached to the intravenous cannula. This chamber is placed completely under the skin so no part is exposed. The chamber can be accessed through the skin.

Suggested analgesia
- Topical local anaesthetic, for example amethocaine or EMLA (lignocaine (lidocaine), prilocaine), for Infusaport access.
- Consider sedation and nitrous oxide in children >2 years.
- A procedural pain management plan should be developed for all children with a central venous access device.

Equipment
Sterile gloves, dressing pack, alcohol-based chlorhexidine, Huber point needle (90° bend) for Infusaport, short three-way tap or minimum volume extension tubing, giving set, sterile adhesive strips, syringe with sterile 0.9% saline flush, additional syringes/blood collection tubes, gauze, two occlusive clear plastic dressings.

Technique
Generic (Hickman, Broviac, Infusaport)
- Strict asepsis is required.
- Central venous access devices are flushed with heparin-containing solutions when not in use.
- For short-term disconnection use 50 units heparin per 5 mL 0.9% saline.
- For long-term disconnection (e.g. on discharge) use 1000 units heparin per 1 mL 0.9% saline ×1 mL diluted to 10 mL with 0.9% saline (i.e. 100 units heparin/1 mL final concentration).
- For both types of flush use 4–5 mL volume. Stop backflow immediately by clamping catheter devices and in Infusaports by turning tap to off (short-term flush) or removing needle (long-term flush).
- Catheter devices require weekly flushing; Infusaports require monthly flushing.
- Catheter devices require dressing changes weekly. The exit site is washed with antiseptic solution (applied radially from centre outwards) and the tubing is also washed. The solution is allowed to dry, then two clear adhesive dressings are used to 'sandwich' the tubing. The distal tubing is then taped to the child's chest wall and the remainder safety-pinned to clothing to avoid pulling on the line. In younger children tape the clamp and tap to avoid little fingers exploring.

Infusaport specific
- Wash the site with antiseptic preparation and allow it to dry.
- Attach Huber point needle to minimum volume extension tubing connected to a three-way tap and prime the line with 0.9% saline.
- Insert Huber point needle into the centre of the port chamber. Aspirate 5 mL of blood back through three-way tap (may be used for blood cultures), then take other bloods using a second syringe as required. Ensure tap is turned to 45° to avoid backflow when connecting/disconnecting syringes. Flush line with 5 mL 0.9% saline.
- Make a pillow of gauze under the Huber point needle and secure with sterile adhesive strips; then apply airtight adhesive clear plastic dressing.

Umbilical vein catheterisation
Indications
Used in neonates up to 7–10 days of age for
- Emergency vascular access for resuscitation
- IV access for exchange transfusion
- Venous access in low-birthweight infants (preferred initial access in infants <800 g)

Equipment
- Sterile drapes, gown, mask and gloves, sterile instrument pack (gauze, forceps, needle holder, scalpel holder), umbilical tape (or rolled gauze), scalpel blade, antiseptic solution, umbilical catheter (baby <1000 g 3.5 FG, >1000 g 5.0 FG), syringe with 0.9% saline flush, three-way tap/connection tubing, suture.
- If no umbilical catheter is available, a sterile 5 FG feeding tube can be used for umbilical vein access in an emergency.

Site
- Measure the distance of a line drawn from the tip of the shoulder to the level of the umbilicus.
- Using Fig. 4.2 determine the catheter length needed to place **the tip between the diaphragm and the right atrium in the inferior vena cava (IVC)**. Add the height of the umbilical stump to obtain the total length.
- In an emergency, short-term access can be obtained with the UVC tip inserted 3–5 cm past the mucocutaneous junction (will not be in portal circulation).

Technique
- Strict asepsis is required.
- Attach a three-way tap to the catheter and flush with sterile saline then close the three-way tap. Throughout insertion the catheter and connection must be kept filled with fluid to prevent air embolism.
- Drape and prepare the skin. Loosely tie a sterile umbilical tape or rolled gauze around base of the cord. Cut through the cord with a scalpel horizontally 1.5–2 cm from the skin; tighten the tape/gauze to prevent bleeding if necessary.
- Stabilize the cord with artery forceps. Identify the single large thin-walled vein and two smaller thick-walled arteries. Clear any thrombi with forceps, gently dilate the vein with curved iris forceps and insert the catheter.
- Gently advance the catheter to the pre-measured distance. Do not force. Aspirate to check position (blood should fill the cannula easily).
- Secure the catheter with both a purse string suture around the cord and a tape bridge. Radiologically confirm that the catheter tip lies above the diaphragm in the IVC; it is not acceptable within the liver.

Umbilical artery catheterisation
Indications
Used in low-birthweight neonates for
- Monitoring blood pressure and arterial blood gases
- Access and infusion site

Equipment
As for umbilical vein access. In addition, blood pressure transducer and heparin solution.

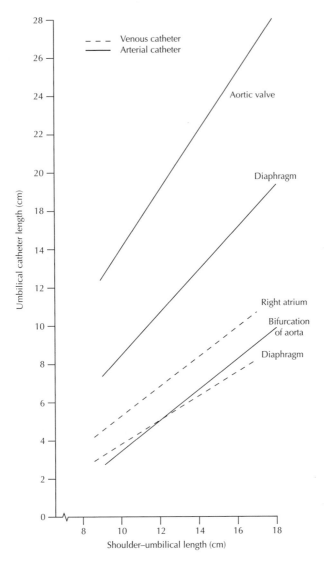

Fig. 4.2 Determining umbilical vein and artery catheter length

Site

- Measure the distance of a line drawn from the tip of the shoulder to the level of the umbilicus. Use Fig. 4.2 to determine the catheter length needed:
  - High line position: between T6–T9; tip above the diaphragm (proximal to the origin of renal and mesenteric arteries).
- The catheter length may also be calculated by formula: (weight (kg) × 3) + 9 cm.

Technique

- Strict asepsis is required.
- Flush the catheter and three-way tap, prepare skin and cord and cut cord as above.
- Identify the arteries, clear any thrombi and dilate the artery with curved iris forceps. Initially one tip of the forceps is inserted, then both, with the tips allowed to spring gently open.
- Insert catheter and advance gently. Aim tip towards the feet. Avoid excessive pressure or repeat probing. Aspirate to check position (blood should fill the cannula easily and pulsations will be seen) then flush line. Arterial lines are heparinised (see Pharmacopoeia).
- Secure the catheter as above and confirm tip position radiologically.
- Check for any complications caused by catheter placement, especially blanching or cyanosis of lower extremities. Nurse infant supine for 24 hours after the procedure.

Arterial puncture

Indications

Suspected hypoxaemia, hypercapnia or severe acidosis with poor peripheral perfusion.

Note: Acid–base status can also be accurately assessed by capillary or venous collection.

Sites

Radial artery

Note: The femoral artery is used only in emergencies when no other arteries are palpable. **Never** use the ulnar artery.

Suggested analgesia

- Sucrose in infants <3 months of age.
- Topical local anaesthetic or injectable local anaesthetic, for example lignocaine (lidocaine) 1%, can be used, but does not prevent pain caused by puncturing the artery.

Equipment

Alcohol wipe, 23 or 25 FG needle (straight or butterfly), syringe (2 mL pre-heparinised syringe for blood gas), cotton ball, band-aid/tape, blood collection tubes.

Technique

- Clean the skin with an alcohol wipe.
- Pierce the skin at a 15–30° angle directly over the artery. On entering the artery, blood will fill the hub; however, gentle aspiration is usually required to fill the syringe.
- If there is no flashback at full depth or when the bone is contacted, withdraw the needle very slowly while aspirating. Blood will often be obtained at this point if the artery has been transfixed. If no blood is aspirated check position of pulse and repeat.
- Only 0.5 mL of blood is required for arterial blood gas, sodium, potassium and haemoglobin measurements.
- After obtaining a specimen, remove the needle quickly and apply firm pressure to the puncture site for 3–5 minutes.

Intra-arterial cannula insertion

Indications

Invasive blood pressure monitoring and frequent blood sampling in the intensive care setting.

Sites

Radial, posterior tibial and dorsalis pedis arteries.

Suggested analgesia

- Sucrose in infants <3 months of age.
- Topical local anaesthetic or injectable local anaesthetic, for example, lignocaine (lidocaine) 1%, can be used, but does not prevent pain caused by puncturing the artery.

Equipment

Dressing pack, antiseptic solution, IV cannula, blood collection tubes and syringe if needed, 0.9% saline flush, three-way tap/connection tubing (primed with 0.9% saline), pressure transducer, heparin solution, splint, tapes, bandage.

Technique

- Do not use a tourniquet. Feel for the pulse of the artery to be cannulated and insert the cannula at an angle of 15–30° to the skin. Once a flashback of blood is obtained reduce the angle (to 10–15°) and advance the cannula gently with the needle *in situ* so it is clearly within the artery before the needle is removed.
- Place a finger proximally over the pulse when withdrawing the needle and attach (primed) connector tubing and transducer quickly.
- Take bloods if required, flush slowly and watch for blanching around the site and distally.
- Arterial lines require continuous heparin infusion.

Intraosseous needle insertion
Indications

For emergency vascular access when efforts to cannulate a vein are unsuccessful.

Sites

Preferred sites of insertion are
- Proximal tibia (depending on size, 1–3 cm inferomedial to tibial tuberosity).
- Distal femur (approximately 3 cm above the condyles on anterolateral surface) (see Fig. 4.4).
- Avoid fractured bones and limbs with proximal fractures.

Suggested analgesia

Performed in emergency situations. Injectable local anaesthetic (lignocaine (lidocaine) 1%) if patient is conscious.

Equipment

Intraosseus needle (if not available a short large-bore lumbar puncture needle or bone marrow aspiration needle are alternatives), syringe with 0.9% saline flush, three-way tap/connection tubing (primed with 0.9% saline), alcohol wipe, syringe, blood collection tubes.

Technique

- Prepare the insertion site.
- Insert the needle at 90° to the skin (see Fig. 4.3). Apply downward pressure with a rotary motion to advance the needle. When the needle passes through the bony cortex into the marrow cavity, resistance suddenly decreases. The needle should stand without support (except in a very young infant).

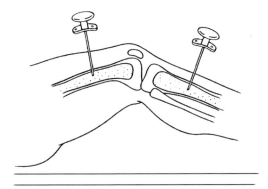

Fig. 4.3 Intraosseous needle insertion sites

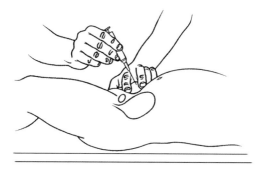

Fig. 4.4 Suprapubic aspiration

- Remove the stylet and attach a syringe; aspirate to confirm that the needle is in the bone marrow (this is not always possible). Flush the needle with saline to confirm correct placement and connect IV tubing. Often fluids will not flow by gravity into the marrow – a three-way tap and syringe or pressure infusion may be needed.
- Watch the infusion site for fluid extravasation, or the calf becoming tense. A pair of artery forceps clamped around the base then taped along the limb (with appropriate padding underneath) can provide stability. The needle should be removed once IV access has been obtained.
- Any fluid or drug that can be given IV can be administered through the intraosseous route.

Suprapubic aspiration

See RCH *Suprapubic aspirate* clinical practice guideline *http://www.rch.org.au/clinicalguide/guideline _index/Suprapubic_Aspirate_Guideline/*

Indications

Sterile urine collection for suspected urinary tract infection (UTI) as part of septic workup.
   Note: Not recommended in age >24 months (unless the bladder is palpable or percussible).
   This is most successfully performed by confirming urine in the bladder with a bed side ultrasound.

Site

- Midline in the skin crease above the symphysis pubis

Suggested analgesia

Topical local anaesthetic. Sucrose if <3 months of age

Equipment

- Alcohol wipe, 23-gauge needle and 2 or 5 mL syringe, cotton ball, adhesive tape, sterile urine collection pot
- Bladder ultrasound if available

Technique

- If multiple procedures are planned, aim to **perform the Suprapubic aspiration (SPA) first** as the child may void whilst having a venepuncture or lumbar puncture.
- Wait at least 30 minutes after the last void.
- Use a bladder ultrasound if possible; attempt SPA only if >20 mL urine present, or bladder size is visualised to be >1 cm in all axes on real time ultrasound.
- Position the patient with legs either straight or bent in the frog-leg position. Have a sterile bottle handy for a midstream clean catch in case the child voids.
- Prepare the skin with an alcohol wipe. Insert a 23-gauge needle attached to a 2 or 5 mL syringe perpendicular to the abdominal wall (see Fig. 4.4). Pass almost to the depth of the needle and then aspirate while

withdrawing. If urine is not obtained, do not remove the needle completely. Change the angle of the needle and insert it again, first angling superiorly and then inferiorly.

- In the event of obtaining no urine, either: (1) perform urethral catheterisation; or (2) wait 30 minutes, giving the child a drink during this time. Repeat the SPA. It is a good idea to put a urine bag on to determine if the child has voided before proceeding with a further SPA.

Urethral catheterisation
Indications
- Suspected UTI where midstream specimen is not possible
- Acute urinary retention

Suggested analgesia
- Local anaesthetic topical gel (e.g. lignocaine (lidocaine) 2% gel) – takes 10 minutes for full effect
- Consider nitrous oxide. Sucrose if <3 months of age

Equipment
- Sterile drapes and gloves, water-based antiseptic solution, catheter, catheter bag and syringe with 0.9% saline (if indwelling catheter), sterile urine collection pot, and bowl/kidney dish (to hold urine).
- For diagnostic catheterisation, use a 5 FG feeding tube (depending on age). For indwelling catheters, use a silastic catheter with an inflatable balloon. Appropriate sizes are: 0–6 months 6 FG, 2 years 8 FG, 5 years 10 FG, 6–12 years 12 FG; this may vary with the size of the patient. Lubricants will aid insertion.

Technique
- The child lies with legs apart in the frog-leg position. Prepare and drape the area, apply local anaesthetic gel and wait.
- Using a sterile technique, locate the urethral orifice (in girls: see Fig. 4.5). In boys the foreskin need not be retracted for successful catheterisation. Gently advance the catheter posteriorly until urine is obtained.
- For indwelling catheters: inflate balloon **only** when urine has been obtained, attach catheter to collection device and tape catheter securely to leg.

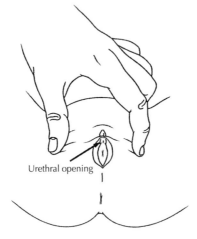

Urethral opening

Fig. 4.5 Urethral orifice in girls

Lumbar puncture
See Lumbar Puncture CPG (http://www.rch.org.au/clinicalguide/guideline_index/Lumbar_Puncture_Guideline/

Indications

- A febrile, sick infant or child with no focus of infection
- Fever with meningism
- Prolonged seizure with fever

Contraindications

- Coma
- Focal neurological signs
- Focal seizures, recent seizures (within 30 minutes) or prolonged seizures (>30 minutes)
- Signs of raised intracranial pressure (ICP): altered pupil responses, decerebrate or decorticate posturing, papilloedema (unreliable and late sign in meningitis)
- Cardiovascular compromise/shock
- Respiratory compromise
- Thrombocytopenia/coagulopathy
- Local superficial infection
- Strong suspicion of meningococcal infection (typical purpuric rash in ill child)

Note:

- Coma – reduced conscious state and absent or non-purposeful responses to painful stimuli. Elicit by squeezing the earlobe hard for up to 1 minute. Children should localise response and seek a parent. If in doubt, do not proceed with lumbar puncture.
- Drowsiness, irritability, vomiting and isolated tonic–clonic, myoclonic, absence or atonic seizures are not in themselves contraindications.
- A bulging fontanelle in the absence of other signs of raised ICP is not a contraindication.

Suggested analgesia

Topical local anaesthetic plus

- Sucrose in infants <3 months of age.
- Injectable local anaesthetic (lignocaine (lidocaine) 1%).
- Consider nitrous oxide.
- Consider sedatives (e.g. midazolam), although this may complicate assessment of conscious state.

Equipment

- Sterile drapes, gown, mask and gloves, antiseptic solution, sterile dressing pack, specimen collection tubes, cotton ball, band-aid/adhesive dressing.
- A lumbar puncture needle with introducing stylet should be used. A 22 or 25 FG needle is usually appropriate. The correct needle length is
  - 20 mm for preterm infants;
  - 30 mm for <2 years old;
  - 40 mm for 2–5 year olds;
  - 50 mm for 5–12 year olds; and
  - 60 mm for older children.
- Longer needles may be required in large adolescents.

Insertion site

- The iliac crests are at the level of L3–L4. Use this space or the space below (see Fig. 4.6).
- At birth the conus medullaris finishes near L3, but in adults it finishes at L1–L2.

Technique

- Using a strict aseptic technique, cleanse the skin and drape the patient.
- Positioning of the patient is crucial and an assistant is needed. Restrain the patient in the lateral position on the edge of a flat surface. A line drawn between the iliac crests should be perpendicular to the table surface. Maximally flex the spine without compromising the airway. In small babies flex from the shoulders only; neck flexion can cause airway obstruction. Alternatively the child can be held in the sitting position with the trunk flexed.

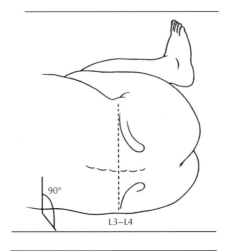

Fig. 4.6 Position for lumbar puncture

- Anaesthetise the area (with injectable lignocaine 1%) until the proximity of the dura (i.e. about two-third the length of the appropriate lumbar puncture needle).
- Grasp the spinal needle with the bevel facing upwards. With the needle perpendicular to the back, insert it through the skin between the spinous processes slowly, aiming towards the umbilicus (i.e. slightly cephalad). Continue advancing the needle until there is decreased resistance (having traversed ligamentum flavum), or the needle has been inserted half its length. Remove the stylet and advance the needle about 1 mm.
- Wait at least 30 seconds for CSF to appear in the hub. Rotation of the needle 90–180° may allow CSF to flow. Advance 1 mm at a time if no CSF has appeared. If no CSF is obtained when bone is contacted or the needle is fully inserted, withdraw the needle very slowly until CSF flows, or the needle is almost removed. Reinsert the stylet, recheck the patient's position and needle orientation, and repeat the procedure.
- Collect 0.5–1 mL of CSF in each of two tubes, for microbiological and biochemical analysis. Remove the lumbar puncture needle swiftly. Press on the puncture site with a cotton ball for about 30 seconds. Cover with a light dressing.

Nasogastric tube insertion
Indications
- Oral rehydration
- Administration of medication (e.g. charcoal, bowel washout solutions)
- Decompression of stomach (e.g. bowel obstruction, abdominal trauma)

Suggested analgesia
Topical anaesthetic spray (e.g. co-phenylcaine) and lubrication with lignocaine (lidocaine) containing lubricant. Sucrose in infant <3 months.

Equipment
- Nasogastric tube, tape or adhesive dressing, litmus paper
- Select the correct tube size (size may vary depending on the use of the nasogastric)
  8 FG for newborns
  10–12 FG for 1–2 year olds
  14–16 FG for adolescents

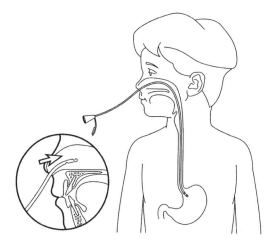

Fig. 4.7 Nasogastric tube insertion

Technique

- Measure the correct length of insertion by placing the distal end of the tube at the nostril and running it to the ear and to the xiphisternum. Add a few centimetres. Mark the tube with permanent marker at this point so the position can be checked.
- If the tube is too pliable, stiffen it by immersing in cold water or freezing briefly.
- Grasp the tube 5–6 cm from the distal end and insert it posteriorly. Advance it slowly along the floor of the nasal passage (see Fig. 4.7). Firm pressure is needed to pass the posterior nasal opening.
- If the child is cooperative, once the tube is in the nasopharynx/oropharynx, ask the child to flex their neck and swallow.
- If the child coughs and gags, their voice becomes hoarse or the tube emerges from the mouth, pull the tube back into the nasopharynx and start again.
- Once the tube has been passed to the measured length, there are two methods for checking the position: (1) by aspirating fluid and testing for an acid pH; (2) with radiograph if necessary.
- Secure the tube to the side of the face using adhesive tape.

Gastrostomy tube replacement

See RCH *Gastrotomy – Acute replacement of displaced tubes* clinical practice guideline *http://www .rch.org.au/clinicalguide/guideline_index/Gastrostomy_Acute_replacement_of_displaced_tubes/*

Indications

- Burst balloon/malfunctioning parts
- Displacement/extrusion of tube

Suggested analgesia

Nitrous oxide or sedation (e.g. midazolam)

Equipment

Gastrostomy tube, syringe and sterile water, lubricant. When a replacement gastrostomy tube is not available, a sterile indwelling urinary catheter can be used as a temporary measure to keep the stoma patent.

Technique

- Check the balloon of the new tube by injecting 3–5 mL of air into the side port. Deflate the balloon fully.
- Slide the skin flange on the new tube to the 8–10 cm mark. Close off the feeding ports and apply a small amount of lubricant to the tube.
- If the old tube is still *in situ*, attach an empty syringe to the side port and deflate the balloon by removing the water. *Note:* There is usually less than the expected 4 or 15 mL of water left in the balloon.
- Gently pull on the tube and rotate it slowly until it is removed.
- Place the tip of the new tube at the opening of the stoma. Hold the distal end of the tube and slowly put pressure on the tube to push it into the hole.
- The new tube should insert easily. Insert it to 6–8 cm.
- Inflate the new tube to either 4 or 15 mL (i.e. not to full capacity) with water. Slowly pull back on the tube until resistance is felt.
- Slide the skin flange down until there is a snug fit, but not too tight. This is usually at the 2–4 cm mark.
- In the case of a MIC key, the correct tube for that patient should be inserted to its full depth before inflating the balloon.
- Gastrostomy buttons or Malecot catheters need introducers and should only be replaced by experienced staff.

Note: If there is any difficulty inserting the tube, a radiographic study (i.e. contrast through the tube) should be performed to check correct positioning.

Tuberculin skin test (intradermal injection)

Indications

Tuberculosis (TB) screening in children.

Sites

By convention: volar surface of left forearm at junction of upper and middle thirds.

Equipment

- Alcohol wipe, short (10 mm) 26-gauge bevelled needle, 1 mL syringe, cotton ball, tape.
- Protective eyewear is essential.
- Dose of 5 TU = 0.1 mL purified protein derivative (PPD).

Contraindications

- Past history active TB or history large reaction.
- Within 3 months of another tuberculin skin test (TST).
- Within 4 weeks of MMR or varicella vaccine (can result in false negatives).

Note: Not reliable in children aged <6 months.

Technique

- TST can only be given by accredited providers. Contact the relevant TB screening program.
- Stretch the skin between a finger and thumb and insert the bevel (facing upwards) 2 mm into the dermis. It will be visible through the epidermis. Inject slowly; there will be considerable resistance. The injection will raise a blanched bleb of about 7 mm with the appearance of *peau d'orange*. Cover with adhesive dressing/cotton ball and tape and advise not to scratch.
- The test should be read at 48–72 hours (up to 5 days). Measure induration (not erythema) in the transverse axis of the forearm. It is helpful to use a pen to draw towards the induration at the same level on either side – it will stop at the edge of the induration and the distance between the points can be measured.
- A large reaction may take days to weeks to disappear.

Immunisation

See Chapter 18, *Infectious diseases and immunisation*.

BCG vaccination is given by intradermal injection (technique as above); by convention it is given in the left upper arm, in the skin over the site of insertion of deltoid into the humerus.

Wound (laceration) management

See RCH *Lacerations* clinical practice guideline *http://www.rch.org.au/clinicalguide/guideline_index/Lacerations/*

Assessment

Lacerations are common in childhood. Most are superficial and tend to occur on the face, scalp and extremities. When assessing a wound consider

- Is the wound contaminated or could it contain a foreign body (e.g. glass)?
- Are there likely to be other associated injuries?
- Is there injury to deeper structures?
- Is blood supply impaired or is this an area of end-arteriolar supply? Do **not** use local anaesthetic with adrenaline on such wounds.

Cleaning wounds

- Superficial wounds can be cleansed with normal saline or aqueous chlorhexidine.
- Adequate analgesia is required for complete examination, cleaning and repair of all but the most superficial wounds.
- Radiograph (particularly for glass and metal objects) or ultrasound is indicated if there is a possibility of a foreign body.

Suggested analgesia

Topical local anaesthetic

- LAT (lignocaine (lidocaine) 4%, adrenaline 1:2000 and tetracaine 2%) or ALA (adrenaline/lignocaine (lidocaine)/amethocaine). Dose = 0.1 mL/kg bodyweight.
- Apply on a piece of gauze or cotton wool placed **inside** the wound and held in place with an adhesive clear plastic dressing.
- Leave for 20–30 minutes. An area of blanching (~1 cm wide) will appear around the wound. Anaesthesia lasts about 1 hour.
- Test the adequacy of anaesthesia by washing and squeezing the wound: if pain free, suturing will usually be painless.
- The sensations of pulling and light touch are preserved. This should be explained to the child and parent.

Injectable local anaesthetic (lignocaine (lidocaine) 1%)

Injectable lignocaine (lidocaine) 1% (max 0.4 mL/kg (4 mg/kg)) can be used

- where LAT/ALA are contraindicated (e.g. areas of end-arteriolar supply);
- in adolescents; and
- to supplement topical local anaesthetic if adequate anaesthesia has not been achieved.

There are several ways to decrease the pain from injecting local anaesthetic:

- Use topical anaesthesia first.
- Use 27 FG needles.
- Inject slowly.
- Place the needle into the wound through the lacerated surface, not through intact skin.
- Pass the needle through an anaesthetised area into an unanaesthetised area.
- Use 1% lignocaine (lidocaine) rather than 2% at body temperature.
- Buffer lignocaine (lidocaine) with sodium bicarbonate (10:1 dilution).

Sedation/other

- Nitrous oxide or sedation (e.g. midazolam).
- Ketamine may be used in children >12 months by staff experienced in its use.

Regional blocks

- Regional blocks provide excellent analgesia. See p. 45.

Wound closure

Tissue-adhesive glues

- Tissue glue (e.g. Dermabond) is an alternative to suturing in wounds that are small (<3 cm), straight, easily approximated and under no tension. It must not be used on mucosal surfaces.
- Topical anaesthesia will reduce bleeding from the wound and the discomfort of gluing.

- Clean the wound with normal saline or aqueous chlorhexidine and let dry. Hold the edges firmly together and apply a small amount of glue (~0.05 mL) to the line of the laceration. Do not allow glue to enter the wound itself.
- Hold the wound edges together for 30 seconds. Steristrips should be applied to prevent the child picking the glue off.
- The wound should be kept dry for 2 days. It then can be washed. The scab will come off in 1–2 weeks.

Suturing

- Rapidly absorbable sutures (e.g. fast catgut, Vicryl rapid) are appropriate for use on areas where the cosmetic advantages of non-absorbable sutures are not required (e.g. scalp and hand). Using absorbable sutures avoids the stress and potential pain of suture removal.
- Non-absorbable sutures (e.g. nylon and polypropylene) are used in areas where cosmetic appearance is important.
- Deep sutures (absorbable) should be used to close deep tissues; this reduces cavitation and dead space, which increase the risk of infection.
- The size of suture and timing of suture removal depends on the area affected.
  - Scalp: 4/0–5/0, 5–7 days.
  - Face: 5/0–6/0, 5–7 days.
  - Arm/hand: 4/0–5/0, 7–10 days.
  - Trunk/legs: 4/0–5/0, 10–14 days.
    Note: Areas of stress (e.g. over joints) need longer.
- Splint any sutured wound that is under tension (e.g. across joints or on the hand), for at least 1 week. This decreases pain and promotes healing.

Special circumstances
Lips

- Accurate approximation of vermilion border and skin is essential.
- May need general anaesthesia and plastic surgical repair in small or uncooperative children.
- Sutures: mucosa/muscle 4/0 gut, skin 6/0 nylon or Fast gut in the young child. Remove sutures in 5 days.
- Lacerations of the inner lip rarely need intervention, but degloving to the gum margin requires specialist referral.

Palate

- Rarely requires suturing unless laceration is wide, extends through posterior free margin or is actively bleeding.
- Beware retropharyngeal injury (needs specialist opinion).

Tongue

- Small lacerations do not require suturing.
- Plastic surgical opinion is required if the laceration is large, bleeding actively, extends through the free edge or is of full thickness.

Finger tips

- Areas of skin loss up to 1 cm^2 are treated with dressings and heal with good return of sensation. Greater areas require specialist referral.
- Involvement of the nail bed requires plastic surgical consultation.

Scalp

For small lacerations suitable for tissue-adhesive glue use hair from each side of the laceration to approximate the wound; twist hair together, pull across the wound and glue over the hair.

Other

Lacerations involving cartilage (e.g. nose, ear) require specialist opinion.

Tetanus prophylaxis

See *The Australian Immunisation Handbook*, 10th edition (http://www.health.gov.au/internet/immunise/publishing.nsf/Content/Handbook10-home)

- For clean minor wounds, if the patient has had a
  - ○ Tetanus course (≥3 doses), last dose within the past 10 years: no requirement.
  - ○ Tetanus course (≥3 doses), last dose >10 years ago: give tetanus toxoid.
  - ○ Unimmunised/incomplete/unknown treatment: give tetanus toxoid.
- For tetanus-prone wounds, if the patient has had a
  - ○ Tetanus course (≥3 doses), last dose within the past 5 years: no requirement.
  - ○ Tetanus course (≥3 doses), last dose >5 years ago: give tetanus toxoid.
  - ○ Unimmunised/incomplete/unknown treatment: full three-dose course and tetanus immunoglobulin.

Note: Tetanus toxoid: give DTPa/DT/Td/dTpa as appropriate.

- Dose of tetanus immunoglobulin is 250 IU <24 hours, 500 IU >24 hours intramuscular injection (21 FG needle).

Antibiotics

- Antibiotics are not indicated for simple lacerations. They are usually given for bites and wounds with extensive tissue damage, but are of secondary importance to the initial decontamination of the wound.
- Recommended antibiotics are amoycillin-clavulanate (400/57 mg per 5 mL), 12.5–22.5 mg/kg per dose, 12 hourly for 5 days.

Femoral nerve block

Indications

- Pain relief for femoral fractures (in addition to other techniques including splinting the fractured leg). It may be appropriate to use nitrous oxide or sedation when giving a femoral nerve block.

Equipment

Dressing pack, antiseptic solution, two 23-gauge needles and syringes, local anaesthetic solution, adhesive tape.

Technique

- This is best performed using ultrasound localisation of the nerve and guided injection.
- If ultrasound guidance is not used:
  After skin preparation, palpate the femoral artery below the inguinal ligament. Raise a wheal just lateral to the artery with local anaesthetic, for example lignocaine (lidocaine) 1%.
- Introduce a short-bevelled needle (such as a lumbar puncture needle or a 23-gauge needle) through this wheal and advance downwards perpendicular to the skin. A characteristic 'pop' or loss of resistance is felt as the needle goes through the fascia lata and again as it penetrates the fascia iliaca (if using a lumbar puncture needle).
- Aspirate to ensure that the needle is not in a blood vessel. Inject local anaesthetic solution (usually bupivacaine 0.5% 2 mg/kg). The anaesthetic should inject smoothly without subcutaneous swelling. Paraesthesia need not be elicited.

Bier's block

Indications

Children over 5 years with forearm fractures requiring manipulation. Consider also intranasal fentanyl (1.5 mcg/kg, half in each nostril) for long bone fractures.

Equipment

Dressing pack, antiseptic solution, two IV cannulae (and associated equipment), lignocaine (lidocaine) 1%, monitored tourniquet system, equipment for plaster application.

Technique

- Keep child nil orally and give adequate pain relief.
- Two trained staff must be present and full resuscitation equipment available. Radiology should be notified.

- Insert an IV cannula into a distal vein on each hand.
- Elevate the affected arm above the level of the heart while compressing the brachial artery for 1 minute.
- Inflate the tourniquet cuff to 200 mmHg. This reading should be maintained throughout the procedure.
- Infuse lignocaine (lidocaine) 0.5% 3 mg/kg (0.6 mL/kg, max 40 mL). Full anaesthesia takes 5–10 minutes.
- Release tourniquet cuff **at least** 20 minutes after lignocaine (lidocaine) infusion, after procedure is complete and position confirmed radiologically.

Digital/proximal nerve block
Indication
Anaesthesia of finger for minor surgical procedures (e.g. suturing, drainage of paronychia).

Equipment
Dressing pack, antiseptic solution, 25-gauge needle and syringe, local anaesthetic.
   Note: Use local anaesthetic, for example lignocaine (lidocaine) 1%. Do **not** use adrenaline.

Technique
Digital nerve block
- With the palm facing up, insert a 25-gauge needle at the base of the finger on either medial/lateral side at a 45° angle to the vertical (see Fig. 4.8).
- Inject when needle hits periosteum.
- Rotate needle to vertical and inject along the side of the finger to at least three-fourth of the depth of the finger.
- Remove needle and repeat on the other side.

Proximal nerve block
- Insert a 25-gauge needle between the fingers at the interdigital fold in line with the web space (see Fig. 4.8).
- Insert until needle tip is level with the head of the metacarpal bone.
- Inject 1–2 mL at this level.
- Repeat on the other side, or for index/fifth finger; inject half ring wheal around the outer side of the finger.

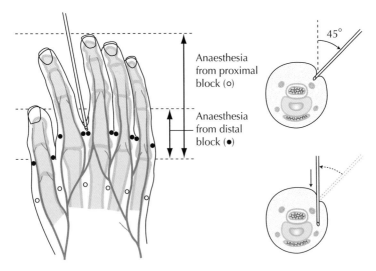

Fig. 4.8 Digital nerve block

USEFUL RESOURCES

- *www.rch.org.au/clinicalguide* [Suprapubic Aspirate Guideline] – Includes video of procedure and flowchart of using a bladder ultrasound.
- *www.rch.org.au/clinicalguide* [Lumbar Puncture Guideline] – Includes video of procedure, interpretation of CSF and patient information handouts.
- *www.rch.org.au/clinicalguide* [Intraosseous Access]
- *www.netsvic.org.au/nets/handbook* [Umbilical Artery/Vein Catheterisation] – Excellent website from the Newborn Emergency Transport Service (NETS) of Victoria.

CHAPTER 5

Poisoning and envenomation

James Tibballs

Poisoning
Background

Poisoning during childhood occurs mainly among 1–3 year olds and tends to follow the ingestion of something that was improperly stored in the home. It should be considered in any child presenting with symptoms that cannot otherwise be explained, such as altered conscious state, fitting, unusual behaviour, hypoventilation, hypotension, tachy- or bradycardia.

Other circumstances of poisoning are iatrogenic (particularly in infants) and the deliberate self-administration of substances by older children. Suicide should always be considered, even in young children. See also Chapter 22, *Adolescent health* and Chapter 25, *Behaviour and mental health*.

Although poisoning in childhood is frequently minor in severity and mortality is low, serious illness may be caused by prescription and over-the-counter drugs as well as non-pharmaceutical products, including complementary medications (see also Chapter 26, *Prescribing for children*). Recovery is expected in the majority of cases if vital functions are preserved and the complications of poisoning and its management are avoided.

Prevention

- Action should be taken to prevent recurrence.
- Parents should be encouraged to store all medicines in childproof cabinets and toxic substances in places inaccessible to young children.
- Urgent psychosocial help should be organised for children who have poisoned themselves intentionally.
- Steps should be taken to ensure that iatrogenic poisoning is not repeated.

General management

In Australia, call Poisons Information on **13 11 26** – a 24-hour nationwide service.
The principles of management for all poisonings are (see Fig. 5.1):
- Resuscitate the patient and remove the poison if indicated.
- Administer an antidote if one exists (see Table 5.1).

A decision to remove the poison from the body should be dependent on the severity of the poisoning and the likelihood of success in removing the poison without further endangering the patient. Most poisonings in childhood are minor and observation alone or non-invasive treatment is indicated.

The severity of poisoning may be assessed by the
- Established and expected effects
- Quantity of the poison(s)
- Preparation of the poison
- Interval since exposure

Removal from the body usually involves gastrointestinal decontamination but occasionally other methods (e.g. dialysis, exchange transfusion, charcoal haemoperfusion, plasmapheresis or haemofiltration) are required.

Gastrointestinal decontamination

If the conscious state is depressed, all methods of gastrointestinal decontamination carry a substantial risk of aspiration pneumonitis, even if the patient is intubated. Hence, the most important factor in determining the technique of decontamination is the conscious state. A guideline for the general management of poisoning using these techniques according to severity of poisoning is shown in Fig. 5.1. The most commonly used method is

Paediatric Handbook, Ninth Edition. Edited by Amanda Gwee, Romi Rimer and Michael Marks.
© 2015 John Wiley & Sons, Ltd. Published 2015 by John Wiley & Sons, Ltd.

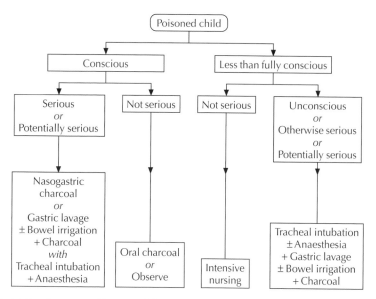

Fig. 5.1 General management of the poisoned child

administration of activated charcoal, with gastric lavage and whole bowel irrigation having limited roles. There is no role for induced emesis in the hospital setting.

Activated charcoal

Activated charcoal is more efficacious than induced emesis or gastric lavage and is currently regarded as a 'universal antidote'. It adsorbs most poisons but not metals, corrosives or pesticides. Like other techniques, however, it is contraindicated if the patient is not fully conscious or has an ileus. If aspirated, charcoal may cause fatal bronchiolitis obliterans. Constipation is relatively common. Addition of a laxative decreases transit time through the gut but does not improve efficacy in preventing drug absorption. It may also upset fluid and electrolyte balance. The initial dose is 1–2 g/kg. Repeated doses of activated charcoal enhance elimination of many drugs, particularly slow-release preparations. A suitable regimen is 0.25 g/kg/h for 12–24 hours.

Gastric lavage

Although gastric lavage appears to be a logical therapy for ingested poisons, it has a limited place in management. Problems include

- Poor efficacy in preventing absorption when done >60 minutes after ingestion.
- Risk of aspiration pneumonitis in the less than fully conscious patient and to a lesser extent in the conscious child.
- In the conscious young child, it is psychologically traumatic and difficult to do.

If it is performed, care should be taken to avoid water intoxication and intrabronchial instillation of lavage fluid.

- Gastric lavage is **contraindicated** after ingestion of corrosives, hydrocarbons or petrochemicals.
- Gastric lavage is **indicated** in serious poisoning when a child is already intubated for airway protection and ventilation. The child should be in the lateral position during lavage. If potentially serious effects of poisoning are expected, gastric lavage should only be done after rapid sequence induction of anaesthesia and tracheal intubation.

Table 5.1 Antidotes to poisons

Poison	Antidotes and doses	Comments
Amphetamines	Esmolol 0.5 mg/kg IV over 1 minute, then 25–200 mcg/kg/min IV.	Treatment for tachyarrhythmia.
	Labetalol 0.15–0.3 mg/kg IV or phentolamine 0.05–0.1 mg/kg IV every 10 minutes.	Treatment for hypertension.
Benzodiazepines	Flumazenil 5 mcg/kg IV repeated at 1 minute, then 2–10 mcg/kg/h by IV infusion.	Specific antagonist at receptor. Titrate to effect. Caution: may precipitate convulsions or arrhythmia in multi-drug ingestion, especially with tricyclics.
Beta-blocker	Glucagon 50–150 mcg/kg IV, then 0.20–2.0 mcg/kg/min IV infusion. Isoprenaline 0.05–2 mcg/kg/min IV. Beware of b_2 hypotension. Noradrenaline 0.05–0.5 mcg/kg/min IV.	Stimulates non-catecholamine cAMP production. Preferred antidote.
Calcium blocker	Calcium chloride 20 mg (0.2 mL of 10%) per kg IV.	
Carbon monoxide	Oxygen 100%.	Hyperbaric oxygen may be required.
Cyanide	Hydroxycobalamin (Vit B_{12}) 70 mg/kg IV plus sodium thiosulfate 25% IV 1.65 mL/kg (max 50 mL) at 3–5 mL/min. Sodium nitrite 3% IV (0.33 mL/kg over 4 minutes) then sodium thiosulfate as above.	Chelates. Give 50 mL 50% glucose after each dose. Nitrites form methaemoglobin–cyanide complex (beware of excess methaemoglobinaemia – restrict to <20%). Thiosulfate forms non-toxic thiocyanate from methaemoglobin–cyanide.
Digoxin	Digoxin Fab. Dose: acute ingestion 1 vial/2.5 tablet (0.25 mg); in steady state vials = serum digoxin (ng/mL) × BW (kg)/100.	

Ergotamine	Sodium nitroprusside infusion 0.5–5 mcg/kg/min.	Treats vasoconstriction. Monitor BP continuously.
	Heparin 100 units/kg IV, then 10–30 units/kg IV per hour according to clotting.	Treatment of coagulopathy.
Lead	If symptomatic or blood lead >2.9 µmol/L, dimercaprol (BAL) 75 mg/m² IM 4-hourly 6 doses, then calcium disodium edetate (EDTA) 1500 mg/m² IV over 5 days. If asymptomatic and blood lead 2.18–2.9 µmol/L, infuse calcium disodium edetate 1000 mg/m² per day for 5 days.	
Heparin	Protamine 1 mg/100 units heparin IV.	Heparin half-life 1–2 hours.
Iron	Desferrioxamine 15 mg/kg/h 12–24 hours if serum iron >90 µmol/L or >63 µmol/L and symptomatic.	Beware of anaphylaxis.
Methanol, ethyleneglycol, glycol ethers	Ethanol, infuse loading dose 10 mL/kg 10% diluted in glucose 5% IV and then 0.15 mL/kg/h to maintain blood level at 0.1% (100 mg/dL).	
Methaemoglobin, e.g. secondary to drug treatment	Methylene blue 1–2 mg/kg IV over several minutes.	
Opiates	Naloxone 0.01–0.1 mg/kg IV, then 0.01 mg/kg/h as needed.	
Organophosphates and carbamates	Atropine 20–50 mcg/kg IV every 15 minutes until secretions dry. Pralidoxime 25 mg/kg IV over 15–30 minutes, then 10–20 mg/kg/h for 18 hours or more. Not for carbamates.	Restores cholinesterase.
Paracetamol	N-acetylcysteine. IV: 150 mg/kg over 60 minutes, then 10 mg/kg for 20–72 hours. Oral: 140 mg/kg, then 17 doses of 70 mg/kg 4 hourly (total 1330 mg/kg over 68 hours).	Give for >72 hours if still encephalopathic.
Tricyclic antidepressants	Sodium bicarbonate IV 1 mmol/kg to maintain blood pH >7.45.	

Whole bowel irrigation

Whole bowel irrigation is done with polyethylene glycol with electrolytes (30 mL/kg/h for 4–8 hours) administered by nasogastric tube. It is useful in delayed presentations and for the management of poisoning by slow-release drug preparations, substances not adsorbed by activated charcoal (e.g. iron) or substances which are irretrievable by gastric lavage.

Induced vomiting

Syrup of ipecacuanha is no longer routinely recommended. Its usefulness in the hospital setting is extremely limited – perhaps only to a case of serious poisoning presenting very early after ingestion when no other effective treatment is possible. It was previously used as a first-aid measure in the home, but it does not reliably empty the stomach and is contraindicated where conscious state is impaired (risk of aspiration pneumonitis) and when the ingested substance is corrosive, hydrocarbon or petrochemical.

Poisoning with unknown or multiple agents

- Suspect poisoning on presentation with convulsions, depression of the conscious state, hypoventilation, hypotension or an illness that is not otherwise readily explained. A urinary drug screen may be useful for diagnosis.
- Multiple poisons may have been ingested. Determine blood levels if there is any possibility of ingestion of paracetamol, iron, salicylate, theophylline, methanol, digoxin or lithium. Blood levels may influence clinical management.
- Contact the Poisons Information hotline for advice (**13 11 26**).

Individual poisons

Thousands of poisons exist. The most common serious poisons in young children presenting to the Royal Children's Hospital have been paracetamol, rodenticides, eucalyptus oil, benzodiazepines, tricyclic antidepressants and theophylline.

Only the most common serious poisonings or poisonings peculiar to children are considered here briefly. Some have antidotes (see Table 5.1). **The general principles of management apply to all individual poisons** (see Fig. 5.1). Details of effects of specific poisons and suggested management should be obtained from a Poisons Information Centre and from appropriate, up-to-date references.

Consider the possibility of intentional drug ingestion. These children are often at 'high risk' for multiple psychological and social reasons. See also Chapter 22, *Adolescent health*.

Paracetamol (acetaminophen)

Paracetamol is the most common pharmaceutical poisoning.

Effects

The liver metabolises it to a toxic product, *N*-acetyl-*p*-benzoquinone imine, which causes hepatic necrosis unless neutralised by the hepatic antioxidant, glutathione. Multi-organ failure and death may occur after 3–4 days if the ingested quantity exceeds 150 mg/kg or with smaller amounts if there is prior hepatic dysfunction or co-ingestion of alcohol or anticonvulsants. Early symptoms are anorexia, nausea and vomiting.

Specific management

N-acetylcysteine (NAC) is an effective antidote if given before hepatic necrosis occurs. Its use is associated with adverse reactions (e.g. rash, bronchospasm and hypotension) that occur more frequently when administered IV. If reactions occur, cease NAC temporarily, give promethazine 0.2–0.5 mg/kg IV (max. 10–25 mg) and recommence the NAC infusion at a reduced rate.

Since the outcome is related to serum levels of paracetamol measured 4–20 hours after ingestion, a decision to administer NAC after a single overdose may be made according to time-related plasma levels. Administer if the level exceeds 1000 μmol/L at 4 hours, 500 at 8 hours, 200 at 12 hours, 80 at 16 hours or 40 at 20 hours (μmol/L × 0.15 = mcg/mL).

- IV NAC: 150 mg/kg in 5 mL/kg of glucose 5% over 60 minutes, then 10 mg/kg/h for 20 hours or longer if the child is encephalopathic, or presentation is 10–36 hours after ingestion; or
- Oral NAC: 140 mg/kg, then 17 doses of 70 mg/kg (4 hourly).
  Note:
- Serum levels >18 hours after a single ingestion are unreliable predictors of risk.

- These recommendations do not apply to multiple smaller ingestions (seek expert advice).
- Presentation <1 hour after significant ingestion may be treated with gastric lavage.
- Monitor liver function tests and serum potassium.

Iron
Small quantities (<20 mg/kg) of elemental iron may be toxic. This is usually ingested as iron tablets/capsules, mixtures or multivitamin preparations.

Effects
- Immediate: nausea, vomiting, abdominal pain and possible gastric erosion
- At 6–24 hours: hypotension, hypovolaemia and metabolic acidosis
- At 12–24 hours: multi-organ failure – gastrointestinal (ileus, gastric erosion), CNS, cardiovascular, hepatic and renal
- At 4–6 weeks: pyloric stenosis

Specific management
- Check serum iron level (mcg/dL × 0.1791 = μmol/L). *Note*: Absorption may be slow.
- Abdominal radiograph may reveal the quantity ingested.
- Whole bowel irrigation (not if ileus, obstruction or erosion is present). Activated charcoal is ineffective.
- Infusion of desferrioxamine no faster than 15 mg/kg/h for 12–24 hours is indicated if
  - patient is clinically hypotensive or has depressed consciousness;
  - >60 mg/kg elemental iron has been ingested;
  - iron level is >90 μmol/L; or
  - iron level is >63 μmol/L and patient is symptomatic.

Tricyclic antidepressants
Sudden death (cardiac arrest) may occur.

Effects
The life-threatening effects are
- CNS depression: coma, convulsions
- Non-cardiogenic pulmonary oedema
- Cardiac depression: hypocontractility, hypotension and sudden dysrhythmias (conduction blocks and ventricular ectopy, including tachycardia/fibrillation)

Specific management
- ECG monitoring: assess heart rate, QRS duration and QT interval.
- Alkalisation of blood to pH 7.45–7.50 with sodium bicarbonate infusion or hyperventilation, or both.
- Anticonvulsant therapy with diazepam 0.1–0.4 mg/kg (max 10–20 mg).
- Antidysrhythmia therapy: give phenytoin slowly (over 30 minutes). Beware of hypotension.
- Treatment of hypotension with an alpha-agonist (noradrenaline 0.01–1 mcg/kg/min). Avoid beta-agonists and drugs with mixed alpha and beta actions.
- Treatment of ventricular tachycardia/fibrillation with DC shock, amiodarone (5 mg/kg IV) and a beta-blocker.
- Treatment of *torsade de pointes* with DC shock, magnesium sulfate (0.1–0.2 mmol/kg IV).

Salicylates
Toxicity is expected if >150 mg/kg is ingested.

Effects
- Coma, hyperpyrexia and respiratory alkalosis followed by metabolic acidosis
- Cardiac depression, pulmonary oedema and hypotension
- Hepatic encephalopathy (Reye syndrome) with chronic use

Specific management
- Serum salicylate level, blood glucose, serum potassium and blood pH
- Correction of dehydration

- Correction of acidosis, maintenance of urine pH >7.5 (with sodium bicarbonate) and correction of hypokalaemia
- Haemodialysis/haemoperfusion if the serum level is >25 mmol/L (mcg/mL × 0.0724 = μmol/L)

Theophylline

Toxicity is related to serum levels and may be delayed with slow-release preparations.

Effects

- Gastrointestinal: nausea, protracted vomiting, abdominal pain
- Metabolic:
  - Hypokalaemia due to migration into cells, diuresis and vomiting
  - Metabolic acidosis
  - Hyperglycaemia, hyperinsulinaemia and hypomagnesaemia
- CNS: seizures, agitation, coma (uncommon)
- Cardiovascular: atrial and ventricular ectopy, hypotension

Specific management

- Prolonged observation if a slow-release preparation is ingested.
- Serum level (anticipate seizures at approximately 300 μmol/L and the need for charcoal haemoperfusion or plasmapheresis at approximately 550 μmol/L, or less if there is protracted vomiting).
- Anti-emetic therapy with metoclopramide 0.15 mg/kg (max 10–15 mg) IV 6 hourly.
- ECG monitoring.
- Beware of early hypokalaemia and late hyperkalaemia when potassium re-enters the blood.

Eucalyptus and essential oils

Effects

- Initial: coughing, choking
- Rapid onset (30 minutes, occasionally delayed): CNS depression (convulsions and meiosis are rare)
- Vomiting and subsequent aspiration pneumonitis

Specific management

- Exclude pneumonitis (perform chest radiograph and measure oxygenation).

Amphetamines and derivatives (e.g. methamphetamine ['ice'] and 3,4-methylenedioxy methamphetamine ['Ecstasy'])

Effects

- CNS stimulation
- Convulsions
- Hyperthermia (with secondary coagulopathy and rhabdomyolysis)
- Hypertension
- Cardiovascular collapse
- Adult respiratory distress syndrome

Specific management

Treatment is largely supportive and may include sedatives (benzodiazepine), anticonvulsants, beta- and alpha-blockade, dantrolene, mechanical ventilation, inotropic and renal support.

Petroleum distillates

Inhaling the fumes of petrol, kerosene, lighter fluid, lamp oils, solvents and mineral spirits is often referred to as 'chroming' or 'sniffing'. There are significant social and cognitive effects of long-term abuse and these children are at high risk because of multiple psychosocial reasons. See also Chapter 22, *Adolescent health*.

Effects

- CNS obtundation
- Convulsions
- Vomiting
- Hepatorenal toxicity

Specific management
- Exclude pneumonitis (perform chest radiograph and measure oxygenation).

Button or disc batteries
- Ingestion may cause electrolysis, corrosion, the release of toxins or pressure effects.
- Impaction in the oesophagus is an emergency – it may cause perforation or an oesophagotracheal fistula and must be removed endoscopically as soon as possible.
- Surgical follow-up is essential.

Caustic substances
- Automatic machine dishwashing detergents, caustic soda, drain cleaners are strong alkalis and cause burns to the gastrointestinal tract when ingested.
- Significant oesophageal damage may occur in absence of proximal injury.
- Arrange surgical oesophagoscopy and follow-up.

Envenomation
The Australian Venom Research Unit (*www.avru.org*) provides a 24-hour advisory service on 1300 760 451.

Snakebite
This section applies to bites by Australian snakes of the family *Elapidae*. Snakebites by species in other countries cause different effects and are not outlined in this handbook. Refer to local publications.

Although not all snakes are venomous and envenomation does not always accompany a bite by a venomous snake, **every snakebite should be regarded as potentially lethal**. In young children, a history of snakebite is often uncertain.

Of the many species of snakes in Australia, the principal dangerous species are from the genera of
- Brown snakes
- Tiger snakes
- Taipans
- Death adders
- Black snakes
- Copperheads
- Several marine genera

Venom from these species contains
- **Neurotoxins** which cause neuromuscular paralysis and subsequent respiratory failure.
- **Procoagulants** that cause disseminated intravascular coagulation (DIC) and depletion of clotting factors, resulting in subsequent haemorrhage (Death adders do not contain significant procoagulant).
- **Rhabdomyolysins** which cause delayed destruction of skeletal muscle (not present in Brown snake or Death adder venoms).

Other less important components are haemolysins and anticoagulants.

Symptoms and signs of envenomation
The bite site may be identifiable by fang or scratch marks surrounded by bruising or oedema. However, note that a bite site may be undetectable and occasionally unnoticed by a victim.
- Headache, nausea, vomiting and abdominal pain may occur within an hour of envenomation.
- Early neurotoxic signs include ptosis, diplopia, blurred vision, facial muscle weakness, dysphonia and dysphagia.
- Advanced neurotoxic signs include weakness of limb, trunk and respiratory muscles.
- Spontaneous haemorrhage may occur from mucous membranes, occasionally into solid organs and from needle puncture sites.
- Hypotension secondary to haemorrhage and respiratory failure.
- Renal failure may occur, secondary to hypotension, haemolysis and rhabdomyolysis, particularly if treatment with antivenom is delayed.

The syndrome culminates in respiratory and cardiovascular failure within several hours after envenomation, but may be accelerated in a small child or after multiple bites.

Suspected envenomation

If there is a suspicious history of snakebite but the patient is asymptomatic, the patient should be observed closely for approximately 12 hours.

- Test blood coagulation, as it is both a sensitive and reliable indicator of envenomation by major species (except death adders).
- Apply a pressure-immobilisation first-aid bandage (Fig. 5.2). It can be removed after ensuring that antivenom is available.
- Perform a venom-detection test (see below). A positive test of a swab from the bite site or of a biological sample (urine or blood) indicates which antivenom to administer, if clinically indicated.

Definite envenomation

A number of measures may be required, depending on the severity of envenomation (see Fig. 5.3):

- Resuscitation with mechanical ventilation, oxygen therapy and fluid volume restoration.
- Application of a pressure-immobilisation first-aid bandage (Fig. 5.2) if not already in place. Do not remove an existing first-aid bandage until antivenom has been administered. Cut a hole in the existing bandage to obtain a bite site swab if needed and then reinforce.
- Perform a venom test of urine (preferred), blood and/or bite site swab.
- Administer antivenom (IV).
- Administer coagulation factors (fresh frozen plasma) after antivenom if haemorrhage present. Occasionally, blood transfusion is needed.

Antivenom therapy

Specific antivenoms are available against Brown snakes, Tiger snakes, Black snakes, Taipans, Death adders and the Beaked sea snake. A polyvalent preparation contains all the above-named antivenoms except the beaked sea snake. All are given IV.

- Antivenom is required for clinical envenomation or for significant asymptomatic coagulopathy that may result in serious (e.g. intracranial) haemorrhage. A mild coagulopathy may resolve but requires repeat testing.
- Monovalent preparations are preferred because of a lower incidence of adverse reaction compared with polyvalent preparations.
- **Always premedicate the patient with SC adrenaline 0.005–0.01 mg/kg (i.e. 0.05–0.1 mL/kg of 1:10,000) or to a maximum of 0.25 mg (0.25 mL of 1:1000) for larger and adolescent patients.**
- This is required only for the first dose of antivenom to prevent or decrease the severity of anaphylaxis.
- A course of prednisolone 1 mg/kg orally, daily for 2–5 days may prevent serum sickness, which may occur after polyvalent antivenom or after multiple doses of monovalent antivenom.
- Selection of antivenom should be based on the result of a venom-detection test or on reliable identification of the snake, as there is little cross-reactivity between antivenoms. Do not rely upon the victim's or witness's identification unless they are an expert.
- If antivenom therapy is required urgently before species identification, administer antivenom according to location. In Victoria, give both Brown and Tiger snake antivenom; in Tasmania, give Tiger snake antivenom; and elsewhere give polyvalent antivenom. All bites by marine species can be treated with Beaked sea snake or Tiger snake antivenom.
- Brown snake, Taipan, Death adder and Black snake antivenoms are only effective against those species, whereas Tiger snake antivenom is effective against Tiger snakes, Copperheads, Red-bellied black snake and many minor species.
- Dilute with crystalloid and infuse IV over 30 minutes (faster in life-threatening envenomation).
- The dose of antivenom cannot be predetermined because the amount of venom injected and the patient's susceptibility to it are unknown. Initially administer 2–4 ampoules of the appropriate antivenom and then titrate additional doses against the clinical and coagulation status. Larger number of ampoules may be required in moderate and severe envenomation.
- Administer antivenom before giving blood or coagulation factors to forestall further DIC.

Venom detection kit

The venom detection kit (VDK) is a bedside or laboratory three-step enzyme immunoassay, able to detect venom in urine, blood or from a swab of the bite site in very low concentration. It takes about 25 minutes to perform.

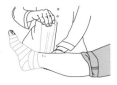

Apply a broad pressure bandage over the bite site as soon as possible. Do not remove clothing, as the movement in doing so will promote the entry of venom into the blood stream. Keep the bitten limb still.

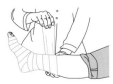

The bandage should be as tight as you would apply to a sprained ankle.

Note: Bandage upwards from the toes or fingers of the bitten limb to help immobilisation. Even though a little venom may be squeezed upwards, the bandage will be far more comfortable than if applied from above downwards; and may be left in place longer.

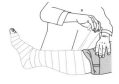

Extend the bandages as far up the limb as possible.

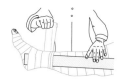

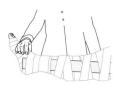

Apply a splint to the leg to immobilise joints on either side of the bite.

Bind it firmly to as much of the leg as possible. Bring transport to the patients.

Hospital staff:
Please note that first aid measures may usually be removed after availability of antivenom is confirmed. Do not leave on for hours.

Bites on the hand or forearm
1. Bind to elbow with bandages.
2. Use splint to elbow.
3. Use sling.

Fig. 5.2   Pressure-immobilisation first-aid bandage

If positive, it indicates which antivenom to administer (if clinically indicated), but not necessarily the species of snake.

Spider bite
Red-back spider
The venom of this spider contains a neurotoxin that causes release of neurotransmitters. Although potentially lethal, the syndrome of envenomation (latrodectism) develops slowly over many hours, and no deaths have been

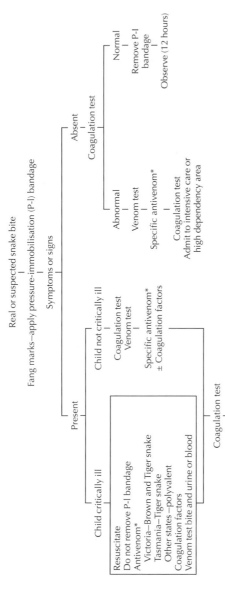

Real or suspected snake bite

Fang marks—apply pressure-immobilisation (P-I) bandage

Symptoms or signs

Present

Child critically ill

Resuscitate
Do not remove P-I bandage
Antivenom*
  Victoria—Brown and Tiger snake
  Tasmania—Tiger snake
  Other states—polyvalent
Coagulation factors
Venom test bite and urine or blood

Coagulation test

Child not critically ill

Coagulation test
Venom test

Specific antivenom*
± Coagulation factors

Absent

Coagulation test

Abnormal

Venom test

Specific antivenom*

Coagulation test
Admit to intensive care or
high dependency area

Normal

Remove P-I
bandage

Observe (12 hours)

Titrate specific antivenom* and coagulation factors against clinical state and coagulation
Admit to intensive care or high dependency area

Dangers and mistakes in management:
- Fang marks may not be visible
- Premature removal of P-I bandage may allow sudden systemic envenomation
- Erroneous identification may cause wrong antivenom (premedicate with adrenaline*)
  to be administered. If in doubt give polyvalent

- Delayed onset of paralysis may be missed
- Insufficient antivenom (premedicate with adrenaline*)
- Antivenom without premedication
- Antivenom without clinical or laboratory evidence of envenomation

* Premedicate with adrenaline 0.005–0.01 mg/kg s.c.; i.e. 0.05–0.1 mL/kg of 1:10,000 or 0.005–0.01 mL/kg of 1:1000 adrenaline.

Fig. 5.3 Management of snakebite

recorded since an antivenom has been available. A similar syndrome is caused by many species of the genus *Latrodectus* worldwide (Australia, *L. hasselti*; New Zealand, *L. katipo*, *L. hasselti*).

Symptoms and signs
- Severe persistent local pain often worsened with movement and referred elsewhere.
- Local erythema, oedema, pruritus, sweating and regional lymphadenopathy.
- Systemic effects may include distal limb and abdominal pain, hypertension, sweating, vomiting, fever and headache.
- Myalgia, muscle spasms, arthralgia, paraesthesia and weakness may last many weeks.

Management
- Do not use a pressure-immobilisation bandage. The symptom onset is slow and immobilisation may exacerbate pain.
- If the effects remain mild and localised up to 24 hours after a bite, treatment may be symptomatic but pain should be treated with antivenom.
- Severe local and systemic effects or prolonged mild effects warrant administration of antivenom IM (occasionally IV). Sometimes several ampoules are needed. Antivenom has been effective even when administered months after envenomation.
- Although the rate of adverse reactions is low (<0.5%), premedication with promethazine may be used. In all cases, adrenaline should be at hand to treat anaphylaxis (see Chapter 1, *Medical emergencies*).

White-tailed spider
Contrary to popular belief, bites by this spider are rarely troublesome, but severe local inflammatory reaction or skin necrosis may occasionally occur.

Funnel-web spiders
Several large aggressive species can threaten life with a venom that releases neurotransmitters and catecholamines. Several dangerous species exist in NSW and Queensland. In some other states (including Victoria), funnel-web species exist but are not known to be dangerous. Envenomation does not always accompany a bite.

Symptoms and signs
Envenomation is indicated by (in approximate sequence)
- Local muscle fasciculation, piloerection, vomiting, abdominal pain, profuse sweating, salivation and lacrimation.
- Hypertension, tachyarrhythmias and vasoconstriction develop.
- The syndrome culminates in coma, respiratory failure and terminal hypotension.

Management
- Apply a pressure-immobilisation bandage.
- Administer funnel-web spider antivenom IV.
- Provide mechanical ventilation, airway protection, atropine and cardiovascular therapy as required.

Jellyfish stings
Chironex box jellyfish
This is the world's most venomous animal. It has a cuboid body, approximately 30 cm in diameter, numerous trailing tentacles and inhabits shallow northern Australian coastal waters. Stings are most common from October to May, but have been recorded throughout the year. Contact with the tentacles leads to the discharge of millions of nematocysts that fire barbs through the epidermis and blood vessels, releasing venom that contain myotoxins, haemolysins, dermatonecrotic toxins and possibly a neurotoxin. Severity of envenomation is related to the length of tentacles contacting the skin.

Prevention is most important. Envenomation is prevented by light clothing. Unguarded waters must not be entered when jellyfish are inshore. Beach warning signs should not be ignored.

Symptoms and signs
Severe pain and possible cardiorespiratory arrest due to direct cardiotoxicity and possible neurological effects causing apnoea.

Management

- Rescue the victim from the water to prevent drowning.
- Cardiopulmonary resuscitation may be required immediately on the beach, en route to hospital and extended as extracorporeal life support.
- Dowse adherent tentacles with vinegar/acetic acid to inactivate undischarged nematocysts (supplies of vinegar are stocked at popular beaches).
- Analgesia: parenteral for extensive stings, cold packs for minor stings.
- Antivenom IV (3 ampoules for life-threatening signs, 1–2 ampoules for analgesia or to prevent skin scarring).

Irukandji jellyfish

This small tropical jellyfish has a bell measuring 2 × 2.5 cm and four tentacles – one from each corner, a few trailing up to 75 cm. It is almost transparent and difficult to see.

Symptoms and signs

Although the sting is only moderately painful, it may be followed within an hour by

- Nausea, vomiting, profuse sweating, agitation and muscle cramps.
- Vasoconstriction and severe systemic and pulmonary hypertension (due to release of catecholamines). This may cause acute heart failure.

Management

- Mechanical ventilation and vasodilators may be required.

USEFUL RESOURCES
- *www.avru.org* – Australian Venom Research Unit. World-renowned Melbourne University unit.
- *www.toxnet.nlm.nih.gov* – Toxicology Data Network. American database containing useful information on toxicology, hazardous chemicals, environmental health and toxic releases.
- *www.toxinology.com* – Excellent clinical toxicology resource from the Women's & Children's Hospital, Adelaide, Australia.
- *www.museumvictoria.com.au/bioinformatics/snake* – Images and ecological data on Victorian Snakes.

CHAPTER 6

Cardiac conditions

Bryn Jones
Michael Cheung

Innocent murmur
Background
At least 50% of school-age children have a systolic cardiac murmur with no structural or physiological cardiac abnormality.

Features of a physiological, functional or 'innocent' murmur

History	Other examination	Murmur
• Asymptomatic • Normal growth • Benign family history	• Normal	• Soft systolic murmur • Continuous • Varies with posture • Normal second heart sound

When to refer for investigation
A cardiac murmur associated with any of the following requires clinical assessment by a specialist.

History
- Family history of cardiomyopathy or sudden unexplained death
- Chromosomal disorder
- Congenital malformation of other organs
- Maternal diabetes
- Exertional syncope or unexplained collapse
- Palpitations
- Symptoms of cardiac failure

Examination
- Cyanosis
- Breathlessness
- Failure to thrive not clearly due to other causes
- Unequal pulses
- Thrill associated with murmur

Murmur characteristics
- Diastolic murmur
- Continuous murmur with no postural variation
- Pan-systolic murmur
- Loud murmur (amplitude grade 3/6 or greater)
- Murmur harsh or high pitched

Paediatric Handbook, Ninth Edition. Edited by Amanda Gwee, Romi Rimer and Michael Marks.
© 2015 John Wiley & Sons, Ltd. Published 2015 by John Wiley & Sons, Ltd.

- Murmur heard best at left upper sternal border
- Abnormal second heart sound
- Early or mid-systolic click

Worrying CXR
- Enlarged heart
- Abnormal cardiac contour
- Pulmonary plethora
- Pulmonary vascular markings

Worrying ECG
- Abnormal QRS axis
- Increased voltages
- Abnormal intervals
- ST/T wave changes

The neonate with symptomatic congenital heart disease
Background
- The greatest mortality risk for a neonate with symptomatic congenital heart disease (CHD) is before diagnosis.
- Critically obstructed systemic circulation (e.g. critical aortic stenosis, coarctation and hypoplastic left heart syndrome) can be indistinguishable from shock due to sepsis.
- CHD should be considered in any unwell neonate, and prostaglandin may be life-saving in duct-dependent lesions.

Clinical syndromes
Clinical syndromes of presentation with symptomatic CHD include
- Shock due to low cardiac output, often with poor peripheral pulses and acidosis
- Persistent cyanosis
- Congestive cardiac failure with respiratory distress and hepatomegaly

Management
Use of prostaglandin (PGE$_1$)
- Dose:
  - Initial dose is 10 ng/kg/min IV; then increase to 20–100 ng/kg/min depending on response
  - Aim for saturations in the 80s and improving systemic perfusion
- Major side effects:
  - Hypotension
  - Apnoea
- Contraindications: There are no congenital cardiac lesions for which PGE$_1$ is absolutely contraindicated.
- The risk–benefit is in favour of PGE$_1$ infusion if
  - Patient is critically unwell
  - Patient is cyanotic with a murmur
  - Patient has poor peripheral pulses

Seek early advice from a specialist centre for support to arrange timely transfer for assessment.

Neonatal cyanosis
Cyanosis in any neonate must be investigated.

Clinical syndromes
- *Cyanotic CHD* is often more likely if there is persistent cyanosis with no respiratory distress and normal CO_2 clearance. The presence of a murmur increases the likelihood of a prostaglandin sensitive lesion.
- *Parenchymal lung disease* is likely if the infant has respiratory distress, elevated Pco_2, lung field changes on CXR and a likely cause (e.g. meconium aspiration).
- *Persistent Pulmonary Hypertension of the Newborn (PPHN)* is difficult to distinguish clinically from cyanotic CHD.

Initial assessment

- Examination: respiratory effort, abnormal pulses and presence of murmur.
- Investigations:
  - Arterial blood gases: look for acidosis, $P\text{co}_2$.
  - CXR: look at cardiac silhouette, pulmonary vascularity and parenchymal lung disease.
  - 12-lead ECG: look at axis, rhythm, presence of sinus P waves, QRS complexes.
  - Echocardiography: diagnostic test of choice.
- Tests:
  - Hyperoxia test: After 10 minutes of breathing 100% O_2, take right arm, preductal (radial artery) arterial blood gas.
    - A $P\text{ao}_2$ <70 mmHg will occur with most major cyanotic defects.
    - A $P\text{ao}_2$ >150 mmHg suggests cyanosis is **not** due to structural heart disease.
  - Trial of prostaglandin (PGE_1).
    - Will generally result in considerable improvement with duct-dependent CHD.

Seek early advice from a specialist centre and neonatal transport service.

Hypercyanotic spells (tetralogy spells)

Severe cyanotic spells are a characteristic feature of tetralogy of fallot (TOF) but may occasionally occur with other cyanotic lesions. The TOF consists of (1) right ventricular hypertrophy, (2) right ventricular outflow tract obstruction, (3) ventricular septal defect, with (4) over-riding aorta.

Clinical presentation and background

- Mechanism probably involves acute reduction in pulmonary blood, peripheral vasodilatation.
- Severe cyanosis with agitation and breathlessness.
- Often precipitated by exertion, feeding or crying, but can be spontaneous.
  - The right ventricular outflow tract murmur becomes softer and may become inaudible.
- Most episodes are self-limiting, lasting 15–30 minutes, but can be prolonged or result in loss of consciousness.

Management
Initial

- Avoid exacerbating distress.
- Give high-flow oxygen via mask or head box.
- Morphine 0.2 mg/kg IM may help in severe cases.
- Continuous ECG and oxygen saturation monitoring; frequent BP monitoring.
- Correct any underlying cause (e.g. arrhythmia, hypothermia, hypoglycaemia).

If prolonged

- IV/Intraosseous (IO) fluids: 0.9% normal saline 10 mL/kg bolus followed by maintenance fluids.
- Correct acidosis: sodium bicarbonate 1–2 mmol/kg IV.
- Beta-blocking drugs: IV esmolol 0.5 mg/kg over 1 minute, then 50–200 mcg/kg/min for up to 48 hours.
- Intubation and positive pressure ventilation may be required in extreme cases.

Longer term

- In most cases, hypercyanotic spells are an indication for palliative or corrective surgery.
- Oral propranolol may be given prophylactically to prevent spells in a child awaiting surgery.

Heart failure after the neonatal period
Main causes

- Congenital heart defects with pressure or volume overload ($\pm$cyanosis)
- Myocardial dysfunction after repair or palliation of heart defects
- Cardiomyopathies
- Tachyarrhythmias
- Rheumatic heart disease (RHD)

Clinical features
- Infants and young children have non-specific symptoms and signs:
  - Dyspnoea, fatigue, feeding difficulties, increased sweating
  - Failure to thrive, poor exercise tolerance
  - Gallop rhythm, hepatomegaly, cardiomegaly
- Older children may have signs more like those in adults:
  - Breathlessness, fatigue, poor exercise tolerance, orthopnoea
  - Nocturnal dyspnoea, venous distension, peripheral oedema

Investigations and management principles
- Seek early advice from a specialist centre.
- Arrange urgent echocardiography to assess cardiac structure and function.
- Oxygen for hypoxia related to pulmonary congestion or respiratory infection.
- Reduce pulmonary and systemic venous congestion:
  - Frusemide: 1 mg/kg per dose (8, 12 or 24 hourly).
  - Spironolactone (dose by weight):
    - 0–10 kg = 6.25 mg/dose oral (12 or 24 hourly);
    - 11–20 kg = 12.5 mg/dose oral (12 or 24 hourly); and
    - 21–40 kg = 25 mg/dose oral (12 or 24 hourly).
- Decrease afterload:
  - Captopril: 0.1–1 mg/kg per dose (max 50 mg) oral 8 hourly.
  - Commence ACE inhibitor in hospital with blood pressure monitoring (every 30 minutes for 2–3 hours after dose).
  - Monitor serum potassium if using spironolactone.
- Inotropes for acute, low-output cardiac failure:
  - Dobutamine: initially 5 mcg/kg/min IV.
  - Dopamine: initially 5 mcg/kg/min IV.
  - Milrinone: 50 mcg/kg over 10 minutes IV then 0.375–0.75 mcg/kg/min.
- Positive pressure ventilation.
- Treat complications:
  - Infection
  - Anaemia
  - Arrhythmia
  - Malnutrition

Supraventricular tachycardia
Seek urgent specialist advice if any tachycardia is broad complex or irregular, or fails to respond to the management.

Definition
Supraventricular tachycardia (SVT) is usually a regular, narrow complex tachycardia, with a heart rate of between 160–300 beats/min.

Differential diagnosis
Sinus tachycardia up to 230 beats/min may occur in the neonate with
- Hypovolaemia
- Hypoventilation
- Pain
- Fever
- Pulmonary hypertension (PH)

Note: Ventricular tachycardia in the neonate can have a relatively narrow QRS complex.

Clinical features
- In utero: may cause hydrops.
- Infancy: irritability, pallor, poor feeding and dyspnoea secondary to congestive cardiac failure.

- Older children: palpitations, chest discomfort.
- Hypotension may be present at any age.

Initial assessment
- Physical examination:
  - Pulse, BP, temperature, heart murmur
  - Signs of cardiac failure (tachypnoea, increased work of breathing, hepatomegaly)
- 12-lead ECG to confirm a narrow complex tachycardia

Management
Patient is normotensive and well perfused
Vagal manoeuvres
- Infant or young child:
  - Ice water in bag or icepack to face for a few seconds only (only try 2–3 times)
  - Oropharyngeal suctioning
  - Gag with spatula
- Older child:
  - Valsalva manoeuvre (e.g. forced blowing through a blocked straw, syringe)

IV adenosine (can be IO if IV access is unsuccessful)
- Full resuscitation facilities should be available.
- IV access in a large, proximal vein.
- Record a continuous ECG rhythm strip throughout administration, to monitor the pattern of reversal.
- Begin with adenosine 0.1 mg/kg as an initial bolus (max 6 mg):
  - Repeat doses can be given at 2-minute intervals increasing by 0.05 mg/kg each dose to maximum 0.3 mg/kg (18 mg).
- Dilute small doses of adenosine with saline to allow rapid infusion.
- Give adenosine quickly, followed immediately by a 5 mL normal saline flush.
- Check patient's vital signs.
  - Rapid re-initiation of the tachycardia may occur due to premature atrial contractions, a repeated and often **lower** dose may be successful in this case.
  - A febrile child should be treated with antipyretics as the fever may make the tachyarrhythmia resistant to treatment.
- Side effects of adenosine: facial flush, chest pain, bronchospasm.

Patient is shocked (hypotensive, poor perfusion, impaired mental state)
- Ensure child is given oxygen and has IV access.
- The airway should be managed by experienced staff.
- Administer midazolam 0.2 mg/kg (max. 10 mg) IV to minimise awareness and fentanyl 1–2 mcg/kg (max 50–100 mcg) if rapidly available for analgesia.
- DC revert using a **synchronised** shock of 1 J/kg.

Subsequent management
After stabilisation of SVT, specialist review is required for
- 12-lead ECG in sinus rhythm (pre-excitation and other abnormality).
- Echocardiogram (structural associations of atrioventricular re-entry SVT, e.g. Ebstein's anomaly, cardiomyopathy).
- 24-hour Holter monitor (intermittent pre-excitation and initiating triggers such as premature atrial contractions).
- Consider prophylaxis, electrophysiological study.

Infective endocarditis
Background
Infective endocarditis is an infection of the endocardial surface of the heart. For it to develop, two independent events are normally required: (1) a damaged area of endothelium and (2) a bacteraemia.

Clinical features

Presentation

- Usually insidious and non-specific presentation.
- Often suggestive of intercurrent viral illness.
- Fever, anorexia, myalgia, arthralgia, headache, general malaise.
  - Splenomegaly, splinter haemorrhages, petechiae and other peripheral stigmata are rarely seen in children but do occur. Careful repeated examination for these signs is necessary as they may not develop until several days into the illness.

Diagnosis

- Suspect endocarditis in any patient with a structural cardiac anomaly and prolonged fever, or who develops fever and a new murmur.
- Multiple blood cultures (at least three) from separate sites and at different times, before antibiotic administration.
- Full blood count.
- ESR and CRP.
- Echocardiogram.

Management

- Admission to hospital.
- Commence empiric antibiotics to cover endocarditis as well as other potentially serious causes for the presenting illness.
  - Native valve/homograft:
    - benzylpenicillin 60 mg/kg (max 2 g) IV 6 hourly **plus**;
    - flucloxacillin 50 mg/kg (max 2 g) IV 6 hourly **plus**;
    - gentamicin 2.5 mg/kg (max 240 mg, synergistic dose) IV 8 hourly.
  - Prosthetic valve:
    - vancomycin 15 mg/kg (max 500 mg) IV 6 hourly **plus**;
    - gentamicin 2.5 mg/kg (max 240 mg, synergistic dose) IV 8 hourly.
- Prolonged antibiotic therapy is required. Specialist consultation is recommended to tailor the antibiotic regimen to individual patients and pathogens.
- Close monitoring of clinical and cardiovascular status including serial echo, blood cultures and inflammatory markers.
- Close monitoring for evidence of other embolic phenomena including cerebral imaging for left-sided lesions.

Endocarditis prophylaxis

- Children at risk should establish and maintain the best possible oral health to reduce potential sources of bacteraemia which includes tooth brushing and regular dental review.
- The following is a suggested guideline for prophylaxis.
  - Recommended only for children with the highest risk of adverse outcome of infective endocarditis (Table 6.1).

Table 6.1 Cardiac conditions for which endocarditis prophylaxis with dental procedures is indicated

Prosthetic cardiac valve or prosthetic valve material used for cardiac valve repair
Previous episode of infective endocarditis
Congenital heart disease (CHD) but only if it involves
Unrepaired cyanotic defects, including palliative shunts and conduits
Repaired congenital heart defect with prosthetic material or device (surgical or catheter intervention) during the first 6 months after the procedure
Repaired defects with residual defect at the site or adjacent to the sire of a prosthetic patch or prosthetic device
Cardiac transplantation recipients who develop cardiac valvulopathy
Rheumatic heart disease in indigenous Australians

○ Give prior to at risk procedures, such as dental procedures involving dental manipulation of gingival tissue, the periapical region of teeth or perforation of the oral mucosa; invasive respiratory procedures (e.g. incision or biopsy of respiratory mucosa including tonsillectomy and adenoidectomy) and invasive genitourinary procedures (see Table 6.1).
○ Give amoxicillin 50 mg/kg oral 1 hour preoperatively (max. 2 g).
○ If unable to take oral medication, give amoxicillin 50 mg/kg IV at induction (max. 2 g).
○ For penicillin-allergic patients, see antimicrobial guidelines.

Pulmonary hypertension
Background
Pulmonary hypertension (PH) is more common in children than adults due to the relative frequency seen in children with CHD and lung problems secondary to prematurity and structural malformations. It is defined as a mean pulmonary artery pressure equal to or greater than 25 mmHg at rest and can be divided into idiopathic pulmonary arterial hypertension (iPAH) and associated pulmonary arterial hypertension (e.g. CHD, liver and lung disease and connective tissue disorders). Without treatment, survival is <12 months in iPAH.

Clinical features
Typical symptoms can be non-specific but a diagnosis of PH should be considered with
● Shortness of breath during mild physical exertion
● Syncope with exertion
● Chest pain

Examination
● Right ventricular lift
● Prominent pulmonary component of second heart sound
● Diastolic murmur of pulmonary regurgitation
● Signs of overt right heart failure are uncommon in children

Investigations
● CXR: enlarged central pulmonary artery arteries.
● ECG: Right atrial enlargement, RVH.
● Echocardiogram: CHD, right ventricular function, estimate right ventricular and pulmonary arterial pressure.
● Cardiac catheterization with pulmonary vasodilator challenge.
● More specific tests may be required to determine any underlying aetiology before a diagnosis of iPAH is made.

Management
Treatment depends on aetiology and severity. The goal of medical therapy is to improve symptoms, quality of life and survival. There are multiple drugs that act to dilate the pulmonary vasculature dilatation and reverse remodeling.

Drug therapy
● Sildenafil (phosphodiesterase inhibitor)
○ Main side effect: systemic hypotension
● Bosentan (Endothelial receptor antagonist)
○ Side effect: elevation of liver enzymes and systemic hypotension
● Epoprostenol (prostacyclin)
○ Short half-life so requires a continuous intravenous infusion
○ Side effects: jaw pain, flushing and diarrhoea

Other
● Home oxygen (if desaturation during sleep)
● Anticoagulation (warfarin or aspirin to prevent thrombosis)
Patients with PH have markedly increased morbidity and mortality with anaesthesia and surgery and should have careful anaesthetic planning.

Table 6.2 Aetiology of dilated cardiomyopathy

Familial
 Sarcomeric protein mutations
 Cytoskeletal genes (Dystrophin, Desmin)
 Nuclear membrane
 Mitochondrial cytopathy

Non-familial
 Myocarditis (infective/toxic/immune)
 Kawasaki disease
 Eosinophilic (Churg Strauss syndrome)
 Drugs
 Endocrine
 Nutritional (thiamine, carnitine, selenium deficiencies)
 Tachyarrhythmia induced

Cardiomyopathies
Background
Cardiomyopathies are structural and functional abnormalities of the myocardium which can affect ventricular systolic and/or diastolic function. There can be both familial (genetic) and non-familial forms.
 Subtypes include
1. Dilated cardiomyopathy
2. Hypertrophic cardiomyopathy
3. Restrictive cardiomyopathy
4. Arrhythmogenic right ventricular cardiomyopathy
5. Unclassified (including left ventricular non-compaction – LVNC)
Potential genetic and non-genetic causes of dilated and hypertrophic cardiomyopathy are listed in Tables 6.2, 6.3 and 6.4.

Syncope and fainting
Background
Syncope is a brief, usually sudden loss of consciousness and muscle tone caused by inadequate oxygen or glucose supply to the brain.

Common causes
- Vasovagal
  - Usually associated with emotional or environmental stressors
- Orthostatic hypotension
  - Usually associated with a sudden change to upright posture

Table 6.3 Aetiology of hypertrophic cardiomyopathy

Familial
 Sarcomeric protein disease
 Glycogen storage disease
 Lysosomal storage disease (Hurler's syndrome, Anderson-Fabry disease)
  Disorders of fatty acid oxidation
  Mitochondrial cytopathies
  Syndromic (Noonan, LEOPARD, Friedreich's ataxia, Beckwith-Wiedemann, Swyer)

Non-familial
 Infant of diabetic mother
 Athletes heart
 Amyloidosis
 Obesity

Table 6.4 Dilated vs. hypertrophic cardiomyopathy

	Dilated cardiomyopathy: (50% of cardiomyopathies)	Hypertrophic cardiomyopathy: (35% of cases)
Incidence	Estimated annual incidence 0.6 per 100,000 children.	3–5 per 1,000,000
Characterised by	Dilatation and impaired contractility of one or both ventricles	Myocardial hypertrophy in the absence of haemodynamic stress (e.g. coarctation of the aorta, hypertension). Commonest cause of sudden cardiac death (SCD) in children
Aetiology	25% are genetic Depends on age at presentation • <12 months: myocarditis and metabolic abnormalities more common • older children: familial forms more common	50% are genetic Can be associated with syndromes (Noonan, Beckwith-Wiedemann. LEOPARD, Friedreich's ataxia)
Clinical features	• Few clinical signs until the degree of ventricular impairment is severe • Possible positive family history • Symptoms: chronic cough, poor feeding, failure to thrive, syncopal episodes, chest pain, decreased exercise tolerance, abdominal pain, palpitations, embolic phenomena • Signs of heart failure	Infants: present with symptoms and signs of congestive heart failure Older children: usually asymptomatic Examination: gallop rhythm; ejection systolic murmur
Investigations	Bloods: screen for general organ function, infective and metabolic cause, Brian Naturetic Peptide (BNP) • CXR • Echo • Catheter	Bloods: FBE, ESR, lactic acid, pyruvate, glucose, LFT's, carnitine and acylcarnitine profile, plasma amino acids Urine: metabolics screen ECG 24-hour Holter monitor Exercise test to assess blood pressure response Echo
Management	• Stabilise heart failure: ACE-I, beta blockers, aldosterone antagonists • IV inotropes • Treat arrhythmias (medications, EP study, implantable defibrillators) • Anticoagulation (poor function or thrombus) • Heart transplantation • Screen family members	• Beta blockers: reduce heart rate. • Assessment of arrhythmia and SCD risk with implantation of implantable cardioverter defibrillator (ICD). • Relief of LVOT obstruction ○ Surgical resection ○ Cardiac pacing ○ Cardiac transplantation • Genetic review • Screen family members
Prognosis	14% mortality in 2 years post diagnosis	Mortality rate of 1% per year

• Cardiac causes (only 2–6% of all cases of syncope)
  ○ Primary electrical (long QT syndrome, Brugada syndrome, catecholaminergic polymorphic ventricular tachy-cardia, short QT syndrome, pre-excitation syndromes)
  ○ Structural (cardiomyopathy (dilated, hypertrophic, arrhythmogenic right ventricular dysplasia), coronary artery anomalies, aortic stenosis, PH, acute myocarditis, CHD)
  ○ Unlikely, if no concerning features on history, examination or ECG

Concerning features on history
• Palpitations or chest pain
• Triggered by fright or auditory stimulus
• No identifiable prodrome
• Brief abnormal motor activity (rapid recovery)

- Syncope during exertion
- Syncope during swimming
- Requiring resuscitation
- History of CHD
- Family history (LQTS, cardiomyopathy, sudden cardiac death (SCD))

Investigations

- All patients presenting with syncope should have a 12-lead ECG performed.

Management

- Most patients with vasovagal syncope or orthostatic intolerance can be managed effectively with simple lifestyle changes and avoidance strategies.
- Any concerning features on history, examination or ECG should result in prompt specialist referral.

Rheumatic fever

Background

Acute rheumatic fever (ARF) is caused by an immunological reaction to an infection with group A streptococcus. In Australia, the highest rates of rheumatic fever are in Aboriginal and Torres Strait Islander people. RHD is a result of damage to the mitral and/or aortic valves during the illness which may persist. Further episodes of ARF can result in cumulative cardiac damage.

Clinical features

For those considered low risk, the diagnosis requires two major or one major and two minor manifestations *plus* evidence of a preceding group A streptococcal infection. (Table 6.5).

Major manifestations:
Carditis (Subclinical carditis for high risk children)
    Polyarthritis
    Chorea
    Erythema marginatum
    Subcutaneous nodules
Minor manifestations:
Monoarthralgia
    Fever (>38°C)
    ESR >30 mm/h or CRP >30 mg/L
    Prolonged PR interval on ECG

Rheumatic carditis

- Inflammation can affect all layers of the heart.
- Involvement of the cardiac valves (particularly mitral and aortic) is the commonest manifestation.
- Can be detected at onset of illness but presentation can sometimes be delayed.
- Clinical findings: pathologic heart murmur, cardiac dilatation, signs of heart failure, pericardial rub. Commonest cardiac lesion is mitral regurgitation.

Investigations

- FBE, ESR, CRP, blood cultures (if febrile)
- ECG
- Throat swab
- Antistreptococcal serology (ASO and anti-DNase B titres)
- All patients with suspected or definite ARF should undergo echocardiography

Management

Acute

- Confirm the diagnosis.
- Admission to hospital for observation and investigation.
- Benzathine penicillin G (BPG) IM or 10 days oral penicillin V (erythromycin if penicillin allergy).

Table 6.5 2012 updated Australian guidelines for the diagnosis of RF

	High Risk Groups[a]	All other groups
Definite initial episode of RF	Two major or one major and two minor manifestations plus evidence of a preceding GAS infection[‡]	
Definite recurrent episode of RF in a patient with known past RF or RHD	Two major or one major and one minor or three minor manifestations plus evidence of a preceding GAS infection	
Probable RF (first episode or recurrence)	A clinical presentation that falls short by either one major or one minor manifestation, or the absence of streptococcal serology results, but one in which RF is considered the most likely diagnosis. Such cases should be further categorised according to the level of confidence with which the diagnosis is made: • highly suspected RF • uncertain RF	
Major manifestations	Carditis (including subclinical evidence of rheumatic valvulitis on echocardiogram)	Carditis (excluding subclinical evidence of rheumatic valvulitis on echocardiogram)
	Polyarthritis or aseptic mono-arthritis or polyarthralgia	Polyarthritis
	Chorea	Chorea
	Erythema marginatum	Erythema marginatum
	Subcutaneous nodules	Subcutaneous nodules
Minor manifestations	Monoarthralgia	Fever
	Fever	Polyarthralgia or aseptic mono-arthritis
	ESR ≥30 mm/h or CRP ≥30 mg/L	ESR ≥30 mm/h or CRP ≥30 mg/L
	Prolonged P-R interval on ECG	Prolonged P-R interval on ECG

[a]High-risk groups are those living in communities with high rates of RF (incidence >30/100,000 per year in 5–14 year olds) or RHD (all-age prevalence >2/1000). Aboriginal people and Torres Strait Islanders living in rural or remote settings are known to be at high risk.

- Simple analgesia and antipyretics (paracetamol and codeine).
- Anti-inflammatory medications (aspirin – high dose, NSAIDs – naproxen and ibuprofen) for arthritis and fever (once diagnosis confirmed).
- Influenza vaccine if receiving aspirin.
- Bed rest with gradual ambulation (if carditis guided by symptoms and inflammatory markers).
- Heart failure treatment (diuretics, ACE inhibitors).

Secondary prophylaxis
- Centralised registries play an important role in ensuring delivery of prophylaxis.
- BPG IMI (450 mg/600,000 units if <20 kg; 900 mg/1,200,000 units if >20 kg) 4 weekly. Phenoxymethylpenicillin 250 mg oral BD if IM not possible.
- Duration of prophylaxis is for a minimum duration of 10 years or until the age of 21 (whichever is longer) with continuation after this time dependant on the severity of residual RHD.
- Optimising oral hygiene and endocarditis prophylaxis for established RHD.

Basic ECG interpretation
ECG interpretation should include a systematic assessment of rate, rhythm, axis, P waves, QRS complex, ST segments, T waves and intervals (PR, QT and QTc).

A normal ECG should have an appropriate rate for age and a P-wave, which should be upright in leads I and aVF, preceding each QRS complex (see Fig. 6.1). There are age-related normal values for axis, P waves, QRS

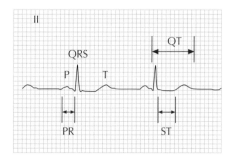

Fig. 6.1 Normal ECG

complexes and all intervals on the 12-lead ECG (see Table 6.6). For children >12 years, adult normals can be used as a guide.

Rate
Calculate as 300/(number of big squares). At a normal paper speed of 25 mm/s, each small square represents 0.04 second, and each big square 0.20 second.

Rhythm
Sinus rhythm is present when there is a P wave with normal axis followed by a QRS complex. Alternatives include:
- Ectopic atrial rhythms: P wave with abnormal axis followed by QRS complex
- AV nodal or junctional rhythm: narrow QRS complexes unrelated to P waves
- Ventricular rhythms: broad often bizarre QRS complexes unrelated to P waves

QRS axis
Normal QRS axis values are listed in Table 6.6. An abnormal QRS axis can indicate ventricular hypertrophy (or hypoplasia with the larger ventricle contributing to relatively greater voltages) or be associated with anatomically abnormal conduction pathways in complex lesions.

P waves
A normal axis sinus P wave is upright in leads I and aVF. Other appearances may result from ectopic atrial foci or structural congenital heart lesions. Tall P waves reflect RA enlargement (P pulmonale), broad P waves LA enlargement (P mitrale). A prolonged PR interval occurs in first-degree heart block.

Table 6.6 Age-related ECG normal values

	Neonate	Young child (1–2 years)	Older child (3–12 years)
Heart rate (per min)	107–182	89–151	62–130
QRS axis (°)	+65–+161	+7–+101	+9–+114
PR (s)	0.07–0.14	0.08–0.15	0.09–0.17
QRS (s)	0.03–0.08	0.04–0.08	0.04–0.09
R V_1 (mm)	3–21	2.5–17	0–12
S V_1 (mm)	0–11	0.5–21	0.3–25
R V_6 (mm)	2.5–16.5	6–22.5	9–25.5
S V_6 (mm)	0–10	0–6.5	0–4
Q V_6 (mm = 98th centile)	3	3	3

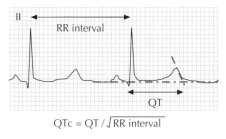

$$QTc = QT / \sqrt{RR \text{ interval}}$$

Fig. 6.2 Bazett's formula for calculating corrected QT interval (QTc)

QRS complexes and T waves

The neonatal ECG shows right-sided dominance with large R waves and upright T waves in leads V1, V2, aVR and V4R. The T waves should have inverted by 1 week of age in the normal child. Persistence beyond this time indicates RVH. The T waves become upright in right-sided leads again in later childhood and the ECG takes on the adult appearance of dominant left-sided forces with small Q waves and large R waves in the lateral leads I, II, aVL, V5 and V6.

ST segments

Normal adolescents and young adults may have sloping elevation of the ST segment due to early repolarisation. Elevation or depression of >1 mm in limb leads and 2 mm in precordial leads is abnormal and occurs in pericarditis, ischaemia or infarction and with digoxin treatment.

Corrected QT interval

The QT interval can be corrected for heart rate by measuring the QT occurring after the shortest RR in sinus rhythm and applying Bazett's formula (all measurements in seconds). The QT is measured to the point where a tangent to its slope crosses the baseline (see Fig. 6.2).

USEFUL RESOURCES

- *www.rch.org.au/cardiology/defects.cfm* – RCH Cardiology Website. Excellent website with pictures and parent handouts regarding the major structural abnormalities.
- www.rch.org.au/cardiology/heart_defects/
- www.rch.org.au/cardiology/howie – interactive website to find out about procedures and tests that you may have on your heart.
- www.rch.org.au/clinicalguide/guideline_index/Supraventricular_Tachycardia_SVT
- www.rch.org.au/rchcpg/hospital_clinical_guideline_index/Peri-operative_management_of_patients_with_pulmonary_hypertension_or_cardiomyopathy
- *www.heartkids.org.au* – parent support organisation

CHAPTER 7

Respiratory conditions

Sarath Ranganathan
John Massie

Respiratory illness accounts for at least 50% of all acute paediatric presentations. Infants and young children tire quickly and can rapidly present in acute respiratory failure.

Respiratory conditions result in
- Airway compromise (e.g. asthma, bronchiectasis, croup). This results in noisy breathing (stertor above the larynx, stridor if extrathoracic or wheeze if intrathoracic).
- Parenchymal compromise (e.g. pneumonia). This may directly affect the blood–gas barrier and result in hypoxaemia.
- Mixed picture of airway and parenchymal compromise (e.g. bronchiolitis).

Asthma
See also Chapter 19, *Allergy and immunology*, p. 311.

Pathology
The two main components include
- Airway inflammation
- Reactive airways (bronchoconstriction and airway hyperresponsiveness)

Risk factors
- Individuals with allergic disease (perennial rhinitis, hay fever, eczema)
- First-degree relatives with asthma and/or atopic disease

Natural history
- Most children with episodic (infrequent or frequent) asthma will improve over time.
- Some will go on to have this condition throughout their life.

Common triggers
- Upper respiratory tract infections (URTIs)
- Exercise
- Exposure to cold air
- Allergen exposure
- Laughing (in preschool children)

Clinical features
- Wheeze
- Shortness of breath
- Chest tightness
- Cough
- Response of symptoms to short-acting bronchodilators
- Interval symptoms may be present, that is symptoms at night (waking the patient), early in the morning, at rest during the day, during physical activity

Note: Cough alone, in the absence of wheeze, is rarely due to asthma.

Paediatric Handbook, Ninth Edition. Edited by Amanda Gwee, Romi Rimer and Michael Marks.
© 2015 John Wiley & Sons, Ltd. Published 2015 by John Wiley & Sons, Ltd.

There may be few physical signs found between acute attacks. Undertreated or chronic asthma may be associated with:

- Hyperinflation
- Chest wall abnormalities, for example pectus carinatum or flaring of the lower ribs (Harrison sulcus)
- Expiratory wheeze (generalised)
- Slowed growth parameters
- Side effects of medication (e.g. oral candidiasis in those taking inhaled steroids)

Other causes of wheeze to consider

- Small airway calibre (usually stops by 6 years)
- Suppurative lung disease (may have clubbing)
- Mediastinal mass (may have tracheal shift)
- Inhaled foreign body (localised wheeze)
- Cardiac failure (may have other cardiac signs)

Diagnosis

The diagnosis of asthma is usually clinical. Occasionally, a therapeutic trial of bronchodilator is required to aid in this diagnosis. Usually no investigations are required, but tests that may help with the diagnosis and management of asthma include

Spirometry

- Children over the age of 5 years can learn to do spirometry accurately. However, it is important to note that peak flow measurements are unreliable in children and have a minimal role in diagnosis or in monitoring progress.
- Airway obstruction is defined as FEV_1 <80% (predicted), FEV_1/FVC <75% (but this figure varies with age), MMEF 25–75 <67% (predicted).
- If there is evidence of airway obstruction, bronchodilator reversibility should be assessed (an improvement of FEV_1 of 12% in absolute values).
- In most cases, spirometry is unhelpful during an acute admission unless there is a difference between the perceived symptoms and objective clinical measures.

Exercise challenge

- 70% of children with asthma have exercise-induced bronchoconstriction.
- Exercise challenge may be used in children who are able to do accurate spirometry.
- 15% reduction in FEV_1 following exercise is considered significant.
- Graded dose inhalation of dry powder mannitol is a new alternative to the exercise challenge.
- Other challenges such as histamine and methacholine are sometimes used for children.

Chest radiograph (CXR)

- CXR is not routinely required in either the acute or interval management of asthma.
- CXR may be required if there is evidence of an acute complication (e.g. mucous plugging) or patients with difficult-to-control, persistent asthma (particularly if they have not had a previous CXR).
- CXR is helpful if symptoms and signs are not wholly explained by asthma and may be caused by another disease (e.g. mediastinal mass, suppurative lung disease or foreign body).

Assessment of the severity of an attack

The severity of acute asthma can be classified as mild, moderate, severe or critical. The most reliable indicators are mental state and work of breathing (comprising accessory muscle use and recession). See Table 7.1.

- The initial arterial O_2 saturation (SaO_2) in air, heart rate and ability to talk should be used as additional features in assessing the severity of acute asthma.

Table 7.1 Assessment of the severity of an acute asthma attack

Sign	Mild	Moderate	Severe	Critical
Mental state	Normal	Normal	Agitated	Confused/drowsy
Work of breathing	Normal	Mildly increased	Moderately/markedly increased	Maximally increased or exhausted

- Wheeze intensity, central cyanosis, pulsus paradoxus and peak expiratory flow are not reliable for the assessment of the severity of acute asthma.
- Arterial blood gases, CXR and spirometry should not be routinely used in assessing the severity of acute asthma.

Management of acute asthma.

The management of asthma is dependent upon its severity (see Fig. 7.1).

Treatment at home

Patients are safe to be treated at home when they

- Require salbutamol 3–4 hourly or less frequently;
- Have adequate oxygenation;
- Have adequate oral intake; AND
- Their carer is well educated in regards to asthma management and has the ability to administer salbutamol via a spacer.

All children being discharged from hospital following an asthma attack should have a plan given to them. The key elements in the plan are

- Daily treatment
- Treatment before exercise (if it is a known trigger)
- Treatment of minor symptoms
- Treatment of acute exacerbation
- Emergency plan

Parents who are familiar with their child's asthma can initiate prednisolone at home at the start of an exacerbation, although there is limited evidence for this practice in children over 5 years old and none in preschool children.

Hospital treatment

Consultation with a paediatrician is recommended if

- The attack is of moderate or severe severity.
- There is poor response to bronchodilators.
- The child has an oxygen requirement.

Drug delivery

- All MDI doses should be given through a spacer, regardless of age. In young children, a mask is firmly applied to the face and in older children (generally greater than 4 years old), their lips should go around a mouthpiece.
- Shake the puffer initially and then after each puff.
- Load with one puff at a time (and repeat).
- If the child uses tidal breathing, allow five breaths.
- Spacers should be washed in household detergent weekly to reduce static and then air-dried (spacers should not be rinsed, rubbed or towel dried).
- All patients using inhaled corticosteroids should rinse their mouths afterwards.

Follow-up

- Determine the pattern of asthma in order to prescribe the appropriate treatment (see Table 7.2).
- Review asthma action plan and medication regimen.
- Check adherence to medication.
- Educate regarding avoidance of precipitants (e.g. allergens).
- Educate regarding avoidance of cigarette smoking (active and environmental).
- Monitor growth and development.

Acute viral bronchiolitis

Aetiology

Bronchiolitis is a generalised lower respiratory tract infection. Respiratory viruses are the most common cause of bronchiolitis in young infants. The most common is respiratory syncytial virus (RSV).

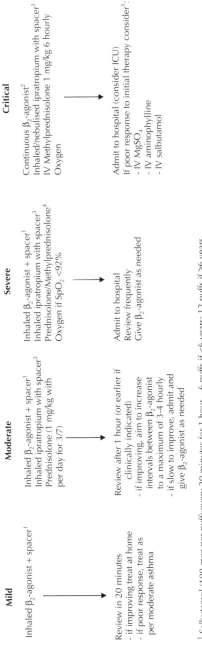

Mild

Inhaled β₂-agonist + spacer[1]

Review in 20 minutes
- if improving treat at home
- if poor response, treat as per moderate asthma

Moderate

Inhaled β₂-agonist + spacer[1]
Inhaled ipratropium with spacer[3]
Prednisolone (1 mg/kg with per day for 3/7)

Review after 1 hour (or earlier if clinically indicated)
- if improving, aim to increase intervals between β₂-agonist to a maximum of 3-4 hourly
- if slow to improve, admit and give β₂-agonist as needed

Severe

Inhaled β₂-agonist + spacer[1]
Inhaled ipratropium with spacer[3]
Prednisolone/Methylprednisolone[4]
Oxygen if SpO₂ <92%

Admit to hospital
Review frequently
Give β₂-agonist as needed

Critical

Continuous β₂-agonist[2]
Inhaled/nebulised ipratropium with spacer[3]
IV Methylprednisolone 1 mg/kg 6 hourly
Oxygen

Admit to hospital (consider ICU)
If poor response to initial therapy consider[5]:
- IV MgSO₄
- IV aminophylline
- IV salbutamol

[1] Salbutamol (100 mcg per puff) every 20 minutes for 1 hour – 6 puffs if <6 years; 12 puffs if ≥6 years
[2] Even in critical asthma, studies have shown inhaled β₂-agonist to be as effective but nebulised β₂-agonist may be considered
[3] Ipratropium (40 mcg per puff) every 20 minutes for the first hour then cease – 4 puffs if <6 years; 8 puffs if ≥6 years
[4] Given prednisolone 1 mg/kg for 3 days; if vomiting give IV methylprednisolone
[5] More evidence is required but a reasonable guideline would be to start with IV MgSO₄; then IV aminophylline (if needed); then IV salbutamol (if needed)

Fig. 7.1 Asthma management flowchart

Table 7.2 Patterns of asthma and interval treatment

Classification of pattern	Common features	Preventer	Symptom controller	Reliever
Infrequent episodic	Episodes 6–8 weeks apart or more Attacks usually not severe Symptoms rare between attacks Normal examination and lung function between episodes	Nil	Nil	Short-acting β₂-agonist as needed*
Frequent episodic	Attacks <6 weeks apart Attacks more troublesome Increasing symptoms between attacks Normal examination and lung function between episodes	Inhaled corticosteroids (most patients will be well controlled on 100–200 mcg/day fluticasone (or equivalent) or montelukast	Nil	β₂-agonist as needed*
Persistent	Daytime symptoms >2 days/week Nocturnal symptoms >1 night/week Attacks <6 weeks apart May have abnormal lung function Multiple emergency department visits or hospital admissions	If mild, montelukast Inhaled corticosteroids (most patients will be well controlled on 100–200 mcg/day fluticasone or equivalent)	If on ≥250 mcg/day fluticasone and poorly controlled, add a long-acting β₂-agonist (maximum effective dose of fluticasone is 500 mcg/day) If symptoms poorly controlled on maximum inhaled therapy, reconsider the diagnosis, adherence, drug delivery and consider referral to a paediatric respiratory physician	Short-acting β₂-agonist as needed*

Clinical features

- Cough, wheeze, tachypnoea, apnoeas, fever and poor feeding in an infant.
- There may be signs of respiratory distress including tracheal tug, recession, use of accessory muscles, grunting.
- Crackles and wheeze on auscultation.
- Severe bronchiolitis is associated with respiratory failure.

Risk factors for severe bronchiolitis

- Young, especially <6 weeks
- Ex-premature infants
- Congenital heart disease
- Neurological conditions
- Chronic respiratory illness
- Pulmonary hypertension

Management

See Fig. 7.2.

- CXR and nasopharyngeal aspirates are not routine investigations for bronchiolitis.
- Fluids can be administered by either NGT or IV.
- Infants <3 months and those with severe bronchiolitis are more likely to become hyponatraemic (due to the syndrome of 'inappropriate' increased ADH secretion (SIADH)) and warrant close attention to fluid balance.

Pneumonia

Aetiology

- Respiratory viruses are the most common cause of pneumonia in young infants in developed countries. There is generally only mild to moderate constitutional disturbance. There may be scattered inspiratory crackles on auscultation.
- *Mycoplasma pneumoniae* is the most common pathogen in children >5 years old and is an under-recognised cause of pneumonia in younger children. Typically, symptoms develop over several days before the cough, often with a systemic illness. Cough is prominent and crackles may be focal or widespread. Children are usually unwell, may have headache and focal signs are present in the chest.
- *Streptococcus pneumoniae* is the most common bacterial pathogen in all age groups, followed by non-typeable *Haemophilus influenzae* and *Staphylococcus aureus*.
- Group A β-haemolytic streptococcus is less common but may cause severe pneumonia.

Clinical features

- Tachypnoea, fever and cough. There may be signs of respiratory distress.
- Focal signs in the chest may be difficult to detect in young infants.

Investigations

- A diagnosis of pneumonia, especially in younger children, can often only be made with radiological confirmation.
- CXR changes do not distinguish viral from bacterial pneumonia, although lobar changes are more likely to be caused by *Streptococcus pneumoniae*.

Management

- Young infants and those with severe disease are at risk of SIADH. Monitor sodium and consider limiting parenteral fluids. See also Chapter 9, *Fluids and nutrition*.

Pharyngitis/tonsillitis, acute otitis media and URTI

See Chapter 16, *Head and neck conditions*.

Laryngotracheobronchitis (croup)

See Fig. 7.3.

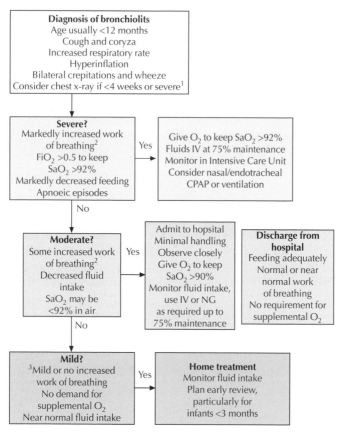

Diagnosis of bronchiolits
Age usually <12 months
Cough and coryza
Increased respiratory rate
Hyperinflation
Bilateral crepitations and wheeze
Consider chest x-ray if <4 weeks or severe[1]

Severe?
Markedly increased work
of breathing[2]
FiO_2 >0.5 to keep
SaO_2 >92%
Markedly decreased feeding
Apnoeic episodes

Yes →

Give O_2 to keep SaO_2 >92%
Fluids IV at 75% maintenance
Monitor in Intensive Care Unit
Consider nasal/endotracheal
CPAP or ventilation

No

Moderate?
Some increased work
of breathing[2]
Decreased fluid
intake
SaO_2 may be
<92% in air

Yes →

Admit to hopsital
Minimal handling
Observe closely
Give O_2 to keep
SaO_2 >90%
Monitor fluid intake,
use IV or NG
as required up to
75% maintenance

**Discharge from
hospital**
Feeding adequately
Normal or near
normal work
of breathing
No requirement for
supplemental O_2

No

Mild?
[3]Mild or no increased
work of breathing
No demand for
supplemental O_2
Near normal fluid intake

Yes →

Home treatment
Monitor fluid intake
Plan early review,
particularly for
infants <3 months

Notes:
[1] Routine CXR is not required for children with typical clinical features.
[2] Use the respiratory rate, accessory muscle use and recessions to judge the work
of breathing.
[3]Very young infants and infants with a co-morbidity (e.g., cardiac disease,
Down syndrome, chronic lung disease etc.) are at greatest risk of severe disease.
These infants may need admission for observation even if they have mild bronchiolitis.
Administration of β2 agonists may be distressing for young infants and is of no
proven value.

Fig. 7.2 Management of bronchiolitis

Epiglottitis
Aetiology
Epiglottitis is usually due to *Haemophilus influenzae* type b (Hib). The incidence of acute epiglottitis has
fallen markedly in countries where Hib immunisation is widespread. However, it continues to occur (child not
immunised, immunisation failure, other bacteria) and if the diagnosis is not made promptly, the child is likely
to die.

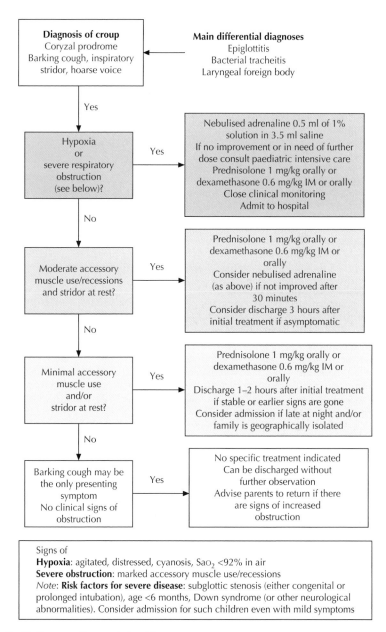

Fig. 7.3 Management of laryngotracheobronchitis

Clinical features

Epiglottitis differs from laryngotracheobronchitis in the following ways:
- The onset is with fever and lethargy, possibly following a URTI.
- Cough is not a prominent feature.
- Most children appear toxic because of the associated sepsis.
- The stridor is soft, and the expiratory element is often dominant with a snoring or gurgling quality.
- Symptoms of respiratory obstruction develop rapidly.
- Difficulty in swallowing with drooling of saliva is common.

Management

- Keep the child as calm as possible in a seated position and administer oxygen by mask.
- Complete obstruction may occur in just a few hours. In general, tracheal intubation under anaesthesia is required and should be arranged promptly.
- If complete obstruction is imminent, summon immediate help from an intensivist or anaesthetist. If inexperienced, do not attempt intubation unless the child becomes comatosed. Intubate orally initially with a relatively small endotracheal tube.
- If intubation proves to be impossible, attempt to ventilate with bag–valve–mask; a good technique may achieve adequate oxygenation and ventilation. If ventilation is impossible, perform cricothyrotomy or tracheostomy.
- Antibiotic therapy: ceftriaxone 100 mg/kg (max 2 g) IV followed by 50 mg/kg (max. 2 g) 24 hours later.
- Treat contacts prophylactically with rifampicin 20 mg/kg (max 699 mg) PO daily for 4 days.

Whooping cough (pertussis)

Whooping cough continues to be widespread in many communities because of suboptimal uptake of childhood immunisation and waning immunity in adolescents and adults who were immunised as children (the current vaccines give protection for only 5 to 10 years).

Clinical features

- Starts with a coryzal illness that resembles a URTI (infectious period).
- The cough may continue for many weeks to months, is paroxysmal and may be associated with facial suffusion and vomiting. In some children, the paroxysm is terminated by an inspiratory whoop. The cough is often only recognised as pertussis at this stage (paroxysmal phase).
- The child appears well between coughing paroxysms.
- In small infants, pertussis can present with apnoea alone.

Diagnosis

- Diagnosis can be made on clinical grounds.
- Lymphocyte count may be markedly elevated ($>20 \times 10^9$/L).
- In the acute phase, the diagnosis can be confirmed by identifying *Bordetella pertussis* from a nasopharyngeal aspirate (culture, immunofluorescence, PCR).
- Pertussis serum IgA is specific (but not sensitive) for past infection. It may be elevated after 3 weeks and persist for 2 years. It is rarely positive in infants <2 years of age.

Management

Pharmacological treatment

- No pharmacological agents improve the clinical course of whooping cough.
- Clearance of nasal carriage of *B. pertussis* with erythromycin estolate for 14 days has been best studied, but the estolate preparation is no longer available in Australia.
- Comparative studies suggest that a shorter course of clarithromycin is as at least as effective as erythromycin. The current recommendation is clarithromycin 7.5 mg/kg (max 500 mg) twice daily for 7 days. Azithromycin is an alternative, and is the preferred treatment for neonates.
- Treatment of household and other close contacts has not been proved to be effective, but contact prophylaxis is recommended if a contact is in the late phase of pregnancy or there is an incompletely immunised child in the family. Use clarithromycin (same dosage) for 7 days.
- Infants with proven pertussis should continue with routine vaccinations (which will include DTPa).

Hospital treatment

- Admit those who are
  - infants <6 months
  - apnoeic
  - cyanotic
  - not coping with the cough
  - feeding poorly
  - systemically unwell
- In hospital, careful observation, including the use of an apnoea monitor.
- If paroxysms occur frequently and are associated with marked cyanosis, nursing in oxygen may be of some help.

Cough

Cough is a common symptom in children. The degree to which a family becomes concerned about the frequency and severity of a child's cough is extremely variable. There is often a poor correlation between a parental report of cough and objective measures.

Acute cough

The cause of an acute onset cough is generally easy to recognise, most commonly with a respiratory infection, asthma or inhaled foreign body.

Persistent or recurrent cough

The history and characteristics of the cough are usually the keys to diagnosis. Whilst asthma, gastro-oesophageal reflux and post-nasal drip are the three favoured diagnoses in adults, these occur less commonly in children. In children think of

- Onset in infancy (and barking): tracheomalacia
- Dry (worse at night): post-viral cough, chronic non-specific cough of childhood, asthma
- Dry (paroxysmal): pertussis
- Wet (productive): suppurative lung disease (chronic suppurative bronchitis, cystic fibrosis (CF), immunodeficiency, primary ciliary dyskinesia, inhaled foreign body)
- Onset in older childhood (honking): psychogenic

Cough due to asthma

Although cough can be a troublesome symptom of asthma, it rarely occurs without some evidence of airways obstruction (e.g. wheeze). There is considerable doubt as to whether the entity of 'cough variant asthma', in which cough is the only symptom of asthma, exists in children. Be very reluctant to diagnose asthma in the absence of evidence of airways obstruction. The management of asthma is based on the severity and duration of the airways obstruction, not on the cough.

Physical examination

This is usually normal, but key findings include

- Poor growth and nutrition
- Digital clubbing (suppurative lung disease)
- Chest wall deformity (pectus carinatum suggesting chronic airway obstruction)
- Localised wheeze (inhaled foreign body)

Investigations

Specific investigations for persistent cough depend on the clinical suspicion after history and examination. In some circumstances, it can be reassuring to the family to have a normal CXR and lung function.

Cough management

- The most important aspect of management is to make a diagnosis and explain its nature to the parents. The effects of passive smoking should be discussed.
- Cough suppressants do not work.
- A foreign body must be removed bronchoscopically.
- It is often much more difficult to control the cough of asthma than the wheeze.

Foreign body in the bronchial tree
Clinical features
Symptoms
- Coughing or choking episodes while eating solid foods (classically nuts), or while sucking a small plastic toy or similar object. This history should never be dismissed.
- Persistent coughing and wheezing.
- Beware of the sudden onset of a first wheezing episode in a toddler in whom there is no history of allergy, especially if it follows a choking episode.
- Parents may not volunteer the history of possible inhalation (many foreign body aspirations are not witnessed).

Signs
- There may be no physical signs or alternatively reduced breath sounds over the whole or part of one lung.
- Wheeze.

Investigations
A CXR is taken in full inspiration and full expiration to exclude obstructive hyperinflation or an area of collapse. The radiograph should include the nasopharynx to the chest. Normal radiographs do not exclude a foreign body.

Management
Bronchoscopy is indicated for all patients with a suspected inhaled foreign body. There should be a high index of suspicion as aspirated foreign body is frequently missed.

- Bronchoscopy in children is difficult and requires an expert paediatric endoscopist teamed with an experienced paediatric anaesthetist. It should only be done in a major children's hospital. Rigid bronchoscopy is the procedure of choice.
- In most cases, the removal of the foreign body improves symptoms and there is rarely an indication for corticosteroids or antibiotics.

Cystic fibrosis
Background
CF is the most common life-shortening inherited disease of childhood. The incidence is 1:2500 and carrier frequency in people of European origin is 1:25.

Screening
- Newborn screening for CF detects 90% of affected babies.
- All babies have a heel prick on day 2 to 4 and the blood placed on a filter paper card. Serum trypsinogen is measured by immunoreactive assay (IRT).
- Babies with an IRT >99th percentile have gene mutation testing for 12 common CF gene mutations (Note: >2000 have been identified). Babies with two CF gene mutations have CF and are referred to the CF clinic. Babies with one CF gene mutation are referred for a sweat test at an approved laboratory. Those with a positive sweat test are referred to the CF clinic. Those with a negative sweat test are healthy carriers and their families referred for genetic counselling.
- Most babies with an elevated IRT and no CF gene mutations do not have CF.
- This screening test can miss babies who have a falsely low IRT or an uncommon gene mutation.
- Screening only began in Australia in the 1980s and many other countries do not have the same screening program. So if there is clinical suspicion, refer for a sweat test.

Diagnosis
- Classic clinical features of CF include
  - Suppurative lung disease
  - Pancreatic exocrine insufficiency (85% of patients), which manifests as steatorrhoea and failure to thrive
  - Multifocal biliary cirrhosis
  - Meconium ileus
  - Male infertility (absent vas deferens)
  - Elevated sweat electrolytes (occasionally presenting as hyponatraemic, hypochloraemic metabolic alkalosis)

Family history
- CF gene mutation analysis.
- Genetic counselling for the extended family of patients with CF is offered routinely but most babies with CF are born to families with no history of CF. For this reason preconceptual and prenatal carrier testing of all prospective parents is available.
- The diagnosis and management of CF is complex and best achieved in a specialist CF centre.

Management
General principles
- Nutrition:
  - High-fat, high-calorie diet.
  - Pancreatic enzyme replacement.
  - Vitamin supplementation (A, E and D).
- Salt supplementation.
- Pulmonary care:
  - Chest physiotherapy, usually at least once daily.
  - Bronchoalveolar lavage is done soon after diagnosis and then annually until the child can expectorate sputum. Cough suction specimens are also taken at each clinic visit.
  - Antibiotics and treatment regimens are largely dependent on which organism colonises and infects the lungs (see Table 7.3).
  - The acquisition of chronic *Pseudomonas aeruginosa* infection is associated with deterioration in lung function and a poorer prognosis. An aggressive antibiotic approach may prevent chronic infection and limit airway disease. **The aim of treating infection early is to eradicate *P. aeruginosa* when first identified.**

Management of upper respiratory tract infections
- A viral infection may predispose CF patients to secondary bacterial infection, so oral antibiotics are used aggressively (Table 7.3).
- For mild URTI, we recommend 2 weeks of anti-*Staphylococcal* and *Haemophilus* cover (e.g. Augmentin).
- If a child who is chronically infected with *Pseudomonas* develops a cold or an infective acute exacerbation, 2 weeks of oral ciprofloxacin is indicated. If symptoms persist, admit for IV antibiotics. It is accepted practice to give two antibiotics – usually combining an aminoglycoside with a penicillin/β-lactam (e.g. Timentin = ticarcillin/clavulanic acid) or third-generation cephalosporin (ceftazidime) to minimise the development of antimicrobial resistance. Nebuliser therapy can be stopped during IV therapy.
- Eradication is considered successful if there is
  - at least three negative cultures one month apart; **or**
  - one negative culture from bronchoalveolar lavage **and** one other negative culture 1 month apart.

Non-pulmonary complications of CF
Distal intestinal obstruction syndrome
- The accumulation of tenacious, muco-faeculent masses in the distal ileum or caecum which may become adherent and calcify.
- The cause is unclear but appears to be associated with dehydration, fever, reduction of enzyme supplementation, liver disease and the use of anticholinergic and opiate drugs.
- Although it occurs most frequently in those >15 years, it can occur at any age.
- Distal intestinal obstruction syndrome (DIOS) presents acutely with signs of abdominal obstruction or more commonly, sub-acutely with cramping abdominal pain and relative constipation.
- A mass is often palpable in the right iliac fossa. The management varies according to severity (see Table 7.4).
- Other conditions which should be considered in the differential diagnosis include
  - Constipation
  - Intussusception
  - Acute appendicitis
  - Acute pancreatitis
  - Volvulus

Table 7.3 Management of bacterial infection in CF

	Staphylococcus aureus	*Haemophilus influenzae*	*Pseudomonas aeruginosa*
Prophylaxis	Antibiotic prophylaxis against infection with *S. aureus* is given soon after diagnosis for 1 year or until cultures in early infancy are clear	Antibiotic prophylaxis against infection with *H. influenzae* non-type B is given soon after diagnosis for 1 year or until cultures in early infancy are clear	Not used
Acute infection	2 weeks oral antibiotics	2 weeks (co-amoxiclav, e.g., Augmentin) if *Haemophilus* is isolated in sputum. Continue for a further 2 weeks if symptoms persist If symptoms persist after a total of 4 weeks, consider IV antibiotics A bronchoalveolar lavage is indicated in patients not responding to treatment	If child is quite well and treatment adherence is good, the initial 2 weeks of intravenous therapy is omitted First-line IV therapy is ticarcillin and tobramycin pending sensitivities
Chronic infection	Patients should remain on prophylactic anti-staphylococcal antibiotics where (1) *S. aureus* is regularly cultured in sputum, (2) annual bronchoalveolar lavage is positive on two consecutive occasions, or (3) symptoms return when anti-staphylococcal antibiotics are stopped If patients develop an intercurrent respiratory tract infection, change to another anti-staphylococcal agent for 2 weeks If this is unsuccessful, IV ticarcillin and gentamicin (pending sensitivities) for 2 weeks may be necessary. Consider a bronchoscopic lavage in patients not responding to rule out *Pseudomonas* infection After treatment, oral antibiotics are recommended	In those patients who repeatedly have *H. influenzae* cultured in their sputum consider long-term prophylaxis (e.g. Augmentin) Augmentin is also the antibiotic of choice for acute exacerbations in those with chronic *H. influenzae* infection	Three consecutively positive cultures obtained at least 1 month apart Long-term nebulised tobramycin is then commenced If patients continue to deteriorate then switch to either nebulised colistin, nebulised preservative-free tobramycin (TOBI), or oral ciprofloxacin alternating with nebulised tobramycin on a monthly basis An exacerbation is characterised by an increase in cough, sputum production, change in sputum colour, loss of weight, decreased activity and deterioration in lung function. Fever may occur but is not typical

Table 7.4 Management of DIOS

Acute presentations	Investigation	Treatment
Mild episodes		
Mild abdominal pain No obstruction May be recurrent (out-patient management)	Nil	Rehydration Lactulose 10–20 mL BD Acetylcysteine 100 mg 3 times daily Consider adding oral gastrografin
Severe episodes		
Abdominal pain with distension and constipation No obstruction No peritonism (consider admission)	Full blood count Urea and electrolytes Abdominal radiograph (classically, speckled faecal gas pattern in right lower quadrant with dilated small-bowel loops)	Rehydration Lactulose 20 mL 3 times a daily Klean-Prep or ColonLytely via NG tube until clear fluid passed PR[a] Consider gastrografin enema (under radiological guidance)
Obstruction present		
Admit to ward	Full blood count Urea and electrolytes Abdominal radiograph	Rehydration 'Drip and suck' Inform surgeons Consider gastrografin enema (under radiological guidance)

[a]Monitor for hypoglycaemia in those with diabetes or liver disease.

- Strictures of the colon or ileocaecal junction
- Obstruction due to adhesions or strictures

Other considerations in DIOS
- Check dose of pancreatic enzymes.
- Check timing of enzymes and consider possible mismatch in gastric emptying between food bolus and pancreatic enzymes.
- Check adherence to medications.
- Ensure adequate dietary fibre and fluid intake.
- Ensure patient has a well-established toilet routine.
- Consider adding ranitidine or omeprazole if evidence of ongoing malabsorption.

Primary spontaneous pneumothorax
This is an air leak into the pleural cavity that occurs in patients without underlying chronic lung disease (CLD), when there is no provoking factor, such as trauma, surgery, or diagnostic intervention.

Incidence
8 to 16 per 100,000 in the general population.

Clinical features
- Acute onset of chest pain that is severe and/or stabbing pain, radiating to ipsilateral shoulder and increasing with inspiration (pleuritic).
- Sudden shortness of breath.
- Anxiety, cough and vague presenting symptoms (e.g. general malaise, fatigue) are less commonly observed.
- General appearance may be normal.
- Sweating, tachypnoea, tachycardia (most common finding).
- Splinting chest wall to relieve pleuritic pain.
- Asymmetric lung expansion – mediastinal and tracheal shift to the contralateral side with a large pneumothorax.

- Decreased or absent breath sounds.
- Hyperresonance on percussion.

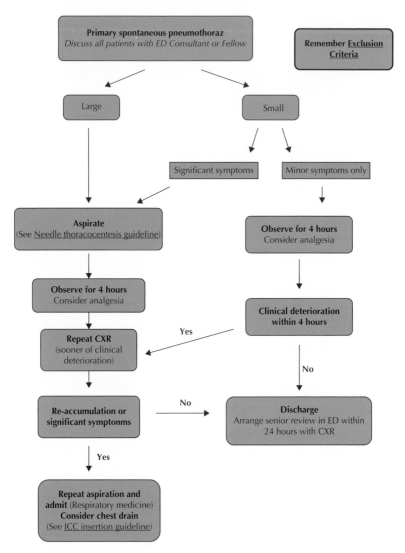

Fig. 7.4 Primary spontaneous pneumothorax

Investigations
- CXR
- CT scan is not recommended

Management

- 100% oxygen may accelerate the resorption of air in the pleural cavity.
- Aspiration
  - recommended for large primary spontaneous pneumothoraces (PSPs) and small pneumothoraces causing symptoms
  - has been shown to have comparable success and recurrence rates to intercostal chest catheter (ICC) insertion and yet is less invasive and more cost-effective
- Surgical Intervention
  - Aims to identify (if possible) and oversew or staple an ongoing leak (if present) and to prevent recurrence.
  - Surgical resection for ongoing leak (leak persisting greater than 4 days) may involve removal of identified blebs (blebectomy) or bullae (bullectomy) or an apical resection.
  - PSP will not usually recur. However, if it does recur on the same side, the majority will occur again if not prevented. Recurrence prevention procedures include pleurodesis or pleurectomy (Fig. 7.4).

Chronic lung disease of prematurity

See also Chapter 21, *Neonatal conditions*

- CLD is a long-term respiratory problem faced by babies born prematurely due the underlying lung pathology of bronchopulmonary dysplasia. It occurs as a result of insults that occur in the immature lung.
- The main insults are secondary to oxygen therapy and barotraumas due to mechanical ventilation but other insults such as perinatal infection are also implicated.

Clinical features

- Difficulty breathing is the main symptom of CLD.
- CLD can be associated with pulmonary hypertension, tracheobronchomalacia and gastro-oesophageal reflux.

Management

- Respiratory support in the form of oxygen therapy, CPAP or mechanical support is needed initially and then weaned as appropriate.
- RSV immunoglobulin is indicated for those in their first year of life who remain oxygen dependent with evidence of pulmonary hypertension.
- These children must be followed up in the long term as lung function and underlying lung developmental abnormalities may persist throughout life.

CHAPTER 8

Gastrointestinal conditions

George Alex
Susie Gibbs
Winita Hardikar
Michael Nightingale

Abdominal pain, vomiting and diarrhoea either in isolation or in combination, is the commonest presentation for most gastrointestinal conditions affecting children. Causes of abdominal pain in childhood are listed in Table 8.1. Vomiting occurs in various gastrointestinal and systemic conditions but importantly, acute surgical conditions need to be excluded. Diarrhoea can also be seen in a variety of gastrointestinal conditions. It is related to the consistency (loose) and frequency of stooling in a 24-hour period (>3 stools). Diarrhoea may be acute or chronic (more than 2–3 weeks).

Acute infectious gastroenteritis

Since the introduction of the rotavirus vaccine into the National Immunisation Program in 2007, the incidence of rotavirus-induced gastroenteritis requiring GP/hospital presentations, and admissions, has fallen dramatically. Other viruses such as adenovirus, norovirus and astrovirus are now the major etiological agents in acute infectious gastroenteritis. Bacterial gastroenteritis is less common, causing 5–10% of all cases; causes include *Salmonella* spp., *Campylobacter jejuni*, *Yersinia enterocolitica* and *Escherichia coli*. Parasites, such as Cryptosporidium, are also a known cause of acute gastroenteritis but mainly in the immunocompromised host.

The two most important issues in the management of acute infectious diarrhoea are

- Exclusion of other important causes of vomiting and diarrhoea such as
  - Appendicitis
  - Urinary tract infection
  - Other sites of infection (including meningitis, sepsis)
  - Surgical conditions including intussusception
  - Haemolytic uraemic syndrome
- Adequate assessment and treatment of dehydration

Clinical features

- Presenting symptoms include poor feeding, vomiting and fever, followed by diarrhoea. Stools are frequent and watery in consistency.
- Bacterial gastroenteritis is suggested by a history of frequent small-volume stools with passage of blood and mucus, and abdominal pain. Be wary of diagnosing gastroenteritis in the child with vomiting alone who is dehydrated or unwell.
- It is essential that all children with acute onset of vomiting, diarrhoea and fever are re-evaluated regularly so as to confirm the diagnosis of acute gastroenteritis and adequacy of rehydration therapy.

Assessment of dehydration

The risk of dehydration is increased with younger age as infants (<6 months) have an increased surface area to body volume ratio. This results in increased insensible fluid losses. Recent change in body weight provides the most accurate indication of fluid depletion:

- <4% body weight loss represents no or mild dehydration

Paediatric Handbook, Ninth Edition. Edited by Amanda Gwee, Romi Rimer and Michael Marks.
© 2015 John Wiley & Sons, Ltd. Published 2015 by John Wiley & Sons, Ltd.

Table 8.1 Causes of abdominal pain in childhood

Common	Uncommon
Gastroenteritis	Peptic ulcer
Appendicitis	Pancreatitis
Mesenteric adenitis	Inflammatory bowel disease
Constipation	Abdominal migraine
Intussusception	Pneumonia
Urinary tract infection	
Gastritis	

- 4–6% body weight loss represents moderate dehydration
- >6% body weight loss represents severe dehydration

Note: These percentages are approximate and serve only as a guide.

Starvation produces no more than 1% body weight loss per day.

Decreased skin turgor and peripheral perfusion accompanied by deep (acidotic) breathing are the only signs proven to discriminate between dehydration and hydration. The actual degree of dehydration may be underestimated with obesity and overestimated with wasting or sepsis.

Biochemical investigations
Glucose, electrolyte and acid–base studies are required in children with

- A history of prolonged diarrhoea with severe dehydration
- Altered conscious state
- Convulsions
- Short-bowel syndrome, ileostomy, chronic cardiac, renal and metabolic disorders
- Infants <6 months of age who are assessed to be dehydrated

Who to admit to hospital
- Infants/children who have moderate or severe dehydration.
- Patients at high risk of dehydration on the basis of young age (<6 months) with a high frequency of diarrhoea (8 per 24 hours) and vomiting (>4 per 24 hours) should be observed for 4–6 hours to ensure adequate maintenance of hydration.
- High-risk infants/children (e.g. ileostomy, short gut, cyanotic heart disease, chronic renal disease, metabolic disorders and malnutrition).
- Infants/children whose parents and carers are thought to be unable to manage the child's condition at home.
- If the diagnosis is in doubt.

Guidelines for management of acute gastroenteritis
Hydration (oral/nasogastric)
For infants/children with dehydration, rapid enteral rehydration over 4–6 hours is now suggested (Table 8.2).

Slower rehydration may be indicated in infants <6 months, children with significant co-morbidities and also those with significant abdominal pain (Table 8.2). Further exception applies to children with significant neurological (altered conscious state) or biochemical disturbance (see sections on hyper- and hyponatraemic dehydration Chapter 9, Fluids and Nutrition).

Most infants/children with dehydration can be safely and adequately rehydrated using oral rehydration solutions (ORS) (Table 8.3). If these are not tolerated by the oral route, nasogastric administration is an alternative. Vomiting is not a contraindication to nasogastric hydration.

ORSs use the principle of glucose-facilitated sodium transport in the small intestine. The solutions currently used in Australia are outlined in Table 8.4.

Table 8.2 Enteral rehydration

Weight on admission	mL/h	Total infusion time (hours)
7 kg	175	4
8 kg	200	4
9 kg	225	4
10 kg	250	4
12 kg	300	4
14 kg	300	4.5
16 kg	300	5
18 kg	300	6
20 kg	300	6.5

Source: RCH gastroenteritis clinical practice guideline.

Table 8.3 Slower nasogastric rehydration. Replacing deficit over first 6 hours and then daily maintenance over the next 18 hours

	Degree of dehydration			
	Moderate (4–6%)		Severe (>7%)	
Weight on admission	mL/h 0–6 hours	mL/h 7–24 hours	mL/h 0–6 hours	mL/h 7–24 hours
3.0 kg	30	20	50	20
4.0 kg	40	30	65	30
5.0 kg	50	35	80	35
6.0 kg	60	40	100	40
7.0 kg	70	45	115	45
8.0 kg	80	50	130	50
9.0 kg	90	55	150	55
10 kg	100	60	165	60
12 kg	120	65	200	65
15 kg	150	70	250	70
20 kg	200	85	285 for 7 hours*	85 for 17 hours**
30 kg	300	90	300 for 10 hours*	115 for 14 hours**

*RCH enteral pumps deliver a maximum of 300mL/h.
**Residual maintenance delivered over a shorter time course.

Table 8.4 Oral rehydration preparations available for use in Australia (concentrations are expressed as mmol/L of made-up solution)

	Na	K	Cl	Citrate	Glucose
Gastrolyte	60	20	60	10	90
Repalyte	60	20	60	10	90
Hydralyte	45	20	35	30	80

Parent education is vital, especially in the outpatient management of children. The important message is the need to drink more fluid more often, which is best given in small volumes frequently.

Hydration (intravenous)

Intravenous rehydration is indicated for severe dehydration and if nasogastric tube rehydration fails (e.g. ongoing profuse losses or abdominal pain). It is also suitable for children who already have an IV in situ. Children with certain co-morbidities, particularly GIT conditions (e.g. short gut or previous GI surgery) should be discussed with senior staff.

- Initial boluses: 20 mL/kg normal saline boluses, repeated until shock is corrected. If >40 mL/kg boluses required, involve senior staff.
- Measure blood glucose and treat hypoglycaemia with 5 mL/kg of 10% dextrose.
- Measure Na, K and glucose at the outset and at least 24 hourly from then on (more frequent testing is indicated for patients with co-morbidities or if more unwell).
- Consider a septic work-up or surgical consult in severely unwell patients with gastroenteritis.
- Ongoing fluids: 5% dextrose + 0.9% normal saline. Use a fluid containing KCl 20 mmol/L if serum K <3 mmol/L or give oral supplements.

  Refer http://www.rch.org.au/clinicalguide/guideline_index/Intravenous_Fluids//

Nutritional management

Early re-feeding (after rehydration) has been shown to enhance mucosal recovery in children/infants with acute gastroenteritis and reduces the duration of diarrhoea. Breastfeeding should continue through rehydration and maintenance phases of treatment. Formula-fed infants and children should restart oral age appropriate formula or food intake after completion of rehydration. Children can have complex carbohydrates (e.g. rice, wheat, bread and cereals), yoghurt, fruit and vegetables once rehydration is complete.

Pharmacotherapy

Infants and children should not be treated with antidiarrhoeal agents, as there is no substantial clinical evidence to suggest that this treatment alters symptoms. Most bacterial infections do not require antibiotics. *Salmonella* or *Campylobacter* gastroenteritis may require antibiotic treatment (see Chapter 18, *Infectious diseases and immunisations*). *Shigella* dysentery requires antibiotic treatment. Ondansetron (in the wafer form) can be administered once in the hospital setting for vomiting in gastroenteritis if symptoms are mild to moderate and if it helps facilitate oral rehydration.

Complications

Hypernatraemic dehydration (Na >150 mmol/L) or hyponatraemic dehydration (Na <130 mmol/L) – see Chapter 9, *Fluids and nutrition*.

Sugar intolerance

Following infectious diarrhoea, infants may have temporary lactose intolerance (due to lactase deficiency). This sequela of acute gastroenteritis used to be prominent in infants <6 months of age, but it is now uncommon. This may be due in part to early oral feeding which aids mucosal recovery.

Clinical features of sugar intolerance include

- Persistently fluid stool.
- Excessive flatus.
- Excoriation of the buttocks.
- Typically, these infants appear well.

Diagnosis is by

- Collection of the fluid stool in napkins lined with plastic. Dilute 5 drops of stool with 10 drops of water. Add a Clinitest tablet. A colour reaction corresponding to ≥0.75% or more reducing substance indicates that sugar intolerance is present.

Treatment:

- Breastfeeding should continue unless there are persistent symptoms with buttock excoriation and failure to gain adequate weight.

- Formula-fed infants should be placed on a lactose-free formula for 3–4 weeks. A clinical response after change to soy formula may indicate either post-infectious lactose intolerance or allergy to cow's milk protein, as soy formulae available in Australia are lactose-free.

Infrequently, infants with severe bowel damage secondary to gastroenteritis may be unable to absorb normal amounts of monosaccharide such as glucose or fructose. Diarrhoea will continue even with a lactose-free formula. Monosaccharide intolerance requires specialist consultation.

Chronic diarrhoea

An increase in stool frequency or fluid content is often of concern to parents, but does not necessarily imply significant organic disease, although this needs to be excluded. In every child who presents with chronic diarrhoea, the decision must be made as to whether further investigation is required. The algorithm (refer Fig. 8.1) outlines an approach to the child with chronic diarrhoea.

Toddler's diarrhoea

This is a clinical syndrome characterised by chronic diarrhoea often with undigested food in the stools of a child who is otherwise well, gaining weight and growing satisfactorily. Stools may contain mucus and are passed 3–6 times a day; they are often looser towards the end of the day. The onset is usually between 8 and 20 months of age and often there is a family history of functional bowel disease, such as irritable bowel syndrome. The treatment consists of reassurance and explanation. No specific drug or dietary therapy has been shown to be of value in toddler diarrhoea. Some toddlers on a high-fructose intake may have ('apple-juice') diarrhoea that responds to dietary change.

Coeliac disease

Coeliac disease is an autoimmune enteropathy triggered by the ingestion of gluten in genetically susceptible individuals, with an approximate incidence of 1:100 in Australia. The prevalence of this disorder amongst first-degree relatives is approximately 10%. The clinical expression of this disorder is more heterogeneous than previously thought and onset may be at any time, after years without symptoms.

Serological screening tests

An IgA antibody to tissue transglutaminase (TTG-IgA), which is over 98% specific and sensitive, has replaced the anti-endomysial antibody test in many hospitals. False-negative results can occur in IgA-deficient patients; hence, all patients will require total IgA levels measured to interpret the results appropriately. At RCH, we now use the combination of the TTG-IgA and the Deamidated gliadin peptide IgG to screen for coeliac disease in suspected cases.

Diagnosis

A small-bowel biopsy remains the gold standard. The need for subsequent biopsies to confirm or refute the diagnosis is dependent upon the clinical response of the patient to a gluten-free diet and subsequent serology or if the patient is <2 years of age at the time of diagnosis. This step needs to be individualised and in discussion with a gastroenterologist.

Management

A lifelong gluten-free diet excluding wheat, barley, rye and oats

Non-IgE-mediated cow's milk protein allergy

Allergic responses to cow's milk protein may result in a rapid (IgE) or delayed (non-IgE or mixed IgE/non-IgE) onset of symptoms. IgE-mediated allergy is characterised by sudden onset vomiting, angio-oedema, urticaria and rarely anaphylaxis. Non-IgE-mediated allergy may be more difficult to diagnose and presents with diarrhoea, malabsorption or failure to thrive, as well as intermittent intestinal loss of protein or blood in a well infant/child (sometimes called allergic proctocolitis). Non-IgE cow's milk protein allergy predominantly affects young infants; prospective studies suggest a prevalence of 2% in this group.

Diagnosis

This form of cow's milk protein allergy can only be diagnosed with a complete and thorough history, and with unequivocal reproducible reactions to elimination and challenge. Blood tests (i.e. RAST) and skin prick testing are generally unhelpful, as the underlying immunological mechanism is usually non-IgE mediated.

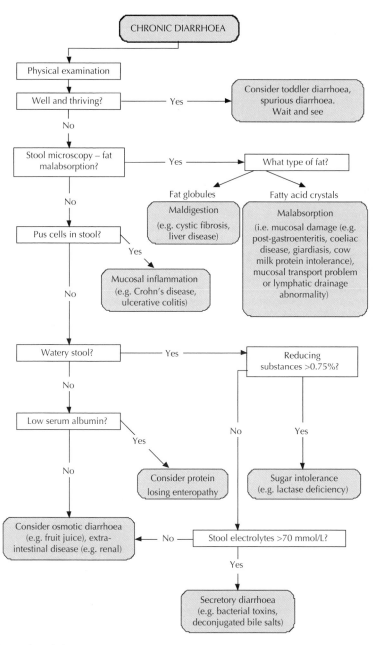

Fig. 8.1 Chronic diarrhoea

Management

After a definitive diagnosis is established, cow's milk protein should be removed from the diet and replaced with an extensively hydrolysed (e.g. Alfare™ or Pepti-junior™) or elemental formula (e.g. Neocate™ or Elecare™). A full soy formula is not recommended in young infants with severe enteropathy, as coexistent soy allergy occurs in 15–20% of such patients. Most food allergies in infants improve or resolve with increasing age.

Inflammatory bowel disease

The incidence of Crohn's disease has increased dramatically in Australian children since the 1970s, with a slower but steady rise in the incidence of ulcerative colitis.

- Crohn's disease can present in several ways including recurrent abdominal pain, weight loss, chronic diarrhoea, mouth ulcers and perianal disease. It may also present with isolated growth failure without any gastrointestinal symptoms.
- Ulcerative colitis is associated with bloody diarrhoea, which extends beyond the time frame of infective colitis.
- Extra-intestinal manifestations can occur in both disorders and include arthritis, erythema nodosum, hepatitis and ophthalmological complications (uveitis and episcleritis).

Diagnosis

Initial laboratory investigations should include

- Full blood count (anaemia and thrombocytosis), ESR (often raised) and albumin level (low with active disease).
- Stool microscopy (looking for WBC and RBC) and cultures for bacterial pathogens; Clostridium difficile and toxin should be collected.

Management

Evaluation and management, including pain management, should occur under specialist guidance.

Rectal bleeding

See Fig. 8.2.

Gastro-oesophageal reflux

Oesophageal reflux of gastric contents occurs normally and is more frequent after meals. It is regarded as pathological if associated with frequent regurgitation, or if it results in clinically significant adverse sequelae. The number of reflux episodes is normally greater in infants than in older children.

Reflux of gastric acid with heartburn may result in episodic irritability, but this is usually associated with obvious regurgitation and is rarely 'silent'. Although gastro-oesophageal reflux may cause infant distress, it is important to consider other possible causes. Both infant distress and frequent regurgitation are common in the first 6 months of life. Coexistence does not prove cause and effect. In selected cases investigations such as 24-hour oesophageal pH monitoring can be useful to correlate any episodes of reflux with irritability.

It is important to recognise that vomiting in infants may result from other causes, and these need to be excluded on the basis of history, physical examination and further tests if indicated.

Complications

- *Peptic oesophagitis:* this usually correlates with an increase in the number and duration of reflux episodes. Blood-flecked vomitus and anaemia may result.
- *Peptic strictures:* these are well recognised in childhood and present with dysphagia and failure to thrive.
- *Failure to thrive:* severe cases of gastro-oesophageal reflux may cause the loss of calories and anorexia.
- *Pulmonary complications:* recurrent or persistent cough and wheeze may be present and can occur without marked vomiting. These symptoms may result from aspiration of refluxed material (inhalation pneumonia) or through reflex bronchospasm. This mode of presentation requires a high degree of clinical suspicion to make the diagnosis.

Management

Regurgitation of gastric contents is common in infancy. In most cases, this 'posetting' does not result in any adverse sequelae and the most appropriate therapy is parental reassurance. 'Physiological' gastro-oesophageal reflux with regurgitation usually resolves by the age of 9–15 months.

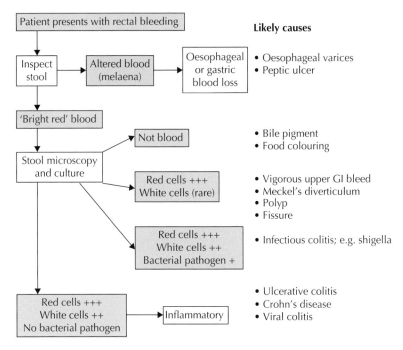

Fig. 8.2 Rectal bleeding

Simple measures

In the absence of signs of significant oesophagitis, aspiration or growth failure, the following should be suggested:

- Avoid excessive handling.
- Posture after feeds: the infant should be placed in a cot in the head-up position at or near 30 degrees.
- Thicken feeds: use a proprietary thickening agent or a prethickened formula if formula-fed.

Medication

Medications are not indicated in otherwise healthy, thriving infants with frequent regurgitation.

- Mylanta may offer relief from symptoms of heartburn (0.5–1.0 mL/kg per dose given 3–4 times a day). There are some concerns about its long-term use because of its mineral content.
- H_2 receptor antagonists such as ranitidine (2–3 mg/kg per dose given 2–3 times a day before meals) will reduce gastric acidity.
- Proton pump inhibitors are prescribed to infants and children with severe oesophagitis that is unresponsive to an H_2 receptor antagonist.

  There may be a role for a brief empirical trial of anti-reflux therapy in infants in whom it is thought reflux is the cause of their distressed behaviour. However, these agents are not without risk and should not be prescribed for prolonged periods without evidence to substantiate the severity of reflux.

Surgery

Laparoscopic fundoplication is indicated for reflux with complications when medical therapy has failed or is inappropriate. The indications include recurrent large-volume regurgitation, hiatal hernia, oesophageal stricture or Barrett oesophagus, growth failure and life-threatening respiratory symptoms.

Recurrent abdominal pain

Recurrent abdominal pain affects about 10% of school-age children. There is usually no specific identifiable cause, though it has been speculated that this condition may be a result of dysmotility of the bowel. Occasionally, it can result from a significant emotional problem.

Recent evidence suggests there may be a subgroup with migrainous abdominal pain (associated with pallor and family history). Emotional factors, lifestyle and temperamental characteristics can modulate the child's response to pain, irrespective of its cause.

It is essential to take a careful history, including psychosocial details. It may be helpful to interview the parents alone, the child alone and the family together. Onset of pain after the consumption of dairy products in older children and young adolescents should be sought, as lactase deficiency can present in this manner. Constipation needs to be excluded.

'*Red flags*' in the evaluation of chronic abdominal pain include pain localised away from the umbilicus, accompanying vomiting, diarrhoea, poor weight gain or linear growth, and pain awakening the patient from sleep. A thorough physical examination is essential and urine microscopy and culture is an appropriate baseline investigation.

Management

The two major causes of recurrent abdominal pain in childhood are constipation and functional pain.

- The treatment of underlying constipation is essential and management of non-organic issues may be required.
- Functional pain may be related to variation in the perception of visceral sensation in the absence of an identifiable organic cause. A detailed explanation to the child and reassurance is often all that is required. The diagnosis of psychogenic recurrent abdominal pain cannot be made simply in the absence of features of an organic disorder; positive evidence of emotional maladjustment is required. If present, referral to a general paediatrician or mental health service is appropriate.

Pancreatitis

Acute pancreatitis has a variable presentation in children and symptoms may range from mild abdominal pain to severe systemic involvement with accompanying metabolic disturbances and shock. The pain is commonly in the epigastrium but may also be in the right and left upper quadrant. Back pain is an uncommon feature in children, unlike in adults. Other accompanying features may include vomiting, anorexia and nausea. Pancreatitis should be considered in children with complex disability, presenting with irritability.

The diagnosis is based on clinical symptoms and signs, accompanied by a threefold increase above the normal range, in either amylase or lipase – serum lipase having the greater sensitivity and specificity of the two.

On examination, the child may appear unwell and features of an acute abdomen may be present.

Management

Is primarily supportive and aims at limiting exocrine pancreatic secretion and managing pain. Most mild to moderate cases will settle with bowel rest, IV fluids and analgesia with early reintroduction of enteral nutrition depending on clinical progress. In children with recurrent attacks and/or a complicated course, specialist input is recommended (see Fig. 8.3).

Chronic constipation and faecal incontinence
Chronic constipation

Constipation is not just hard or infrequent stools but a symptom complex that reflects difficulty passing bowel motions, that is at least two of the following problems within the previous 8 weeks:

- <3 bowel motions per week
- >1 episode of faecal incontinence (FI) per week
- Large stools in the rectum or palpable on abdominal examination
- Passing of stools so large that they obstruct the toilet
- Retentive posturing and withholding behaviour
- Painful defecation

In most children, chronic constipation is due to functional faecal retention (withholding of stool). Painful or fear of painful defecation are the most common triggers, leading to apprehension about defecation and a cycle of withholding and passage of hard retained stool.

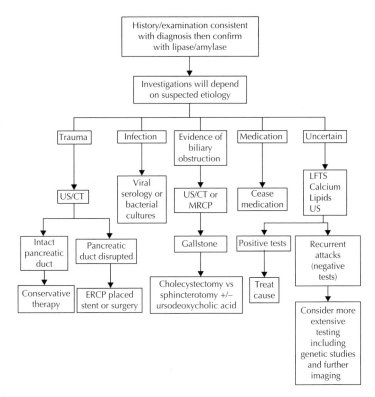

Fig. 8.3 Pancreatic algorithm flowchart

Organic causes of chronic constipation are rare. They include
- Cow's milk protein allergy (non-IgE) which may manifest as constipation in the first 3 years of life
- Hirschsprung's disease usually causes failure to pass meconium in the first 48 hours of life, and virtually never causes faecal soiling
- Coeliac disease
- Hypothyroidism
- Hypercalcemia
- Drugs (codeine, antacids)
- Spinal cord lesions
- Anorectal malformations

Lack of dietary fibre and poor fluid intake rarely contribute to childhood chronic constipation. Inappropriate emphasis on diet and fluid serve to lay blame on the child or parents, while deflecting attention from treatments that do work.

Dyschezia (a healthy infant, straining and crying before passing soft stool) is normal but can be mistaken for constipation.

Faecal incontinence
This is a common consequence of chronic constipation. It is defined as the passage of stool in an inappropriate place. The term FI supersedes the terms encopresis and faecal soiling.

Most FI is functional and is associated with constipation (see above). Other causes include functional non-retentive FI (i.e. not constipated), and organic causes such as neurological damage or anal sphincter anomalies.

Several conditions are associated with FI:

- Nocturnal enuresis and daytime detrusor overactivity. When all three occur together, it is known as 'dysfunctional elimination syndrome' – perhaps linked through pelvic floor dysfunction. About 30% of children with FI also have nocturnal enuresis. Many have a family history of nocturnal enuresis.
- Behavioural problems are common but most are secondary to FI rather than the cause.
- Genetics: a family history of FI is common.

The majority of children with FI have significant faecal retention causing in turn, chronic rectal dilatation, hyposensitivity to stretching of the rectal ampulla, loss of the normal urge to pass stool and further retention. When the external anal sphincter relaxes, the stool accumulated in the rectal ampulla leaks. Unaware of the full rectum, the child may only sense the passage of stool by its contact with external skin, initiating an urgent rush to the toilet and a false impression that the child has 'waited until the last minute' – leading to inappropriate blaming.

Assessment of chronic constipation and faecal incontinence

A history and examination should be performed to exclude organic causes. Symptoms and signs to beware of include

- Delayed passage of meconium stool (>48 hours) or neonatal onset
- Regression of motor skills/neurological signs lower limbs/foot deformity
- Faecal or urinary incontinence, day or night
- Significant abdominal distension
- Poor growth
- Lower back abnormalities: dimples, pigmented lesions, hair tufts

Inspection of the perianal area for painful conditions is needed but rectal examination is not usually required and most often does not change management. Abnormal neurological findings are rare but must be investigated urgently. An abdominal radiograph is rarely required.

Management

The aim of management is to empty the bowel, and to keep it empty and with soft lubricated stools. This needs to be maintained for a long period in order for the child to overcome the apprehension about defecation.

Disimpaction

This may be used for severe symptoms or to kick-start long-term management.

Rectally instilled medication (suppositories or enemas) may add to the child's fearfulness. If using medications per rectum, consider sedation with nitrous oxide or midazolam.

Suggested medications (singly or in combination) include

- Osmotic laxative: Macrogol 3350 (Movicol or Osmolax) disimpaction regime.
- Gut stimulant: Senokot granules $\frac{1}{2}$–1 teaspoon per day or Dulcolax drops.

For children refusing oral medication: sodium sulfate (Colonlytely) 1–3 L per day, via nasogastric tube in hospital may be required.

Surgical disimpaction can be considered if medical therapy fails.

Follow-on treatment

A long-term approach is needed, often for months to years. The physician, child and family need to work together and design an individualised treatment plan.

Behaviour modification is the mainstay of treatment. This involves regular sitting on the toilet and pushing, three times a day for 3–5 minutes. Use of a timer can be helpful to avoid arguments. Attention to the sitting position: feet supported, hips flexed and encourage 'bulging' of the abdomen. Reinforce desired behaviour with stickers on an age-appropriate chart. Reward achievable goals such as good compliance with sitting programme rather than clean pants.

Medications are an adjunct to a toileting regimen. Paediatricians usually start with a single agent, most commonly paraffin oil or macrogol.

- Stool lubricants/softeners: paraffin oil 15–25 mL per day (see below).
- Osmotic laxatives:
  - Movicol 1 sachet per day.
  - Lactulose: <12 months, 5 mL per day; 1–5 years, 10 mL per day; >5 years, 15 mL per day.

- Stimulants:
  - Senokot: 2–6 years, $\frac{1}{4}-\frac{1}{2}$ teaspoon per day; >6 years, 1 tab per day (7.5 mg).
  - Bisacodyl: >4 years – 1 tablet per day (5 mg).

Paediatric follow-up is advisable. Consider referral to a sub-specialist continence clinic if combined faecal/urinary incontinence, suspected organic cause, complex or difficult cases.

- Long-term use of most of these medications is safe and does not render the bowel 'lazy' or make the child 'dependent'. Only when defecation has been effortless for many months and toileting behaviour is consistent should one try to gradually withdraw adjunct medications.

Medication notes

- *Paraffin oil* is a stool lubricant that is colourless, odourless and almost tasteless. It is easily camouflaged in many foods. In liquids, it will float and disperse into droplets without changing the taste of the liquid.
- *Parachoc* is paraffin oil with soluble fibre, flavour and sweeteners which children often find too sweet. *Agarol* is similar, but with flavourings that some will prefer. Parachoc carries a warning about risks of aspiration and lipoid pneumonia. Although this complication is not seen in practice, it seems reasonable to avoid using Parachoc in children <6 months, and those with swallowing difficulty (lactulose may be a helpful alternative).

Liver disease

For causes see Table 8.5.

Table 8.5 Causes of liver disease

Mode of presentation	Time of presentation	
	Infancy	**Older child**
Acute	Infectious	Infectious
	● Urinary tract infection	● Viral hepatitis (A to E)
	● Bacterial sepsis	● Non A-E hepatitis
	● Congenital (TORCH)	Biliary/obstructive
	Biliary/obstructive	● Cholelithiasis
	● Inspissated bile	Drug toxic
	● Cholelithiasis	● Paracetamol intoxication
	Metabolic	● Antibiotics, tuberculostatics, anticonvulsives, anticonceptives
	● Galactosemia	Metabolic
	● Niemann-Pick C disease	● Wilson disease (acute-on-chronic)
	● Fatty acid oxidation defect	
	● Mitochondrial disease	
	Immunologic	
	● Neonatal hemochromatosis	
Chronic	Biliary/obstructive	Infectious
	● Extrahepatic biliary atresia	● Chronic hepatitis B/C
	● Alagille syndrome	Biliary/obstructive
	metabolic	● Sclerosing cholangitis (prim./sec.)
	● α1-antitrypsin deficiency	Drug toxic
	● Cystic fibrosis	● Methotrexate (e.g. chemotherapy)
	● Tyrosinemia type 1	Metabolic
	● Glycogen storage disease	● α1-antitrypsin deficiency
		● Cystic fibrosis
		● Wilson disease
		● Non-alcoholic fatty liver disease
		Immunologic
		● Celiac disease
		● Autoimmune hepatitis

Source: This table was originally published in South & Isaacs, Practical Paediatrics, 7th Edition, Elsevier: 2012, Chapter 20.5, pp. 744–754. (South 2012. Reproduced with permission of Elsevier.)

Liver disease in infants

There are a large number of significant and treatable conditions which present with jaundice in infancy. Successful management relies on a prompt diagnosis and early referral to a specialist.

Clinical presentation:

- Jaundice (usually conjugated hyperbilirubinaemia).
- Passage of pale grey or white stools and dark tea-coloured urine.
- Hepatosplenomegaly.
- Failure to thrive.
- Bleeding diathesis.
- Hypoglycaemia.

Biliary atresia is an important cause of conjugated hyperbilirubinaemia which presents with jaundice in the first 4–6 weeks of life. Infants may appear well on clinical examination, with conservation of growth. Stools are usually acholic (pale white). If untreated, biliary atresia is fatal, however, the natural history of this condition can be modified by early surgery (Kasai portoenterostomy).

Other important causes of conjugated hyperbilirubinaemia, many of which may have dire consequences if not recognised or treated adequately, include congenital infections, galactosaemia, tyrosinaemia, fructosaemia and hypothyroidism. Unconjugated hyperbilirubinaemia may be due to breast milk jaundice, haemolysis (immune or breakdown of a haematoma) or rare inherited conjugation defects. See Fig. 8.4.

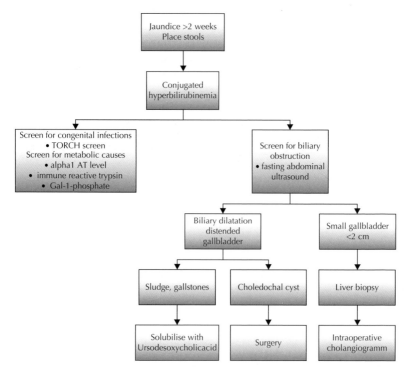

Fig. 8.4 Liver disease in children. This figure was originally published in South & Isaacs, *Practical Paediatrics*, 7th edition, Elsevier: 2012, Chapter 20.5, pp. 744–754. (South 2012. Reproduced with permission of Elsevier.)

Table 8.6 Gastronomy tube management

Problem	Clinical features	Management
Infection at skin site	Erythema weeping at insertion site	Kenacomb ointment to site
Granulation tissue	Tissue growth at insertion site with bleeding	Kenacomb ointment and silver nitrate sticks
Migration of tube either towards pylorus or out of stomach	Enlargement of entry site visible retention device peritonitis, vomiting	Urgent gastroenterology/surgery referral
Blocked tube	Unable to pass feed	Check location, try inserting cola

Liver disease in children

Important causes of liver disease in children include autoimmune hepatitis, α1-antitrypsin deficiency, viral hepatitis (hepatitis A, B, C, EBV, CMV), non-alcoholic steatohepatitis, Wilson disease and drug-induced. Children may present with a history of jaundice, dark urine, pale stools, pruritus, abdominal pain or abnormal liver function tests found incidentally. The clinical signs of chronic liver disease include spider naevi, palmar erythema, dilated abdominal veins and splenomegaly.

Investigations:

- Viral serology as above
- Autoantibodies (ANA, LKM, SMA)
- Serum copper and caeruloplasmin
- Iron studies
- α1-antitrypsin level and Pi type
- Liver ultrasound

In general, prompt specialist consultation is required, as both acute and chronic liver disease require urgent investigation and treatment.

Gastrostomy care and problems

Gastrostomies are now used frequently to nourish children who are either unable to eat or are at risk of aspiration from oral feeding. During a percutaneous endoscopically placed gastrostomy tubes (PEGs), the initial gastrostomy tube is usually long and is subsequently replaced by a low profile device or 'button'. If a gastrostomy is formed during a surgical procedure, a button is commonly placed initially. Certain types of buttons require changing every 4 to 6 months and certain types may be replaced in an outpatient setting by suitably qualified staff or parents.

Common issues with gastrostomy tubes and their management are listed in the Table 8.6. It is best to consult with a gastroenterologist, surgeon or stoma nurse experienced in the care of these tubes as inappropriate management can be fatal.

Umbilical hernia

This is a common finding in newborn children and usually resolves in the first 12 months of life. Parents will often note the hernia becomes tense during crying, but this is a consequence of increased abdominal pressure rather than the cause of discomfort. If a hernia persists beyond the age of 2 years, an operation as a day case is recommended before starting school. The operation is primarily cosmetic, although strangulation can occur during adult life (particularly during pregnancy).

Appendicitis

Appendicitis is the most common abdominal condition requiring surgery in childhood. It is unusual in patients less than 5 years of age, but it is in this age group where misdiagnosis is most likely to occur.

The symptoms and signs of appendicitis are related to the degree of peritoneal irritation and the position of the appendix. The classical description is of colicky periumbilical pain migrating to a continuous pain in the right iliac fossa with associated anorexia, fever, nausea. Mild vomiting and loose stools are frequently seen.

Examination is straightforward if there is localised peritonitis with guarding in the right iliac fossa; however, peritonitis may not occur in retrocaecal appendicitis and in pelvic appendicitis there may be only vague supra-pubic tenderness. Gastrointestinal infections often produce a local ileus but no peritonitis and are frequently distinguished by 'squelchiness' (secondary to air and fluid) in the right iliac fossa on examination. Rectal examination should not be done in children.

Management

Repeated clinical examination is the most sensitive test for appendicitis. Routine blood tests should not be performed. An abdominal ultrasound may be helpful in difficult cases.

It is important to refer a child who complains of persistent abdominal pain, even if this is associated with vomiting or diarrhoea. In particular, suspect significant peritonitis if the child does not allow abdominal examination.

Intussusception

This condition is where one segment of bowel telescopes inside the adjacent distal bowel causing intestinal obstruction. It should be considered in children aged 3 months to 2 years presenting with vomiting, intermittent abdominal pain and lethargy/pallor. These early symptoms should be acted on, rather than awaiting the classic 'red currant jelly stool', which is a feature of advanced disease.

Children with intussusception have an abdominal mass which is central, beneath the rectus abdominis on the right side. This is often difficult to feel.

Management

- Ultrasound should be done to confirm the diagnosis and is highly sensitive and specific.
- Contrast air enema is required to reduce the intussusception, but should not be used in the presence of peritonitis or significant dehydration. If a contrast air enema does not fully reduce an intussusception, it may need to be repeated. If there is a contraindication to air enema, or if multiple attempts fail, surgical correction may be required.

These procedures should only be undertaken by experienced radiologists with a surgical team immediately available at a tertiary centre.

Pyloric stenosis

Pyloric stenosis is an acquired thickening of the gastric outlet which results in the gastric outlet becoming obstructed. The aetiology is unclear but includes a genetic component. It usually presents between 2 and 6 weeks of age; that is chronological age, regardless of prematurity. The classical symptoms are of progressive milky vomits becoming projectile, with associated loss of weight and continual hunger. It may be difficult to diagnose. Gastric peristalsis occurs due to pyloric obstruction and is clearly visible on the baby's abdominal wall. When seen, it should prompt surgical referral. If the stomach is not grossly distended, the pyloric tumour is readily palpable in experienced hands. Ultrasound is only required if the diagnosis is unclear and the pyloric tumour cannot be felt.

Metabolic complications

Vomiting in these infants results in loss of gastric fluid (water and HCl). The kidneys can initially conserve H^+, but once the baby becomes dehydrated, water and Na^+ are conserved in exchange for K^+ and H^+. The resulting condition is hypovolaemia with alkalosis, low chloride and potassium. Even if serum K^+ is normal, there is a total body potassium deficiency.

A metabolic alkalosis (chloride <100 mmol/L, pH >7.45, bicarbonate >32 mmol/L and sodium <130 mmol/L) is present only in severe cases.

Inappropriate rehydration with low-sodium-containing fluids can result in cerebral oedema.

Management

Early surgical consultation is recommended.

An appropriate fluid for resuscitation is 0.45% (1/2 normal) saline with 5% dextrose. Potassium should be added once the baby is passing urine. If the baby's weight before the onset of symptoms is known, fluid deficit is easily calculated. Maintenance requirements may be calculated at 100 mL/kg per 24 hours.

For example: a baby normally weighing 3 kg now weighs 2.7 kg.

- Deficit 300 g (10% dehydration): replacement required 300 mL.
- Maintenance required: 300 mL per 24 hours.
- For resuscitation over 12 hours, 450 mL is required in this period, that is 48 mL/h

Pyloric stenosis is not a surgical emergency. The priority is the gentle correction of dehydration. Surgery is only undertaken in fully rehydrated babies with no biochemical abnormalities.

CHAPTER 9

Fluids and nutrition

Sarah McNab
Julian Kelly
Trevor Duke
Zoë McCallum
Michele Meehan
Liz Rogers

Fluids

Sick children should be given enteral fluids/feeds where possible. If oral fluids are not tolerated, consider giving fluids/feeds via a nasogastric (NG) or nasojejunal (NJ) tube. Clear intravenous (IV) fluids provide no nutrition.

Oral rehydration and feeds

Dehydration without shock can generally be managed with oral rehydration fluid and solid or semi-solid feeds, unless there is a contraindication (e.g. imminent surgery). Even where vomiting is present, frequent administration of small volumes of fluid are often sufficient. In gastroenteritis, ondansetron may be given to facilitate this.

Fluid with high sugar content (e.g. undiluted juice or soft drink) should not be given and fortification of formula feeds should cease during the acute illness.

Nasogastric feeds

NG or NJ fluids may be given where oral feeds have been unsuccessful. NG fluids are less likely to be associated with electrolyte imbalances compared with intravenous (IV) fluids, but an NG tube tends to be poorly tolerated in older children.

Rapid NG rehydration using oral rehydration solution at 25 mL/kg/h may be given over 4 hours for most children with gastroenteritis and moderate dehydration.

NG rehydration should be slower in infants <6 months old, children with comorbidities, complications such as hypernatraemia and those with significant abdominal pain.

An NJ tube is usually only used for children at high risk of aspirating or with delayed gastric emptying. NJ fluids/feeds are used for long-term feeding rather than acute rehydration.

Intravenous fluid (outside neonatal period)

Intravenous fluids are used where enteral fluids are not tolerated or contraindicated. They are more likely to be associated with electrolyte imbalances and other adverse effects. Children receiving intravenous fluid should be clinically assessed and have electrolytes checked regularly (see *Principles of safe fluid management*, p. 108).

Hypovolaemic shock

Children with shock (hypotension and acidosis) caused by hypovolaemia should be given parenteral fluid immediately: **administer 20 mL/kg of an isotonic fluid such as 0.9% sodium chloride (NaCl), Plasma-lyte148 or Hartmann's solution repeatedly until plasma volume is restored** (20–100 mL/kg may be required). Fluid can be given IV or via an intraosseous needle. NG fluid is not effective in shock. Any child with shock who requires more than 40 mL/kg in fluid boluses should be urgently reviewed to consider the need for vasopressor or inotropic support. It is important to also consider the adverse effects of additional fluid boluses on lung function.

Paediatric Handbook, Ninth Edition. Edited by Amanda Gwee, Romi Rimer and Michael Marks.
© 2015 John Wiley & Sons, Ltd. Published 2015 by John Wiley & Sons, Ltd.

Replacement and maintenance therapy

Four basic aspects are considered.

- Existing deficit
- Continuing losses
- Maintenance requirements
- Principles of safe fluid management

Fluid deficit/dehydration

The fluid deficit is most reliably estimated from the loss of body weight if a recent pre-illness weight is available. Any loss of weight is equal to the fluid deficit. (e.g. if 600 g have been lost, there is a fluid deficit of 600 mL, which represents 6% dehydration in a 10 kg child.)

Clinical signs may be used to determine approximate fluid deficit, but are not precise. These include
Mild dehydration (<4%)

- Usually no clinical signs

Moderate dehydration (4–6%)

- Delayed capillary refill time
- Increased respiratory rate
- Mildly decreased tissue turgor

Severe dehydration (≥7%)

- Very delayed capillary refill >3 seconds, mottled skin
- Other signs of shock (irritable or reduced conscious level, hypotension)
- Deep, acidotic breathing
- Decreased tissue turgor

In children, hypotension is a late sign. Normal blood pressure does not exclude severe dehydration or shock.

Less reliable markers of mild–moderate dehydration include

- a history of oliguria;
- lethargy;
- sunken eyes;
- dry mucous membranes;
- sunken fontanelle; and
- absence of tears.

The child's weight as well as the estimated degree of dehydration can be used to calculate an approximate fluid deficit. (e.g. a 10 kg child who is 7% dehydrated has lost 700 mL of fluid.)

In general, intravenous fluids to replace the existing deficit are given over the first 24 hours using an isotonic fluid with a similar sodium concentration to plasma. But, for hypernatraemic or hyponatraemic dehydration, they should be given over at least 48–72 hours (see *hypernatraemia* and *hyponatraemia*, pp. 111–112).

Continuing losses

Fluid balance charts should accurately record – volumes of vomitus, gastric aspirates, drainage from fistulae/stoma, diarrhoea, urine output and other fluid losses to guide fluid replacement. In practice, it can be difficult to accurately measure all losses; body weight should be measured regularly (at least daily), as this is an important marker of ongoing losses and hydration status.

Maintenance requirements

Maintenance fluid requirement is the daily water requirement for well children to excrete an iso-osmotic urine. This is high (per kg of bodyweight) in infancy and gradually decreases throughout childhood. Tables 9.1 and 9.2 indicate the maintenance volumes required in well children. This volume differs in disease states.

Many acutely ill children have high levels of **antidiuretic hormone (ADH)**, resulting in reduced free water excretion. This particularly occurs in postoperative children and those with brain or lung disease (meningitis, encephalitis, bronchiolitis, pneumonia), although any hospitalised child is at risk. As urinary output is reduced, the total fluid required to maintain normal intravascular volume is reduced. If these children receive maintenance IV fluid at standard rates, fluid overload and hyponatraemia may occur. Hence, in children at particular risk, a total fluid intake (TFI) of about 60% of the usual maintenance volumes should be the starting point for IV-administered fluid.

Table 9.1 Daily maintenance intravenous fluid requirements

Bodyweight	Requirements
3–10 kg	100 mL/kg per day
10–20 kg	1000 mL + (50 mL/kg per day for each kg over 10 kg)
20 kg and over	1500 mL + (20 mL/kg per day for each kg over 20 kg)

In contrast, some sick children will have increased fluid requirements (e.g. those with high fever, capillary leak, third-spacing of fluid into the abdomen or those with continuing losses). These children may need more than the standard maintenance fluid rate to maintain normal intravascular volume.

Prescribing fluid volumes can be complex; some ill children have clinical features that imply a need for increased *and* decreased fluids. These children need regular assessments, including weight, to ensure adequate hydration is achieved.

In general, maintenance fluids should be isotonic, containing a similar sodium concentration as plasma (see Table 9.3 – commonly prescribed intravenous fluids). Glucose concentrations between 2.5–5% are recommended.

Maintenance fluid containing <75 mmol/L of sodium should never be used. 0.18% NaCl (or 1/5 saline) contains only 30 mmol/L of sodium and is **not** appropriate for maintenance hydration.

Principles of safe fluid management
Calculate the total fluid intake (TFI)
At least once a day the TFI in mL/h and in mL/kg/day should be calculated. The prescribed intravenous TFI should take into account: deficit replacement + maintenance + estimation of continuing losses.

Remember to factor in the following:

- IV fluid for drug lines
- Blood products
- Enteral feeds
- Other

The balance of enteral and parenteral fluid should be adjusted around this prescribed TFI.

Regular monitoring
The key to good fluid management is regular clinical monitoring. Signs of dehydration should be corrected, but signs of overhydration, such as rapid weight gain and eyelid oedema, avoided.

- Children receiving IV fluids must be weighed at least every day. Children receiving deficit replacement fluid should be weighed at least every 6 hours. An increase in weight of 5% or more over 24 hours is likely to indicate fluid overload. Manage by stopping IV fluids, measure serum sodium and consult senior medical staff. A decrease in weight of 5% or more is likely to indicate dehydration.
- Assess for oedema every day. Check for eyelid and lower limb swelling. If either is present, stop IV fluids and consult senior medical staff.
- Check serum electrolytes and glucose at least daily. Senior medical staff should be consulted if
  - serum sodium is ≤130 mmol/L or has fallen by >5 mmol/L
  - serum sodium is ≥150 mmol/L or has risen by >5 mmol/L.

Table 9.2 Hourly maintenance intravenous fluid requirements

Bodyweight	Requirements
3–10 kg	4 mL/kg/h
10–20 kg	40 mL + (2 mL/kg/h for each kg over 10 kg)
20 kg and over	60 mL + (1 mL/kg/h for each kg over 20 kg)

Table 9.3 Commonly used intravenous solutions

	Na+ mmol/L	Cl− mmol/L	K+ mmol/L	Lactate mmol/L	Ca2+ mmol/L	Glucose g/L
0.9% NaCl (isotonic)	154	154	–	–	–	–
0.9% NaCl with 5% glucose and 20 mmol/L of potassium chloride (isotonic)	154	174	20			50
0.45% NaCl with 5% glucose (hypotonic)	77	77	–	–	–	50
Plasmalyte148 solution (isotonic)	130	110	5	30	2	–
Plasmalyte148 solution with 5% glucose (isotonic)	130	110	5	30	2	50
Hartmann's solution (similar in ionic composition to Ringer's lactate) (isotonic)	131	111	5	–	2	29

Acid–base problems

The maintenance of pH within narrow limits is a result of two mechanisms.

- Buffer systems: the bicarbonate system is quantitatively the most important in plasma (70% of total).
- Excretory mechanisms: via the kidneys and lungs.

Acidosis (low pH) and alkalosis (high pH) may be respiratory or metabolic in origin.

The four primary disorders are:

1. Metabolic acidosis. Due to
   - increased production of acid (e.g. ketoacids and lactic acid);
   - failure of the kidney to excrete acid or conserve base; and
   - excess loss of buffer base (e.g. gastroenteritis or intestinal fistula).
2. Metabolic alkalosis. Due to
   - excess loss of acid (e.g. pyloric stenosis);
   - excess intake of buffer (e.g. bicarbonate infusion); and
   - conditions where hydrogen ions are lost in the urine (e.g. renal tubular syndromes, diuretic therapy) or from vomiting (e.g. pyloric stenosis).
3. Respiratory acidosis
   - Hypercapnia is the result of alveolar hypoventilation from any cause (e.g. central, neuromuscular or pulmonary disease).
4. Respiratory alkalosis.
   - This is caused by hyperventilation.

See Table 9.4.

In practice, isolated metabolic and respiratory disorders are uncommon. Most disorders have a metabolic and a respiratory component. Usually one is the primary disorder and the other occurs secondarily and tends to

Table 9.4 Changes in arterial capillary blood (before compensation)

	pH (mmol/L)	Pco$_2$ (mmHg)	Base excess (mmol/L)	Actual bicarbonate (mmol/L)
Normal reference range	7.36–7.44	36–44	−5 to +3	18–25
Metabolic acidosis	Decrease	Normal	Decrease	Decrease
Metabolic alkalosis	Increase	Normal	Increase	Increase
Respiratory acidosis	Decrease	Increase	Normal	Normal
Respiratory alkalosis	Increase	Decrease	Normal	Normal

Table 9.5 Change in indicators of acid–base status seen in combined disorders

	pH (mmol/L)	$P\text{co}_2$ (mmHg)	Base excess (mmol/L)	Actual bicarbonate (mmol/L)
Normal reference range	7.36–7.44	36–44	−5 to +3	18–25
Primary metabolic acidosis + compensatory respiratory alkalosis (e.g. gastroenteritis, diabetic ketosis)	Decrease or normal	Decrease	Decrease	Decrease
Primary metabolic alkalosis + compensatory respiratory acidosis (e.g. pyloric stenosis)	Increase or normal	Increase	Increase	Increase
Combined primary respiratory and metabolic acidosis (e.g. respiratory distress syndrome)	Decrease	Increase	Decrease	Normal or low

correct the change in pH. However, sometimes primary metabolic and respiratory disturbances occur together; for example in respiratory distress syndrome, acidosis is contributed by both hypoxia leading to lactic acid accumulation and subsequent metabolic acidosis, whilst carbon dioxide retention results in respiratory acidosis (see Tables 9.4 and 9.5).

Hyperkalaemia

Potassium may be elevated as an artefact where haemolysis is present. This is more common on a capillary specimen or where venepuncture has been difficult. If hyperkalaemia is an unexpected finding, consider repeating the sample using venepuncture.

The management of hyperkalaemia depends on the underlying cause. Causes include

- Decreased excretion (e.g. renal failure, mineralocorticoid deficiency)
- Transcellular shift (e.g. acidosis)
- Increased production (e.g. trauma, rhabdomyolysis)
- Exogenous source (e.g. ingestion, iatrogenic)
- Medication (e.g. potassium sparing diuretic)

A 12-lead ECG should be obtained. Indications of a conduction disturbance include

- Peaked T wave (early)
- Prolonged PR, flattening of P wave, widening of QRS (increased risk of arrhythmia)
- Absence of P wave, sine wave (fusion of QRS and T wave)
- Ventricular arrhyhyperkathmia, asystole

A normal ECG does not eliminate the risk of arrhythmia (Fig. 9.1).

–See http://www.rch.org.au/clinicalguide/guideline_index/Hyperkalaemia/

If cardiac arrhythmias or severe hyperkalaemia are present, rapid but temporary benefit may be achieved by giving (while arranging dialysis)

- Salbutamol nebuliser
- IV sodium bicarbonate 2 mmol/kg
- Short-acting (regular) insulin 0.1 unit/kg given with 10 ml/kg of IV 10% dextrose
- IV calcium gluconate 10% 0.5 mL/kg, given slowly

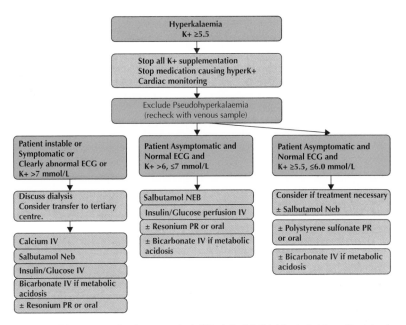

Fig. 9.1 Hyperkalaemia support algorithm. *Source*: Royal Children's Hospital Clinical Practice Gudelines – Hyperkalaemia. Reproduced with permission of the Royal Children's Hospital.

Rectal or NG sodium polystyrene sulfonate (Resonium) 1 g/kg may also be given to reduce total body potassium, but has a longer onset of action.

Hypokalaemia

Metabolic alkalosis may cause hypokalaemia, but this resolves if alkalosis is treated. Severe hypokalaemia causes long QT interval, often with prominent U waves. Management is usually sufficient with supplementation of oral potassium or by adding potassium to IV maintenance fluid.

Potassium should rarely be given faster than 0.2 mmol/kg/h and never faster than 0.4 mmol/kg/h. ECG monitoring should be considered in massive potassium replacement and infusions of concentrated solutions should be controlled with the use of a pump.

Concentrated potassium infusions can cause chemical burns if extravasation occurs. Concentrations of potassium >40 mmol/L should be used with extreme caution, generally only through a central line. Infusions of potassium at concentrations of ≥60 mmol/L should only be given in the intensive care unit.

In hyperkalaemia and hypokalaemia the causes should be identified and treated.

Hypernatraemia

Hypernatraemia is most frequently due to a water deficit (e.g. increased losses or reduced intake). In rare cases it is due to an increase in total body sodium (e.g. ingestion of large quantities of sodium, incorrect preparation of formula).

If the patient is shocked, provide volume resuscitation with an isotonic fluid as required in 20 mL/kg boluses (see *hypovolaemic shock*, p. 106).

After the correction of shock, the aim is to lower the serum sodium slowly at a rate of no faster than 12 mmol/L in 24 hours (0.5 mmol/L/h). This should be even slower if the hypernatraemia is chronic. **If sodium is corrected too rapidly, cerebral oedema, seizures and permanent brain injury may occur.** Monitor and manage for concurrent hyperglycaemia and other electrolyte abnormalities.

Moderate hypernatraemic dehydration, [Na$^+$] 150–169 mmol/L
After initial resuscitation, replace the deficit plus maintenance **over 48 hours**.
- Use nasogastric oral rehydration solution (Gastrolyte) where possible, but remember that Gastrolyte has a low sodium concentration of 60 mmol/L. Electrolytes will need to be monitored.
- If requiring IV rehydration use **an isotonic fluid with glucose**. Add maintenance KCl if required once urine output is established.
  Initial daily volume (mL) = Daily maintenance fluids (mL) + (remaining fluid deficit (mL)/2)
  Initial hourly rate (mL/h) = Daily volume (mL)/24(h)
- Check urea, electrolytes and glucose every hour – if serum sodium is falling faster than 0.5 mmol/h, slow down rate of infusion by 20%. Recheck the serum sodium in 1 hour.
- If after 6 hour of rehydration therapy the sodium is decreasing at a steady rate then check the U&Es and glucose 4 hourly.
- If there are persistent neurological signs, consider cerebral imaging.

Severe hypernatraemic dehydration, [Na$^+$] >169
- Consult with intensive care.
- After initial resuscitation, replace deficit and maintenance with **an isotonic fluid with glucose over 72–96 hours**.
  Initial daily volume (mL) = Daily maintenance fluids (mL) + (remaining fluid deficit (mL)/3)
  Initial hourly rate (mL/h) = Daily volume (mL)/24 (h)

Hyponatraemia
Hyponatraemia may be caused by excessive water intake or salt loss.

Hyponatraemia is frequently iatrogenic, caused by the administration of hypotonic intravenous fluid (fluid containing less sodium than plasma). This is worsened when ADH levels are elevated, leading to reduced excretion of water.

Hyponatraemia with seizures or decreased conscious state
Resuscitation should occur, including the use of anticonvulsants, where indicated. The sodium level should be increased using 4 mL/kg of 3% NaCl intravenously. If central access is readily available, this should be used. Ongoing seizures with persistent hyponatraemia will require further 3% NaCl.

Hyponatraemia without symptoms
A low serum sodium should be corrected slowly, especially if the abnormality is long-standing. It should never be increased faster than 0.5 mmol/L/h and usually an increase of 0.25 mmol/L/h or less is more appropriate.

If sodium is corrected too rapidly in hyponatraemia, cerebral (especially pontine) demyelination and permanent brain injury may occur.

Management of asymptomatic hyponatraemia depends on the hydration status and severity of sodium imbalance.

If the child has a *normal or increased volume state*, restrict fluids to slowly remove excess water.

If the child is *moderately dehydrated with a serum sodium of 130–135 mmol/L*, aim to rehydrate orally or via a nasogastric tube. Note that the sodium concentration of gastrolyte is low (60 mmol/L) – **rapid nasogastric rehydration is not appropriate where hyponatraemia is present**. If it is not possible to give enteral fluid, use isotonic fluid with glucose.

Where there is *severe dehydration with a serum sodium of <130 mmol/L*, isotonic fluid should be administered.

Electrolytes should be monitored regularly (at least every 4 hours) until stable.

The newborn
Babies are different from older children because they have
- Proportionately more body water in all compartments
- Greater insensible water losses
- Higher metabolic requirements
- Reduced renal capacity to compensate for biochemical abnormalities
- Less integrated and responsive endocrine controls
  Any baby needing IV therapy should be in a level 2 or level 3 nursery.

Table 9.6   Water requirements in well neonates

Age	mL/kg per day	
	Pre-term >32 weeks or low birth weight 1500–2500 g	Term/birth weight >2500 g
Day 0/1	60–80	40–60
Day 2	90–110	90
Day 3	120–150	120

As with older children, an isotonic fluid without glucose at 20 mL/kg should be used for hypovolaemic shock. The rest of this section refers to maintenance hydration for neonates.

Water requirements for neonates

Babies' water and milk requirements are different. For normal nutrition, babies need 150–200 mL/kg per day of milk. This is substantially more than their water or IV fluid requirements (see Table 9.6). Newborns who are fasted should *not* be given the volume of fluid required for nutrition intravenously as this invariably leads to water overload. This difference is of greatest importance in babies suffering illnesses that are made worse by excess water administration, for example acute and chronic lung disease, heart failure or renal impairment.

Water requirements may differ depending on

- *Gestational age*: the earlier the gestation, the greater the skin losses and the poorer the renal concentrating ability. Insensible water losses can vary from around 20–30 mL/kg per day at term to more than 60–80 mL/kg per day at <27 weeks' gestation.
- *Postnatal age*: skin losses decrease and renal function increases steadily from day 1.
- *Nursing condition*: naked babies under radiant heaters lose water. Humidified respiratory circuits (e.g. ventilators) reduce respiratory losses.

Electrolyte requirements for neonates

Babies are less able to conserve sodium and excrete excess sodium loads. All neonates on intravenous fluids will need electrolytes performed at least daily, as well as regular clinical assessment, including hydration status and weight.

In general, newborns should receive 10% dextrose as a starting maintenance intravenous fluid for the first 48 hours of life.

After 48 hours, if intravenous hydration is still required, electrolytes should be added. Electrolytes should be added earlier, if required, on the basis of serum electrolyte results.

Glucose requirements for neonates

Both hypoglycaemia and hyperglycaemia are associated with adverse outcomes. Glucose requirement for neonates is around 6–8 mg/kg/min. Ten per cent dextrose solutions at 2.5 mL/kg/h (suggested initial maintenance rate for the first day of life) provide only 4.1 mg/kg/min, so on the first or second day of life, a higher concentration glucose solution may be required to maintain the blood glucose. Sick neonates should have blood glucose measured at admission and then every 4–24 hour depending on severity of illness, risk factors for hypoglycaemia, presence of clinical signs of hypoglycaemia and changes made to glucose infusions.

Infants at high risk of hypoglycaemia include macrosomia, infants born to diabetic mothers (hyperinsulinaemia) and those with intrauterine growth restriction (low glycogen stores). Concentrated glucose solutions (>12.5%) require central venous access.

Nutrition
Breastfeeding

Breastfeeding is the best means of feeding babies, and all efforts should be made to promote, encourage and maintain breastfeeding. Exclusive breastfeeding is recommended for the first 4–6 months of life. Breastfeeding can be continued for as long as mother and baby prefer (see Table 9.7).

Table 9.7 How to assess good breastfeeding

	Good	Problem
Baby's body position	On side – chest to chest	On back – angled away from mother
Mouth	Open wide	Lips close together
Chin	Touching or pressing into the breast	Space between chin and breast
Lips	Flanged out	Tucked in, inverted
Cheeks	Well rounded	Dimpled or sucked in
Nose	Free of or just touching the breast	Buried in breast, baby pulls back
Breast in mouth	Good mouthful, more of bottom part of breast in mouth	Central, little breast tissue in mouth or only nipple in mouth
Jaw movement	Rhythmic deep jaw movement	Jerky or irregular shallow movement
Sounds	Muffled sound of swallowing milk	No swallowing, clicking sounds
Body language of the baby	Peaceful, concentrated	Restless, anxious
Body language of the mother	Comfortable, relaxed	Tense, hunched, awkward
Awareness of feelings during feed	Pain free, may feel a drawing feeling deep in breast or 'let down'	Nipple or breast pain
Nipple, post-feed	Nipple elongated, well-shaped	Not elongated, compressed 'stripe' or blanched

Source: Murray S. *Breast Feeding Information and Guidelines for Paediatric Units*, Royal Children's Hospital, Melbourne, Australia, 1992.

Normal variations in breastfeeding
Frequency of feeds
Breastfed infants usually feed every 2–5 hour from both breasts each feed. Young babies feed frequently, but demand feeding (i.e. feeding when hungry) will usually have the baby settle into a fairly predictable pattern of feeds. The frequency of feeds is determined by the baby's appetite and gastric capacity, as well as the amount of mother's milk available.

Length of feeds
The duration of the feed is determined by the rate of transfer of milk from the breast to the baby, which, in turn, depends on the strength of the baby's suck and the force of the mother's 'let down' or flow of milk. This may vary from 10–30 minutes. Young infants tend to feed for longer. It is the cessation of strong drawing sucks and the appearance of shorter-duration bursts of sucking that indicate the 'end' of the feed – not the time.

If the mother feels the baby is on the breast 'all the time', rather than focusing on the sucking alone, it is more important to look for longer duration of pauses between bursts of sucking, indicating less milk transfer. At this point, either take the baby off the breast or swap to the other side.

Appetite spurts
Babies seem to experience appetite spurts at 2 weeks, 6 weeks and 3 months. During a growth spurt, a baby will suddenly begin to feed more frequently. It is crucial that parents are aware of this or the baby's natural increase in feed frequency may be mistaken for diminution of milk supply. This is especially true at 6 weeks when breasts are no longer carrying extra fluid and the supply is settling to the demands of the baby. Unfortunately, many women wean at this time through poor advice. During appetite spurts, let the baby feed on demand, even 2 hourly, and this pattern should settle in 48 hours.

Qualities of breast milk

Breast milk is naturally thinner in consistency than an artificial formula and may have a bluish tinge – this is normal, healthy and nutritious. The composition of breast milk varies during the feed. The fat content of milk varies diurnally: it is lowest at about 6 a.m. and gradually increases to its peak at about 2 p.m. At any one feed, the highest concentration of fat is at the end of the feed in the 'hind milk'. The change in concentration is a gradual merging over the feed and is part of the feeding process. Hind milk is not 'better' than the early 'fore milk'; fore milk is higher in water and lactose and provides liquid to quench the baby's thirst and a quick surge of energy.

The presence of blood in the milk may cause a red or pinkish-brown discoloration. If this is present when the mother first starts expressing colostrum it may be due to duct hyperplasia. This gradually disappears and is of no significance. The most common cause of blood-stained milk (usually first noticed when the baby possets) is trauma to the nipple.

Bowel actions

The motions of breastfed infants are normally bright yellow and soft to loose. The normal frequency varies, ranging from a bowel action with every feed (strong gastrocolic reflex) or up to once every 5–8 days.

Temporary cessation of breastfeeding

If the feeding pattern is interrupted because of illness, a planned fast for a procedure or the mother's absence, the mother will need to express to maintain milk supply.

- Milk can be expressed by hand or by pump.
- Express as often as the baby would normally feed (i.e. 6–8 times a day). Several volumes of expressed milk can be added to the same bottle or storage bag (available from commercial pharmacies), but a new container should be used every 24 hours.
- Milk may be kept in the freezer section of the refrigerator for 2 weeks or in the deep freeze for 3 months.
- To thaw frozen milk, place a bag/bottle in a container of cool water and run in hot water until the bag/bottle is standing in hot water. When the milk is thawed, it will be cold; continue to heat in hot water or place in the fridge until required for a feed.
- Thawed milk should be used within 24 hours.

How much milk to express?

If the mother wants to express to give a feed by bottle or to substitute a feed as she is weaning, how much will the baby need?

Daily requirements of milk are
- From 0–6 months: 150 mL/kg
- >6 months: 120 mL/kg

Divide this amount by the usual number of feeds to calculate the amount required per feed.

Growth in breastfed infants

Growth patterns differ between breastfed and artificially fed infants. Average weights of breastfed babies are similar to or higher than formula-fed babies until 4–6 months, after which breastfed babies slow significantly in their weight gain. Length and head circumference remain similar.

Growth charts are now available for fully breastfed infants. The naturally slower weight gain of breastfed infants should not be taken in isolation as abnormal.

Maternal illness

When the mother is unwell, breastfeeding should continue. In the case of maternal infection, antibodies will pass through the breast milk to protect the baby.

Mastitis is a common reason for early weaning. Any reports of pain by the mother should be actively addressed (see Chapter 21, *Neonatal conditions*).

Maternal drugs

If the mother has to take medication, the risk–benefit ratio should be weighed carefully by the prescriber. The mother should continue to breastfeed unless use of the drug is absolutely contraindicated during lactation and there is no safe alternative. There are very few drugs in this category and almost all have a safe alternative. If the mother is concerned about continuing breastfeeding, even if the drug is safe, suggest taking the drug after a feed to minimise the concentration, or dividing the dose if possible.

Vitamin D

A baby's vitamin D stores increase during pregnancy and decrease after birth until the baby starts getting vitamin D from sunlight along with diet. If a pregnant woman has low levels of vitamin D, her infant will also have low vitamin D. Breast milk has many benefits, but it is generally not a rich source of vitamin D.

Women with risk factors for low vitamin D should have their vitamin D levels checked at the first antenatal visit and should be treated with daily supplements (1000–2000 IU D3 daily) to ensure their vitamin D levels are >50 nmol/L. Exclusively breastfed infants of vitamin D deficient mothers should be supplemented with 400 IU vitamin D3 daily for at least the first 12 months of life.

Formula feeding

If breast milk is not available, either from the breast or as expressed milk, a commercially prepared formula should be chosen. These are based on cow's milk, modified to lower the protein, calcium and electrolytes to levels better suited to the human infant and contain added amino acids, vitamins and trace minerals. A 'from-birth' formula should be selected for infants from birth to 6 months. For infants >6 months, follow-on formulas may be used – these have a higher protein and renal solute load (RSL) and are not suitable for infants <6 months of age.

The introduction of some formula need not mean the end of breastfeeding. A combination of breast and formula may be quite suitable for the infant.

Cow's milk-based formulas

- The range of formula options has increased in recent years, with options now including specifically modified proteins, long-chain polyunsaturated fatty acids (LCPUFA) and probiotics. All formulas meet the Australian Food Standards code and are suitable choices, although some are more expensive.
- Changes between types of formula are made for a variety of reasons, including irritability, poor sleep and possetting. In the normal thriving infant there is little indication to change the type of formula.
- Care should be taken when changing between formulas to use the correct scoop and dilution (as these vary significantly between brands). A history for a formula-fed infant with possible feeding problems should include a review of formula preparation technique.

There are a number of special types of formulas available over the counter including soy, AR (anti-reflux), low-lactose and hypoallergenic or partially hydrolysed formulas. They have specific indications and should not be encouraged unless there is evidence that they are required. That is low-lactose formula for proven lactose intolerance.

Introduction of whole cow's milk

The introduction of cow's milk products as part of an expanding diet is appropriate, but the main milk intake should be breast milk or formula until 12 months of age because of the risk of iron deficiency. Small amounts of cow's milk can be used on cereal, in custard and yoghurt from about 6 months.

Full-cream dairy products should be used for children up to 2 years; reduced-fat milk can be used from 2 years. Skim milk (essentially no fat) should not be used for children under 5 years.

Introduction of solids

Breast milk (or formula) will meet all nutrient needs until infants are 6 months old. This also corresponds to the age when most infants develop head control and oropharyngeal function sufficient to allow introduction of solids. From around 4–6 months solids can be introduced, to increase the intake of nutrients, such as iron, and as part of the educational process of learning to eat.

Babies show they are ready to start solids when they

- Start showing interest when others are eating
- Start making gestures that seem to say 'feed me too'
- Stop pushing out any food put in their mouth (disappearance of the tongue-thrust reflex)
- Start being able to hold their head up and sit without support

Solids can be iron-fortified baby cereal, smooth vegetables or fruits, followed by meat and chicken. Foods should be introduced one at a time to allow observation of tolerance. Texture should be increased so that by about 8–9 months the infant is managing lumps and varying textures, and is starting to manage finger foods.

The 2012 NHMRC recommendations on solids introduction state that high allergen foods such as fish, eggs, do not need to be delayed after 6 months as there is little evidence that this will reduce the likelihood of food allergies

By about 12 months, most family foods can be offered. Increasing intake of solids should result in a reduction of milk intake to about 600 mL per day by 12 months. Higher intake of cow's milk limits the intake of other foods and is associated with iron deficiency.

Iron deficiency and associated anaemia is the most common nutrient deficiency in children in Australia. It is associated with the early introduction of cow's milk, high intake of cow's milk in the second year and low intake of iron-rich foods, such as meat and pulses.

Weaning

There is no set rule for weaning age. Solids should be introduced at around 4–6 months and cup-drinking of breast milk, formula or water should start by 7–9 months. There is no need for the baby to be weaned to a bottle – if they are old enough they can go straight to a cup. Most babies can manage adequate fluid from a cup by 12–15 months.

Some babies decrease the number of breastfeeds as they begin to be able to digest solid food.

Sudden cessation of breastfeeding leaves the mother at risk of developing mastitis. Ideally, weaning is achieved by reducing the feeds by one a week. Start by offering a drink in a cup or bottle instead of a breastfeed at midday, and gradually increase these other drinks. Many mothers retain the early morning feed or the last feed at night for longer.

Persistent difficulty in weaning usually requires someone to support the mother, giving the baby a feed and allowing the baby some time away from the mother to help with mutual separation. Specialist lactation advice may be needed.

Toddler Food Refusal

An assessment of the toddler who refuses food (who seems otherwise healthy) includes the following steps:

- Clarify the dietary history, exploring intake, volume, pattern, mealtime routine, and battles around food. Many children are given milk, juice or foods (e.g. yoghurt, banana) if they do not eat their meals and will 'hold out' for these options.
- Plotting weight and height and head circumference to assess the child's growth, and reassure the parents where appropriate.
- Using the growth chart to demonstrate that the growth rate normally slows in the second year.
- Linking this to a lessened need for food and subsequent drop in appetite.
- Emphasising developmental progress.

Advise parents that:

- A healthy child will eat when hungry – *quit the fight!*
- Avoid arguments over food. Remember: 'It's the parent's job to offer food, it's the child's job to eat it!'
- Showing independence is an important part of toddler development – choosing and refusing food is an expression of independence.
- Educate regarding appropriate portion size – this is usually smaller and lowers expectations.
- Allow the child to choose among the healthy (limited) options.
- Include some healthy food choices that they like. Offering cereal at lunch is okay! A lack of variety is not a major worry at this age.
- Avoid filling up on milk and juice – large volumes of milk (>600 mL a day) can make the child feel full. Juice is not necessary in the child's diet.
- Give the child time to enjoy the meal without comment. Remove the food after 30 minutes or if they dawdle or lose interest.
- Learning to eat is fun. Switch to finger food if they refuse to be fed.
- Do not use food as a punishment or reward. It only increases its potential power.

Daily food needs of preschoolers

The following is a guide to the quantities suitable for 2–5 year olds. Many parents are surprised at how little children of this age need. However, because total needs are small there is relatively little place for high-fat, high-sugar extras.

- **Milk group:** two servings
  One serving = 250 mL of milk, 200 g of yoghurt or 35 g of cheese.
- **Bread and cereal group:** four to five servings
  One serving = one slice of bread, half cup of pasta or two cereal wheat biscuits.
- **Vegetable and fruit group:** four or more servings
  One serving = one piece of fruit or two tablespoons of vegetables – focus on variety of different vegetables and fruits rather than quantity.
- **Meat or protein group:** two servings
  One serving = 30 g of lean meat, fish or chicken, half cup of beans or one egg.

Feeding the sick infant and child
Nutritional assessment

A thorough nutritional assessment should be undertaken taking into account

- Medical history
  Type and duration of illness
  Degree of metabolic stress
  Treatment (medications or surgery, or both)
- Dietary assessment
  24-hour dietary recall
  3-day food record
- Physical examination
  General assessment: wasting, oedema, lethargy and muscular strength
  Specific micronutrient deficiencies: pallor, bruising, skin, hair, neurological and ophthalmological complications
  Anthropometry – weight, length, head circumference – serial measurements plotted. Correct for age for preterm infants
  Growth velocity
  Skinfold thickness, mid-arm circumference
- Fluid requirements
  Take into account intravenous and enteral fluids
  Any restrictions as per medical team
- Laboratory data
  Assessment of GI absorptive status – stool microscopy, pH and reducing sugars
  Protein status: albumin, total protein, pre-albumin, urea, 24-hour urinary nitrogen
  Fluid, electrolyte and acid–base status: serum electrolytes and acid–base, urinalysis
  Iron status: serum ferritin and full blood examination
  Mineral status: calcium, magnesium, phosphorus, alkaline phosphatase, bone age and bone density
  Vitamin status: vitamins A, C, B_{12}, D, E/lipid ratio, folate and INR
  Trace elements: zinc, selenium, copper, chromium and manganese
  Lipid status: serum cholesterol, HDL cholesterol and triglycerides
  Glucose tolerance: serum glucose, HbA1 c

Establishing a nutrition treatment plan
Calculating nutritional requirements
Energy

Estimated energy requirements for the sick infant or child can be calculated by using either

- the requirements of a normal well child of the same sex and age, or
- an estimate of basal requirements with additional stress and activity factors.

Less common, but the most accurate method to calculate energy requirements in very sick infants and children, is via measurement of energy expenditure using indirect calorimetry.

Energy requirements can be expressed as kilocalories (kcal) or as kilojoules (kJ). The conversion equation is kJ = kcal × 4.2.

Energy requirements are increased in the following conditions:

- Very low birthweight (VLBW) infants
- Chronic lung disease
- Cardiac defects
- Cystic fibrosis
- Diseases causing malabsorption, that is liver, intestinal failure, allergic enteropathy
- Burns
- Tumours

Energy requirements are decreased in

- Critically ill patients who are ventilated.

Protein

Increased protein intake is recommended in

- Protein-losing states, that is enteropathy and nephrotic syndrome
- Chronic malnutrition
- Burns
- Renal dialysis
- HIV
- Haemofiltration (~2 g/kg per day)

Reduced protein intake is recommended in

- Hepatic encephalopathy
- Severe renal dysfunction (not dialysed)

Fat

- Concentrated source of energy and essential for transport of fat-soluble vitamins and hormones.
- Deficiency can occur rapidly in neonates and will manifest as reduced growth rate, poor hair growth, thrombocytopenia, susceptibility to infection and poor wound healing.

Micronutrients

Special consideration is needed when estimating the micronutrient requirements of sick children (see Table 9.8).

Feeds for sick infants

See Table 9.9.

- Breast milk, including expressed breast milk (EBM).
- Infant formulas, including 'low birthweight (LBW)' formulas.
- Specialised feeds for specific disease states, for example inborn errors of metabolism, renal, complex malabsorption and liver conditions.

Breast milk

Breast-milk feeding should be the primary aim for very sick babies. When babies are too ill or too premature to suckle at the breast, most mothers can establish lactation by expression. EBM can be fed via a tube until the baby is well enough to be placed on the breast. In this way breast-milk feeding can be achieved in extremely premature babies and in babies with serious illness. The only situations where breast-milk feeding is not possible are

- When an informed mother chooses not to express
- Some inborn errors of metabolism, which require specific formulas
- Complex malabsorption syndromes

Table 9.8 Diseases that increase micronutrient requirements

Disease	Increased requirement
Burns	Vitamins C, B complex, folate, zinc
HIV/AIDS	Zinc, selenium, iron
Renal failure: dialysis	Vitamins C, B complex, folate (reduce or omit copper, chromium, molybdenum)
Haemofiltration	Vitamins C, B complex, trace elements
Protein–energy malnutrition	Zinc, selenium, iron
Refeeding syndrome	Phosphate, magnesium, potassium
Short bowel syndrome, chronic malabsorption states	Vitamins A, B_{12}, D, E, K, folate, zinc, magnesium, selenium
Liver disease	Vitamins A, B_{12}, D, E, K, zinc, iron (reduce or omit manganese, copper)
High fistula output, chronic diarrhoea	Zinc, magnesium, selenium, folate, B complex, B_{12}
Pancreatic insufficiency	Vitamins A, D, E, K
Inflammatory bowel disease	Folate, B_{12}, zinc, iron

Table 9.9 Appropriate feeds at different ages

Age	Normal gut function	Impaired gut function
0–12 months	Expressed breast milk (EBM) standard infant formula or follow on formula (>6 months) ± Fortifiers • Formula • Carbohydrate powder • Fat Infatrini (420 kJ/100 mL)	EBM All formula below can be fortified: lactose free formula S-26 LF, De-Lact Soy formula (>6 months) S26 Soy, Karicare soy Partially hydrolysed formula Nan HA, Karicare HA Extensively hydrolysed formula Peptijunior, Alfare Elemental formula Neocate, Elecare Modular feed
1–6 years (8–20 kg)	Standard paediatric formulas: Nutrini, Pediasure, resource for kids 420 kJ/100 mL (1 kcal/mL) Nutrini Energy, Pediasure Plus 630 kJ/100 mL (1.5kcal/mL) ± fibre	Concentrated hydrolysed infant formula Peptijunior, Alfare Hydrolysed Paediatric formula MCT Peptide 1+, Peptamen Junior, Paediatric Vivonex Elemental paediatric formula Neocate Advance, Elecare 1+
>6 years (>20 kg)	Paediatric feed may still be appropriate Standard adult formula: Nutrison Standard, Osmolite, Ensure, Resource 420 kJ/100 mL (1 kcal/mL) Nutrison Energy, Ensure Plus, Fortisip, Resource Plus 630 kJ/100 mL (1.5 kcal/mL) Nutrison Concentrated, NovaSource 2.0, TwoCal HN 840 kJ/100 mL (2 kcal/mL) ± fibre	Concentrated hydrolysed infant formula may still be appropriate Hydrolysed Paediatric formula Elemental Paediatric formula Adult Elemental Formula Vivonex TEN, Peptamen OS

Breast-milk fortifiers

Breast-milk fortifiers are available to add to EBM to increase its content of protein, energy and other nutrients. The addition of fortifier should be delayed until feeds are fully established (i.e. at 150–200 mL/kg per day), unless babies have a condition requiring fluid restriction, for example congestive cardiac failure or chronic lung disease.

Babies who may benefit from fortifiers are those with increased nutritional requirements (e.g. VLBW babies) and those requiring fluid restriction (as listed above).

In addition, VLBW babies require higher levels of phosphorous, folate, iron, sodium and vitamins C, D, A, K and E. Iron supplementation should begin between 4–8 weeks. VLBW babies who receive multiple blood transfusions may not need supplemental iron.

Infant formulas

When breast milk is not available, an infant formula is required. LBW formulas are designed for very premature (<32 weeks) babies. In general, these contain more energy, protein, calcium, phosphorus, trace elements and certain vitamins than standard formula. They include LCPUFA as part of their fat content, based on evidence that this improves the developmental outcomes in premature infants. Generally LBW formulas are used until a weight of 2.5 kg is achieved. Babies are then fed with a standard infant formula, which can be fortified if necessary.

Fortification of standard infant formulas

Standard formulas provide approximately 280 kJ/100 mL (20 kcal/30 mL) and 1.5 g protein/100 mL. Fortification should only be implemented under the supervision of a paediatrician or dietitian.

- To increase energy to 350 kJ/100 mL (25 kcal/30 mL)
  Use *additional* formula powder, that is for formulas where the standard dilution is 1 scoop/30 mL of water, use 1 scoop/25 mL of water, or for formulas where the standard dilution is 1 scoop/60 mL of water use 1 scoop/50 mL of water.
  This will also increase protein and other nutrient intakes.
  Care should be taken in infants with renal or liver impairment.
- To increase energy to 420 kJ/100 mL (30 kcal/30 mL):
  Concentrate the formula further with additional powder (e.g. 1 scoop/30 mL to 1 scoop/20 mL). This provides an improved energy/protein ratio and additional nutrients, which can be beneficial in fluid restricted infants and those with high catch-up growth requirements. Use of this formula needs to be monitored carefully due to its higher RSL and osmolality.

Specialised feeds can also be fortified in similar ways to the above.

- Infants and young children who develop an intercurrent gastroenteritis must have all fortification ceased until vomiting and diarrhoea resolve, to avoid the potential complication of hypernatraemic dehydration.
- VLBW babies require 180–200 mL/kg per day of EBM or standard formula, or 150–180 mL/kg per day of fortified EBM or LBW formula, starting at 20–30 mL/kg per day at birth and increasing by 30 mL/kg per day as tolerated. Regimens should be modified according to condition and stability in VLBW infants. Initial feed frequency should be 1–2 hourly. Hourly feeds may be necessary in babies <1000 g.
- Orogastric tubes should be used in babies <1250 g, as nasogastric tubes cause significant airways obstruction. Continuous intragastric infusion of feed rather than intermittent boluses may help if reflux, gastric distension or apnoea is persistent.
- Term infants require 150 mL/kg per day. This is usually reached over 5–7 days, starting at 30–40 mL/kg per day and increasing by 30 mL/kg per day as tolerated. Feed frequency should be 3–4 hourly, although with reflux or abdominal distension, smaller volume and more frequent feeds may help.

Feeds for children

Young children often maintain oral intake when they are ill. In some cases additional supplements should be added to oral feeds to maintain nutritional status.
  These include
- Energy supplements, for example glucose polymers (Polyjoule) or fat emulsions (Calogen (long-chain fats), Liquigen (medium chain fats)) added to normal foods and fluids to increase energy intake.

- Complete supplements, for example Pediasure, Fortisip or Sustagen drinks, which can be used in addition to usual foods to increase energy, protein and nutrient intake.

Enteral feeding

Enteral nutrition is the provision of nutrients to the alimentary tract through a feeding tube. It can be used to provide the total nutritional needs of a patient (either short or long term), or to provide additional nutrients when voluntary oral intake is inadequate. See nutritional support algorithm, Fig. 9.2.

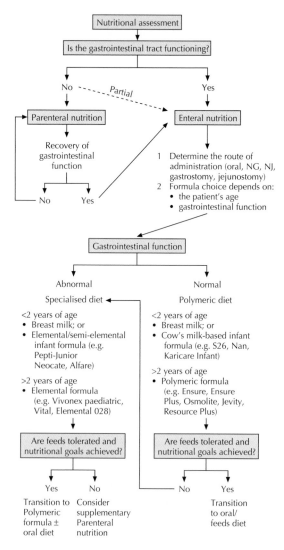

Fig. 9.2 Nutrition support algorithm.

Table 9.10 Types of enteral feeding regimens

	Advantages	Disadvantages
Bolus feedings	Most closely mimics physiological feeding increases patient mobility Little equipment is needed. Volume given can be precisely measured	Can be time-consuming for caregiver May decrease voluntary oral intake
Gravity drip	Little equipment needed Feeding most likely to be tolerated	Rate of delivery cannot be closely monitored
Pump-assisted continuous	Feeding can be delivered while patient sleeps Larger volumes can be tolerated than if given by bolus method	Requires feeding pump

Enteral feeding has certain advantages over parenteral nutrition.

- Lower risk of serious infection (central line infection)
- Lower risk of metabolic abnormalities
- Nutrients provided to the alimentary tract enhance intestinal growth and function
- Inexpensive

Administration

The most commonly used route for enteral feeding is nasogastric, the main benefit being ease of insertion. When long-term feeding is required, a gastrostomy tube may be indicated.

When gastric motility is poor, or when gastric residues are persistently high, a nasojejunal tube may be of benefit.

Feeding method

When choosing a method consider the feeding route, the expected length of time the feed will be required and the type of feeding regimen to be used (see Table 9.10).

Selection of feed

A full nutritional assessment (current nutritional status, current intake, requirements and the consideration of medical condition/fluid restrictions) should be completed by a paediatric dietitian to establish which feed will be optimal. See Table 9.9 for appropriate feeds to use in different age groups.

It is **inappropriate** to administer puréed foods down feeding tubes as the amount of fluid required to achieve a suitable consistency dilutes the energy and nutrient content, while increasing the risk of microbial contamination and tube blockage.

Monitoring enteral nutrition

Monitoring patients on enteral feeds requires regular assessment of mechanical, metabolic, gastrointestinal, nutritional and growth parameters. In the early stages of feeding, the patient's tolerance of the feeding regimen is critical to the success of feeding.

Once the feeding plan has been fully implemented, regular assessment of the patient's nutrient requirements is needed to ensure that nutritional support has been adequately maintained and to indicate when enteral feeding can be reduced or ceased.

From enteral to oral feeding

Once the patient is able and willing to eat by mouth, enteral feeds can be reduced in proportion to the amount consumed orally. Transition from continuous feeds to overnight feeds may help establish oral intake while ensuring the patient is not nutritionally compromised.

Common problems with enteral feeding

- **Gastrointestinal disturbance.** This is the most common problem (diarrhoea, cramping, nausea and vomiting) and can be minimised by correct formula selection and review of medications. High gastric residues should be managed by reducing the rate of feeds, feeding smaller volumes, reassessing the concentration of feed and GI function. Jejunal feeding alleviates the problems caused by slow gastric emptying.

- **Food aversion.** Non-nutritive sucking and mouth contact or taking small amounts of appropriate food/fluid orally will help establish or maintain eating and feeding skills. A speech pathologist may be of assistance.
- **Malnutrition** is associated with major changes in electrolyte balance. Enteral feeding should be initiated with caution in patients with significant and long-standing under nutrition. (See Refeeding syndrome, Chapter 22).

Parenteral nutrition
General indications for parenteral nutrition
- Recent weight loss of >10% of usual body weight and a non-functional GI tract.
- No oral intake for >3–5 days in a patient with suboptimal nutritional status and a non-functional GI tract.
- Anticipated need for parenteral nutrition for a minimum of 3–5 days.

Medical/surgical conditions that may require parenteral nutrition.
- Patients unable to tolerate enteral feeding because of GI dysfunction; that is postoperative neonates, extensive short-bowel syndrome or severe malabsorption.
- Patients with increased metabolic requirements that may not be adequately treated with enteral therapy; that is severe burns, cystic fibrosis or renal failure.

Refeeding syndrome
After a period of prolonged starvation, aggressive nutritional therapy may precipitate a cascade of potentially fatal metabolic complications. These include
- Hypokalaemia
- Hypophosphataemia
- Hypomagnesaemia
- Glucose intolerance
- Cardiac failure
- Seizures
- Myocardial infarction/arrhythmias

Patients at particular risk are those with
- anorexia nervosa;
- classical marasmus;
- kwashiorkor;
- no nutrition for 7–10 days in adolescents (much less in infants and children) with significant metabolic stress;
- acute weight loss of ≥10–20% of usual body weight and possible metabolic stress, or weight loss of >20% of usual body weight; and
- morbid obesity with massive weight loss (i.e. postoperative).

Management
- Identify risk and chronicity.
- Identify and treat metabolic stress if present (e.g. infection).
- Establish baseline status: weight, height/length, head circumference, fluid status, electrolytes, urea, creatinine, calcium, phosphate and magnesium, liver function and albumin, blood sugar, lipid status and acid base balance prior to commencing nutritional rehabilitation.
- Assess micronutrient and trace element status at baseline.
- Establish modest nutritional goals initially (e.g. basal requirements until stability is assured), then aim to provide for catch-up growth. During the first week of nutritional therapy, weight gain may not be seen or, if present, may reflect fluid gain rather than muscle or fat gain. Patients at high risk for refeeding syndrome are often started on less than 50% of their estimated energy requirements.
- Monitor closely over the first week until a nutritional plan is established with pulse rate, fluid balance, weight, caloric intake, glucose, electrolytes, urea, creatinine, calcium, phosphate and magnesium. Bloods are required daily for the first 3 days.

- Administer vitamin and mineral supplements. Patients who are severely malnourished may require on spec supplementation with folate, vitamin A, thiamine and a multivitamin, and consideration of prophylactis antibiotics, iron therapy should be avoided in initial management in this situation.

USEFUL RESOURCES

Fluids
- http://www.rch.org.au/clinicalguide/guideline_index/Gastroenteritis/
- http://www.rch.org.au/clinicalguide/guideline_index/Dehydration/
- http://www.rch.org.au/clinicalguide/guideline_index/Intravenous_Fluids/
- http://www.rch.org.au/clinicalguide/guideline_index/Hyperkalaemia/
- http://www.rch.org.au/clinicalguide/guideline_index/Hyponatraemia/
- http://www.rch.org.au/clinicalguide/guideline_index/Hypernatraemia/
- http://ww2.rch.org.au/pharmacopoeia/pages/guideNeonatalFluid.html
- http://www.netsvic.org.au/nets/handbook/index.cfm

Nutrition
- www.breastfeedingbasics.org – Breastfeeding Basics. Academic, web-based short course on breastfeeding fundamentals. Aimed at the medical practitioner, with useful revision of anatomy and physiology and a number of case studies.
- www.lalecheleague.org – LaLeche League. International breastfeeding advocacy/support group. Excellent FAQs for breastfeeding mothers.
- www.raisingchildren.net.au – Raising children network. Commonwealth government parenting site – contains comprehensive information.
- www.rch.org.au/nutrition – RCH Nutrition Department. Resources section contains useful fact sheets and links.

Growth charts: http://www.cdc.gov/growthcharts/who_charts.htm

Treatment of severe malnutrition: http://www.who.int/nutrition/publications/severemalnutrition/guide_inpatient_text.pdf

- www.breastfeedingbasics.org – Breastfeeding Basics.
- http://www.rch.org.au/rchcpg/hospital_clinical_guideline_index/Parenteral_Nutrition_PN

CHAPTER 10

Genitourinary conditions

Amanda M. Walker
John Hutson
Mike O'Brien
Sonia Grover

Continence
Nocturnal enuresis

Nocturnal enuresis (NE) is (arbitrarily) defined as bedwetting in a child ≥ 5 years of age. It affects 20% of 5-year olds, 5% of 10-year olds and up to 1% of adults. Bedwetting in the absence of daytime urinary symptoms is called 'monosymptomatic' nocturnal enuresis (MNE) whereas if day symptoms occur it is 'non-monosymptomatic' nocturnal enuresis (NMNE). Primary NE refers to a child who has never been dry for at least 6 months. Secondary NE refers to children who have become wet after a period of at least 6 months of dryness. Although secondary NE may suggest an organic or psychological cause, in practice most secondary NE is simply primary NE that never fully resolved.

Aetiology and pathophysiology

NE is usually inherited as an autosomal dominant trait with variable penetrance. The pathophysiology involves a combination of
- Poor arousal to stimulus of full bladder.
- Nocturnal polyuria – relative deficiency of vasopressin at night.
- Overactive bladder with reduced nocturnal functional bladder capacity.

Other factors may be involved in a way as yet unexplained. NE is more common in children with developmental delay, clumsiness, short stature or low birthweight. Most psychological problems in children with NE are likely to be the result of the wetting rather than the cause, and usually resolve with resolution of the wetting.

Children with NMNE have daytime symptoms such as wetting, jiggling, urgency, frequent passage of small volumes of urine. Parents of such children often mistakenly think their child preoccupied simply habitually 'waits until the last minute'. In fact they have an overactive detrusor muscle (irritable bladder) resulting in a small functional bladder capacity and small urgently voided volumes. The jiggling represents tightening of pelvic floor muscles in an attempt to defend against the forceful bladder contraction, so that wetting may be prevented or minimised. These children often have NE that is refractory to alarms and desmopressin, and persists beyond 10 years of age. Some also develop faecal incontinence (see Chapter 8, *Gastrointestinal conditions*). Rare physical causes include UTI, diabetes mellitus/insipidus, epilepsy, ectopic ureter, obstructive sleep hypoventilation, neurogenic bladder. Sexual abuse will occasionally first present as NE.

Management

The spontaneous remission rate is approximately 15% per year. Those least likely to resolve spontaneously are those with NMNE. Treatment should be offered to children ≥ 6 years for whom wetting has become a problem. See Fig. 10.1 for management algorithm.

Monosymptomatic NE

- *Alarms:* First line treatment is with a pad and bell alarm or personal (body-worn) alarm, used nightly for 8–12 weeks. Relapses may be minimised by 'overlearning' – using a fluid load before bed for the last

---

Paediatric Handbook, Ninth Edition. Edited by Amanda Gwee, Romi Rimer and Michael Marks.
© 2015 John Wiley & Sons, Ltd. Published 2015 by John Wiley & Sons, Ltd.

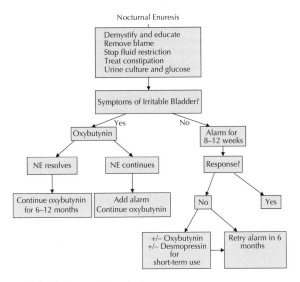

Fig. 10.1 Management algorithm for nocturnal enuresis

1–2 weeks of treatment. A wetting diary may help in motivation and monitoring. When symptoms are refractory to treatment, unsuspected nocturnal bladder dysfunction with detrusor overactivity is often the cause.

- *Desmopressin (DDAVP):* A synthetic analogue of vasopressin. In Australia it is available on authority prescription for those who have not responded to or are unsuitable for an alarm. While not curative, it can nonetheless serve a purpose for the short-term (school camps and sleepovers) and medium-term (adolescents who are fed up). Side effects are uncommon and include nose bleeds, sore throat and abdominal pain. Hyponatraemia with convulsions has been reported and it is important to ensure that appropriate advice regarding fluid intake is given to minimise this risk. The child should **not** drink for 1 hour before and 8 hours after the administration of DDAVP. The oral dose of DDAVP is 120–240 mcg (1–2 melts) at night. These should be placed under the tongue 1 hour before sleep. Nasal spray is still available in Australia: the dose is 10–40 mcg per night (1–4 sprays).

- *Other treatments:* Imipramine should no longer be used. It has an unacceptably high relapse rate and there is an ever-present danger of accidental or intentional overdose causing cardiotoxicity. There is no evidence to suggest that fluid restriction or liberalisation influences outcome. There is insufficient evidence to recommend lifting or waking the child, psychotherapy, hypnosis, acupuncture, rewards, chiropractic or bladder training.

Non-monosymptomatic NE

- *Treatment plan*
  - ○ Treat constipation/faecal incontinence first (see Chapter 8, *Gastrointestinal conditions*, Faecal incontinence) and exclude UTI.
  - ○ Use anticholinergics to treat detrusor instability (see Anticholinergics).
  - ○ Then use alarm if needed as above.
  - ○ Frequent, regular voiding may help.
- *Anticholinergics*
  - ○ Oxybutynin (Ditropan). Dose: 2.5–5 mg b.i.d. Dry mouth is common. Less common side effects include rash, mood changes, constipation, headache, epistaxis, blurred vision. Treatment is often needed for many months to years.
  - ○ Tolterodine (Detrusitol) is a more bladder-specific anticholinergic. There is currently little experience with the use of this drug in childhood.

Daytime wetting without NE
The following classification is useful in determining appropriate investigations and management.

Urge incontinence
The condition is caused by overactivity in the detrusor muscle during bladder filling.
- Symptoms include urgency, frequency, posturing (squatting) and wetting.
- There is an association with recurrent UTI, vulvovaginitis and constipation.
- Management includes treating any coexistent UTI and constipation, regular voiding, and anticholinergic medication to reduce detrusor spasm.

Dysfunctional voiding
- There is a lack of coordination between detrusor and bladder neck activity with poor relaxation of the external sphincter during voiding.
- The condition is associated with increased intravesical pressure, high residual urine volumes and, at times, upper tract dilatation.
- Management relies on teaching sphincter relaxation (i.e. pelvic floor relaxation) and ensuring optimal voiding techniques.

Neurological and urological pathology
- These children do not have jiggling, urgency or frequency and *they may wet at night.*
- Ectopic ureter and fistulae cause constant rather than episodic dribbling. Bladder neck and urethral obstruction and neurogenic bladder may have large or expressible bladders.

Investigation
NE alone does not usually require investigation. Children with NE and day-wetting (PNE) should have a urine microscopy, culture and glucose. Where there is diagnostic uncertainty or a poor response to treatment, a renal and bladder ultrasound including an assessment of residual urine volume will exclude major structural pathology. A 2-day voiding volume diary, uroflow (volume/time) measurement and post-void bladder scan can provide information about detrusor overactivity, outflow obstruction, polyuria and further guide management.

Urinary tract infections
Symptomatic lower urinary tract infections (UTIs) during childhood are common and generally carry little long-term risk.

Important but uncommon associations of febrile UTIs during childhood include pyelonephritis, renal impairment and hypertension (HTN). The primary aim of investigation of childhood UTIs is to reduce the risk of sepsis and identify children at risk of chronic renal impairment.

Clinical features
- UTIs may present with nonspecific clinical features. Fever may be the sole symptom. This is more common in younger children.
- Cystitis refers to urinary infections limited to the bladder and urethra. It may present with dysuria, frequency, wetting, urgency, cloudy or malodorous urine and lower abdominal pain. Fever is often absent although irritability and other minor constitutional symptoms are common in young children.
- Pyelonephritis usually presents with additional symptoms of fever, lethargy, vomiting, loin or generalised abdominal pain. Pyelonephritis in neonates and infants may present as an undifferentiated fever.
- Offensive urine is neither sensitive nor specific for UTIs in children.
Remember that finding a UTI in a sick child does not exclude another site of serious infection (e.g. meningitis).

Pathogens
- *Escherichia coli* (80%).
- *Enterococcus faecalis* (10%).
- Other gram-negatives – *Klebsiella* spp., *Proteus* spp., *Enterobacter* spp., *Citrobacter* spp.
- Other gram-positives – *Staphylococcus saprophyticus.*

Diagnosis of UTI

The most reliable collection technique appropriate to the clinical setting should be used. This may be suprapubic bladder aspiration (SPA), in/out catheter specimen urine, clean catch or midstream urine sample. Urine bag samples should be used only in specific settings as contamination risk is high.

Urine 'ward test' strips

These are useful as a screening test in a child with low suspicion of a UTI (>6 months, without known renal tract abnormality and with an alternative focus for fever). Ward test should not be used in a child with a high chance of a UTI. If leukocyte esterase and nitrites are both positive then a UTI is likely. The ward test strips for leucocytes or nitrites are negative in up to 50% of UTIs in children. This is because the production of nitrites by bacteria is time-dependent and infant bladder capacity necessitates frequent voiding.

Bag urine specimen collection

- Do not send for culture.
- Use for chemical strip screening only.
- In sick infants or those where the suspicion of UTI is high (e.g. renal tract anomaly or previous UTI), a bag specimen should not be taken, as it only delays the diagnosis. An SPA (preferred) or CSU sample should be obtained as part of the septic workup.

Midstream urine specimen collection

This can be obtained from children who are able to void on request (usually by 3–4 years of age). The child's genitalia are first washed with warm water. In girls the labia should be separated. The child is asked to void. After passing the first few millilitres, a specimen is collected.

- A pure growth of 10^8 c.f.u./L in an MSU is proof of a UTI.
- A pure growth of $>10^5$–10^8 c.f.u./L in an MSU is suggestive of a UTI (correlate with clinical setting).

Catheter specimen collection

See Chapter 4, *Procedures*.

- These are useful in infants after a failed SPA or in older children who are unable to void on request. A pure growth of $>10^5$ c.f.u./L indicates infection.

Suprapubic aspirate collection

See Chapter 4, *Procedures*.

- This is the preferred method of urine collection in infants. Aspirated urine should be sterile; hence any pure growth of bacteria indicates infection.

It is important to identify bacteraemia, meningitis and sepsis in neonates and young infants with UTI. Additional investigations to consider include

- Blood culture and electrolytes.
- Lumbar puncture. Do not omit a lumbar puncture in a sick child just because a UTI has been diagnosed. Collection of CSF should be undertaken in infants <3 months with UTI and considered in children <2 years.

Treatment of UTI

- Will be directed by clinical severity, ability to tolerate oral medications and previous antibiotic sensitivities.
- Most infants <12 months of age with a UTI require benzylpenicillin 60 mg/kg IV (max. 2 g) 6 hourly and gentamicin 7.5 mg/kg IV (<10 years) or 6 mg/kg IV max. 240 mg (>10 years) daily.
- In children who are well and not vomiting (even those with clinical pyelonephritis), a course of oral antibiotics has been shown to be as effective as IV antibiotics (see Appendix 3, *Antimicrobial guidelines*). Antibiotic sensitivity should be checked when available (usually at 48 hours).

Recurrence of UTIs

Ten to thirty per cent of children with a UTI will have a recurrence, usually within 12 months. A greater risk of recurrence is associated with the first UTI occurring <6 months of age, dysfunctional voiding, constipation, the presence of dilating VUR or evidence of renal parenchymal loss on initial scanning.

Approach to identifying children with a UTI who are at renal risk. This varies across different units which is reflective of patchy evidence to guide decision making.

- Clinical history
  - Likely site of infection (cystitis vs. pyelonephritis)
  - Factors contributing to risk of infection
    - Voiding pattern (wetting, infrequent voider, dysfunctional voiding)
    - Constipation
  - Factors contributing to kidney vulnerability and risk of CKD
    - Family history of kidney disease
    - Structural renal disorders, chronic systemic illnesses
- Investigations
  - Confirm UTI by urine m/c/s
  - Screened population: antenatal ultrasound known to be normal
    - First infection
      - Lower tract, afebrile UTI in peri-continent or primary school aged girl. Consider renal ultrasound.
      - Lower tract, afebrile UTI in toddler or boy. Arrange renal ultrasound.
      - Unusual microbiology or clinical features. Investigate more thoroughly including renal ultrasound.
      - Upper tract febrile UTI
        - Renal ultrasound followed by dimercaptosuccinic acid (DMSA) scan at 3–6 months. This nuclear medicine scan looks for renal parenchymal defects (primarily renal scarring).
        - Consider micturating cystourethrogram (MCU) if presenting during infancy. Radiographic contrast is instilled in the bladder via a urethral catheter and subsequent radiographs taken to image the bladder and urethra to evaluate bladder emptying, exclude PUV and vesicoureteric reflux.
    - Recurrent UTIs
      - Lower tract: bladder function evaluation by 2-day voiding volume diary and renal ultrasound.
      - Upper tract: as per lower tract, then DMSA at 3–6 months, consider referral to nephrologist or urologist.
  - Unscreened population: antenatal scans not performed
    - Earlier renal ultrasound

Management of recurrent UTIs
- Manage wetting and voiding dysfunction
- Manage constipation
- If >3 UTI's in 12 months then review history and management adherence, consider referral and prophylactic antibiotics

Renal conditions
Abnormalities of urinary sediment
Isolated microscopic haematuria

Isolated microscopic haematuria may be observed in febrile children with normal renal tract, following vigorous exercise, or may be familial (thin membrane disease). It is important to differentiate these from the patients whose haematuria represents more significant renal pathology. Concerning features are listed below and should be followed by investigation

- persisting microhaematuria (three separate occasions when the child is well) or recurrent macrohaematuria;
- the presence of proteinuria ($\geq+$), confirm by morning urinary protein: creatinine (UPr:Cr) ratio;
- high-level microhaematuria (>50 RBC/mL) particularly if associated with casts;
- HTN, oliguria or oedema: would suggest acute glomerulonephritis;
- features suggesting systemic or chronic illness; and
- painful haematuria suggests involvement of bladder (e.g. UTI), renal calculi or other urologic disorders.

Investigation should follow confirmation of isolated haematuria on three separate occasions when the child is well. Patients with heavy isolated microhaematuria (>50 dysmorphic (glomerular) RBC/µL) should be referred. If low-level haematuria only is present then these patients may potentially be followed clinically. Blood pressure, general, pubertal and genital examination should be performed and abnormalities managed. If these are normal then the following management plan may be followed:

- If proteinuria (≥++) is present then consider acute nephritis and refer paediatrician/paed. nephrologist for further evaluation.
- If proteinuria is absent then the following should be performed:
  - Urinary calcium:Cr ratio. If ≥0.7 mmol/mmol on more than one morning sample then hypercalciuria-likely diagnosis, arrange renal ultrasound and refer for further evaluation.
  - Urinalysis or urine M&C on immediate family members. If isolated microhaematuria identified, then consider familial haematuria and refer.
  - Renal ultrasound. If abnormalities identified then refer.
- If screening investigations are normal then annual review with general heath check, BP, urine M&C and Pr:Cr ratio is appropriate until haematuria has been absent for 2 years. Patients should be referred if they demonstrate persistence of haematuria for 4–5 years or into adolescence or if heavy microhaematuria (>50 dysmorphic (glomerular) RBC/μL) is consistently noted.

Macroscopic haematuria without proteinuria

Bleeding from any site within the renal tract may present with macroscopic haematuria. Generally glomerular inflammation (glomerulonephritis) presents with both haematuria and proteinuria although IgA nephropathy may commonly present with recurrent episodes of painless macroscopic haematuria without proteinuria.

Pain associated with macro/microhaematuria may be helpful in directing investigations (Table 10.1).

Haematuria with proteinuria

The presence of both haematuria and proteinuria suggests pathological changes within the glomerulus (glomerulonephritis), endothelium (haemolytic uraemic syndrome) or renal interstitium.

The most common cause is glomerulonephritis. Associated features may include tea coloured urine, oliguria, fluid retention with oedema and HTN (nephritic syndrome). Renal function may be impaired and electrolyte abnormalities are common.

Table 10.1 Causes of haematuria

Symptoms	Causes	Clinical examples
Painless	Glomerular inflammation Tumour cell infiltration	Glomerulonephritis Wilm's tumour
Loin pain + haematuria	Renal engorgement with stretch of renal capsule	*Blood* ● Renal vein thrombosis ● Nutcracker syndrome ● Cortical necrosis ● Renal trauma ● Haematoma *Inflammatory infiltrate* ● Glomerulonephritis ● Interstitial nephritis *Infection* ● Complicated pyelonephritis *Tumour* ● Wilm's (may be painless)
	Renal pelvis obstruction	Obstructing calculi
Renal colic	Ureteric obstruction/peristalsis	● Obstructing calculi ● Upper tract bleeding → clot colic
Suprapubic pain	Bladder mucosa	*Infection* ● Haemorrhagic cystitis (bacterial/viral) *Cytotoxic agents:* ● Cyclophosphamide cystitis

Evaluation should include careful history for antecedent infections, systemic illnesses and medication exposure. Examination should evaluate aetiology and consequences of acute kidney injury (AKI). Management should be discussed with a nephrologist.

Considerations should include

- Assessment of AKI: refer 'Acute kidney injury' section, p. 135.
- Aetiology of acute glomerulonephritis: C3,C4, ASOT, ANA, ± ANCA, ± AntiGBM Ab
  - Post infectious GN: nephritic syndrome typically follows throat or skin infection
  - HSP nephritis: palpable purpura, arthralgia
  - IgA nephritis: microhaematuria with episodic macrohaematuria coincident with mucosal infection
  - SLE nephritis: nephritic or mixed nephrotic/nephritic picture, multisystem disorder
  - ANCA associated and anti-GBM diseases: often associated with respiratory tract involvement. ANCA or Anti-GBM Ab positive
- Other pathologies presenting with microhaematuria and some proteinuria
  - HUS: Coombs negative haemolytic anaemia, thrombocytopaenia, increased LDH, low haptoglobin, AKI, HTN common. May or may not be associated with bloody diarrhoea
  - Acute interstitial nephritis: haematuria, low-grade proteinuria, WBC casts ± eosinophiluria, eosinophilia, AKI. Commonly due to medications or infection

Isolated low-level proteinuria

Isolated proteinuria (+ or >0.3 g/L) is commonly detected on routine health checks, following exercise, during unrelated febrile illnesses or with UTIs. It is important to differentiate this transient physiologic proteinuria from persistent pathological causes.

When *low grade (+) proteinuria without haematuria* is detected, a thorough history and physical examination including measurement of BP should be performed. An early morning urine M&C and protein:Cr (UPr:Cr) ratio should be checked when systemically well. If examination and urine investigations are normal, transient physiological proteinuria is the likely diagnosis. No further investigation is required in this setting.

If *high-grade proteinuria* (+++ or >1.0 g/L) *without haematuria* is identified, then careful examination for evidence of generalised oedema suggestive of nephrotic syndrome should be performed (see Heavy isolated proteinuria and Nephrotic syndrome section below).

If *proteinuria with haematuria* is noted then patient should be investigated further as outlined above.

If isolated proteinuria is persistent then orthostatic proteinuria or pathological proteinuria needs to be considered:

- A normal early morning UPr:Cr ratio (after recumbent overnight) and elevated UPr:Cr ratio in afternoon after being upright during the day is indicative of *orthostatic proteinuria*. This diagnosis carries a good long-term renal prognosis and reflects alteration in glomerular haemodynamics with changes in body position.
- *Pathologic proteinuria* demonstrates a similar diurnal pattern. It may be differentiated from orthostatic proteinuria by the presence of elevated UPr:Cr ratio in an early morning sample. Daily protein excretion measured by 24-hour urine collection will be elevated in pathological proteinuria. Long-term renal prognosis will be determined by underlying renal pathology; thus persisting proteinuria requires further investigation and management.

Preliminary evaluation should include careful history of renal symptoms, medication exposure and family history. Thorough physical examination including growth, BP and general examination followed by repeat urine M&C, UPr:Cr, serum U&E, Cr, FBE, LFT and renal ultrasound. Patients with screening test abnormalities or persisting proteinuria should be referred for further targeted evaluation and management.

Heavy isolated proteinuria and Nephrotic syndrome
Nephrotic syndrome

Nephrotic syndrome is characterised by heavy isolated proteinuria (≥+++ or UPr:Cr ≥200 mg/mmol), hypoalbuminaemia (≤25 g/L) and generalised oedema. Renal function is usually preserved. It is usually idiopathic and steroid sensitive.

Initial evaluation and management should be directed towards confirming the diagnosis, optimising fluid status, management of complications, followed by specific treatment and family education.

- Confirming the diagnosis of idiopathic nephrotic syndrome (INS)
  - Generalised oedema
    - Usually dependent oedema. Scrotal/labial oedema is common and secondary cellulitis can occur in the setting of skin breakdown.
    - Ascites and pleural effusions indicate significant oedema.
    - Clinical monitoring of oedema and daily weighs are required.
  - Hypoalbuminaemia
    - Although less common consider nutritional or gastrointestinal protein loss on history and examination.
  - Proteinuria without significant haematuria
    - Confirm on formal measurement: UPc:Cr ratio $\geq$200 mg/mmol. Timed urinary excretion is not usually required in most cases of childhood nephrotic syndrome.
    - Haematuria should be mild (+/++) or absent.
    - Hyaline casts may be present but granular or RBC casts should alert to the diagnosis being acute glomerulonephritis (GN) rather than INS.
    - Macroscopic haematuria should alert to possible renal vein thrombosis or acute GN.
  - Preserved renal function
- Optimisation of fluid status
  - Extravascular fluid/oedema
    - Monitor oedema, body weight (daily or b.i.d.), BP, fluid balance chart, urine output.
    - No added salt diet is appropriate during oedematous state.
    - Fluids may be restricted to 1.0 L/m^2 per day.
    - IV 20% albumin (1 g/kg = 5 mL/kg) over 4–6 hours with frusemide 1 mg/kg at midway and end of infusion, may be considered if gross oedema, evidence of imminent skin breakdown, symptomatic pleural effusions.
  - Intravascular volume depletion
    - Should be considered if cool extremities, postural hypotension, oliguria, abdominal cramps (may represent bowel wall oedema or peritonitis.).
    - If evidence of severe hypoalbuminaemia and proteinuria, may consider IV albumin supplementation (IV 20% albumin 1 mg/kg over 6 hours $\pm$ frusemide 1 mg/kg).
- Recognition and management of complications
  - Primary peritonitis or sepsis
    - Multifactorial including loss of complement factors, immunoglobulins and impaired T cell function in addition to bowel wall oedema, venous stasis and bacterial translocation into ascitic fluid.
    - Most common organisms: *Streptococcus pneumoniae* or Gram negative organisms.
    - Initial therapy should cover resistant pneumococci and bowel organisms, (e.g. cefotaxime, amoxicillin and metronidazole). Advice should be sought from a nephrologist and infectious disease physician.
  - Thromboembolism
    - Contributing factors include intravascular depletion, haemoconcentration, urinary loss of antithrombin III and increased hepatic synthesis of clotting factors.
    - May occur as lower limb or pelvic deep venous thrombosis (80%), venous sinus thrombosis (seizures or altered conscious state), renal vein thrombosis (macrohaematuria) or arterial thrombosis.
    - Evaluation and management should be in consultation with haematologist and nephrologist.
  - Skin breakdown and cellulitis
  - Induction of remission and adjunct therapy
    - Prednisolone is first-line therapy for INS. Should commence at 60 mg/m^2 per day (max 70–80 mg) orally. Remission would be expected by 7–10 days. If failure to remit, discussion with a nephrologist is appropriate.
    - Phenoxymethylpenicillin 12.5 mg/kg (max. 1 g) orally b.i.d until gross oedema clears.
    - Aspirin (2–5 mg/kg per day) until gross oedema clears.

○ Management once into remission
  ▪ Prednisolone therapy
    – Weaning schedules may vary across nephrology services. It is clear that a duration of 6 months induction therapy reduces risk of relapse to approximately 30%.
      ● 60 mg/m^2 per day (max. 70–80 mg) for a total of 4 weeks
      ● 40 mg/m^2 per day for 4 weeks
      ● 20 mg/m^2 per day for 4 weeks
      ● 15 mg/m^2 per day for 4 weeks
      ● 10 mg/m^2 per day for 4 weeks
      ● 5 mg/m^2 per day for 4 weeks
  ▪ Low salt diet
    ● Until oedema has resolved and high-dose prednisolone reduced.
  ▪ Aspirin, penicillin and fluid restriction (if used)
    ● May be ceased once ascites and gross oedema resolved.
  ▪ Immunisation
    ● Should receive the 13-valent conjugate pneumococcal vaccine (13vPCV) once in remission if no previous booster given after 12 months age. A follow-up dose should be given if the patient did not complete primary vaccination.
○ Interim therapy and follow-up
  ▪ Patients should be monitored regularly for steroid side effects including HTN, obesity, poor growth and mood disturbance whilst receiving steroids.
  ▪ 23-valent polysaccharide pneumococcal vaccination should be given at 4–5 year of age and ≥2 months after 13vPCV. Ideally this should be given after cessation of steroids.
  ▪ Home monitoring for recurrence of proteinuria by daily urinalysis should be continued for several months after cessation of steroids. Recommendations regarding frequency of subsequent monitoring varies across different centres but often continues beyond 6–12 months.
○ Management of relapse
  ▪ Relapse is defined as recurrence of proteinuria (UPr:Cr >200 mg/mmol or >++ protein or urinary protein >40 mg/m^2/h) on three consecutive days.
  ▪ Relapse may be precipitated by infectious or immunologic factors or may occur without a clear trigger.
  ▪ There is no consensus regarding use of prophylactic penicillin; however, our usual practice is to recommend it when children have significant ascites. It is continued until ascites or gross oedema has resolved.
  ▪ Low-dose aspirin (2–5 mg/kg per day) is usually recommended when patients have significant oedema. There have been no controlled studies of aspirin to demonstrate efficacy in reducing the incidence of thromboembolism.
  ▪ Prednisolone therapy is of shorter duration when treating relapse. Again, there is some variation across centres but a suitable weaning program is outlined below:
    ● 60 mg/m^2 per day (max 70–80 mg) until proteinuria resolves (this may be continued for an additional week in many cases)
    ● 40 mg/m^2 per day for 2 weeks
    ● 20 mg/m^2 per day for 2 weeks
    ● 15 mg/m^2 per day for 2 weeks
    ● 10 mg/m^2 per day for 2 weeks
    ● 5 mg/m^2 per day for 2 weeks
○ Indications for referral
  ▪ Uncertain diagnosis
    – Acute nephritis features
    – Other multi-systemic features
  ▪ Complications of nephrotic syndrome
  ▪ Failure to respond by 2 weeks
  ▪ Frequent relapses or steroid dependence

Abnormalities of renal function
Estimation of GFR
Schwartz formula allows for estimation of renal function: *eGFR (mL/min/1.73 m^2) ≈ (36 × Ht (cm))/sCr (umol/L).*

Acute kidney injury
An acute decline in renal function may be evidenced by inability to maintain normal chemical homeostasis and fluid balance. Definitions vary but all highlight the importance of recognising mild changes in sCr and urine output as early signs of AKI. Evaluation of fluid status, nephrotoxins etc. should be undertaken even with small changes.

Evaluation of AKI (see table 10.2 Aetiology of AKI)
- Assess kidney function
  - U&E, Cr, calcium, magnesium, phosphate, FBE, LFT and urine output
- Acute or chronic kidney disease?
  - Clinical indicators of CKD (growth, Hb, baseline sCr, PTH)
  - Anuric non-catabolic acute renal failure
    - Serum urea (sUrea) usually rises 3–5 mmol/L per day
    - Serum creatinine (sCr) usually rises 50–100 μmol/L per day
    - Does the serum urea and Cr match with known duration of current kidney injury?
- Nephron number
  - Renal ultrasound: kidney number, size, cortical thickness, echotexture, cortico-medullary differentiation
- Glomerular blood flow
  - Hypoperfusion: often sUrea (μmol/L) >100 × sCr (μmol/L)
  - Renal Doppler ultrasound
- Glomerular permeability and surface area: markers of specific disease entities
  - HUS: haemolytic anaemia, thrombocytopaenia, LDH, haptoglobin, complement (if atypical)
  - Glomerulonephritis: haematuria, proteinuria, urinary casts, complement, GN serology

Table 10.2 Aetiology of AKI (GFR = nephron number × single nephron GFR)

Nephron number	
Reduced renal mass	Underlying structural renal disease Solitary kidney Ex IUGR Previous renal injury Chronic systemic disorders Chronic renal impairment
Single nephron GFR	
Reduced glomerular blood flow	Dehydration, hypotension Renal arterial embolism or obstruction Capillary endothelial damage; for example HUS, acute severe HTN Renal vein obstruction
Reduced glomerular permeability and surface area	Capillary endothelial cell damage; for example HUS, acute severe HTN Glomerular pathologies; for example glomerulonephritis
Reduced glomerular–tubular pressure difference or tubular damage	Tubular obstruction; for example calculi, tumour lysis, rhabdomyolysis Tubular swelling and damage; for example ATN, nephrotoxins, interstitial nephritis, pyelonephritis Tubular ischemia; for example hypoxic injury
Distal tubule obstruction (tubular–glomerular feedback)	Obstruction at pelviureteric, ureter, vesicoureteric junction, bladder wall, bladder outlet

- Loss of glomerular–tubular pressure differences or tubular damage
  - Nephrotoxic drug levels, contrast exposure, rhabdomyolysis, interstitial nephritis
  - Urine M&C including eosinophils
- Distal tubular obstruction
  - Renal ultrasound: hydronephrosis, hydroureter, bladder wall thickness

Management of AKI

- Minimisation of primary insult
- Minimisation of secondary insult
  - Careful fluid management, avoid fluid overload or dehydration.
  - Avoid hypoxia.
  - Maintain normotension.
  - Remove nephrotoxin exposure, minimise diuretic exposure.
  - Treat infection.
- Maintain metabolic homeostasis: careful fluid balance, electrolyte and glucose balance
  - Limit fluids to insensible losses (300–400 mL/m^2) plus urine output.
  - Sodium
    - Anuric: minimal intake
    - Polyuric: measure UNa and volume of urine. Often 75 mmol/L required.
  - Potassium: monitor for ECG changes of hyperkalaemia (decreased P waves, prolonged PR interval, widened QRS, decreased Q wave, depressed ST segment, peaked T waves, prolonged QT interval).
  - Hypocalcaemia: usually due to hyperphosphataemia. Correct before correcting acidosis.
  - Acidosis: correct with sodium bicarbonate (mmol = base deficit × weight (kg) × 0.3). Take care with correction if the patient is fluid overloaded (excess sodium) or hypocalcaemic (will be lowered further with correction of acidosis).
  - Hyperphosphataemia: low phosphate diet, phosphate binders (calcium carbonate).
  - Uraemia: acute rise to >30 mmol/L may cause CNS symptoms. Protein restrict if able, consider dialysis if nutrition is restricted by this. If unable to be easily corrected, consider dialysis.
- Enhance recovery
  - Provide adequate nutrition for recovery.

Hypertension
Measurement of BP in childhood

- Children >3 years of age should have BP measured.
- Children <3 years should have BP measured if risk factors have been identified. They include
  - Prematurity, VLBW or NICU graduate
  - Congenital heart disease
  - Recurrent UTIs, haematuria, proteinuria
  - Known personal or family history of congenital renal disease or urologic malformations

Definitions and measurement of blood pressure in children

- HTN in childhood is defined as the 95th percentile for gender, age and height. This is a statistical definition. It differs from the definition used in adulthood which is based on the risk of adverse cardiovascular outcomes. Nevertheless significant sustained elevation of blood pressure in childhood is associated with end organ damage and should be treated.
- Blood pressure should be measured when the child is quiet and cooperative. The widest BP cuff that can fit around the arm should be used. The cuff bladder should cover at least 80%, preferably 100% of arm circumference.
- Oscillometric BP measurements may overestimate BP and few are validated for use in young children.
- Always check high results especially if oscillometric measurements used. Check blood pressure cuff size is appropriate. A smaller cuff size is associated with higher readings.
  See table 10.3 Interpretation of BP measurement.

Table 10.3 Interpretation of BP measurement

Classification	Definition	Management
Normal BP	Systolic BP (SBP) and diastolic BP (DBP) <90th percentile	Check 1 year
Prehypertension	SBP or DBP ≥90th percentile but <95th percentile BP >120/80 to <95th percentile	Recheck 6 months and begin weight management if appropriate
Stage 1 hypertension (HTN)	SBP and/or DBP ≥95th percentile to ≤99th percentile plus 5 mmHg	Recheck 1–2 weeks, if remains high then begin evaluation and treatment including weight management if appropriate
Stage 2 HTN	SBP and/or DBP >99th percentile plus 5 mmHg	Begin evaluation and treatment within 1 week, more rapidly if symptomatic

Source: www.nhlbi.nih.gov.

For BP reference values
- See *http://www.rch.org.au/uploadedFiles/Main/Content/clinicalguide/bp˙charts˙boys.pdf*
- See *http://www.rch.org.au/uploadedFiles/Main/Content/clinicalguide/bp˙charts˙girls.pdf*

Rough rule of thumb
- BP systolic approximates 99% $\approx$ 100 +2 × age in years
- BP diastolic 99% $\approx$ 60 +2 × age in years (<10 years) or 70 + 2 × age in years (>10 years)
- Systolic and diastolic BP 95% $\approx$ 0.95 × 99%

Aetiology of HTN during childhood
- HTN in young children and infants warrants thorough investigation for secondary causes. HTN in adolescents, however, is not uncommon and may be primary in nature, related to obesity or may be due to secondary causes (see table 10.4 Causes of secondary HTN).

Evaluation and management of childhood HTN
- Aetiology and consequences of HTN should be evaluated. The extent of investigations will be determined by severity, likely aetiology and clinical findings.

Table 10.4 Causes of secondary HTN

Obesity

Renal
- Acute glomerulonephritis
- Cystic kidney disease – ADPCKD, ARPCKD, syndromic
- Renal dysplasia – reflux nephropathy
- Haemolytic uremic syndrome
- Renal artery stenosis – idiopathic, fibromuscular dysplasia, NF1

CVS
- Coarctation of aorta
- Mid-aortic syndrome
- Renal artery stenosis

Endocrine
- Aldosterone mediated – CAH, primary aldosteronism
- Glucocorticoid mediated – exogenous steroids and Cushing syndrome
- Catecholamine mediated – phaeochromocytoma, neuroblastoma, medications
- Thyroid mediated – hyperthyroidism

CNS
- Raised intracranial pressure

Medications

- Stage 1 and 2 HTN should be investigated. Aetiologic evaluation should include
  - Careful history including sleep (OSA), drugs, FHx, risk factors
  - Thorough examination including evaluation of obesity, 4-limb BP and pulses
  - Renal function, electrolytes, FBE
  - Urine M&C, UPr:Cr
  - Renal ultrasound with Doppler
  - Lipids, fasting glucose if overweight or family history
  - Drug screen/sleep study as appropriate
- Additional investigations for young children with Stage 1 and all children stage with 2 HTN
  - Plasma renin and aldosterone: low renin suggests mineralocorticoid-mediated HTN
  - Renal Doppler
  - Plasma and urinary steroid profile
  - Plasma and urinary catecholamines
- End organ evaluation in Stage 1 and 2 HTN should include
  - Echocardiogram: LVH and exclude coarctation of aorta
  - Retinal examination: acute and chronic HTN changes

Management of HTN in childhood

- Prehypertension
  - Recommend physical activity, dietary management and weight reduction if overweight
  - Pharmacologic therapy only if significant additional CVS risk factors
- Stage 1 HTN
  - General management as per Pre-HTN
  - Pharmacologic therapy if symptomatic, secondary cause or additional risk factor (diabetes mellitus, chronic kidney disease, LV hypertrophy, heart failure, or persists despite general measures)
- Stage 2 HTN
  - General management as per Stage 1 HTN
  - Commence antihypertensive therapy
- Pharmacologic treatment of HTN
  - Commence low-dose single agent to avoid rapid fall in BP then increase over several weeks to full mg/kg or adult dose, whichever is lower.
  - Short-acting agents allow more rapid changes in dosing, once HTN is controlled then change to a single daily medication in the same drug group.
  - Choice of agents may be guided by aetiology in cases of secondary HTN, however, generally HTN in children responds well to agents that block the renin system (ACE inhibitors, angiotensin II receptor blockers (ARB)) and β blockers. Ensure renin and aldosterone levels are collected prior to commencement. If there is a delay in this, then consider a calcium channel blocker.
    Note: ACE inhibitors and ARB are teratogenic (renal dysplasia) and problematic in patients with renal impairment. Patients should be counselled about the risks of these medications prior to commencement.
  - If a second agent is required add a calcium channel blocker then, after this, diuretics may be considered.
  - Referral to nephrologist should be considered if HTN is not well controlled on a single agent.
- Symptomatic HTN / HTN urgencies
  - Management should be discussed with an appropriate specialist with the aim to reduce BP by ≤25% over first 6–8 hours followed by a further reduction over the next 1–2 days.
  - HTN emergency is severe HTN with acute target organ dysfunction (CNS, CVS, renal)
    - Management should be in ICU usually with infusions (e.g. labetalol, nitroprusside)
  - HTN urgency is severe HTN without acute target organ dysfunction
    - Management should be in conjunction with nephrologist and usually involves oral and bolus IV agents
    - This may include
      - Short-acting nifedipine
      - Frusemide
      - Captopril
      - Hydralazine

- Propranolol
- Prazosin (oral)
- Clonidine
- Labetalol

Urological conditions

Antenatal hydronephrosis

A detailed antenatal scan and report will allow for stratification of post-natal investigations. It is important to review the antenatal ultrasound results. Hydronephrosis (HN) is graded according to renal pelvis AP diameter and calyceal changes (see Table 10.5).

Assessment and management

Perform a post-natal renal ultrasound (US) day 4–7 or within 24 hours if severe Antenatal hydronephrosis (ANH) in boy. If the ultrasound shows

- Abnormal kidney → refer to Nephrology for prompt management.
- Two kidneys present and either severe unilateral ANH or moderate bilateral ANH →
  - If severe post-natal hydronephrosis (HN4) then refer to Urology for prompt management.
  - If HN less severe, repeat US at 6 weeks.
- Solitary kidney with mild (4–7 mm second trimester or 7–8 mm third trimester) or greater ANH →
  - If HN mild (5–7 mm with normal calyces = HN1) or more then refer to Urology for prompt management.
  - If HN less severe, repeat US at 6 weeks.
- Oligohydramnios, ureteric dilatation or ureterocoele or other organ anomalies →
  - Manage according to kidney findings outlined above.
- If none of above apply → then renal ultrasound at 6 weeks is recommended.

Management after 6 week renal ultrasound

- No post-natal hydronephrosis: significant renal pathology unlikely, counsel regarding symptoms of UTI. If UTI develops then reimage.
- Persisting HN1 or HN2 with two normal kidneys, normal ureters and normal bladder: renal US at 6 months and follow below with reinvestigation or referral if UTI, loin pain or HTN occurs. DTPA/MAG3 if HN3 or renal AP diameter ≥15 mm at any time.

Table 10.5 Antenatal hydronephrosis grading[a]

	Pelvis AP diameter (mm)	
	Second trimester (T2)	Third trimester (T3)
Normal	<4	<7
Mild	4–7	7–9
Moderate	7–10	9–15
Severe	>10	>15

Post-natal hydronephrosis (HN) grading[a]

Grade		Pelvis AP diameter (mm)	Calyces
HN1	Mild	5–7	N
HN2	Mild–moderate	7–10	N
HN3	Moderate–severe	>10	Dilated
HN4	Severe	Gross	Dilated

[a]Note difference between antenatal and post-natal measurements.

- If N at 6 months: discharge.
- If HN1 at 6 months: US at 2 years.
- If HN2 at 6 months: US at 12 months, 2 years, 5 years, ±10 years.
- Persisting ≥HN2 with two normal kidneys and any distal hydroureter or abnormal bladder wall (≥3 mm beyond bladder base):
  - MCU under antibiotic cover.
  - If VUR, normal urethra and normal drainage film on MCU → manage for vesicoureteric reflux.
  - If abnormal urethra on MCU: refer to Urology for specialist management.
  - Normal or VUR with poor drainage: exclude VUJ obstruction by MAG3/DTPA and refer to Urology if abnormal. If nuclear study normal then follow up renal ultrasound as outlined above.
- Persisting ≥HN3 without hydroureter
  - MAG3/DTPA to exclude obstruction. If abnormal refer to Urology.

Posterior urethral valves and obstructive uropathy

Posterior urethral valves affect 1 in 8000 newborns and accounts for less than 1% of ANH. Epithelial folds in the posterior urethra form a 'valve' which prevents flow of urine. Severe obstruction results in foetal death. Less severe cases are at risk of UTIs and renal failure. The clinical features include an enlarged bladder and a poor urinary stream. The diagnosis is confirmed on an MCU.

Inguinoscrotal conditions

The underlying pathological basis of an inguinal hernia, an encysted hydrocele of the cord or a scrotal hydrocele is the persistence of a patent processus vaginalis after the completion of testicular descent.

The causes of groin lumps in neonates are

- Inguinal hernia – if lump is irreducible, irritable baby, tender lump in the groin, unable to get above it.
- Encysted hydrocele of the cord – unable to be reduced but a well baby and a mobile lump.
- Undescended testes.
- Lymphadenitis with abscess formation – rare condition, often not diagnosed until operation.

Inguinal hernia

Occurs when the patent processus vaginalis is large enough to allow bowel, omentum or ovary (in females) to protrude through the inguinal canal and sometimes, in males, down to the scrotum. The younger the child, the greater the risk of bowel or ovary becoming strangulated. Bowel strangulation in boys compresses the testicular vessels and may result in testicular ischaemia. Surgery is always required to prevent strangulation and this is done as a day case, except when the baby is <6 weeks of age.

Irreducible inguinal hernia

Urgent surgical referral is indicated. Most irreducible inguinal hernias can be manually reduced by a surgeon and surgery carried out within 48 hours. Pain relief is appropriate to aid with reduction but the use of ice packs or traction is inappropriate.

Scrotal hydrocele, encysted hydrocele of the cord

In these conditions, the patent processus vaginalis is narrow and enables peritoneal fluid, but not abdominal contents, into the cord structures. A patent processus vaginalis often closes of its own accord in the first 18 months of life.

The important clinical signs of a scrotal hydrocele are:

- Brilliantly transilluminable swelling.
- Narrow cord above the swelling.
- Swelling does not empty on squeezing and a normal testicle is felt in it.
- Non-tender.

If a hydrocele persists beyond 1 year of age, surgery is recommended and an inguinal herniotomy (i.e. division of patent processus vaginalis) is done as a day case.

Varicocele

A varicocele feels like 'a bag of worms' in the scrotum, best felt when a patient stands. It is caused by enlargement of veins in the pampiniform plexus. It is almost always on the left side and is associated with a dragging ache in the scrotum, though some cases are noticed incidentally. Varicoceles can cause relative infertility and should have a surgical assessment.

Undescended testis

Undescended testes can be

- Congenital: When the testis cannot be brought to the bottom of the scrotum, it is 'undescended'. This is caused by incomplete migration of the gubernaculum to the scrotum. An assessment should be made by a paediatric surgeon between 3–6 months of life and an orchidopexy done at 6–12 months of age.
- Acquired: Some boys present with undescended testis later in childhood (4–10 years). This is the result of failure of elongation of the spermatic cord with age, caused by persistence of a fibrous remnant of the processus vaginalis. Surgery is recommended if the testis does not remain in the bottom of the scrotum, to optimise fertility.

Genital conditions

Ambiguous genitalia

Genitalia that are frankly ambiguous need urgent consultation with an experienced paediatric endocrinologist or surgeon on the first day of life (see Chapter 13, *The endocrine system*).

- An enlarged clitoris in an apparent female is also abnormal and needs immediate referral.
- Hypospadias (see below) may overlap with ambiguous genitalia. This needs a careful initial assessment; if the diagnosis of hypospadias has been made, someone has already assumed the gender is male.
- If one or both testes are undescended, or the scrotum is bifid, or both, the baby should be treated as having ambiguous genitalia until proven otherwise, with immediate referral for further investigation.

Male genital tract

Hypospadias

Hypospadias is caused by the impaired development of the tissues forming the urethra. It affects 1 in 350 boys. The clinical features of hypospadias are

- The urethral orifice (meatus) opens on the ventral surface of the penis and does not reach the end of the glans.
- There is deficiency of the ventral foreskin known as a 'dorsal hood'.
- There is ventral bending of the penis known as chordee.

These features cause several functional problems and in severe cases can result in ambiguous genitalia. Surgical correction is performed between 6 and 12 months of age.

Smegma deposits

- Present as firm yellow–white masses beneath the prepuce in non-retractile foreskins (see Fig. 10.2). This is caused by peeling skin accumulating under the foreskin when separation is incomplete.
- Often confused with tumours or cysts of the penis, but are a normal variant and require no treatment.

Balanitis

- This is an infection under the foreskin with redness, inflammation, swelling and sometimes a white exudate (see Fig. 10.2).
- Immediate treatment with local penile toilet, that is soaking in an antiseptic solution, local antiseptic ointment (e.g. neomycin eye ointment) beneath the foreskin and topical hydrocortisone 1% are used in mild cases. Oral antibiotics (e.g. co-trimoxazole) may also be added.
- If the whole penile shaft skin is red and swollen to the pubis, IV antibiotics may be required.

Phimosis

- Phimosis is scarring of the preputial opening (Fig. 10.2). This causes
  - Urinary obstruction
  - Ballooning of the foreskin on micturition
- Phimosis usually requires circumcision or preputioplasty if severe, although mild cases respond to topical 0.5% betamethasone valerate cream applied four times daily for 14 days.

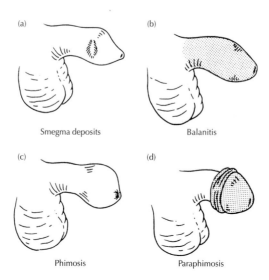

Fig. 10.2 Conditions of the penis. (a) Smegma deposits, (b) balanitis and (c) phimosis (d) paraphimosis

Paraphimosis

- This is an acutely painful condition, which results from a retracted foreskin trapped behind the glans, forming an oedematous ring constricting the exposed and swollen glans penis.
- Manual reduction should be attempted in all cases. To facilitate the procedure, use topical local anaesthetic cream (e.g. EMLA cream) 5 minutes before reduction, and consider the use of nitrous oxide. Ice and adrenaline-containing creams should not be applied. Failure to reduce the paraphimosis requires urgent surgical consultation.

Circumcision

- The indications for circumcision are phimosis and recurrent balanitis. There is no indication for neonatal circumcision.
- Hypospadias is an absolute contraindication, as the foreskin may be required for penile reconstruction.
- Circumcision is not required for cleanliness and <10% of Australian boys are currently being circumcised.
- It is an unnecessary operation with complications of surgery and anaesthesia.

Female genital tract
Ovarian cysts

Ovarian cysts can be detected antenatally and are likely to be physiological. Follow-up ultrasounds post-natally usually demonstrate reduction in size and resolution. Torsion can occur, and the development of complex changes in a previously documented simple ovarian cyst, particularly in the setting of an unsettled baby should raise concerns regarding this diagnosis.

Labial adhesions

Occur in infancy and often resolve by late childhood. They may persist through to puberty, but will resolve around the time of menarche under the influence of oestrogenisation. The adhesions are not congenital, but occur secondary to adherence of the atrophic surfaces of the labia minora presumably as a result of irritation.
Treatment

- Uncomplicated labial adhesions do not require any intervention due to the natural history of spontaneous resolution.
- Refer only if recurrent UTIs.
- Treatment with lateral traction to separate the labia is often distressing and is associated with a high recurrence rate.

- Treatment with topical oestrogen is unnecessary and is also associated with a significant failure rate and high recurrence rate.

Vulvovaginitis

This is the most common gynaecological problem in prepubertal girls. The vagina in prepubertal girls is relatively thin and atrophic due to the low oestrogen levels. The normal flora of the non-oestrogenised vagina is bowel flora. Overgrowth of this flora results in a discharge which is irritant to the labial skin (which is also atrophic) causing a reddened appearance. The moist environment between the opposing skin surfaces may also be exacerbated by urine, particularly in obese girls. Consideration of potential sexual abuse needs to occur.

Presentation
- Erythema/irritation of the contact skin between the labial surfaces
- Burning/pain with micturition
- Itch
- Offensive vaginal discharge

Management
- Simple measures – protecting the atrophic skin with Bepanthen or zinc/castor preparations.
- Ensure adequate hygiene, bathing daily.
- Avoidance of irritants such as soaps.
- Do not take vaginal swabs – they are distressing and painful. Swabs will generally culture mixed enteric flora. An introital swab is useful when there is profuse discharge or where there is marked inflammation beyond the labial contact surfaces in which case the overgrowth of one organism may be present (e.g. group A streptococcus). Thrush (candida infection) is rare in prepubertal girls as it thrives in an oestrogenised environment and vaginal pessaries should never be prescribed in prepubertal girls.

Natural history: symptoms fluctuate over time – until onset of puberty.

Vaginal bleeding

Causes of vaginal bleeding in children include
- In the neonate a vaginal bleed caused by the fall in maternal oestrogen levels is relatively common.
- Vulvovaginitis.
- Trauma (including straddle injury and sexual assault).
- Vaginal foreign body. A persistent vaginal discharge (often blood-stained) can occur. An examination under anaesthesia with vaginoscopy is required to exclude this.
- Urogenital tumours (vaginal bleeding or mass).
- Urethral prolapse may present as 'vaginal bleeding'. The red prolapsed tissue at the site of the urethra is diagnostic. Treatment is with topical oestrogen.

Vulval itch

Causes of vulval itch include
- Eczema. If this occurs elsewhere on the body, this can be superimposed on the symptoms of vulvovaginits. Treatment is then as for vulvovaginits and topical steroids.
- Threadworms (particularly if nocturnal itch).
- Lichen sclerosis. Whitened skin changes with associated splitting, blistering and resorption of labial skin. Referral to a specialist is appropriate. Treatment is with topical steroids.

Vaginal pain

Vaginal pain is distressing. Nocturnal vaginal pain usually occurs due to 'lost' threadworms in the vagina. Movement of the worms on the sensitive hymen and introital area cause a shooting vaginal pain. Treatment includes repeated doses of pyrantel (Combantrin) or mebendazole (Banworm) to ensure clearance of the worms and their eggs.

USEFUL RESOURCE
- Pocket guide to blood pressure measurement in children: National Institute of Health (*http://www.nhlbi.nih.gov/health/public/heart/hbp/bp̈child̈pocket/bp̈child̈pocket.pdf*)

CHAPTER 11

Neurologic conditions

Andrew Kornberg
Mark Mackay
Wirginia Maixner

Febrile convulsions

- Febrile convulsions (FC) are usually brief, generalised seizures associated with a febrile illness, in the absence of any CNS infection or past history of afebrile seizures.
- Occur in 3–4% of children aged 6 months to 5 years.
- Recurrent in one-third (more likely if seizures occur in early infancy or if there is a family history).
- They can be divided into
  - *Simple* = brief, generalised and single.
  - *Complex* = either focal, >15 minutes, or multiple in a 24-hour period.
- In otherwise healthy children, FC are not accompanied by an increased risk of intellectual disability, cerebral palsy, other neurological disorders or death. However, there is a modest increase in the risk of epilepsy.

Management

- A careful search for the cause of fever is required. Most will be due to viral respiratory infections.
- A lumbar puncture need not be done routinely following a simple FC, but meningitis should be considered in any unwell child, especially when there is a persistently depressed conscious state and in children with multiple or prolonged convulsions. The younger the child, the higher the index of suspicion of meningitis.
- General temperature-lowering measures such as removing clothing and administering paracetamol 15 mg/kg may help reduce symptoms of fever. It will not, however, minimise the risk of recurrence.
- Stop a continuing convulsion (>10-minute duration) with IV or rectal diazepam 0.2–0.4 mg/kg (max. 10 mg).
- Given that FC are usually benign and anticonvulsants may have significant side effects and do not alter long-term prognosis, they are not routinely recommended for children with recurrent FC. In some circumstances (e.g. children with a history of prolonged FC) parents may be taught to administer rectal diazepam or buccal or intranasal midazolam.

About 3% of children with FC subsequently develop afebrile seizures (epilepsy), as opposed to 0.5% of children in the general population. The risk is greater with

- Previous abnormal neurological development.
- A history of epilepsy in first-degree relatives.
- Prolonged (>10 minutes) FC.
- Focal features present during, or after, the FC.
- Multiple convulsions during a single febrile episode.

When counselling parents, remember that many will have felt that their child nearly died. It is important to emphasise the very low risk of neurological complications and excellent prognosis for eventual remission of FC, as well as the 1:3 risk of recurrence. Advice on the management of future febrile illnesses and FC is required. A follow-up visit is recommended to discuss what happened and help prevent the development of 'fever phobia' in parents. An electroencephalogram (EEG) is of little value in single or recurrent, simple or complex FC.

Paediatric Handbook, Ninth Edition. Edited by Amanda Gwee, Romi Rimer and Michael Marks.
© 2015 John Wiley & Sons, Ltd. Published 2015 by John Wiley & Sons, Ltd.

Epilepsy

Epilepsy (defined as two or more unprovoked seizures) occurs in approximately 0.5–1% of children. Seizures may be focal (partial) and/or generalised and the aetiology may be idiopathic (genetic) or symptomatic (malformation, tumour, scar, degenerative).

Benign focal (idiopathic partial) epilepsies of childhood

- Onset is typically in mid-childhood (peak 7 years).
- Seizures are commonly nocturnal or early morning. In the centrotemporal (Rolandic) variety, they are usually focal motor or sensory phenomena related to the face, mouth or jaw. The occipital variety may have visual manifestations. Secondary generalised tonic–clonic seizures may occur.
- On EEG, spike discharges typically occur in the centrotemporal or occipital region.
- Imaging is only necessary if clinical or EEG features are atypical or if seizure control is difficult.
- The prognosis is excellent as the seizures are usually infrequent and remit before the teenage years.
- Treatment is only indicated in children with frequent or prolonged seizures. Low-dose carbamazepine or sodium valproate is used for 1–2 years given the spontaneous remission of seizures.

Idiopathic generalised epilepsies

- Characterised by recurrent generalised tonic–clonic, absence or myoclonic seizures of presumed genetic cause.
- The first seizure usually occurs at 4–16 years of age, in an otherwise normal child who may have a history of prior FC.
- The EEG shows intermittent generalised spike wave patterns.
- The prognosis is generally good for seizure control and remission in later childhood or adulthood.

Symptomatic focal epilepsies

- This term describes a heterogeneous group of seizure disorders in which children have focal (partial) seizures from particular brain regions.
- Usually due to an underlying developmental (congenital) or acquired lesion.
- Complex partial seizures and focal motor seizures are the main seizure type.
- Complex partial seizures usually manifest by arrest of activity, staring, autonomic disturbances, semi-purposeful automatic movements (automatisms) and altered conscious state, sometimes preceded by an aura. Specific seizure manifestations depend on the brain region involved. Seizures may secondarily generalise.
- Seizures typically occur in clusters and may be difficult to treat.
- Children may have associated learning and behavioural problems, due to dysfunction in the affected brain region or the pervasive effect of uncontrolled seizures and medications.
- An EEG may show localised epileptic activity. Structural pathology is sought using MRI.

Symptomatic generalised epilepsies

- These are usually severe seizure disorders affecting infants and young children in which uncontrolled generalised seizures are associated with generalised epileptic disturbances on EEG and global developmental delay or regression.
- Examples include West and Lennox–Gastaut syndromes. The characteristic seizures in these syndromes are epileptic spasms (clusters of brief tonic seizures that are usually generalised and in flexion), drop attacks and tonic–clonic seizures, generally difficult to control with medication.
- West syndrome is also known as infantile spasms and refers to the triad of seizures (appearing usually in the third to fourth month), with a specific EEG pattern (hypsarrhythmia) and developmental regression. Infantile spasms are seen more frequently in association with other conditions, for example Down syndrome, Tuberous sclerosis, CNS abnormality.

Investigation

The decision to investigate a child following a seizure depends on many factors.

- Children with FC do not generally need EEG or imaging investigation.

- An EEG should generally be done in any child with a definite, non-febrile seizure, whether generalised or partial. EEG aids in the characterisation of seizures and epilepsies, but should not be used to distinguish seizures from non-epileptic events.
- Brain imaging is reserved for children with epilepsy in whom there is suspicion from history, examination or EEG that there may be an underlying cerebral lesion.
- Children with typical forms of uncomplicated and well-controlled idiopathic focal or generalised epilepsy do not require imaging. MRI is more sensitive than CT scan in identifying cerebral lesions, particularly subtle abnormalities of the cerebral cortex.

Management

- After the first afebrile seizure, only one-third of children experience further episodes. Therefore treatment is not normally commenced unless there are features to suggest a significantly increased risk of recurrence.
- Children with absence, myoclonic, complex partial seizures and epileptic spasms have usually had multiple seizures at presentation and require treatment.
- It is important to characterise the epileptic syndrome from history, EEG and sometimes imaging. This guides prognosis and the need for treatment, including choice of anticonvulsant.
- About 50% of childhood epilepsies have a favourable course from the outset, 25% gradually improve with time, and 25% are refractory to treatment.

Antiepileptic medication is only indicated in children at risk of recurrent epileptic seizures (see Table 11.1).

Principles of anticonvulsant therapy

- *Monotherapy:* most patients are well controlled with one anticonvulsant.
- *Titrate slowly:* most antiepileptic medications are commenced at a low dose and titrated up to the maintenance dose, to avoid side effects during their introduction (start low and go slow).
- *Changing medications:* introduce or change one anticonvulsant at a time, except in emergency situations.
- *Dosage variation:* individuals vary greatly in dosage requirements and tolerance. Young children and infants typically require relatively large doses.
- *Monitoring:* if seizure control is inadequate, or non-adherence or clinical toxicity is suspected, anticonvulsant blood levels may be measured for phenytoin, phenobarbitone, carbamazepine and valproate. Routine monitoring of phenytoin and phenobarbitone levels are indicated, especially in young infants and intellectually disabled older children in whom side effects may not be identified as easily. Other drugs are generally monitored with attention to usual prescribed doses and clinical markers.
- *Poor response to medication:* if seizure control is poor, the diagnosis and the choice of medication should be reviewed. Always consider non-adherence to therapy.

Depending on the type of epilepsy, one to several years free of seizures are generally required before anticonvulsants are withdrawn. This is done gradually over several months.

Parents also need to be instructed in the first aid management of seizures, and be given a plan for what to do when seizures recur. Safety precautions such as supervision in water and avoidance of heights need to be discussed. Driving and other lifestyle and vocational restrictions apply to older teenagers and adults with epilepsy.

Status epilepticus

A convulsion involving the respiratory musculature and upper airways that does not cease within a few minutes may cause hypoventilation with hypoxaemia and hypercarbia. Refer to Fig. 11.1 for proposed algorithm on acute seizure management.

- Seek senior assistance early.
- Support airway and breathing, apply oxygen by mask, monitor.
- Be prepared to give mechanical ventilation, particularly if the child has meningitis.

Table 11.1 Guidelines for the use of common anticonvulsants

	Generalised tonic–clonic seizures	Partial: simple, complex or 2° generalised	Absence (typical and atypical) myoclonic, tonic	Spasms and tonic seizures	Side effects (common or severe)
Carbamazepine (Tegretol, Tegretol CR)	++	+++	Avoid	Avoid	Drowsiness, irritability, GIT, rash
Clobazam (Frisium)	+	+	+	+	Drowsiness, irritability
Clonazepam (Rivotril)	+	+	+	+	Irritability and behaviour disorder, increased secretions
Diazepam (Valium)	–	–	–	–	Drowsiness, respiratory depression
Ethosuximide (Zarontin)	–	–	+	–	GIT, thrombocytopenia
Gabapentin (Neurontin)	–	++	Avoid	Avoid	Drowsiness, dizziness, ataxia, fatigue
Lamotrigine (Lamictal)	++	++	++	+	Skin rash (3%) – may be severe. Increased risk if rapid introduction or on concurrent sodium valproate
Levetiracetam (Keppra)	+	++	–	–	Behaviour disturbance
Nitrazepam (Mogadon)	–	–	–	+	Drowsiness, increased bronchial secretions
Oxcarbazepine (Trileptal)	+	++	Avoid	Avoid	Drowsiness, hyponatraemia
Phenobarbitone	++	+	–	–	Cognitive, irritability, overactivity or drowsiness
Phenytoin sodium (Dilantin)	++	++	–	–	Gum hyperplasia, ataxia, nystagmus, serum sickness-like illness, cognitive, rash
Pregabalin (Lyrica)	–	+	–	–	Weight gain
Sodium valproate (Epilim)	+++	++	++	+	Nausea, anorexia, vomiting, weight gain, severe hepatotoxicity (rare)
Tiagabine (Gabitril)	–	+	Avoid	Avoid	Headache, dizziness
Topiramate (Topamax)	+	++	–	+	Weight loss, sedation, cognitive nephrolithiasis, paraesthesia
Vigabatrin (Sabril)	–	+	Avoid	++	Excitation, agitation, drowsiness, dizziness, headache, weight gain, visual field constriction

Table shows relative effectiveness of each drug against each of the major seizure types. It does not represent a comparison of one drug against another.
Table represents suggestions only. Final decision of most appropriate anticonvulsant should take into consideration the patient's age, neurological status, co-morbidities, epilepsy syndromes, EEG, patient and parent attitudes and potential side effects.
Anticonvulsants listed as to "avoid" can potentially exacerbate seizures.
Sodium valproate should be used with caution in children >3 years old, particularly if multiple anticonvulsants are used and underlying cerebral pathology is present.
Cognitive side effects are seen with all anticonvulsants (particularly benzodiazepines and barbiturates).
For status epilepticus, refer to Chapter 1, Medical emergencies.

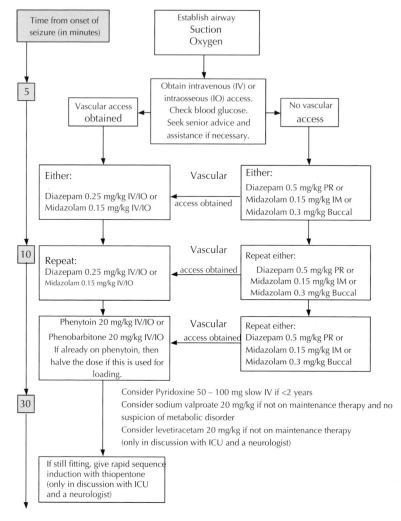

Fig. 11.1 Acute seizure management

- Secure IV access. Check blood glucose, electrolytes/calcium, blood gas. Consider blood culture if indicated
- If hypoglycaemia present – correct low blood sugar. See http://www.rch.org.au/clinicalguide/guideline_index/Hypoglycaemia_Guideline/
- Anticonvulsant choices include the following:
  - Initial treatment – Benzodiazepines
    - Midazolam: 0.15 mg/kg IV/IO/IM. Intranasal 0.2–0.5 mg/kg (max 10 mg) or buccal 0.3 mg/kg (max. 10 mg) can be given if no IV access.
    - Diazepam: 0.1–0.3 mg/kg (max 10–20 mg) IV/IO. May be given per rectum 0.3–0.5 mg/kg (max. 10 mg) if there is no IV access.

- o If the seizure does not terminate after two appropriate doses of benzodiazepines consider the following:
  - ▪ Phenobarbitone 20 mg/kg IV over 20 minutes in a monitored patient. Beware of hypotension.
  - ▪ Phenytoin 20 mg/kg (max. 1.5 g) IV over 20 minutes in a monitored patient. Beware of negative inotropic effect – infuse under ECG monitoring.
- o For refractory status epilepticus
  - ▪ Midazolam infusion 1–5 mcg/kg/min IV/IO. This should only be given in a high-dependency setting with senior staff involvement and can serve as an alternative to rapid sequence induction (RSI) and ventilation.
  - ▪ Propofol 2.5 mg/kg stat followed by 1–3 mg/kg/h IV for no longer than 48 hours.
  - ▪ Thiopentone titrate dose slowly to effect (usually 2–5 mg/kg) slowly stat. Beware of hypotension and be ready to control the airway and breathing before administration. This should only be undertaken with ICU support.
- ● Consider IV ceftriaxone (100 mg/kg max. 2 g) if meningitis suspected.
- ● Consider pyridoxine (100 mg IV) in young infants with seizures refractory to standard anticonvulsants.

  Prolonged convulsions may require large and repeated doses of anticonvulsant drugs or infusions and, consequently, mechanical ventilation. Suspect hyponatraemia as the cause of convulsions in meningitis and severe gastroenteritis-related dehydration.

Non-epileptic paroxysmal events

- ● Many children referred for assessment of epilepsy do not have epilepsy, but rather a non-epileptic paroxysmal disorder such as syncope, breath-holding spells, parasomnias or non-epileptic staring.
- ● In differentiating epileptic from non-epileptic events, the description of the event is important, including the circumstances in which the event occurred and the details of what the child was doing immediately before the event.
- ● Most non-epileptic paroxysmal disorders can be diagnosed on history alone, or with the aid of a home video recording of a typical event. In some circumstances video-EEG monitoring may be required.
- ● The long Q–T syndrome should be considered in any episode of fainting or seizure that is not clearly due to typical breath-holding, vasovagal syncope or a definable epilepsy syndrome (11.2).

  Table 11.2 lists some of these events and their salient features.

Weakness of acute onset

The acute onset of symmetrical limb weakness usually has a peripheral neuromuscular or spinal cord origin. Toxins (e.g. snake or tick bite), metabolic disturbance, systemic illness and psychogenic causes need to be considered under appropriate circumstances. Oral polio vaccine is a rare cause of acute flaccid paralysis.

Two key questions require urgent consideration:

- ● Is there a treatable cause?
- ● Is there respiratory or bulbar dysfunction of sufficient degree to warrant management in an intensive care unit?

Myasthenia gravis

- ● This diagnosis should be considered in any child with relatively acute-onset limb weakness, particularly if accompanied by ptosis, eye movement disorder, pharyngeal or respiratory insufficiency.
- ● A diagnostic/therapeutic trial of parenteral anticholinesterase is warranted if myasthenia is a possibility.

Guillain–Barré syndrome

- ● Presents with weakness (ascending progression may be less clear in young children), pain and sensory loss. Weakness may be misinterpreted as ataxia.
- ● The child should be transferred to a tertiary referral centre at the time of diagnosis, as respiratory weakness may occur rapidly.
- ● Intravenous gammaglobulin or plasma exchange need to be commenced early if they are to be effective.

Infant botulism

- ● Suspect in children 2–9 months of age with constipation and rapid onset of weakness, particularly with ophthalmoplegia and bulbar/respiratory weakness.

Table 11.2 Non-epileptic paroxysmal events

	Syncope	Breath-holding attacks	Shuddering	Benign paroxysmal vertigo	Self-stimulation	'Daydreams'	Confusional arousals[a]	Nightmares
Age	All ages	Infancy	Infancy	Preschool	Preschool	School	Preschool/school age	All ages
Circumstances	Always triggering factor or situational	Always upset or a trigger is needed	Any time, anywhere	Any time, anywhere	Any time, anywhere	Commonly school, watching TV, times of inactivity	First one-third of sleep (non-REM)	Second half of sleep (REM)
Frequency	Occasional	Varies greatly	Sometimes many per day	1/month or less	Daily or less	Varies, but not large numbers per day	Nightly or less. Rarely >1/night	Nightly or less
Onset	Gradual or sudden	Sudden, with or without crying	Sudden	Sudden	Sudden	Vague	Sudden	Sudden
Recovery	Gradual	Slow if hypoxic seizure occurs	Rapid	Rapid	Rapid	Vague. May be 'snapped out'	Returns to sleep	Remains asleep
Duration	Seconds to minutes	Seconds to minutes	Seconds	1–5 minutes	Minutes to hours	Seconds to minutes	Minutes	Minutes
Impairment of consciousness	Yes	Usually	No	No	No	Apparent but not real	Apparently awake but does not respond	Asleep
Observations	May describe light-headedness, dizziness or loss of vision. Tonic or tonic-clonic seizure may occur at end	Cyanotic or pale, limp, may develop opisthotonos /seizure	Rapid shivering movement maximal in head, trunk and arms	Frightened, pale, holds on to objects to maintain balance or falls	Posturing with stiffening and while lying on side or supine, leaning against firm edge. Irregular breathing, flushing, sweating	Blank staring but no motor automations or blinking despite long episodes. Not precipitated by hyperventilation	Screaming, crying inconsolably, may get out of bed. Appears terrified	Nil
Post-event impairment	Minimal	Mild unless hypoxic seizure occurs	No	No	No	No	No recollection of event	Good recall of event

[a] Including sleep-walking and night terrors.

- A child with suspected infant botulism should be transferred urgently to a centre capable of undertaking long-term ventilation and providing specific therapies.

Spinal cord compression
- Persistent or severe back pain and stiffness are ominous symptoms requiring prompt attention.
- Myelopathy should always be considered when there is paraparesis or quadriparesis without neurological dysfunction at higher levels.
- Brisk deep tendon reflexes or extensor plantar responses may not be prominent early and a sensory level is often the most important clue to a myelopathy.
- The confirmation or exclusion of trauma, tumour, abscess, haematoma or skeletal pathology is an urgent priority.
- Spinal imaging with MRI is required urgently even when acute 'transverse' myelopathy is suspected.
- Steroid therapy is important in spinal cord compression, before decompression.

Encephalopathies
- Encephalopathies are characterised predominantly (but not exclusively) by cerebral hemispheric dysfunction producing at least two of the following:
  - Altered conscious state.
  - Altered cognitive state/personality.
  - Seizures.
- The onset can be acute, subacute or chronic.
- Causes can be grouped into infective (or post-infective), hypoxic, traumatic, epileptic, metabolic, migrainous, raised intracranial pressure and drug or toxin exposure. The primary cause may be systemic or originate in the CNS (see also Chapter 18, *Infectious diseases and immunisation*, Encephalitis, p. 289).

Examination
Impaired conscious state or cognitive function is the cardinal sign. There may be widespread upper motor neuron signs. Meningism may or may not be present.

Investigations
Investigations are guided by history and examination. Consider the following:

- Electrolytes
- Toxin and metabolic screen
- Lumbar Puncture (microscopy and culture; viral and mycoplasma PCR)
  Note: For contra-indications to lumbar puncture see Chapter 4, *Procedures*.
- EEG.
- Neuroimaging: CT can exclude a mass lesion or acute bleed, but MRI is preferable in most circumstances. MRI of the brain and spinal cord may show multifocal demyelination in acute disseminated encephalomyelitis (ADEM).

Management
- Early specialist referral – early neurosurgical referral if raised intracranial pressure is suspected.
- Seizure control.
- Identify and treat the primary cause.
- Consider empiric antimicrobials, for example cefotaxime and aciclovir.
- If ADEM is suspected, consider high-dose IV corticosteroids.

Acute disseminated encephalomyelitis
ADEM is a monophasic inflammatory condition of the CNS that most commonly affects children and young adults. The usual presentation is with altered conscious state and multifocal neurological disturbance. It typically occurs following a viral prodrome and has been described following a variety of infections including measles, varicella, EBV, *Mycoplasma pneumoniae* as well as with non-specific febrile illnesses.

Clinical

- A prodrome of ataxia before onset is typical.
- Encephalopathy may vary in severity from irritability to coma.
- Multifocal neurological abnormalities such as ataxia, hemiparesis, optic neuritis, cranial nerve palsies and bladder dysfunction.
- A characteristic feature of ADEM is the evolution of symptoms and signs over time. New neurological symptoms and signs appear over the first few days (compared to other types of encephalitis where the onset is usually explosive without new manifestations after 24–48 hours).

Investigation

MRI is the investigation of choice and usually demonstrates white matter changes (although grey matter involvement is not uncommon).

Management

- General principles as above.
- Steroids are used in the treatment of ADEM despite the lack of controlled studies to prove their efficacy. Anecdotal evidence of their benefit is now strong. Steroid therapy may improve the patient's condition but withdrawal of treatment while the disease is still active may result in the return of original symptoms, or the development of new symptoms.

Prognosis

Early studies found a mortality rate of up to 20% with a high incidence of neurological sequelae in those who survived. Recent case reports and small series suggest a more favourable prognosis, with most individuals recovering fully. Residual deficits in higher cognitive function may occur.

Chronic and recurrent headache

- Migraine is the most common identifiable cause of recurrent or chronic headache in childhood.
- In adolescence, muscle contraction (tension-type) headache is also common.
- Although rare, raised intracranial pressure and systemic illness must also be considered.

History

- Determine the location of the headache and its quality, duration, frequency and time of onset.
- Identify trigger factors (food, sleep deprivation), associated symptoms (e.g. nausea or vomiting, visual disturbance and localising or focal symptoms) and the disruption to normal activities.
- Inquire as to whether the symptoms are progressive and if there is a history of recent head injury; development of visual, gait or coordination difficulties; or changes in personality or intellectual functioning; or a family history of migraine or cerebral tumours.
- Take a detailed social history.
- Consider recording symptoms in a 'headache diary'.

Distinguishing features

- *Tension headache:* tends to be persistent but usually does not interfere with sleep.
- *Migraine:* tends to have a fluctuating temporal pattern.
- *Migraine without aura:* usually frontotemporal or bilateral in older children. It is frequently accompanied by nausea and vomiting, followed by lethargy or sleep. Marked pallor is common and there is commonly a positive family history.
- *Migraine with aura or prolonged neurological symptoms:* uncommon in young children. Note that aura is not often reported by young children.
- *Intracranial pathology:* suggested by recurrent morning headaches; headaches that are intense, prolonged and incapacitating or that show a progressive change in character over time. Other features include abnormal examination findings, unusual migraine description and failure to respond to simple treatment measures. Such patients require urgent specialist referral.

Examination

- Do a thorough neurological examination, including visual acuity and fields, eye movements, optic fundi, coordination and gait. Measure head circumference and blood pressure.

- Assess the child's growth and pubertal status
- Inspect the skin for neurocutaneous stigmata.
- Palpate over the sinuses, cervical spine and teeth.
- Auscultate the skull for intracranial bruits.

Management of migraine

- Reassure the child and parents that migraine is not usually a serious condition.
- In an acute attack, all that is usually required is trigger avoidance, stress management and the early use of paracetamol 15 mg/kg per dose orally, 4 hourly (max. 90 mg/kg per 24 hours). NSAIDs (e.g. ibuprofen 2.5–10 mg/kg per dose (max. 600 mg) oral 6–8 hourly) can also be useful. In children with severe vomiting who are unable to tolerate oral agents consider ondansetron, metoclopramide and chlorpromazine.
- Prophylactic therapy for those with severe or frequent attacks is best used in consultation with a specialist. Propranolol or pizotifen are commonly used. Sodium valproate, cyproheptadine, verapamil, clonidine and amitriptyline can also be effective in some children.
- Two-thirds of children cease having attacks but 50% of these have recurrences in adult life.

Abnormal head shape

Craniosynostosis is an uncommon disorder of childhood affecting 4/10,000 children. It is a condition of pre-mature fusion of the cranial sutures resulting in an abnormal head shape. The resulting head shape depends on which suture fuses. The common shapes are scaphocephaly (sagittal suture), brachycephaly (coronal suture) and plagiocephaly (lambdoid suture).

Most children with plagiocephaly have a postural deformation rather than craniosynostosis. The incidence of postural (positional or deformational) plagiocephaly has increased with changes in sleeping position to prevent SIDS.

Management

- Frank sutural synostosis requires surgical correction.
- Postural lambdoid plagiocephaly is not associated with fusion of sutures and does not require surgery. It may partially correct spontaneously with changes in sleeping position. The asymmetric head shape becomes less obvious with hair growth.

Childhood stroke
Background

Childhood stroke is more common than brain malignancy and is among the top ten causes of morbidity in childhood.

Subtypes include
- Arterial ischaemic stroke (AIS)
- Cerebral sinovenous thrombosis (CSVT)
- Haemorrhagic stroke (HS)

Aetiology

- Arteriopathies
  - Transient; for example post varicella, dissection
  - Progressive; for example Moya Moya disease in AIS
- Congenital heart disease in AIS and CSVT
- Thrombophilias in AIS and CSVT
- Head and neck/ENT infections in CSVT
- Metabolic/mitochondrial disorders; for example homocystinuria
- Genetic conditions; for example Down Syndrome
- Haematological conditions; for example sickle cell disease

Clinical features
Common presentations
- Neonates
- Non-specific presentation with seizures, lethargy, apnoea. Focal neurological signs are rarely evident.

- Older infants and children
- Typically present with hemiplegia, early hand preference and lateralized neurological deficits.
- Patients with CSVT commonly present with seizures and signs of raised intracranial pressure.

Diagnosis
Urgent imaging is required for diagnosis
- CT head – will exclude haemorrhage but may miss AIS or CSVT.
- MRI or MRA head – within 48 hours.
- ECG and transthoracic echocardiogram – to look for structural cardiac defects including patent foramen ovale (PFO) with paradoxical embolization.
- Prothrombotic workup – should be done before anticoagulation, and includes antithrombin, protein C, protein S, plasminogen, activated protein C resistance (APCR), prothrombin gene 20210 A, anticardiolipin antibody (ACLA), lupus anticoagulant, serum homocysteine.

Management
Measures that have been shown to improve outcome in adults are likely to be beneficial in children.
  These include
- Correct fever, maintain normal glycaemia and normal blood pressure.
- Keep SaO$_2$ >95% in the first 24 hours.
- Close observations (initially hourly neurological observations).
- Maintain nil by mouth until assessment by speech pathologist.
- If seizures are occurring, load with IV phenytoin (or phenobarbitone in neonates).
- Early referral to a rehabilitation team should be made once the child is stable.
- Discuss acute antiplatelet/anticoagulant treatment with the Neurologist and Haematologist on call.
  For neonates with AIS
- Cardioembolic AIS: Aspirin or anticoagulation is recommended for 6–12 weeks.
- Non-cardioembolic AIS: Do **not** use anticoagulation or aspirin unless there are recurrent events.
  For children with AIS
- Initial treatment with aspirin, 1–5 mg/kg per day, UFH or LMWH for 5–7 days whilst being investigated for cardioembolic sources and vascular dissection.
- Treatment should be continued with LMWH or warfarin for another 3–6 months if dissection or cardioembolic source are confirmed.
- Conversion to aspirin, 1 to 5 mg/kg day is recommended for all other children for a minimum of 2 years.
  For children with CSVT
- Anticoagulation is usually recommended, except if associated with a significant haemorrhage, patient is hypertensive or other risks for bleeding are present.
- For CSVT **without** significant intracranial haemorrhage anticoagulation
  ○ Initially with UFH or LMWH.
  ○ Subsequently with LMWH or warfarin for a minimum of 3 months (neonates 6 weeks to 3 months).
- For CSVT **with** significant intracranial haemorrhage
  ○ Radiological monitoring at 5–7 days and anticoagulation if thrombus propagation occurs.

Head injuries
Assessment
- Determine the nature of the injury, its severity, the time of occurrence and the clinical course before the consultation.
- Always consider inflicted injury (child abuse) in infants and young children with head injury (see Chapter 29, *Forensic medicine*).
- Assessment using the Glasgow coma chart is essential (see Table 11.3).
- General and neurological examination findings will provide a baseline for further assessment and must be carefully recorded. In the unconscious patient the presence of brain stem signs must be assessed.
- In all but minor cases of head injury, cervical spine injury must be assumed until excluded.

Table 11.3 Level of consciousness – Glasgow coma scale

Eye opening		Verbal response (modifications for small children in italics)		Motor response	
Spontaneous	4	Orientated *Appropriate words or social smile, fixes, follows*	5	Obeys commands	6
To speech	3			Localises to stimuli	5
		Confused *Cries but consolable*	4	Withdraws to stimuli	4
To pain	2			Abnormal flexion	3
		Inappropriate words *Persistently irritable*	3		
Nil	1			Extensor responses	2
		Incomprehensible words *Restless and agitated*	2		
		Nil	1	Nil	1

Radiological examination

- Skull radiograph: not done routinely.
- Cervical spine radiograph: necessary when there is a suggestion that the spine may have been injured and in all patients with moderate-to-severe head injuries.
- Brain CT scan: indicated in all patients with significant head injury, particularly if there is the possibility of an intracranial haematoma, as suggested by severe headache and vomiting, a depressed conscious state or focal neurological signs.
- Brain MRI: indicated if there is suspicion of a spinal cord injury or a vascular injury or anomaly.

Blunt head injury

This form of injury is due to an impact on a flat surface that produces an acceleration–deceleration type of injury.

Effects

- *Scalp haematomas*: are common in the infant or young child. They may be responsible for a significant reduction in the circulating blood volume.
- *Skull fracture*: significant injuries may not necessarily have a skull fracture, but the majority do. Conversely, a skull fracture may not be associated with significant brain injury. The fracture is usually linear and it may extend to the skull base. The involvement of the nasal, paranasal or middle ear spaces implies that the injury is compound, with a risk of infection. Check for CSF rhinorrhoea or otorrhoea.
- *Concussion*: the most common and least serious type of traumatic brain injury. Involves transient loss of brain function, such as loss of awareness or memory of the event. The duration of unconsciousness is an indicator of the severity of the concussion.
- *Localised brain damage*: this is due to either local deformity at impact (which is not generally an important factor except for some injuries in infancy) or surface laceration of the brain due to brain movement within the skull.
- *Intracranial haemorrhage*: subarachnoid and subdural haemorrhages are usually due to a surface laceration of the brain. In extradural haemorrhage, a dural vessel is torn by distortion at or near the point of impact, especially if on the lateral aspect of the head.
- Intracerebral haemorrhage may result from local damage or a shearing injury within the brain.

Clinical course

Most patients rapidly recover from the effects of concussion in 12–24 hours. A delay or reversal of recovery suggests haemorrhage, brain swelling, infection or an extracranial complication – most commonly an impairment of ventilation, with hypercarbia leading to brain swelling.

Management
Mild
- A brief loss of consciousness (<5 minutes) without other neurological symptoms or signs suggests a mild injury and these patients can be sent home after an initial 4-hour observation in emergency.
- Explanation and written information must be given to the parents regarding signs suggesting deterioration and indications for re-presentation (see below).
- The patient should be reviewed the following day, either by the local medical officer or in the ED.
  Blows to the side of the head are potentially serious and these patients should be admitted.
See Box 11.1 Minor head injuries: discharge instructions for parents.
Serious
A more serious head injury is indicated by
- A longer period of unconsciousness.
- Increasingly severe headache with or without vomiting.
- A deterioration in the conscious state, behaviour or vital signs.
- Neurological defects.
- Bleeding or CSF leak from the nose or ear.
- Severe bleeding from a scalp wound.
- A superficial haematoma on the side of the head. This may be associated with an extradural haematoma, even if no fracture is seen on the radiograph.

Children with these signs will require admission and must be observed carefully for at least 48 hours.

Delayed presentation
This can be grouped into four categories:
- Clinical features of potentially serious head injuries – admit.
- Patients with a wide linear fracture and a large scalp haematoma – admit.
- Patients with a skull radiograph showing a narrow linear fracture, but who do not require admission on clinical grounds – discuss with a neurosurgeon and consider early involvement of a paediatrician.
- Apparently well patients – send home after appropriate advice, with instructions to return immediately if there is any deterioration.

Localised head injury
In these injuries the damage is predominantly confined to a focal area of the head. Injuries of this type are relatively more common in children than in adults.

Effects
- Simple or compound depressed fractures are common.
- Infection may occur with compound injuries.
- Focal contusion or laceration of the brain may be present to a varying size or depth, and may produce neurological signs or seizures.
- Concussion may be absent.

Management
- Radiographs are always required and should be done as part of the admission including, where indicated, tangential views. CT is indicated in focal injuries.

Box 11.1 Minor head injuries: discharge instructions for parents

For the next 24 hours keep a careful watch over the patient, who should be roused at least every 2 hours. The child must be reassessed immediately if you notice any of the following:
- The child becomes unconscious or more difficult to rouse.
- The child becomes confused, irrational or delirious.
- There are convulsions or spasms of the face and limbs.
- The child complains of persistent headache or has neck stiffness.
- Repeated vomiting.
- Bleeding from the ear or recurrent watery discharge from the ear or nose.

- Admission for neurosurgical assessment and monitoring is required in most cases.
- Prophylactic antibiotics are not indicated.
- All patients with external compound head injuries should receive antibiotics (flucloxacillin IV; also add gentamicin IV and metronidazole IV if there was contamination) and the wound covered by a head dressing.
- All patients with internal compound fractures (base of skull) with CSF leaks should be observed closely and given empirical antibiotics (e.g. flucloxacillin 50 mg/kg (max. 2 g) IV 4–6 hourly and cefotaxime 50 mg/kg (max. 2 g) IV 6 hourly) if they develop a fever with no obvious focus.

Care of the unconscious patient
General management
- Maintain the airway.
- Observe for vital and basal neurological signs.
- Protect the cervical spine.
- Ensure temperature regulation.
- Fluid and electrolyte balance.
- Nasogastric aspiration to avoid the inhalation of gastric contents (orogastric if the base of the skull is definitely or possibly fractured).

Anticipate complications
Early evaluation is essential to assess the development of complications, such as compression and infection. Observing for complications associated with extracranial injury is also important. The patient who is not improving should be referred to a neurosurgeon.

Cerebrospinal fluid shunt problems
Subacute shunt obstruction
Cause
- *Upper end block*. The tube is too long or blocked by the choroid plexus.
- *Lower end block*. The tube is too short or blocked by abdominal tissues.
- *Fracture/disconnection*.

Symptoms
- Headache
- Drowsiness
- Vomiting
- Seizures
- The same as a previous episode

Signs
General

- Increased fontanelle tension
- Abnormal cranial percussion note
- Focal neurological signs
- Change in vital signs
- Deterioration in the conscious state
- Recent increase in head circumference in infants
  Specific
- *Upper end block*. The pump depresses but it does not refill.
- *Lower end block*. The pump is difficult to depress. A radiograph of the chest or abdomen will give an indication of the length of the tube.
- *Fracture/disconnection*. The signs depend on the site of the disconnection. Ventricular tube disconnection is unusual and has the same signs as upper end block. Pump disconnection produces local swelling. Fracture along the course of the tubing may produce local swelling. Radiographs may demonstrate a disconnection.

Assessment

The neurosurgeon will want to know
- Type of shunt: atrial or peritoneal.
- Symptoms and signs, including the state of the pump and shunt tubing.
- Findings on plain radiograph, CT head or ultrasound.

Shunt infection

These infections are often indolent and should be suspected in any child with a shunt who is constitutionally unwell with fevers. There may be associated obstruction, with symptoms and signs as above.

USEFUL RESOURCES
- *http://www.rch.org.au/cep/* – Children's epilepsy program includes information about epilepsy, tests, treatments; proformas for seizure diary and management plan and links to other resources.
- *http://www.pedisurg.com/PtEduc/Craniosynostosis.htm* – Texas Pediatric Surgical Associates – includes diagrams and discussion about surgical management.
- *http://www.headaches.org/education/Educational_Modules* – A series of education modules provided by the US National Headache Foundation.

CHAPTER 12

Haematologic conditions and oncology

Anthea Greenway
Diane Hanna
Francoise Mechinaud
Yves Heloury

Haematology
Anaemia
Anaemia is defined as having a haemoglobin (Hb) less than the lower limit of the reference range for age (Table 12.1).

Causes can be broken down into

- Inadequate production
  - Bone marrow failure/replacement such as TEC (transient erythroblastopenia of childhood), aplastic anaemia, leukaemia/ tumour infiltration, metabolic disorders
  - Haematinic deficiency such as iron deficiency, B12/folate
  - Haemoglobinopathies such as sickle cell anaemia/thalassaemia
- Excessive destruction
  - Haemolysis
  - Bleeding
  - Sequestration into an enlarged spleen

Clinical features suggestive of anaemia
- Pallor
- Poor growth
- Pale conjunctivae
- Signs of cardiac failure – tachycardia, flow murmur, S3
- Fatigue, anorexia, postural hypotension, fainting
- Lethargy, reduced exercise tolerance
- Shortness of breath

Investigation
If anaemia is suspected, begin with a full blood examination (FBE), blood film, ferritin and reticulocyte count. The initial classification is based on the mean corpuscular volume (MCV) (see Fig. 12.1) (Table 12.2).

Iron deficiency
Iron deficiency is common among Australian children, but it is often subclinical. Anaemia only occurs in those with more severe deficiency. Iron deficiency may be present in 10–30% of children in high-risk groups. Iron deficiency may lead to impaired cognitive and psychomotor performance, even in the absence of anaemia.

Most cases of iron-deficiency anaemia in young children are due to inadequate dietary intake, although faecal blood loss may be provoked by cow's milk protein or rarely gastrointestinal diseases, including Meckel diverticulum. In older children consider recurrent epistaxis and in adolescent girls, blood is lost through menstruation. Consider urinary blood loss also. A full dietary history is essential.

Paediatric Handbook, Ninth Edition. Edited by Amanda Gwee, Romi Rimer and Michael Marks.
© 2015 John Wiley & Sons, Ltd. Published 2015 by John Wiley & Sons, Ltd.

Table 12.1 Haemoglobin reference ranges for age

Age	Lower limit of normal range of Hb (g/L) MCV (fL)	
2 months	90 (80–110)	
2 years	110 (75–90)	
6 years	115 (77–95)	
12 years	Male 135 (80–97)	Female 120 (80–97)
>12 years	Male 130	Female 120

Risk factors for iron deficiency include:
- exclusive breast feeding beyond 6/12, delayed introduction of iron containing solids;
- excessive cow's milk (particularly <12/12);
- vegetarian/vegan diet; and
- exclusion diet in association with allergic diseases.
See Table 12.3 for the variation in findings during stages of iron deficiency.

Diagnosis requires measurement of serum ferritin; however, ferritin is an acute phase reactant and may be misleadingly normal/high during an acute febrile illness. In such circumstances, a repeat measurement a month later (if not anaemic), or a limited empiric trial of iron therapy, is an alternative strategy. Measurement of soluble transferrin receptors can provide additional information, particularly in the setting of chronic disease. Serum iron concentration varies considerably throughout the day in normal individuals, is low in chronic disease and does not reflect iron stores. It can be used as a measure of compliance.

Remember that iron-deficiency anaemia secondary to a poor diet may be associated with other macro- and micronutrient deficiencies.

Prevention of iron deficiency
- Introduce iron-containing solids from 4–6 months.
- Avoid cow's milk in the first 12 months of life (apart from small amounts in custards and cereals).
- Cow's milk should only form a small part of the diet <2 years of age.
- Ensure that formulas and cereals are iron fortified.
- Consider supplementation in high-risk groups.

Good sources of iron for children
See also Chapter 9, *Fluids and nutrition*.
- Infant milk formulas.
- Fortified breakfast cereals.
- Meat (including red meat, chicken and fish).
- Green vegetables (especially legumes; e.g. peas and beans).
- Dried beans and fruit.
- Egg yolk.

Note: Iron absorption from non-meat sources is increased when taken with foods high in vitamin C (citrus fruit, strawberries, cauliflower and broccoli). Absorption is impaired if taken with calcium containing foods such as milk.

Management
- Dietary advice should be given in all cases. This includes increasing the amount of iron-containing foods and limiting the intake of cow's milk. Parents often need considerable support to manage behavioural issues around the diet, especially in the toddler age group.
- Supplemental iron should be recommended for any child with documented iron deficiency, even in the absence of reduced haemoglobin, because it takes a long time to replenish iron stores by dietary change alone. Behavioural changes and an improved energy levels and appetite are often noted with iron replacement even in children who were not anaemic.

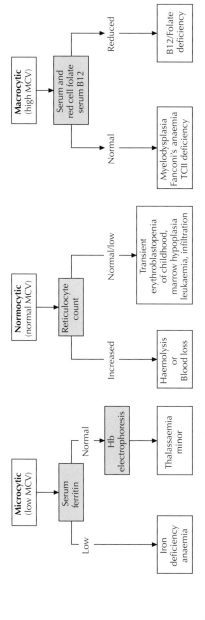

Fig. 12.1 Classification of anaemia; TCII, transcobalamin II deficiency.

Table 12.2 Classification of anaemia

Size of red cells	Causes	Relevant features
Reduced MCV	Iron deficiency Thalassaemia Lead Sideroblastic anaemia/CDA	Relevant dietary history Ethnicity/ family history
Normal MCV	Anaemia of chronic disease Acute blood loss/haemolysis Transient erythroblastopenia of childhood Mixture nutritional deficiency (iron plus B12/folate) Blackfan–Diamond anaemia (with other congenital anomalies) Aplastic anaemia/marrow infiltration	Poor growth Bleeding history Features of malabsorption Extreme dietary restriction Dysmorphic features – cardiac, renal, neuro, typical facies
Increased MCV	B12/folate deficiency Drugs Thyroid disease Myelodysplasia/Fanconi's anaemia	Neurological features – floppy, regression, seizures Dysmorphic features

- For young children, supplemental iron should be given at a dose of 2–6 mg/kg per day elemental iron and should be continued for 3 months after the Hb has returned to normal to replenish stores. The stools may become black/grey. As iron overdose can be fatal, supplements should be stored in a locked cabinet. In older children Fefol spansules may be used as the spansules can be broken apart or given as alternate day dosages.
- Parenteral (IV) iron supplementation may be used in certain circumstances (such as inflammatory bowel disease, extreme cases of oral aversion or if severe side effects with oral iron). There is a small but well recognized risk of anaphylaxis with parenteral iron.
- Blood transfusion should be avoided wherever possible but may be used if a very anaemic child requires urgent surgery or if cardiac failure is present. Transfusion should be administered slowly and only raise the Hb to a safe level such as 60–80 g/L (see calculating the blood transfusion volume, Chapter 12, *Haematologic conditions and oncology*, Transfusion therapy).

Vitamin B12 deficiency
Vitamin B12 is essential for DNA synthesis in rapidly dividing cells such as bone marrow and neuronal tissue. B12 deficiency is therefore associated with anaemia/cytopenias and neurological symptoms.

Table 12.3 Stages of iron deficiency

	Features on FBE and iron studies
Iron deficiency anaemia	Low haemoglobin
	Low ferritin
	Low MCV
	Low MCHC
Iron deficiency	Normal haemoglobin
	Low ferritin
	Low MCV
	Low MCHC
Iron depletion	Normal haemoglobin
	Low ferritin
	Normal/low normal MCV
	Normal MCHC

Table 12.4 Causes of B12 deficiency

Classification	Cause	Investigations
Dietary deficiency	Severe FTT/ food refusal, vegetarian diet	FBE, ferritin, active B12, homocysteine, MMA
Maternal B12 deficiency	− Autoimmune gastritis − Dietary deficiency − vegetarian − GI disorders − IBD, ileal resection, *Helicobacter pylori*, gastric bypass − Drugs − PPI, antacids	Maternal testing FBE Active B12 Homocysteine/MMA Anti-parietal cell and intrinsic factor AB ↑fasting serum gastrin, H. pylori serology
Malabsorption	Terminal ileal disease, Crohn disease	
Metabolic	Inborn errors of metabolism − cobalamin disorders	Guthrie card Urinary metabolic screen − organic acids
Genetic	− Immerslund-Grasbeck syndrome − TCII deficiency (transcobalamin II) − Juvenile pernicious anaemia	Associated with proteinuria Genetic testing − cubilin mutation, TCII

B_{12} deficiency in childhood most commonly presents during the first 2 years of life. The most common cause is nutritional, due to undiagnosed maternal B12 deficiency in a fully breastfed child. Dietary sources of B12 include animal protein such as meat, chicken, eggs and milk, therefore infants of vegan mothers or strict vegetarians with inadequate intake are most at risk.

Earlier age of presentation, absence of proven maternal deficiency or failure to maintain B12 levels after initial replacement should trigger assessment for metabolic/syndromic/genetic causes. Early involvement of a haematologist/metabolic physician is imperative for timely diagnosis of these rare conditions.

Any child with failure to thrive or neurodevelopmental abnormalities (particularly developmental regression) with an associated haematological abnormality (any cytopenia, macrocytosis or hypersegmented neutrophils) should be suspected of B12 deficiency and investigated urgently. The urgency relates to the potential for rapid neurological deterioration (seizures, apnoea, choreoathetosis) and the lack of reversibility if treatment is delayed. See Table 12.4 for a list of causes.

Investigations
- FBE − macrocytic anaemia, neutropenia/pancytopenia, hypersegmented neutrophils.
- Active B12 level (if serum B12 only is available and the result is normal/borderline but clinical suspicion is high request active B12 level).
- Serum homocysteine and urinary methylmalonic acid are essential to establish cellular vitamin B12 deficiency and to allow monitoring of response to therapy.
- Ferritin (coexistent iron deficiency is common).
- Maternal investigations − FBE, active B12, serum homocysteine, urinary MMA, anti-parietal cell/intrinsic factor AB, fasting serum gastrin.

Treatment
With proven deficiency and neurological features commence parenteral therapy with IM B12 (Hydroxycobalamin) 500–1000 mcg daily to second daily for 1 week until maternal/dietary deficiency proven. Ongoing oral supplementation can then be used once stores replete.

If there is diagnostic uncertainty, without proven maternal deficiency parenteral supplementation should be continued indefinitely.

Seek advice for frequency of treatment for metabolic causes.

Regular testing and clinical monitoring is essential.

Haemoglobinopathies
β-thalassemia
β-thalassemia minor is common and causes hypochromic microcytosis without significant anaemia or clinical symptoms. It is most common in children of Mediterranean descent (Greek, Italian families). One clue is an

elevated red cell count on the FBE (this will not usually be seen with iron deficiency anaemia). The diagnosis is confirmed by Hb electrophoresis (or high performance liquid chromatography, HPLC) demonstrating an elevated HbA_2 +/− elevated haemoglobin F. Iron deficiency obscures the diagnosis by reducing HbA_2 levels, so underlying β-thalassaemia may be missed therefore if the microcytosis persists after adequate iron therapy consider repeating the thalassaemia screen.

Thalassemia major is now uncommon because of the increased use of antenatal screening. However, the diagnosis should be considered in the context of hypochromic microcytic anaemia presenting in the second 6 months of life (i.e. after β-globin chain switch has occurred at 6 months). Hepatosplenomegaly, marked erythroblastosis with frontal bossing and bizarre red cell forms with significant anaemia on the blood film are usually diagnostic.

α-thalassemia

α-thalassemia traits are relatively common in Asian populations.

Children with α-thalassemia traits (one- or two-gene deletions) may be microcytic (from birth) although they will not be significantly anaemic and are asymptomatic throughout life (silent carriers). HbH disease (three-gene deletion) usually presents with mild-to-moderate microcytic anaemia plus splenomegaly. When physiologically stressed (fever/intercurrent illness/rapid growth/pregnancy), they can become more significantly anaemic due to haemolysis and may require transfusion support.

Hb Barts (four-gene deletion) classically presents with hydrops fetalis antenatally or at birth.

Note: The thalassaemia screen will not be abnormal in α-thalassaemia trait (as no abnormal haemoglobin is produced). Confirmation requires DNA testing to document the mutation and number of genes involved, and to provide antenatal counselling.

Sickle cell anaemia

Homozygous SS or compound heterozygous sickle thalassaemia (such as HbS/β-thalassaemia trait or Hb S/C) usually presents after 6 months of age (after β-globin chain switch).

Clinical presentations include

- Anaemia (haemolysis or ineffective erythropoiesis).
- Joint/bone pains due to dactylitis in infants (small joints of hand/foot) or vaso-occlusive crises.
- Acute chest syndrome (fever, chest pain, hypoxia and new pulmonary infiltrate).
- Arterial ischaemic stroke.
- Acute splenic sequestration (rapidly progressive anaemia with shock and splenic enlargement).
- Painful crisis (usually bone or abdominal pain).
- Asymptomatic diagnosis when parents are known carriers.
- Sepsis, especially encapsulated organisms in young infants.

Diagnosis

Diagnosis is made by blood film examination (anaemia, polychromasia, sickle cells, hyposplenic changes) and Hb electrophoresis (Hb S will be 70–90%). Sickle trait (Hb S trait) is usually an incidental diagnosis but essential to document for future antenatal counselling.

Management

Acute management of sickle crisis includes hydration, analgesia, transfusion support and often antibiotics. Chest syndrome and stroke usually require exchange transfusion. Specialist consultation is required for each presentation.

Long-term management includes folate supplementation, penicillin prophylaxis, vaccinations to prevent opportunistic infection due to asplenia.

Hydroxyurea can reduce frequent acute sickle crisis, and prevent recurrent chest crisis.

Chronic red cell transfusion may be required for stroke prevention, severe failure to thrive, recurrent chest crisis or frequent sickle complications requiring recurrent hospitalisation. Complications of chronic transfusion include iron overload with significant cardiac/endocrine/rheumatological/hepatic complications, risk of transfusion transmissible infections, and complications of recurrent venous access. Effective iron chelation therapy is essential.

Haemolysis

Acute haemolysis in childhood is a life-threatening disorder that usually requires admission, thorough investigation and potentially transfusion support. Severe anaemia can develop quickly over hours and frequent clinical review of vital signs and monitoring of Hb is required.

Clinical features include anaemia with pallor/fatigue/cardiac instability plus jaundice with dark urine. Additional features may suggest the underlying cause such as recent viral illness/vomiting/diarrhoea, transfusion history, family history/ethnicity.

Laboratory features of haemolysis include anaemia, polychromasia on the blood film, reticulocytosis and hyperbilirubinaemia. Other biochemical features include elevated LDH and low haptoglobin (haptoglobin is unhelpful in infants as hepatic synthesis is reduced).

Causes include

- Extrinsic to red cell
  - Immune mediated – autoimmune haemolytic anaemia (AIHA), drug induced
  - Consumptive, that is DIC
  - Fragmentation/mechanical – HUS/TTP/vascular malformation, prosthetic cardiac valve
- Intrinsic to red cell
  - Red cell membrane disorders such as hereditary spherocytosis/hereditary elliptocytosis, hereditary pyropoikilocytosis
  - Haemoglobinopathies – sickle, Hb E or β-thalassaemia, unstable haemoglobins
  - Enzymopathies – G6PD, PK deficiency

Investigations

First-line investigations include

- Blood film examination looking for
  - Spherocytes: hereditary spherocytosis, Coombs positive AIHA, ABO in compatibility in neonates
  - Fragments: microangiopathic haemolysis (DIC/TTP/HUS)
  - Blister/bite cells: oxidative haemolysis (drug induced or G6PD)
  - Sickle cells, bizarre red cells: sickle cell anaemia, thalassaemia, disorders of red cell membrane
- Reticulocyte count: indicates marrow response if low consider parvovirus/aplastic anaemia
- Direct Coombs test (IgG and IgM/complement)
- Blood groups and antibody screen
- Hb electrophoresis/isopropanol test for unstable Hb
- Bilirubin (unconjugated hyperbilirubinaemia), low haptoglobin, elevated LDH
- G6PD assay/red cell enzyme assays
- Eosin-5-maleimid (E5M) flow cytometry test for hereditary spherocytosis

Further investigation is often required once the acute episode has resolved, and usually requires input from a specialist.

Potential causes of acute haemolysis are shown in Fig. 12.2.

Treatment modalities vary according to aetiology above but include

- Haematinics such as folic acid, rarely iron replacement
- Transfusion support as required for severe uncompensated haemolysis
- Steroid therapy/immunosuppression
- IVIG
- Splenectomy
- Anti-CD20 monoclonal AB

Transient erythroblastopenia of childhood

This is a form of acquired red cell aplasia predominantly affecting children between 2 and 7 years old.

Anaemia is normochromic, normocytic and there is no reticulocyte response until the recovery phase commences. Jaundice is absent. A history of a recent viral illness may precede the presentation by several weeks. Bone marrow aspirate may show red cell aplasia with preservation of other cell lines. The prognosis for previously normal children is excellent, with recovery for most within 2 months. No specific therapy is warranted and blood transfusion is best avoided if possible (consider if Hb <50 g/L and no reticulocyte response with haemodynamic

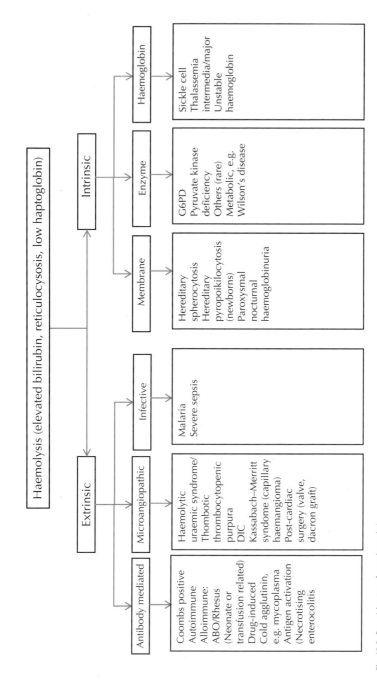

Fig. 12.2 Potential causes of acute haemolysis

compromise). The differential diagnosis is Blackfan–Diamond anaemia (DBA), which usually occurs at a younger age, but may be indistinguishable on peripheral blood and bone marrow aspirate findings. DBA is commonly associated with a range of dysmorphic features and typical facial appearance. A significant number of these patients will respond to steroid therapy, specialist consultation is required.

Coagulation abnormalities

Severe bleeding disorders in childhood can present at any time, however abnormal bleeding and bruising in the newborn period should raise a high suspicion. Severe spontaneous bleeding or bruising of multiple ages in unusual sites such as the chest/face or proven haemarthrosis should raise suspicions of a bleeding tendency. Severe mucosal bleeding (such as epistaxis/menorrhagia) resulting in anaemia should prompt further investigation and consideration of specialist consultation. Often coagulopathy screening is required to differentiate a bleeding diathesis from non-accidental injury.

Family history (including consanguinity), drug history and history of previous surgical challenges (including tooth extraction) are important. Routine coagulation screening preoperatively in well children is rarely indicated and coagulation testing should be guided by the clinical history.

Investigation

Knowledge of the variation of reference range for age is essential to avoid unnecessary anxiety and investigation in a normal child.

First-line investigations of a suspected bleeding disorder include

- Platelet count and blood film
- Activated partial thromboplastin time (APTT)
- Prothrombin time (PT) or international normalised ratio (INR)
- Fibrinogen

Interpretation of these investigations is shown in Table 12.5. Further investigations should usually be done in discussion with a haematologist.

Fibrinogen is an acute-phase reactant. In severe sepsis, when fibrinogen should be elevated, a normal level is still consistent with disseminated intravascular coagulation (DIC).

If the APTT or INR are prolonged a mixing study is performed. If full correction is seen a factor deficiency is likely and the appropriate factor assays should be done. If there is incomplete correction an inhibitor such as a transient lupus anticoagulant (which is not associated with bleeding or thrombosis and is likely temporary in association with a viral illness) is probable.

If the investigations above are normal in the setting of clinically abnormal bleeding, consider factor XIII deficiency (AR), von Willebrand disease, platelet function defects or a capillary fragility syndrome/collagen vascular

Table 12.5 Investigation of coagulation abnormalities

Screening test result	Causes
Low platelet count	Idiopathic thrombocytopenic purpura (ITP) Neonatal alloimmune thrombocytopenia (NAITP) Congenital thrombocytopenia syndromes Chemotherapy/marrow replacement
Isolated prolonged APTT	Factor XI, IX, VIII deficiency von Willebrand disease Heparin Factor XII (no clinical bleeding)
Isolated prolonged PT/INR	Factor VII deficiency Warfarin
Prolonged APTT, PT Low fibrinogen	Liver disease Disseminated intravascular coagulation (DIC) ± also low platelets Vitamin K deficiency, factor II, V, X deficiency (normal fibrinogen)

disorder. Specific investigations such as a PFA100, von Willebrand screen, formal platelet aggregometry may be required.

In the setting of acute severe bleeding, if the diagnosis of a specific bleeding disorder is unclear, consider treatment with 10–20 mL/kg of fresh frozen plasma (FFP) ± platelets. If fulminant DIC is suspected with low fibrinogen (<1.0 g/dL) give cryoprecipitate (5–10 mL/kg) as well as FFP, platelets and red cells as above.

Generally, children presenting acutely with a possible bleeding disorder should be discussed with a haematologist as specific treatment/factor replacement may be available/required.

General measures
These are applicable to all congenital bleeding disorders.

RICES: Rest, Ice, Compression (gentle compression bandage), Elevation, Splinting
- Analgesia
  - Do not give aspirin or other NSAIDs.
  - Narcotic analgesics should only be given as part of a comprehensive pain management plan.
- Do not give intramuscular injections. Do not do arterial puncture.
- Lumbar punctures should only be done after haematological consultation and appropriate factor replacement.
- Splinting limbs reduces pain.

Beware of the risk of
- Compartment syndromes such as Volkmann's ischaemic contracture in forearm bleeds or with severe calf bleeds.
- Femoral nerve palsies with retroperitoneal bleeds tracking underneath the inguinal ligament.
- Potential for massive blood loss with shock due to psoas/retroperitoneal bleeding.

Haemophilia A
X linked factor VIII deficiency: severe <1% FVIII, moderate 1–5% FVIII, mild 5–40% FVIII.

Management of bleeding
- Recombinant human factor VIII is used to treat all boys with haemophilia A. Dosage is usually 30–50 units/kg, which increases factor VIII levels by 60–100%. Note that 1 unit/kg of factor VIII raises levels by 2%. Repeat doses are usually required 8–12 hourly.
- Most bleeding can be controlled with one to two doses calculated to increase the factor VIII level to at least 50%. Higher doses are required for joint bleeding, major muscle bleeds, head injury with potential central nervous system (CNS) bleeding or prior to surgery where a continuous factor infusion may be required. A minor head injury can become serious; treatment with factor concentrate should not be delayed while waiting for diagnostic imaging if suspected bleeding of head/neck/chest or abdomen.
- Up to 30% of boys with severe haemophilia may develop a factor VIII inhibitor, such that they will fail to respond to usual factor replacement. On demand treatment for bleeding episodes then requires recombinant factor VIIa (Novoseven). The usual dose of factor VIIa is 90–180 mcg repeated in 2 hours. Specialist consultation is required.

Mouth bleeding
Use tranexamic acid tablets (antifibrinolytic), stabilizes clot formation (see Appendix 2, *Pharmacopoeia*).

Haemophilia B (Christmas disease)
X linked factor IX deficiency: severe <1% FVIII, moderate 1–5% FVIII, mild 5–40% FVIII.

Management of bleeding
Bleeding is treated with recombinant factor IX concentrate.
- Dose: in general 1 unit factor IX/kg increases levels by 1.6%.
- Frequency: injections at 24-hour intervals (the half-life for factor IX is 24 hours).

von Willebrand disease
The most common inherited bleeding disorder.

Clinical features include platelet type bleeding with bruising, epistaxis, menorrhagia or bleeding with injury/trauma/surgery.

Subtypes

- Type 1 is a quantitative reduction in von Willebrand factor.
- Type II is due to qualitative dysfunction.
- Type III is due to a severe quantitative lesion.

Treatment

Depends on subtype, extent of bleeding/type of surgery.

If von Willebrand factor replacement is required human-derived factor VIII (Biostate®) contains VW factor.

Many patients respond to desmopressin/DDAVP for minor bleeding/minor surgery (see Appendix 2, *Pharmacopoeia* – DDAVP) (see Appendix 2, *Pharmacopoeia*).

Idiopathic thrombocytopenic purpura

Idiopathic thrombocytopenic purpura (ITP), also known as immune thrombocytopenic purpura, is an acquired thrombocytopenia due to shortened platelet survival (immune mediated) in the absence of other disturbances of haemostasis or coagulation.

The most common age of presentation is 2–10 years where ITP usually presents with bruising and petechiae, often with a history of recent viral infection. In some instances there is oral bleeding, epistaxis, rectal bleeding or haematuria. Presentation <12 months of age is rare and should prompt consideration for other diagnosis (congenital platelet disorders).

Bone marrow biopsy is not necessary where the clinical features are consistent with ITP including previously well child (absence of fever, loss of weight, bone pain) with recent onset of symptoms, FBE and blood film is consistent (no anaemia, leucopenia nor blasts), no hepatosplenomegaly or lymphadenopathy.

Although bruising and petechiae can present dramatically, morbidity in ITP is usually minimal. Intracranial haemorrhage is the most concerning risk but the incidence is low (3 per 1976) or <1%. Evidence of mucosal bleeding may indicate an increased risk of serious bleeding associated with ITP.

Management

Controversy surrounds the indications and best form of treatment for children with acute ITP. Without active treatment, most patients' platelet counts return to normal within 3–6 months. Common treatment modalities including steroids and IVIG have been shown to increase the platelet count more quickly but do not alter the natural history of the disease including rate of remission. Bleeding complications have been observed equally in children on treatment and in those conservatively managed with observation only.

Therefore careful observation without specific treatment may be appropriate in milder cases, in older children where activity can be modified, and where close clinical surveillance is possible. Patients with active bleeding (e.g. mucosal and gastrointestinal) should receive treatment to increase their platelet count more rapidly.

When treatment is indicated, corticosteroids are often first-line therapy. Immunoglobulin (IVIG) has similar efficacy with more rapid onset of action. IVIG may be an appropriate choice if there are concerns about steroid side effects, if more rapid improvement in platelet count is required or to avoid steroids if there is diagnostic uncertainty.

Various steroid regimens have been used. Doses from 1–4 mg/kg per day (prednisolone) with rapid taper (over 4 weeks) after documented response have been used with no specific regime found to be superior. The following has been demonstrated to raise the count almost as quickly as IVIG: prednisolone 4 mg/kg for 1 week (maximum 75 mg per day), then 2 mg/kg for 1 week followed by 1 mg/kg for 1 week.

Modification of activity to avoid contact sports and rough physical activity should be discussed with the child and family. Avoidance of aspirin/NSAIDs is recommended. Intramuscular injections and other invasive procedures should be deferred until thrombocytopenia remits or treatment should be considered.

Following recovery, relapse may occur with future viral infections usually in the year after diagnosis.

Chronic ITP (lasting >12 months) occurs in <10% and requires specialist management. Treatment options include therapy as for acute ITP or splenectomy, or the use of monoclonal anti-CD20 antibody. The risk–benefit ratio of these second-line treatments should be carefully considered and discussed with a paediatric haematologist.

Neutropenia

Neutrophil count lower than the reference range for age.

General definitions

Mild neutropenia $>1.0 \times 10^9$/L

Moderate $0.5–1.0 \times 10^9$/L

Severe $<0.5 \times 10^9$/L

Very severe $<0.2 \times 10^9$/L

Interpretation with knowledge of reference range for age is essential, also racial variation with lower counts in African American and Middle Eastern populations is well described.

Causes can be generally divided into two mechanisms: Failure of production (bone marrow disorders) versus immune-mediated peripheral destruction.

- Transient neutropenia associated with infection (days to weeks)
- Immune neutropenia (months to years) – NAIN (neonatal alloimmune neutropenia) or autoimmune (older children)
- Cyclical neutropenia (may be familial)
- B12 or folate deficiency
- Drug induced
- Associated with autoimmune disorders – SLE, IBD
- Marrow infiltration – leukaemia/lymphoma, neuroblastoma (NB), aplasia
- Splenic sequestration
- Severe congenital neutropenia – Kostmans syndrome
- Syndromic – Schwachman–Diamond syndrome (FTT, exocrine pancreatic insufficiency, associated congenital anomalies), Fanconi's anaemia, dyskeratosis congenita, Chediak–Hiagashi, reticular dysgenesis, Pearson syndrome

Clinical features

- Family history, birth history/maternal history, early/unusual bacterial infections, poor growth/FTT, dysmorphic features.
- Periodic symptoms with fever, mouth ulcers, infections suggestive of cyclical neutropenia (cycles often occur every 3–4 weeks, lasting 3–6 days at a time).
- Suspicious infections include chronic diarrhoea, recurrent sinopulmonary infections/pneumonia, periodontitis, cellulitis, bone/joint infections such as osteomyelitis.
- Long-standing neutropenia is associated with risk of fungal infection.

Baseline investigations

- FBE and film, consider weekly FBE for 6 weeks for cyclical neutropenia
- Maternal FBE/NAIN screen in neonates
- Hepatic and renal function, active B12/ folate
- Consider immune markers if suggestive features: ANA, ENA, DSdna, Rh Factor
- Consider immune function – immunoglobulins, lymphocyte subsets
- Bone marrow aspirate – essential for severe, early onset neutropenia with significant infections or prior to GCSF therapy
- Genetic testing – known mutations such as ELANE (neutrophil elastase) particularly in the congenital group

Treatment

- For non-neonatal cases that are well close clinical surveillance with neutropenic precautions (assessment/admission to hospital for septic work up and parenteral antibiotics until cultures negative) may be adequate.
- Avoid PR medications, care with dental procedures as risk bacteraemia.
- Consider vaccination status (care with live vaccines).
- If significant infections/severe congenital neutropenia/possible syndromic diagnosis specialist input is required with consideration of GCSF therapy after bone marrow aspirate.

Anticoagulation therapy in children

Thromboembolic disease is increasingly frequent in neonates and children, presumably because of increased survival of children with previously fatal primary disorders and the increased use of invasive arterial and central venous catheters (CVCs), as well as extracorporeal circuits. Consequently the frequency of anticoagulant use in children is increasing, for both treatment and prophylaxis.

The coagulation systems of children and adults are physiologically different, which impacts the use of investigations, and the action/pharmacokinetics of anticoagulant medications in children. Current literature suggests children receiving anticoagulant therapy appear to have higher treatment failure rates and more bleeding complications than adults. Anticoagulation in children should be managed by or in consultation with specialist paediatric haematologists.

The most commonly used anticoagulant agents in children are unfractionated heparin (UFH), low-molecular-weight heparin (LMWH) and warfarin.

- UFH is given by continuous IV infusion and is advantageous because of its rapid onset of action, short half-life and reversibility. However, there is controversy over appropriate therapeutic ranges in children and the interpretation of currently available monitoring tests including the APTT and anti-Xa. Heparin-induced thrombocytopenia appears to be significantly less frequent in children than in adults.

- LMWH is frequently used because of its more predictable bioavailability and weight-adjusted dosing schedules, and reduced need for therapeutic monitoring. A number of LMWH preparations are available, but most experience in children is with enoxaparin (Clexane). Twice daily subcutaneous dosing is recommended, but the inability to completely reverse LMWH once given, limits its use in very sick children. Extreme care must be taken when children are having procedures (e.g. lumbar puncture), and at least two doses should be omitted before any procedure. Monitoring of LMWH is via the anti-Xa assay. The generally accepted therapeutic range is 0.5–1.0 anti-factor Xa units/mL (4–6 hours after the dose). Like UFH, LMWH is excreted via the kidneys and half-life may be prolonged in renal disease. APTT does not reflect the anticoagulant activity of LMWH and may be normal in a fully anticoagulated child.

- Warfarin is the agent of choice for long-term therapy, but there is a multitude of paediatric-specific issues. There is no paediatric preparation, resulting in complicated dosing schedules. Avoidance of half or quarter tablets can be achieved by variable daily doses (e.g. alternating daily doses, 1 mg one day and 2 mg the next). Dietary variation and the effect of intercurrent illness on stability of anticoagulation is a significant issue in paediatric patients. Warfarin is particularly difficult to manage in infants <6 months due to variable concentrations in breast milk, supplementation of formula and variability of oral intake in this age group.

  Monitoring is now significantly easier with 'point of care' capillary blood monitors, although the accuracy is operator dependent and technical limitations remain (especially at higher therapeutic ranges).

  Lifestyle restrictions are necessary for children on long-term warfarin (avoidance of contact sports), which may impact on adherence. Long-term issues include reduced bone density, which requires ongoing surveillance.

- Thrombolytic therapy (tPA) in children is reported to cause major bleeding (intracranial or shock requiring transfusion) in >10%, with variable treatment success rates reported. Consideration may be necessary in the setting of life- or limb-threatening thrombosis. Specialist management with a paediatric haematologist is essential.

See RCH *anticoagulation* clinical practice guideline *http://www.chestnet.org/Guidelines-and-Resources/Guidelines-and-Consensus-Statements/Antithrombotic-Guidelines-9th-Ed*

Transfusion therapy

Blood transfusion is common in the tertiary paediatric setting. The most common blood product transfused is packed red cells.

Indications for red cells include

- acute restoration of oxygen-carrying capacity (i.e. to relieve symptomatic or predictably progressive anaemia);
- to achieve marrow suppression in chronic ineffective erythropoiesis (e.g. thalassemia major, sickle cell anaemia).

Transfusion should only occur when expected benefits outweigh the potential risks. Nutritional anaemia rarely, if ever requires transfusion as the onset is chronic and usually well tolerated. Knowledge of the expected time course of recovery with appropriate nutritional supplementation is important to discuss with the family.

To calculate the desired transfusion volume, the following formula can be used:

Packed red cells (mL) = weight (kg) × Hb rise required (g/L) × 0.4

See RCH *Blood product transfusion* clinical practice guideline *http://www.rch.org.au/clinicalguide/guideline_index/Blood_product_transfusion/*

Indications for platelets may include
- severe thrombocytopenia platelet count $10–50 \times 10^9/L$
- assess additional risk factors which lower bleeding threshold such as fever, sepsis, coagulopathy, known CNS lesion, surgery/invasive procedure
- platelet function defect with bleeding or surgery/trauma
- thrombocytopenia associated with massive transfusion
  To calculate dose the following formula can be used:
  Platelet volume to be transfused = 5–10 mL/kg (expected to raise platelet count by $50–100 \times 10^9/L$).
Indications for FFP include
- coagulopathy due to liver disease;
- bleeding associated with warfarin therapy, rapid reversal of warfarin (prothrombin complex concentrates such as Prothombinex® may also be used);
- disseminated intravascular coagulation; and
- massive transfusion.
  To calculate dose of FFP the following can be used:
  FFP volume to be transfused = 10–20 mL/kg
Indications for cryoprecipitate (concentrated source of fibrinogen)
- Low fibrinogen – associated with DIC/massive transfusion/liver disease
- Dysfibrinogenaemia
  To calculate dose of cryoprecipitate the following can be used:
  Cryoprecipitate = 5–10 mL/kg
Also consider the specifics of paediatric blood products (such as paediatric platelets, FFP and red cells) when prescribing blood products to avoid unnecessary donor exposure, transfusion complications and wastage.
  Special requirements may include
- Irradiated blood products (to reduce the risk of graft vs. host disease)
- CMV seronegative products (leukodeplete products are considered to be CMV safe for the majority of patients)
  Further information is available at Blood products CPG
Informed consent must be obtained and documented in the medical record, including
- indication for transfusion, risks if transfusion not undertaken;
- type of blood product, calculation of volume and expected outcome;
- potential alternative if any; and
- discussion of risks of transfusion.
  Positive patient identification, correct specimen labelling and careful checking of the blood prescription and product to be transfused is essential to prevent near miss or adverse events such as wrong blood in tube (WIBIT) or incompatible transfusion.

Adverse reactions of blood transfusion
Management of a potential transfusion reaction involves the 3 Rs:
- Recognise
- React
- Report
  See Table 12.6

Oncology
Cancer in childhood is relatively rare. Approximately 1 in 600 children will develop a malignancy before the age of 15 years.

Presentation of childhood malignancies
Malignancy should be considered in children presenting with any of the following:
- Fever, pallor, bruising or petechiae, and bone pain
- Lymphadenopathy – marked, progressive or persistent, localised or generalised
- Hepatosplenomegaly
- Recurring morning headache, particularly if associated with vomiting or visual disturbance

Table 12.6 Adverse effects of transfusion

Type of reaction	Symptoms	Treatment
Allergic reactions (1–3%)	Hives/urticaria, rash, itch, wheeze	Antihistamine, steroids
Febrile, non-haemolytic transfusion reaction (0.1–1%)	Fever, chills, (release of cytokines for residual lymphocytes) No haemodynamic instability, no haemolysis	Anti-pyretic, antihistamines, consider blood cultures +/− antibiotics (Reduced by pre-storage leukodepletion)
Sepsis/bacterial contamination (1 in 75,000 to 1 in 500,000)	Fever, hypotension, haemodynamic instability	Resuscitation, blood cultures, antibiotics Prevention, correct storage of blood, completion of transfusion within 4 hours of issue
Acute haemolytic transfusion reaction – incompatible transfusion	Haemodynamic instability, pain, coagulopathy, dark urine, jaundice, fear/sense of impending doom	Resuscitation, supportive care
Transfusion associated cardiac overload (TACO) <1%	Hypertension, shortness of breath, oedema	Supportive care, diuretics
TRALI: transfusion related acute lung injury, 1 in 5000 to 190,000	Respiratory symptoms <4/24 of transfusion, hypoxia, white out on CXR	Supportive care, notify haematologist for further investigation
TAGVHD – transfusion associated graft versus host disease		Specialist consultation Avoid with appropriate irradiation of blood products
Transfusion transmitted Infections	HIV <1 in a million Hepatitis B and C <1 in a million HTLV I/II <1 in a million Malaria <1 in 10 million Bacterial infection 1in 500,000 (red cells); 1 in 75,000 (platelets)	Surveillance, specialist consultation and management required

- Ataxia, cranial nerve palsies, or other neurological signs, particularly when associated with headache or back pain
- New onset of dry cough, or stridor, without other symptoms of respiratory infection, particularly if associated with orthopnoea
- Any unusual mass or swelling
- Persistent severe unexplained pain, especially bone or joint pain
- Unexplained weight loss
  When a suspicion of a malignancy arises, investigation should be done in consultation with a paediatric oncologist.
  Types of emergencies (see Table 12.7)
- Mass lesions: mediastinal masses (solid or liquid tumours), spinal cord compression, increased intracranial pressure (ICP)
- Haematologic/metabolic: hyperleukocytosis, tumour lysis syndrome (TLS), cerebrovascular accident (CVA)
- Immunosuppression: typhlitis

CNS tumours
Background and aetiology
CNS tumours comprise approximately 20% of all childhood cancers, gliomas being the most common. Most CNS tumours (80–90%) originate in the supratentorial area (cerebral hemispheres or midline), but are infrequently located in the posterior fossa (3–12%) and spinal cord (5–10%).

The causes of brain tumours remain largely unknown. Certain familial cancer predisposition syndromes are associated with an increased risk including neurofibromatosis type I (NF1), Li-Fraumeni syndrome (p53), and

Table 12.7 Oncologic emergencies

Emergency	Presentation	Differential diagnosis	Management
Superior medistinal syndrome (SVC)	Orthopnoea Cough, shortness of breath, respiratory arrest Venous engorgement: facial swelling, plethora, syncope	NHL – B or T Hodgkin lymphoma Acute lymphoblastic leukaemia (ALL); rarely acute myeloid leukaemia (AML) Germ cell tumour Thymoma Neuroblastoma Sarcoma	*Investigations:* CXR – wide mediastinum, tracheal deviation, narrowing CT chest Echocardiogram *Treatment:* Airway – use least invasive method with minimal sedation. VC – heparinisation/thrombectomy, IV access (femoral) Tumour – steroids and chemotherapy (CTx).
Spinal cord compression	Back pain (80%) – especially if pain has radicular component or is not relieved in supine position Neurologic signs - weakness, sensory abnormalities, urinary and faecal incontinence or retention	Any tumour type. Most commonly: Neuroblastoma Sarcoma Leukaemia/lymphoma CNS tumour/ metastases	*Investigations:* MRI spine – contrast will show intra-spinal lesion. *Treatment:* Dexamethasone 0.25–0.5 mg/kg q.i.d. – If <80% compression: dexamethasone + radiotherapy (XRT) or CTX – If ≥80% compression: dexamethasone + XRT or surgery (laminectomy)
Hyperleukocytosis (WCC >100,000 cells/mm^3)	CNS leukostasis: headache, mental status change, seizures, coma, death *Note:* risk of intracranial haemorrhage if thrombocytopenic or coagulopathic. Pulmonary leukostasis: Triad of respiratory symptoms, hypoxia and infiltrates on CXR. *Note:* risk of pulmonary haemorrhage.	ALL – higher risk of tumour lysis syndrome AML – higher risk of hyperviscosity	*Treatment:* Hyperhydration (decrease hyperviscosity) Avoid diuretics initially Avoid PRBCs (increases hyperviscosity) Keep plts >20,000/mm^3 and treat coagulopathy *Note:* FFP/cryoprecipitate do not increase overall viscosity Cytoreduction (lower WCC): CTx Leukapheresis is less commonly used as it produces a transient effect and does not reduce the risk of TLS
Tumour lysis syndrome Dying cell release their contents into the blood stream spontaneously or in response to therapy	Hyperuricaemia → renal uric acid deposition, lethargy, nausea/vomiting, renal toxicity, CNS dysfunction Hyperkalaemia Hyperphosphataemia Hypocalcaemia These electrolyte abnormalities can result in renal insufficiency, cardiac arrhythmias, seizures and death due to multiorgan failure.	Tumours with a high rate of cell death: Burkitt lymphoma ALL ≫AML	*Investigations:* Frequent blood monitoring *Treatment:* Hydration (with no potassium) at 1.5–2X maintenance or 125 ml/m^2/h ± NHCO3. Urine alkalinisation: aim for urine pH 7–8. CaPO4 Low risk: Allopurinol (xanthine oxidase) prevents hypoxanthine becoming xanthine and in turn, uric acid. High risk/established TLS: urate oxidase/rasburicase breaks down uric acid to allantoin which can be easily excreted.

Table 12.7 (*Continued*)

Emergency	Presentation	Differential diagnosis	Management
Typhlitis (neutropenic enterocolitis)	Nausea, diarrhoea Fever	Most common in patients with leukaemia or lymphoma, especially after cytarabine.	*Investigations:* AXR/abdominal US: pneumatosis, paucity of air, bowel wall oedema ± Abdominal CT *Treatment:* Nil orally IV antibiotics (to cover enteric organisms)

Turcot syndrome, which are autosomal genetic conditions associated with mutations in the NF1, TP53, and adenomatous polyposis coli (APC) genes, respectively. The most significant association linked to the development of malignant gliomas, however, is previous exposure to ionising radiation.

Clinical features

The presentation of brain tumours varies and depends largely on the age of the patient and the tumour location. Compared with low-grade tumours, high-grade tumours tend to have a shorter interval of symptoms. Children with high-grade tumours frequently also present with symptoms related to raised ICP, including headache, nausea, and vomiting, which are classically worse in the morning. Infants present with non-specific symptoms, particularly developmental delay or regression of previously attained developmental milestones. If an infant's cranial sutures have not fused, they may present with an increasing head circumference and/or hydrocephalus.

- *Supratentorial tumours*: localized signs, such as hemiparesis or seizures; alterations in personality, mood changes, and declining school performance.
- *Posterior fossa tumours*: symptoms of raised increased ICP due to compression of the fourth ventricle, including headache, emesis, lethargy, behavioural changes and deterioration in school performance, and signs of obstructive hydrocephalus such as ataxia or torticollis.
- *Brainstem tumours*: cranial nerve palsies (VI and VII are the most commonly affected; infants with bulbar nerve involvement may present with failure to thrive); signs of long tract involvement; ataxia. Hydrocephalus is rare (<10%).
- *Cervicomedullary tumours*: signs of long tract involvement; no ataxia or cranial nerve involvement.

Leukaemia and lymphoma
See Table 12.8.

Bone tumours
See Table 12.9.

Abdominal tumours in children

The two most common abdominal tumours in children are neuroblastomas (tumour of the sympathetic chain and adrenal gland) and Wilms tumour (WT) (renal tumour). See Table 12.10.

Neuroblastomas
Background
- NB are mainly localised in the abdomen but can occur anywhere along the sympathetic chain (neck, thorax, pelvis).
- It is the most common solid tumour outside the brain, most frequent in infants.
- Some tumours in infants demonstrate spontaneous regression even if metastatic (Stage 4 S).

Risk stratification
- The main prognostic factors are the age (better prognosis before 18 months), the stage (localised or metastatic NB), the biology (amplification of MYCN, ploidy).

Clinical features
- If localized: abdominal mass, signs of spinal cord compression.
- In infants, the metastases are localised in the skin (blue tumours) and the liver (hepatomegaly).
- In older children, their symptoms are related to the metastasis in bone marrow/bone (pain, fever, anaemia).

Table 12.8 Leukaemia and lymphoma

	Acute lymphoblastic leukaemia (ALL)/Non-Hodgkin lymphoma (NHL)	Acute myeloid leukaemia (AML)
Background	ALL and NHL constitute a family of genetically heterogeneous lymphoid neoplasms derived from B- (80%) and T-lymphoid progenitors (15%). Lymphoblastic leukaemia implies >25% bone marrow involvement whereas lymphoma is <25%. ALL is the most common cancer (30%) in children with a peak age of 2–5 years.	AML consists of a group of relatively well-defined haematopoietic neoplasms involving precursor cells committed to the myeloid line of cellular development (i.e. those giving rise to granulocytic, monocytic, erythroid, or megakaryocytic elements). Childhood AML is a rare disease occurring in children younger than 15 years.
Aetiology	• Clonal proliferation of lymphoid progenitor cells. Accumulation of leukemic blasts or immature forms in the bone marrow, peripheral blood, and occasionally in other tissues results in variable reduction in the production of normal red blood cells, platelets, and mature granulocytes. • Cause is unknown. • Certain genetic syndromes have a higher incidence: including trisomy 21 (T21), neurofibromatosis type 1 (NF1), Bloom syndrome and ataxia-telangiectasia.	• Clonal proliferation of myeloid precursors with reduced capacity to differentiate. Accumulation of blasts as described in ALL. • Associated with genetic abnormalities including T21 and Fanconi anaemia. *Note:* 5% of newborns with T21 have transient leukaemia (aka transient abnormal myelopoiesis or transient myeloproliferative disorder) which usually resolves spontaneously. Within the first 4 years of life 10–20% of these infants will develop myeloid leukaemia.
Clinical features	*ALL:* Presenting symptoms and signs reflect bone marrow infiltration and extramedullary disease. History: • Bone pain, limp, refusal to weight bear • Fatigue, pallor • Easy bruising, bleeding, petechiae and fever/infection • If CNS involvement – headache, nausea, vomiting, irritability Examination • Lymphadenopathy >1 cm, hepatosplenomegaly • Testicular involvement (painless, unilateral enlargement) *Note:* T-ALL often occurs in older boys with a large anterior mediastinal mass. *NHL:* mediastinal mass and/or matted lymphadenopathy	See ALL *Note:* Palpable lymphadenopathy and hepatosplenomegaly is uncommon (<20%)

Investigations	• FBE + film – anaemia, thrombocytopenia, neutropenia, peripheral blasts.
	• Bone marrow aspirate +/− trephine (BMAT). Indications:
	  • Atypical cells in peripheral blood film
	  • Depression of >1 cell line
	  • Unexplained lymphadenopathy/hepatosplenomegaly
	• CXR – to determine presence of mediastinal mass.
	• If suspected NHL – excisional biopsy of the abnormal lymph node.
	• Consider LP
		See ALL

Table 12.8 (*Continued*)

	Acute lymphoblastic leukaemia (ALL)/Non-Hodgkin lymphoma (NHL)	Acute myeloid leukaemia (AML)
Treatment	Current chemotherapy protocols achieve an overall cure rate >80% in children ALL: Patients with ALL require prolonged chemotherapy (2–3 years) Pre-B ALL, T ALL/NHL: Tumour lysis syndrome or the presence of a mediastinal mass should be regarded as medical emergencies (refer to oncologic emergencies Table 12.7)	Improvements in supportive care have had a major impact on increased survival rates in childhood AML. Immunosuppression due to intensive chemotherapy can be associated with significant morbidity and mortality from infection. Hyperleukocytosis and APML should be regarded as medical emergencies due to the risk of haemorrhage (see oncologic emergencies Table 12.7).

Investigations
- Urinary catecholamines (24 hours collection) are positive in 90% of the cases.
- CT/MRI.
- A biopsy (or a surgical resection) of the primary tumour is needed to obtain a definitive diagnosis and determine prognostic factors (histology, biology).

Treatment
- Surgical resection ± chemotherapy.
- The prognosis is good in localised NB with favourable biology with a 5-year overall survival (OS) greater than 90%. In infants, with a small tumour detected by systematic ultrasound, NB may be safely observed as spontaneous regression can occur.

Wilms tumour
Background
- WT is the second most common abdominal tumour and the most common renal tumour in children.
- 10% of children with WT have other abnormalities. Syndromes associated with WT include the overgrowth syndromes (Beckwith–Wiedemann syndrome, isolated hemihypertrophy, Sotos syndrome) and non-overgrowth syndrome (WAGR syndrome – Wilms tumour, aniridia, genitourinary malformation and mental retardation).

Clinical features
- Well child with massive abdominal tumour.
- Severe hypertension.

Investigations
- On ultrasound, the tumour arises from the kidney
- The local and metastatic evaluation is done by a thoraco-abdominal CT scan. It confirms the renal tumour and assesses the contralateral kidney, patency of renal vein and inferior vena cava, lymph nodes, lungs and liver.
- Tumour markers (AFP, HCG, urinary catecholamines) are negative.

Treatment
- Chemotherapy + surgery at week 4.

Supportive care guidelines
Aggressive supportive care improves clinical outcome.

Blood products
- Blood products should be irradiated and leukodepleted.
- Transfusion with red blood cells is indicated to correct severe Hb <80 g/L or symptomatic anaemia or acute blood loss.

Table 12.9 Bone tumours in children

	Osteosarcoma	Ewing's sarcoma
Background	Most common primary bone tumour. Predilection for age of pubertal growth spurt and sites of maximum growth. Cause: • Unknown in most • Exposure to radiation or alkylating agents • Increased risk with some hereditary disorders associated with alterations of tumour suppressor genes (hereditary retinoblastoma, Li-Fraumeni syndrome)	Second most common primary bone tumour. Aggressive form of childhood cancer. A quarter of ES arise in soft tissues rather than bone. Unknown cause
Clinical features	• Can occur in any bone – most commonly metaphyses of long bones (distal femur, proximal tibia, and proximal humerus). • 85% have localised disease and present with pain, swelling, limitation of joint movement, pathological fractures. • 15% of patients present with radiographic metastases (lung, bone and rarely lymph nodes and soft tissue).	• Most common sites – bones of the pelvis, lower extremities, chest wall, axial skeleton. In long bones, they tend to arise from the diaphyseal–metaphyseal portion. • 75% localised disease. • 25% present with metastases (lung, bone, bone marrow most commonly). • Constitutional symptoms due to metastatic disease (malaise, fever, anorexia and weight loss).
Diagnosis	• X-ray – osteoblastic, osteolytic or mixed appearance of bone. Soft tissue patchy calcifications. A triangular area of periosteal calcification at the border of tumour and healthy tissue is known as *Codman triangle* – this is typical for osteosarcomas. • MRI – this should include the entire involved bone as well as the neighbouring joints, so as to not miss skip lesions. • Open or imaging guided biopsy.	• MRI – this threshold include the entire involved bone or compartment. • Imaging-guided core biopsy without fixation.
Treatment	• Local therapy alone is insufficient, as 80–90% of all patients with seemingly localised disease will develop metastases. • Current treatment regimens include – primary (preoperative; neoadjuvant) induction chemotherapy – definite surgery – aim for complete tumour removal – postoperative (adjuvant) chemotherapy lead to cure in approximately two-thirds of patients with seemingly localised disease Approximately 30% of all patients with primary metastatic osteosarcoma and >40% of those who achieve a complete surgical remission can become long-term survivors.	• Complete local control with surgery (preferred) and/or radiotherapy is imperative for curative treatment + chemotherapy. The use of chemotherapy has greatly improved survival rates for patients with localised ES from about 10 to 70–80%.

Packed red blood cells
• Formula: amount required in mL = desired rise in Hb (aim for 100–120) × wt (kg) × 0.4.
• Each unit is 200–250 mL.
Platelets (plts)
• Transfusion with platelets is indicated to correct bleeding manifestations. Indications may include
  ○ Plts <10,000/L without bleeding.
  ○ Plts <20,000/L if febrile or mucosal bleeding.

Table 12.10 Wilms tumour versus neuroblastoma

	Wilms tumour	Neuroblastoma
Symptoms	Abdominal mass	Pain, anaemia
Mean age (months)	39	22
Predisposing syndromes	Frequent	Rare
Frequency metastasis	10%	70%
Site metastasis	Lung, liver	Bones, bone marrow
Prognostic factors	Stage, histology	Age, biology, histology, stage

- ○ Plts <30,000/L prior to lumbar puncture or if brain tumour.
- ○ Plts <70,000/L prior to any other surgical procedure.
- Use apheresed platelets only if you anticipate the need for long-term support to minimise exposure to multiple donors.
- *Formula: one pedipack per 10 kg up to 40 kg or 10–15 mL/kg.*

Infection

Risk factors for infection in immunocompromised patients are

- Neutropenia: A neutrophil count of <0.5 × 10^6/L is associated with a significantly increased risk of bacteraemia. This risk is markedly increased with a neutrophil count <0.1 × 10^9/L. The longer the duration of neutropenia, the higher the risk of infection.
- Lymphopenia is associated with increased risk of opportunistic infection such as *Pneumocystis jirovecii* and reactivation of herpes simplex and herpes zoster viruses.
- Steroid therapy is a risk factor for invasive fungal infection.
- CVCs: Most children receiving chemotherapy have either a Hickman catheter (externalised central venous catheter, CVC) or an infusaport (subcutaneous catheter).
- Breaches of the normal skin and mucosal barriers, particularly in heavily colonised sites around the perineum, in the mouth, nose and lower gastrointestinal tract, allow organisms' access to the bloodstream.

Febrile neutropenia

Fever and neutropenia (FN) are common complications in children who receive chemotherapy for cancer. It is associated with significant morbidity and mortality. Causes of an initial fever in a neutropenic child may be bacterial, viral, or fungal.

Definition

- A temperature between 38.0–38.5°C twice in 1 hour, or ≥38.5 °C on a single occasion and ANC <500/μL or 1000/mm^3.

Assessment and Management

- Initial management of paediatric FN is influenced by many factors, such as patient characteristics, clinical presentation, drug availability and cost, and local epidemiology, including resistance patterns.
- Careful clinical assessment and blood cultures are essential.
- *Empiric antibiotics* are routinely indicated and should be administered down all lumens of the CVC without delay (see Fig. 12.3). Also see RCH *febrile neutropenia* clinical practice guidelines *http://www.rch.org.au/clinicalguide/guideline_index/Febrile_Neutropenia/.*
- Initial empiric antibiotics should be rationalised to include the clinically or microbiologically documented infection. It is reasonable to cease antimicrobials when the child is afebrile, there is platelet recovery and the absolute neutrophil count >100/μL and rising.
- Empiric antifungal therapy should be initiated for invasive fungal disease (IFD) in high-risk neutropenic patients after 96 hours of fever in the setting of broad-spectrum antibiotics. It should be continued until resolution of neutropenia (ANC >100–500/μL) in the absence of documented or suspected IFD.

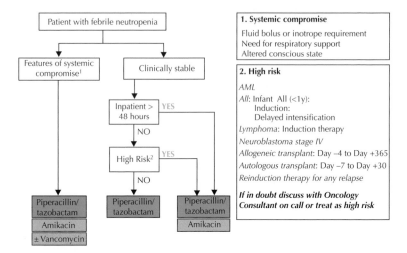

Fig. 12.3 Febrile neutropenia guideline – initial management. *Source*: the Royal Children's Hospital Clinical Practice Guidelines. Reproduced with permission of the Royal Children's Hospital.

Pneumocystis jirovecii pneumonia

- All patients should receive trimethoprim/sulfamethoxazole (TMP/SMX) at a dose of TMP 2.5 mg/kg/dose (maximum dose 160 mg/dose) orally twice daily on 2 or 3 sequential days per week.
- Consider *Pneumocystis jirovecii* pneumonia in an at-risk patient who presents with tachypnoea, lowered oxygen saturations and/or diffuse opacities on chest radiograph.

Infectious disease contacts in immunosuppressed patients

- Varicella and measles may lead to very severe illness in immunocompromised children.
- No effective antiviral agent is available for measles, and it may cause fatal pneumonitis. Although immunity may wane during chemotherapy, prior vaccination or infection is usually protective.
- If the patient's immune status is not known or negative, give zoster immunoglobulin (ZIG) for varicella contact or normal human immunoglobulin (NHIG) for measles contact within 72 hours (see Australian immunisation handbook http://www.health.gov.au/internet/immunise/publishing.nsf/Content/Handbook10-home).

ZIG dose for varicella contact

- Weight <20 kg or <5 years of age: 250 mg IM (1 × 2 mL/125 IU vial).
- Weight, 20–40 kg or 5–10 years of age: 500 mg IM (2 × 2 mL/125 IU vial).
- Weight >40 kg or age >10 years: 750 mg IM (3 × 2 mL/125 IU vials).

Immunoglobulin for measles contact

- 0.25 mL/kg IM daily for 2 days.

Management of mucositis/perirectal cellulitis

- IV hydration and/or parenteral nutrition
- Effective analgesia (topical lignocaine gel and opioids such as oxycodone or morphine)
- Anti-infective therapy as indicated
- Salt baths
- Strong barrier cream (Calmoseptine cream)
- Mouthcare with Curasept

Table 12.11 Anti-emetics options

Emetic risk	Antiemetics
High	Ondansetron, dexamethasone (small doses) and aprepitant
Moderate	Ondansetron, dexamethasone (small doses) and aprepitant
Low	Ondansetron alone
Minimal	Nil
Anticipatory	Addition of lorazepam or promethazine

Antiemetic Protection

- Chemotherapy-induced nausea and vomiting (CINV) are classified as acute, delayed or anticipatory.
- Anticipatory nausea and vomiting is reported by 30% of patients and is a conditioned response that usually occurs prior to the actual administration of chemotherapy based on previous experiences of nausea and vomiting. It may be triggered by factors, such as tastes, odours, sights, thoughts or anxiety associated with the treatment, and is usually more difficult to control than acute or delayed CINV.
- Actinomycin, cisplatin, carboplatin, cyclophosphamide/ifosfamide and doxorubicin/daunorubicin-based regimens are moderate/highly emetogenic agents.

Anti-emetics options (see Table 12.11):

- Ondansetron is a potent 5-HT3 receptor antagonist of 5-HT. Dosages up to 0.15 mg/kg QID orally or IV.
- Aprepitant is a potent, central nervous system-penetrant, selective NK-1 receptor antagonists of SP. Aprepitant is administered as a 3-day regimen: 125 mg orally 1 hour prior to chemotherapy administration (day 1) and 80 mg per day orally in the morning on days 2 and 3.
- D2 receptor antagonists include promethazine and metoclopramide.
- Anti-histamines include promethazine and cyclizine.
- The steroid dexamethasone, while not an anti-emetic, can potentiate the effect of Ondansetron.

Constipation

- Constipation is a known side effect of vincristine therapy and can be particularly troublesome when the drug is used frequently.
- Commence prophylaxis with laxatives or stool softener at the beginning of therapy.
- If severe constipation persists despite prophylaxis ± addition of other agents, nasogastric colonic lavage solutions (e.g. Golytely) are usually successful.
- **Suppositories and enemas must not be used** because of the risk of causing small abrasions, which can predispose to secondary local infection and/or septicaemia.

Extravasation of chemotherapy

- Depending on the volume and type of drug extravasated, untreated damage can vary from mild irritation and erythema (irritant) to severe necrosis of the dermis and subcutaneous tissues (vesicant). These effects may be immediate or delayed.
- Vesicants include vincristine/vinblastine, anthracyclines, actinomycin-D.
- Treatment includes ceasing infusion, topical application of dimethyl sulphoxide (DMSO), and plastic surgery review if extensive.

Osteonecrosis or avascular necrosis

- May develop during or following steroid therapy in ALL.
- Often involves multiple joints over time, not limited to weight-bearing joints. Common sites include hip, knee, ankle, heel, shoulder and elbow.
- Symptoms and examination findings may include joint pain, joint stiffness, limited range of motion (e.g. pain with internal rotation of the hip), limited mobility or ambulation and/or gait abnormalities.
- MRI is superior in sensitivity and specificity to other modalities, especially with early bone changes.

Immunisation during and after chemotherapy

- Response to routine immunisations will not be optimal during therapy. Hence, routine immunisation programs should be interrupted while the child is on therapy.
- If required for treatment of a tetanus prone wound, tetanus toxoid can be safely given but concurrent use of tetanus immunoglobulin should also be considered.
- **Live virus vaccines must not be given to immunocompromised children.**
- **Siblings of patients should not receive oral polio vaccine (Sabin); give injectable polio vaccine inactivated instead.**
- It is strongly advised that unimmunised, non-immune siblings receive MMR and varicella vaccine.
- All family members including the immunocompromised child should be encouraged to have annual influenza vaccination.
- Approximately 6 months after completion of chemotherapy, interrupted immunisation programs should be completed. A booster dose of ADT or CDT, Sabin and MMR should be given to those who have previously been fully immunised. Hepatitis B immunisation should be commenced if not previously given.
- Consult with a specialist regarding immunisation after an allogeneic bone marrow transplant.

Late effects

- As a result of advances in treatment, almost 80% of children and adolescents who receive a diagnosis of cancer become long-term survivors.
- Damage to the organ systems of children caused by chemotherapy and radiation therapy may not become clinically evident for many years.
- Survivors of childhood cancer have a higher rate of illness owing to chronic health conditions and many? Die prematurely.
- The risk of chronic health conditions is high and increases over time.
- Long-term follow-up of survivors of childhood cancer is necessary with an emphasis on surveillance for:
  ○ second cancers (e.g. breast and colorectal cancer, melanoma, and non-melanoma skin cancer);
  ○ coronary artery disease;
  ○ late-onset anthracycline-related cardiomyopathy; and
  ○ pulmonary fibrosis;
- Endocrinopathies (e.g. premature gonadal failure, thyroid disease, osteoporosis, and hypothalamic and pituitary dysfunction).
- Follow-up care of survivors should also include secondary and tertiary prevention (e.g. strategies to promote tobacco cessation or avoidance, physical activity, and proper weight management) and management of chronic disease.
- Bone-tumour survivors are most likely to have severe limitations in activity, which may further compound the risk of cardiovascular disease.
- Survivors of CNS tumours are most likely to be functionally impaired.
- Hodgkin's disease survivors have the highest risk of second cancers and heart disease.

USEFUL RESOURCES

Haematology
Haemophilia
- *http://www.rch.org.au/clinicalguide/guideline_index/Haemophilia/*
- *http://www.rch.org.au/clinicalguide/guideline_index/Von_Willebrand_Disease_vWD/*
Anticoagulation
- *http://www.rch.org.au/clinicalguide/guideline_index/Anticoagulation_Therapy_Guidelines/*
Transfusion
- *http://www.rch.org.au/clinicalguide/guideline_index/Blood_product_transfusion/*
- *http://www.rch.org.au/rchcpg/hospital_clinical_guideline_index/Blood_Transfusion_Informed_Consent_and_Consumer_Information_/*

ITP

- *http://www.rch.org.au/clinicalguide/guideline_index/Immune_Thrombocytopenic_Purpura/*

Sickle cell

- *http://www.rch.org.au/clinicalguide/guideline_index/Sickle_Cell_Disease_Guideline/*

Other websites

- *ITP: www.itpsupport.com.au*
- *Thalassaemia: www.cooleysanaemia.com*
- *Sickle Cell Anaemia: www.cdc.gov/ncbddd/sicklecell/index.html*
- *Thrombosis and haemostasis: www.isth.org/*
- *http://www.chestnet.org/Guidelines-and-Resources/Guidelines-and-Consensus-Statements/Antithrombotic-Guidelines-9th-Ed*

Haemophilia

- *www.haemophilia.org.au*

Transfusion

- *www.transfusion.com.au*

Oncology

- *www.childrensoncologygroup.org*
- *www.cure4kids.org*

CHAPTER 13

The endocrine system

Margaret Zacharin
Fergus Cameron
George Werther
Michele O'Connell

Type 1 diabetes mellitus
Diagnosis
Diagnosis is made by either
- Random blood glucose measurement ≥11.1 mmol/L in the presence of symptoms of diabetes, or
- Fasting blood glucose ≥7.0 mmol/L.

Note:
- In the absence of symptoms, hyperglycaemia detected incidentally or under conditions of stress may be transient and should not in itself be regarded as diagnostic of diabetes.
- An elevated blood glucose reading should be confirmed with a repeat test performed in a laboratory (as opposed to capillary blood test sampling only).
- There is rarely a need for oral glucose tolerance testing to diagnose Type 1 diabetes (T1DM); symptomatic hyperglycaemia (± presence of ketones) is invariably present.
- Blood ketones can now be tested on a bedside glucometer (Optium™), with a normal reading being <0.6 mmol/L. At diagnosis of T1DM, levels of >1.0 mmol/L are common. Any patient with ketone levels >1.0 mmol/L should have a blood gas assessment to check for acidosis. Serial monitoring of blood ketone levels in addition to capillary blood glucose levels (BGLs) is very useful in assessing response to insulin therapy.

Clinical features
- Typical symptoms are polyuria, polydipsia or weight loss. Glycosuria and ketonuria are often present.
- There may be a family history of diabetes or other autoimmune disease.
- Children presenting with diabetes may range from being mildly unwell to severely unwell in diabetic ketoacidosis (DKA).

Differential diagnosis
Transient hyperglycaemia
Transient elevation of blood glucose and glycosuria (and possibly ketonuria) may occur in children with an intercurrent illness or with therapy such as glucocorticoids. The risk of later developing diabetes mellitus is about 3%, but it is approximately 30% if these findings are picked up in an otherwise well child. Check HbA1 c and diabetes-related autoimmune markers (antibodies against insulin, glutamic acid decarboxylase (GAD) and islet cells) and discuss with a specialist.

Type 2 diabetes mellitus
This form of diabetes is rare in children. It is being seen increasingly in children who are overweight, those with a family history of Type 2 diabetes mellitus (T2DM) and in some specific ethnic groups. An oral glucose tolerance test is often required for diagnosis as symptoms of hyperglycaemia are less common in the early stages.

Monogenic diabetes
Monogenic diabetes results from the inheritance of a mutation or mutations in a single gene. It may be dominantly or recessively inherited or may be a de novo mutation and hence a spontaneous case. In children, almost

Paediatric Handbook, Ninth Edition. Edited by Amanda Gwee, Romi Rimer and Michael Marks.
© 2015 John Wiley & Sons, Ltd. Published 2015 by John Wiley & Sons, Ltd.

all monogenic diabetes results from mutations in genes that regulate beta cell function, although diabetes can rarely occur from mutations resulting in very severe insulin resistance. It is important to correctly diagnose monogenic diabetes as it can predict the clinical course of the patient, explain other associated clinical features and most importantly guide the most appropriate treatment (e.g. in the most common form, due to HNF1α mutations, affected individuals respond exceptionally well to oral sulfonylureas).

New presentation of T1DM, mildly unwell

Refer http://www.rch.org.au/clinicalguide/guideline_index/Diabetes_Mellitus/

Assessment

Less than 3% dehydration, no acidosis and not vomiting.

Management

The decision about the individual insulin regimen should be made by the paediatric team in discussion with the family and child. The regimens outlined below are a guide only and individual clinicians may recommend an alternative approach.

Initial treatment

- 0.25 units/kg of quick-acting insulin s.c. stat.
- If within 2 hours prior to a meal defer and give mealtime dose only.
- Give reduced dose if ≤4 years old. Dose may also be lower if not ketotic.

Ongoing treatment

At diagnosis, standard insulin regimens in newly diagnosed patients may comprise either of the two regimens below:

- Twice daily injections of a mixture of short- and intermediate-acting insulins
- Multiple daily injections (MDI) of insulin using a long-acting insulin analogue at night and pre-meal injections of rapid-acting insulin analogue

In Australia, insulin pump therapy is rarely commenced at the time of diagnosis in children and adolescents, but may be an option at a later stage. Insulin pump therapy is an intensive means of managing diabetes requiring ≥6 BGLs and regular data entry from the young person each day; it therefore won't be suitable or a preferred method for many young people (see Continuous subcutaneous insulin infusion use in children and adolescents, p. 192).

Management of hyperglycaemic and ketotic mildly ill patients with established diabetes

Patients with established T1DM who present with hyperglycaemia and ketosis but normal pH, will need additional s.c. insulin to clear their ketones.

i Patients on intermittent daily injections of insulin (BD or MDI)

Give 10% of the patient's total daily insulin dose (TDD) as an s.c. injection of rapid-acting insulin (this is in addition to the usual insulin regimen). Monitor BGL and ketones 1–2 hourly. This dose of rapid-acting insulin can be repeated after 2–4 hours if blood ketones are not <1.0 mmol/L.

ii Patients on insulin pump therapy

Need to assume line failure/blockage has interrupted insulin delivery. Give 20% of the patient's TDD as an s.c. injection of rapid-acting insulin. (This is a higher dose relative to the above patient group because there is no longer-acting insulin 'on board' in pump patients). Once s.c. insulin has been given, ask the patient or family to resite the pump cannula and commence delivery at usual settings. Monitor BGL and ketones 1–2 hourly. For patients on pump therapy, ketones should clear to <0.6 mmol/L.

Diabetic ketoacidosis

DKA is the combination of hyperglycaemia, metabolic acidosis and ketonaemia. It may be the first presentation for a child with previously undiagnosed diabetes (>30% present in DKA at diagnosis). It can also be precipitated by illness, or poor compliance with taking insulin in any child or adolescent with established Type 1 diabetes. Rapid onset is more likely in patients with poor underlying control or in patients on an insulin pump.

All patients presenting with a BGL ≥11.1 mmol/L should have blood ketones tested on a capillary sample using a bedside Optium™ meter. If this test is positive (>0.6 mmol/L), assess for acidosis to determine further management. Urinalysis can be used for initial assessment if blood ketone testing is not available.

The biochemical criteria for DKA are

- Venous pH <7.3 or bicarbonate <15 mmol/L
- Presence of blood or urinary ketones

Causes

- Delayed diagnosis of T1DM
- Omission of insulin in a patient with established diabetes
- Acute stress (infection, trauma, psychological)
- Poor management of intercurrent illness
- Mechanical factors obstructing insulin delivery by an insulin pump, for example line occlusion/failure

Assessment of children and adolescents in DKA

- Degree of dehydration (often overestimated)
  - None/mild (<4%): no clinical signs
  - Moderate (4–7%): easily detectable dehydration, for example reduced skin turgor, poor capillary return
  - Severe (>7%): poor perfusion, rapid pulse, reduced blood pressure, that is shock
- Level of consciousness – Glasgow Coma Scale
- Investigations – Take venous blood sample (place an IV line if possible as this will be needed if DKA is confirmed) for the following:
  - FBC
  - Blood glucose, urea, electrolytes (sodium, potassium, calcium, magnesium, phosphate)
  - Blood ketones (bedside test)
  - Venous blood gas (including bicarbonate)
  - Investigations for precipitating cause: if clinical signs of infection consider septic workup
  - For all newly diagnosed patients: insulin antibodies, GAD antibodies, coeliac screen (total IgA, anti-gliadin Ab, tissue transglutaminase Ab) and thyroid function tests (TFTs) (thyroid stimulating hormone (TSH) and FT_4)
- Urine – Ketones (if capillary testing not available), culture (if clinical evidence of infection)
- Calculate:
  - Serum osmolality = $2Na^+$ + glucose + urea
  - Corrected serum Na^+ = plasma Na^+ + 0.3 (plasma glucose – 5.5)

Management

Fluids

Initial fluid requirements

- Not all patients in DKA require fluid boluses. Remember, acidosis itself results in poor peripheral perfusion and confounds accurate assessment of dehydration. Peripheral perfusion will improve with correction of the acidosis (with insulin).
- If hypoperfusion is present, give normal saline at 10 mL/kg stat.
- Repeat until perfusion is re-established (warm, pink extremities with rapid capillary refill).
- Commence rehydration with normal saline and potassium as below (see Table 13.1 for appropriate rates depending on fluid status).
- Keep nil by mouth (except ice to suck) until alert and stable.
- Insert a nasogastric tube if patient is comatose or has recurrent vomiting; leave on free drainage.

Subsequent fluid adjustments

Fluid replacement with normal saline and potassium should continue for at least the first 6 hours. If the blood glucose falls very quickly within the first few hours, or if the BGL reaches 12–15 mmol/L, change to normal saline with 5% dextrose and potassium.

Choice of fluid after the initial 6 hours will be influenced by the corrected serum sodium (see above for calculation) and the BGL. Corrected sodium should remain stable or rise as BGL falls. Fluids with a tonicity of <0.45% saline should not be used.

Beyond the initial 6 hours, 0.45% NaCl with 5% dextrose and potassium *may* be used once the BGL is <12–15 mmol/L. However, if hyponatraemia is present, if the corrected serum sodium fails to stabilise or rise as

Table 13.1 Diabetic ketoacidosis fluid rates (mL/h) including deficit and maintenance fluid requirements, to be given evenly over 48 hours

Weight (kg)	Mild/Nil	Moderate
5	24	27
7	33	38
8	38	8
10	48	54
12	53	60
14	58	67
16	64	74
18	70	80
20	75	87
22	78	91
24	80	95
26	83	100
28	86	104
30	89	108
32	92	112
34	95	116
36	98	120
38	101	125
40	104	129
42	107	133
44	110	137
46	113	141
48	116	146
50	119	150
52	122	154
54	124	158
56	127	162
58	130	167
60	133	171
62	136	175
64	139	179
66	142	183
68	145	187
70	148	191

Note: Include fluids given as a bolus and deduct these from ongoing rate.

the BGL decreases, or if hyperosmolar and concerned about rapid shifts in osmolality, 0.9% saline + dextrose and potassium should be continued.

Aim to keep the BGL between 6 and 12 mmol/L.

If the patient is still acidotic, and the BGL is <5.5 mmol/L or is falling rapidly within the range of 5.5–15 mmol/L, increase the dextrose concentration in the fluid to 10%. The insulin infusion rate should only be turned down if BGL continues to fall despite use of 10% dextrose. In such patients, a reduction in the rate of insulin to 0.05 unit/kg/h may be used, provided that metabolic acidosis continues to improve. In this circumstance this should be discussed with a paediatric endocrinologist.

If the patient becomes hypoglycaemic, manage as per hypoglycaemia section below.

Rehydration may be completed orally after the first 24–36 hours if the patient is metabolically stable (this usually coincides with insulin therapy being switched to s.c. injections).

Insulin

- Commence after initial fluid resuscitation.
- Add 50 units of clear/rapid-acting insulin (Actrapid or Humulin R) to 49.5 mL 0.9% NaCl (1 unit/mL solution).
- Ensure that the insulin is clearly labelled.
- Start at:
  - 0.1 unit/kg/h in newly diagnosed children, and those with established diabetes who have glucose levels >15 mmol/L.
  - 0.05 unit/kg/h for children with established diabetes who have had their usual insulin and whose BGL is <15 mmol/L. This rate should also be considered in young children and may be appropriate during inter-hospital transfer when biochemical monitoring is more limited. Note: a doctor should accompany any patient in DKA requiring insulin infusion during transfer.
- Adequate insulin must be continued to clear ketones and correct acidosis.
- Insulin infusion can be discontinued when the child is alert and metabolically stable (pH >7.30 and HCO_3 >15 mmol/L). The best time to change to s.c. insulin is just before meal time.
- The insulin infusion should only be stopped 30 minutes after the first s.c. injection of insulin.

Potassium

Potassium replacement therapy is required for treatment of DKA. This is because a total body deficit of potassium occurs in DKA and correction of the acidosis in the absence of potassium therapy will usually rapidly result in hypokalaemia. Patients may have hyperkalaemia, hypokalaemia or normokalaemia at presentation, depending on the total body potassium deficit and the degree of acidosis. Management includes

- Defer initial potassium replacement if the serum level is >5.5 mmol/L or if the patient is anuric (until K^+ is <5.5 mmol/L or urine output documented respectively).
- Start KCl at a concentration of 40 mmol/L if body weight <30 kg, or 60 mmol/L if ≥30 kg; subsequent replacement is based on serum potassium levels.
- Measure levels 1 hour after starting therapy and 2–4 hourly thereafter.
- Potassium replacement should continue throughout IV fluid and insulin therapy.

Bicarbonate

- Bicarbonate administration is <u>not</u> routinely recommended as it may cause paradoxical CNS acidosis. Continuing acidosis indicates insufficient fluid and insulin replacement.
- In extremely sick children (with pH <7.0 ± HCO_3 <5 mmol/L), small amounts may be given. Liaison with paediatric intensive care unit is advisable.
- The HCO_3 dose (mmol) = 0.3 × body weight (kg) × base deficit. **Infuse half** over 30 minutes with cardiac monitoring. Reassess acid–base status. Remember risk of hypokalaemia.

Sodium

- Measured serum sodium is depressed by the dilutional effect of hyperglycaemia. To "correct" sodium concentration, use the following formula:
  Corrected (i.e. actual) Na = measured Na + 0.3 (glucose − 5.5) mmol/L, that is 3 mmol/L of sodium to be added for every 10 mmol/L of glucose above 5.5 mmol/L.

- Beware of falling adjusted sodium levels as glucose declines – hyponatraemia may herald cerebral oedema. If the sodium level falls, consider decreasing the rate of fluid administration to replace over 72–96 hours; see hypernatraemia section below.

Ongoing monitoring and management

Clinical

- Strict fluid balance
- Hourly observations: pulse, BP, respiratory rate and neurological observations
- 2–4 hourly temperature

  Note: Any headache or altered behaviour may indicate impending cerebral oedema.

Biochemical

- Hourly capillary glucose and ketones (bedside meter) while on insulin infusion.
- Venous blood gas and laboratory BGLs, serum corrected sodium, potassium, chloride performed 2 hourly for the first 6 hours and 2–4 hourly thereafter. More frequent (hourly) measurements may be necessary in those with severe acidosis or as clinically indicated.

Other instructions

- Intensive care admission is required if age <2 years, coma, cardiovascular compromise or seizures.
- Patient should remain nil orally until alert and stable.
- Nurse the patient in a head-up position and in good light.

Hazards/complications of diabetic ketoacidosis

Hypernatraemia

If Na is >160 mmol/L, discuss with a specialist. Sodium should rise as the glucose falls during treatment. If this does not happen or if **hyponatraemia** develops, it usually indicates overzealous volume correction and insufficient electrolyte replacement. This may place the patient at risk of cerebral oedema (see below).

Hypoglycaemia

If blood glucose falls below 4.0 mmol/L and patient is still acidotic, give IV 10% dextrose 2–5 mL/kg as a bolus and use a 10% dextrose concentration for ongoing IV fluids (with 0.45% NaCl and K^+ supplements). Do not discontinue the insulin infusion.

If hypoglycaemia occurred despite use of 10% dextrose in the preceding 2 or more hours, the rate of the insulin infusion may be decreased to 0.05 unit/kg/h as long as ketosis and acidosis are clearing. Continue with a 10% dextrose concentration in IV fluids until BGL stable.

If blood glucose falls below 4.0 mmol/L and most recent pH is >7.30, oral treatment for hypoglycaemia (4–5 jelly beans followed by 15 g of complex carbohydrate) can be used instead of an IV bolus of dextrose 10%.

Hypokalaemia

Monitor frequently and adjust potassium concentration in the infusate. Children at particular risk of this complication are those who are very acidotic or have low potassium levels at presentation.

Cerebral oedema

This is an uncommon (0.5–3.0%) but extremely serious complication of DKA in children, usually occurring 6–12 hours after commencement of therapy. Mortality or severe morbidity is very high without early treatment.

Prevention

Slow correction of fluid and biochemical abnormalities. Optimally, the rate of fall of blood glucose and serum osmolality should not exceed 5 mmol/L/h, but in children there is often a quicker initial fall in glucose. Patients should be nursed head up.

Risk factors

- Newly diagnosed diabetes, young age (<5 years), poorly controlled diabetes
- Excessive fluid rehydration, particularly with hypotonic fluids
- Severe initial acidosis
- Hyponatraemia or hypernatraemia and negative sodium trend during the therapy

Signs
- Early: negative sodium trend, headache, behaviour change (sudden irritability, depression of conscious state) thermal instability and incontinence
- Late: bradycardia, elevated blood pressure and depressed respiration

Treatment
Cerebral oedema is a medical emergency.
- Administer 0.5 g/kg (2.5 mL/kg) of 20% mannitol IV as a bolus dose (range 0.25–1.0 g/kg). This can be repeated if the response is inadequate.
- Nurse the patient in a head-up position, maintain the airway.
- Severely restrict fluids (reduce by one-third in the first instance).
- Transfer to an intensive care unit for further management.
- **Do not delay treatment for radiological confirmation – diagnosis is clinical**.

Hypoglycaemia in children with diabetes
Common causes
- Missed meal/snack
- Vigorous exercise (can be during exercise or hours afterwards)
- Alcohol
- Too much insulin

Management
See Table 13.2

Sick day management during intercurrent illness in the child with diabetes
Principles
- Frequent testing of blood glucose and ketones (Table 13.3).
- The meal plan may temporarily be dropped – replace with fluids and easily digested carbohydrates.
- Ensure good fluid intake – alternate sugar and non-sugar-containing fluids depending on blood sugar levels (water is best if high).

Table 13.2 Management of hypoglycaemia in children with diabetes

Awake	~15 g of fast-acting carbohydrate e.g. 150–200 mL lemonade; 4–5 jelly beans; honey (1 tbs); condensed milk in tube Repeat in 10–15 minutes if no improvement Follow with 'sustaining serve' ~15 g of complex carbohydrate, for example bread, milk[a] If awake and alert but unable to eat (e.g. vomiting due to viral illness), mini-dose glucagon rescue may be appropriate[b]
Drowsy/uncooperative/unconscious/fitting (at home)	Glucagon IM injection 1 mg (1 ampoule) if >15 kg or >6 years old (0.5 mg if <15 kg or <6 years) Blood glucose should rise in 5–10 minutes. Give sips of sugar-containing fluid when awake; contact diabetes team for advice
Uncooperative/unconscious/fitting (in hospital)	Glucose 2–5 mL/kg of 10% dextrose IV over 2 minutes, then infuse 3–5 mg/kg/min until awake and able to eat/drink

[a]Sustaining serve not needed in patients using pump therapy.
[b]Mini-glucagon rescue is used when vomiting is associated with hypoglycaemia or for persistently low blood glucose levels resistant to oral therapy. The doses vary with age: ≤2 years 0.02 mg; 2–15 years 0.01 mg per year of age; >15 years 0.15 mg. These doses are given subcutaneously using an insulin syringe (0.01 mg of reconstituted glucagon = 1 'unit' on insulin syringe). BGL should be checked 20–30 minutes later; if BGL is <5.5 mol/L, repeat mini-dose glucagon giving double the original dose.

Table 13.3 Sick day management

Group	1	2	3
Blood glucose	High	High	Normal/low
Blood ketones	0.6–1.0 mmol/L	>1.0 mmol/L[a]	<1.0 mmol/L
Urine ketones	0–trace	>1+	0–trace
Vomiting	±	none or occasional[b]	±
Potential danger	Progress to group 2	DKA	Hypoglycaemia
Insulin	Increase normal dose by ~10% at next injection	Give rapid acting insulin at 10–20% total daily dose[c] Repeat 2–4 hourly if ketones persist	Reduce normal insulin by 10–25% in first instance
Monitor BGL and ketones	2–4 hourly	1–2 hourly until ketones clear	2–4 hourly
Further action	If ketones increasing, move to group 2	If not improving admit	If BGL low, manage as hypoglycaemia If BGL high move to group 2

[a] A threshold of 0.6 mmol/L is used for those on insulin pump therapy (as ketosis develops more rapidly) – see p. 192.
[b] If hyperglycaemic and ketotic with vomiting on >1 occasion, may need to be assessed in the emergency department (may be in DKA).
[c] Hyperglycaemia + blood ketone level >1.5 mmol/L likely to need 20% of total daily dose as extra rapid-acting insulin.

- Insulin doses usually need to be increased, although additional doses of insulin may be needed if ketones are present. Never omit insulin.
- Keep in touch with diabetes team.

Testing ketones
Blood ketone testing gives a more accurate picture of current ketone levels and is recommended for monitoring during sick days. Urinary ketone strips are cheaper and are adequate to use as an initial screen to check whether ketosis is present. If urinary ketones are present (1+ or more), blood ketone testing is advised for further monitoring.

A 'normal' blood ketone level is 0–0.6 mmol/L. For children on injected insulin regimens, a level 0.6–1.0 mmol/L can generally be managed with additional insulin at the next dose. If ketones are >1.0 mmol/L, an additional injection of rapid acting insulin may be warranted (see Table 13.3).

For children using insulin pump therapy, ketosis may develop more quickly as there is no longer-acting insulin circulating. A blood ketone level of >0.6 mmol/L requires extra insulin.

- Blood ketone level 0.6–1.0 mmol/L, an insulin bolus is given through the pump: add 50% to the correction dose calculated by the pump.
- If ketones are >1.0 mmol/L, the patient should assume a line failure/blockage and give rapid-acting insulin by a subcutaneous injection (20% of usual TDD). They should then resite their insulin pump cannula and recheck BGL and ketones in 1–2 hours.

Management of children with diabetes undergoing surgery or a procedure that requires fasting
The main aims are to prevent hypoglycaemia before, during and after surgery and to provide sufficient insulin to prevent the development of ketoacidosis. Factors that must be considered are
- Time of surgery
- Duration/type of surgery:
  ○ 'Major': GA of >2 hours or prolonged period of fasting anticipated in the post-operative period
  ○ 'Minor': GA of <2 hours duration; anticipated to resume oral intake prior to discharge on the same day
- Current insulin regimen
- Urgency of surgery
  Refer: http://www.rch.org.au/clinicalguide/guideline_index/Diabetes_Mellitus_and_Surgery/

Emergency and major surgery

- Urgent clinical and biochemical assessment as for DKA.
- Rehydrate and start IV insulin. Initial dose will be 0.02–0.03 unit/kg/h with adjustments made based on trend in BGLs.
- Maintain IV 0.45% saline with 5% dextrose and insulin infusion post-operatively until the patient is able to resume oral feeding.

Continuous subcutaneous insulin infusion use in children and adolescents

Continuous subcutaneous insulin infusion (CSII), or insulin pump therapy, is increasingly used in the treatment of Type 1 diabetes in children and adolescents. It relies on the continuous delivery of rapid-acting insulin into the subcutaneous tissues by an insulin pump, which is commonly worn on the belt/waistband or carried in a pocket. The insulin pump is connected to a subcutaneous cannula. The subcutaneous cannula is resited and the pump reloaded with insulin every 3 days. Insulin pumps can be disconnected for 1–2 hours at a time for bathing, swimming or contact sports.

Indications

- CSII can be used at any age but in preschool and young children it requires adult supervision of the numerical data entered into the pump.
- Although it offers benefits in terms of reduction of hypoglycaemia, improved glycaemic stability and improved quality of life, it is not suitable for all patients.
- At a minimum, patients must do 4–6 finger-prick blood glucose measures per day, be able to carbohydrate count accurately and be cognitively able to cope with the challenges of operating the insulin pump.

Calculating dose

Insulin is delivered in two ways:

- A continuous background delivery (*basal delivery*). Basal delivery is preprogrammed for a given patient and is delivered automatically.
- An intermittent meal or correction-based insulin delivery (*bolus delivery*). Bolus delivery is manually undertaken by the patient at the time of meals or when BGLs are to be corrected. Omission of bolus doses of insulin at meals or snacks will result in hyperglycaemia as there is no long-acting insulin to 'cover' food.
- Recurrent missed boluses or infrequent BGL testing are common reasons for failure to achieve good glucose control on CSII.
  Initial TDD at commencement of CSII is derived from pre-existing insulin requirements or based on weight.
- 40–50% of the TDD is given as basal insulin and the remainder given as bolus insulin.
- Patients may have multiple basal rates at varying times of the day and according to the varying levels of activity.
- Bolus insulin doses are calculated using the '500' rule (500 ÷ TDD = the number of grams of carbohydrate covered by 1 unit of bolus insulin). Correct calculation of the amount of bolus insulin requires that the patient is able to accurately 'carb count' their meals.
- The amount of insulin given to correct a high BGL (correction factor) is calculated using the '100' rule (100 ÷ TDD = the number of mmols drop in blood glucose that will result from a correction bolus of 1 unit of insulin).
- Current insulin pumps will automatically calculate bolus doses after they have been configured and a BGL has been entered into the pump software.
  Note: Infants and toddlers will usually require lower insulin bolus doses than are indicated by the '500' and '100' rules.

Complications

DKA is the most concerning acute complication of CSII use (Table 13.4). These patients are at higher risk of DKA because they do not use any long- or intermediate-acting insulin.
  Useful diabetes resources:

- NHMRC evidence based guidelines for Type 1 diabetes in children, adolescents and adults (2011)
- ISPAD clinical practice guidelines (2009)
- RCH clinical practice guidelines and parent manual (http://www.rch.org.au/diabetesmanual/)

Table 13.4 Complications of CSII use

Complication	Causes	Management
Hyperglycaemia ± ketosis ±Diabetic ketoacidosis	When insulin delivery is disrupted or when requirement increases. Ketosis ensues within 2–3 hours. • Cannula dislodgement • Tube kinks • Pump malfunction • Infected insertion site • Intercurrent illness	All patients receiving CSII therapy should also carry a back-up insulin pen containing rapid-acting insulin. **Hyperglycaemia only** – give correction bolus using pump. • Recheck blood glucose in 1–2 hours. **Hyperglycaemia and ketones ≥0.6 mmol/L** – disconnect pump and give injection of rapid acting insulin (one-sixth of usual pump total daily dose) using insulin pen. • Insert a new pump cannula. • Check BGL and ketones 1–2 hourly. **Hyperglycaemia, ketones ≥0.6 mmol/L and vomiting/abdo pain or otherwise unwell** – come to ED for assessment of DKA. If living >1 hour from hospital, can give NovoRapid injection as above (one-sixth of TDD) at home.
Hypoglycaemia	• Excessive basal rate • Excessive bolus insulin • Increased physical activity	Mild symptomatic hypoglycaemia: • Give one serve (15 g) of rapid acting CHO. Severe hypoglycaemia: • Give glucagon injection IM and call diabetes team; pump may be temporarily disconnected (e.g. for 20 minutes).

Hypothyroidism
Congenital hypothyroidism
Incidence is 1 in 3–5000 births.

Causes
• Thyroid dysgenesis (absent or ectopic thyroid gland) 75%
• Abnormal function (dyshormonogenesis) 10–15%
• Transient hypothyroidism (iodine exposure, maternal anti-thyroid antibodies etc.) 10%
• Hypothalamic pituitary deficiency (central, secondary or tertiary hypothyroidism) 5%

Clinical features
• Unusually sleepy baby
• Jaundice
• Large anterior fontanelle, persistent posterior fontanelle
• Coarse features
• Dry skin
• Periorbital oedema
• Umbilical hernia
• Harsh or hoarse cry
• Slow feeding
• Distal femoral epiphysis that is not ossified

Investigations
• Most cases are detected by neonatal screening (high TSH).
• Confirmation of the diagnosis on whole blood TFTs is essential.
• Technetium (Tch) scanning for position, function, size (presence of goitre, Tch uptake).
• Consider genetic studies if familial (e.g. NKX2.1 gene sequencing etc.)

Management

Thyroxine therapy (10–14 mcg/kg per day) must be started as early as possible – before 2 weeks. Evidence suggests better outcome if treatment started at 10 days and T_4 in upper range. At the time of retesting (2–3 weeks after commencing therapy) aim for

- FT_4 at the upper limit of normal range for age or just above
- Normalisation of TSH

Ongoing 3 monthly clinical reviews with repeat TFTs

Acquired hypothyroidism

Prevalence between 1 and 18 years of age is 1.2%.

Causes

- Chronic lymphocytic (Hashimoto) thyroiditis.
- Late appearing congenital dyshormonogenesis.
- Exogenous causes (radiation, high dose iodine exposure (Wolff Chaikov effect), etc.).
- Severe iodine deficiency.
- Central (secondary or tertiary) hypothyroidism.

Clinical features

Hypothyroidism is often very difficult to detect clinically in children. Growth retardation may be the only sign, often with a relative excess weight for height. The classical signs are usually absent when the cause is hypothalamic pituitary.

- Growth retardation
- Weight gain
- Lethargy
- Constipation
- Cold intolerance
- Goitre
- Dry cool skin, dry hair
- Prolonged ankle-jerk relaxation time

Investigations

- FT_4 and TSH
- Thyroid autoantibodies (thyroglobulin and thyroid peroxidase)
- Technetium thyroid scan
- Thyroid ultrasound where indicated (for assessment of gland structure)

Management

Referral to a specialist is important for the management of hypothyroidism.

Replacement thyroxine therapy (single daily dose usually starts with 50–100 mcg per day). Caution should be taken when correcting profoundly hypothyroid patients – initial doses may be somewhat lower. Recheck TFTs 2–3 weeks after commencing therapy and 3–4 monthly thereafter.

Hyperthyroidism

Whilst hyperthyroidism can present in the neonatal period due to maternal Graves disease it is almost always an acquired event later in life. Females are affected six times more commonly than males.

Causes

- Autoimmune hyperthyroidism (Graves disease, rarely a transient "toxic" phase of Hashimoto thyroiditis)
- Thyroid adenoma (rare in childhood)
- Exogenous (e.g. thyroxine consumption for weight loss)

Clinical features

- Goitre (nearly all), diffuse, with bruit
- Weight loss, heat intolerance, tiredness
- Warm sweaty hands, tremor, tachycardia

- Irritability and restlessness
- Proximal muscle weakness and wasting, accelerated ankle-jerk relaxation time
- Thyroid ophthalmopathy (30% of cases): lid lag, lid retraction, chemosis, exophthalmos, ophthalmoplegia
- Accelerated growth velocity

Investigations
- FT_4, FT_3
- TSH should be suppressed to undetectable (<0.01 mU/L)
- TSH receptor antibodies
- Bone age (usually advanced)
- Technetium thyroid scan – expect diffuse increased uptake
- Thyroid ultrasound if adenoma suspected

Management
Antithyroid drugs are used for long-term treatment of autoimmune hyperthyroidism in childhood and adolescence. Note: Propylthiouracil should only be used in case of allergy to carbimazole due to potential for hepatotoxicity. The long-term remission rate in this age group is 20–50%. Management by a specialist is necessary.

Antithyroid drugs
- Carbimazole: 0.2 mg/kg (max 30–60 mg per day depending on age, size) oral 8–12 hourly for 2 weeks. Recheck TFTs 2–3 weeks after commencing therapy. Then continue at least 18–24 months. If remission is to occur, this usually happens after approximately 24 months.
- Beta blockers may be considered as an additional initial therapy if cardiac compromise is suspected. This is contraindicated in children who suffer from asthma.
  Idiosyncratic reactions may occur to carbimazole with urticaria and/or neutropenia. This can occur at any time during treatment but is more common with high doses early in treatment. There is approximately 40% crossover intolerance between carbimazole and propylthiouracil.

Surgery
Used for
- Non-compliance
- Allergy to drugs
- Large goitre, increasing in size
- Long-term patient choice
  This should only be recommended in consultation with an experienced paediatric thyroid surgeon.

Radioactive iodine
Radioactive iodine is the treatment of choice for adults, however, its use in children remains variable around the world. Many centres only use I^{131} ablative therapy at >15 years of age but some centres consider its use over the age of 10–12 years.

Thyroid storm
Thyroid storm is a rare complication of untreated primary hyperthyroidism or non-compliance with thyroid medication. It is characterised by tremor, anxiety, tachycardia, fever and confusion. It requires treatment (usually in ICU), with IV beta blockade, sedation, Lugol iodine and propylthiouracil.

Adrenal hypofunction
Primary adrenal insufficiency
This is rare in childhood and adolescence, but should be considered in the presence of unexplained:
- vomiting
- weight loss
- increasing pigmentation
- chronic tiredness
- low serum sodium
- high serum potassium

Autoimmune destruction (Addison disease)

The commonest cause of primary adrenal insufficiency in the developed world.

- *Autoimmune:* This is usually presents as part of the autoimmune polyglandular syndrome although it often can be the sole manifestation of the condition. In autoimmune polyglandular syndrome is can present in combination with either chronic mucocutaneous candidiasis, primary hypoparathyroidism, or both. Presenting in later childhood or adolescence, it may also be associated with thyrotoxicosis, diabetes mellitus, Hashimoto thyroiditis, coeliac disease, Graves disease, Sjögren syndrome, rheumatoid arthritis and less commonly with T or B cell deficiency.
- *Infective:* Worldwide, the commonest cause of Addison disease is TB, followed by HIV infection.

X-linked adrenoleukodystrophy

This rare condition manifests in boys from early childhood to late adolescence. Milder forms may not be detected until adulthood – careful family history for neurologic disorders should be sought. Carrier females may develop adrenomyelopathy.

Clinical features

- Hyperpigmentation of the skin (ACTH-mediated).
- Tiredness, nausea, anorexia and weight loss.
- Adrenal features are usually, but not always, preceded by the development of a neurological disability (e.g. memory loss, sleep disturbance or ataxia).

Investigations

- Test blood and skin fibroblasts for very-long-chain fatty acids.

Management

- Dietary modification has been used.
- Bone marrow transplantation may be helpful in cases when repeated MRI evaluation demonstrates very early changes of leukodystrophy.

Congenital adrenal hyperplasia

Due to

- 21-hydroxylase deficiency (95% of all congenital adrenal hyperplasia (CAH))
- Other rare types

Clinical features

- In severe deficiency, signs of androgen excess are usually obvious with ambiguous genitalia and precocious sexual development.
- Milder forms present in early-mid childhood with premature pubarche and escalating linear growth.

Investigations for adrenal insufficiency

- Serum electrolytes (low sodium and high potassium).
- Simultaneous serum cortisol and plasma ACTH.
- Specific investigations if CAH is suspected: 17-OH progesterone, urine steroid profile. Tandem mass spectrometry is also used.

Management

- Hydrocortisone 10–14 mg/m^2 BSA per day in divided doses.
- Fludrocortisone 0.05–0.2 mg daily, orally.
- Steroid cover for stress (see below).
- NaCl tablets are useful to reduce salt loss in hot weather.

'Secondary' adrenal insufficiency (due to ACTH deficiency)

Causes

Hypothalamic pituitary failure due to tumour, trauma, post surgery, cranial irradiation (where it may be subtle) or Langerhan's histiocytosis.

Clinical features
- Not usually associated with salt-wasting
- No hyperpigmentation of the skin

Management
- Treat with hydrocortisone alone; fludrocortisone is unnecessary.
- Prednisolone may be used after growth is complete.

Steroid cover for stress in all patients with Adrenal insufficiency
- **All patients with adrenal insufficiency of any cause are at risk for adrenal crisis during periods of severe stress → all need extra steroid cover.**
- In cases of acute medical illness (e.g. gastroenteritis, influenza), any surgery requiring general anaesthetic and any major fracture:
  - Hydrocortisone 0.2–0.3 mg/kg (usually 25–100 mg) IM/IV stat.
  - Repeat every 4–6 hours until recovery.
  - Follow by triple the usual daily doses of hydrocortisone for 2 days, then double for 3 days.

Adrenal hyperfunction
Adrenocortical tumours
- This may manifest as Cushing syndrome, virilisation, hypertension, abdominal mass or pain.
- These tumours are rare. Cushing disease in infancy or early childhood is usually due to an adrenal tumour, compared to older children where a secondary cause is far more common.

Adrenocortical hyperplasia
- This is usually secondary to a pituitary adenoma secreting ACTH (Cushing disease). Such lesions are usually very small (2–3 mm).
- A primary bilateral micronodular form (genetic cause: Carney complex) is rarely seen. A macronodular form is seen in patients with McCune Albright syndrome.

Clinical features
- Cortisol excess is more difficult to detect clinically in children than in adults.
- It is characterised by poor growth velocity and excessive weight gain. The child usually looks obese but the clinical features of moon face, thin limbs and striae may be absent.
- Hypertension is also frequently absent.

Investigation
- 24 hours urinary free cortisol. Plasma cortisol is often abnormal in obesity and may give a spurious result. Loss of diurnal variation of plasma cortisol may be helpful.Overnight dexamethasone suppression (1 mg dexamethasone given at 2400 hours and a plasma cortisol at 0800 hours the following day) will differentiate Cushing syndrome from obesity.

Further investigation for origin and type of cortisol excess is by a specialist. Treatment is surgical.

Adrenal medullary tumours
- Neuroblastoma usually occurs in very young children, but may present in adolescence.
- Phaeochromocytoma occurs in older children and causes hypertension. Phaeochromocytoma may be associated with various genetic conditions – multiple endocrine neoplasia (MEN), neurofibromatosis, von Hippel Lindau, SDH mutations.
- Paraganglioma is increasingly recognized – mass occurs in the adrenal gland or anywhere along the aortic chain, without hypertension (SDH mutation).

Diabetes insipidus
Background
Diabetes insipidus (DI) is an uncommon condition with either relative or absolute lack of anti-diuretic hormone (ADH) leading to an inability to concentrate the urine. The loss of free water and subsequent polyuria/polydypsia can potentially lead to fluid and electrolyte imbalance.

There are a number of potential causes of DI in a paediatric population. It most commonly occurs post-neurosurgical procedures, or secondary to cerebral malformations/tumours.

Clinical features

When assessing a patient with DI, the following features should be considered:

- Hydration status, fluid balance, urine output (strict fluid balance is the key in identifying DI). Change in weight as marker of fluid status
- Presence of intercurrent illness, for example UTI
- Causes of excess fluid loss, for example gastroenteritis, surgical drains
- Past history of DI

Investigations

- Urea and electrolytes
- Full ward test of urine
- Paired serum and urine osmolality

DI is present when the serum osmolality is raised (>295 mOsmol/kg) with inappropriately dilute urine (urine osmolality <700 mOsmol/kg). The serum sodium is often elevated due to excess free water losses.

If baseline tests are equivocal, the patient may require a water deprivation test to exclude DI. This should ONLY be performed as an inpatient in a controlled, well-monitored environment – withholding fluids from a patient with DI can lead to rapid decompensation of fluid and electrolyte status.

Management

Rehydration

Use the degree of dehydration and ongoing losses to calculate rehydration therapy.

- If the serum Na is >150 mmol/L, rehydration should occur over 48 hours (see management of hypernatraemia Chapter 9, *Fluids and nutrition*, Hypernatraemia).
- If Na >170 mmol/L, contact the intensive care unit/specialist team.

Desmopressin administration

Desmopressin (DDAVP, trade name: Minirin®) acts on the distal tubules and collecting ducts of the kidney to increase water reabsorption. It is a long-acting analogue of ADH.

Discussion with an endocrinologist is advised prior to the commencement of desmopressin therapy.

There are several formulations available:

- Minirin melts 60 or 120 mg – roughly 120 mg is equivalent to 10 mcg nasal spray
- Intranasal solution (100 mcg/mL)
- Intranasal spray (10 mcg per spray)
- Parenteral (IV/IM) (4 mcg/mL) – used rarely
- Oral (200 mcg per tablets) – roughly 10 mcg intranasal is approximately equivalent to 200 mcg orally

The following criteria should be met prior to dose administration:

- Serum sodium is >145 mmol/L (reference range 135–145 mmol/L)
- Urine output exceeds 4 mL/kg/h (calculated 6 hourly)
- Urine specific gravity is 1.005 or less (dilute urine output)

If desmopressin has been prescribed but the child does not meet all three criteria, consult with senior staff prior to administration of desmopressin (to prevent fluid overload and hyponatraemic seizures).

Dose:

- <1 year old – discuss with endocrinologist/specialist
- <2 years old – dose is usually 2–5 mcg intranasal
- 2 years and over – dose 5–10 mcg per day

Administration issues:

- Dosage effect is all or nothing – in general, the dose determines the duration of action NOT the degree of response.
- Oral dose has slower onset/offset of action, therefore NOT useful in acute situation.
- Nasal administration is operator dependent – also need to consider effectiveness if problems with nasal mucosa, for example intercurrent URTI, hay fever, post-operative.
- Careful fluid balance needs to be maintained to prevent fluid overload/hyponatraemia.

Ongoing management of patients on desmopressin – general principles:

- At a minimum, serum electrolytes and osmolality and urine osmolality should be tested daily until stable. Consider more frequent electrolytes if hypernatraemic, if there are concerns about fluid state or if the child is fasting for a procedure.
- Ensure most recent serum sodium result is above 145 mmol/L prior to administration of desmopressin.
- Need to have 1–2 hours of diuresis (greater than 4 mL/kg/h) prior to administration of next dose to allow free water clearance and avoid hyponatraemia – may need to withhold dose if inadequate diuresis.
- All urine specific gravity should be checked and documented.
- Strict fluid balance chart with output totalled 6 hourly.
- Daily weighs.

Disorders of calcium metabolism/bone health
Hypocalcaemia
Background
For causes, see Table 13.5.

Clinical features
- Rachitic changes in long bones (swollen wrists, etc.), rachitic rosary
- Tetany (may be demonstrated using sphygmomanometer cuff above systolic pressure for up to 2 minutes – Trousseau sign)
- Facial nerve twitching when tapping over parotid gland – Chvostek sign
- Laryngeal stridor
- Seizure
- Weakness, tiredness, irritability
  Note: even extreme hypocalcaemia may be asymptomatic in an infant.

Investigations
- Total and ionised calcium
- 25-OH vitamin D
- Renal function, lipase, albumin
- Magnesium, phosphate
- Alkaline phosphatase
- Parathyroid hormone (PTH)
- 1,25-diOH-vitamin D if non-vitamin D deficient rickets is suspected
- Radiographs of wrist, knee (metaphyseal splaying)
- Malabsorption studies

Table 13.5 Causes of hypocalcaemia

Neonatal presentation	Infant/childhood presentation
Prematurity/IUGR/birth asphyxia	Vitamin D deficiency
Hypoparathyroidism ±	Hypoparathyroidism
Di George syndrome	Association with autoimmune polyglandular syndrome.
Phosphate load (high phosphate milk)	Look for mucocutaneous candidiasis and/or Addison
Low magnesium	disease in a young child
Maternal gestational diabetes	Pseudohypoparathyroidism
	Albright hereditary osteodystrophy
	Chronic renal failure
	Pancreatitis
	Organic acidaemia
	Critical illness
	1-α-hydroxylase deficiency (rare)
	Vitamin D resistant rickets (VDR receptor mutation)
	Post cardiac surgery (citrate binding during cardiac bypass)

Table 13.6 Causes of hypercalcaemia

Neonatal	Infant/childhood
Hyperparathyroidism (rare)	Primary hyperparathyroidism
Iatrogenic	Familial hypocalciuric hypercalcaemia
Subcutaneous fat necrosis Familial hypocalciuric hypercalcaemia – severe form Hypophosphatasia William syndrome (elfin face, supravalvular aortic stenosis)	1,25-diOH-D excess (nutritional, inflammatory disease, for example sarcoidosis, leukaemia) Neoplasia (lytic bone lesions or humoral hypercalcaemia PTHrP) Immobilisation, for example burns (severe), quadriplegia – can be very severe and cause renal calculi, pancreatitis Drugs (lithium, thiazides) Endocrine disorders: hyperthyroidism (mild, usually asymptomatic), phaeochromocytoma, adrenal insufficiency Vitamin D/Vitamin A intoxication

- Urinary calcium/creatinine ratio
- ECG (prolonged QT interval)

Management
Emergency/symptomatic
Only use IV treatment if symptomatic (tetany, seizures) – ideally requires central access due to the risk of calcium burns if extravasation occurs.

- IV calcium chloride 10% infusion – 1 mmol/kg per 24 hours in 5% dextrose. Monitor calcium levels 6 hourly.
- Occasionally IV calcium chloride 10% – 0.2 mL/kg stat may be required for severe tetany.
- Correct magnesium if low.
- ECG monitor.
- 25-OH-vitamin D if nutritional rickets is suspected – consider megadose therapy (100,000 to 150,000 units cholecalciferol stat)
- 1,25-diOH-vitamin D (calcitriol) if parathyroid disorders suspected or if severe vitamin D deficiency and waiting for 25OH vitamin D treatment to take effect: 0.01–0.02 mcg/kg per day starting dose (may need to be increased).
- Treatment of underlying condition.
  Note: In the first days to weeks after treatment is begun for rickets, bones are 'hungry' – large doses of calcium supplements (and possibly calcitriol) may be required to maintain normocalcaemia and prevent carpopedal spasm once vitamin D is started.

Maintenance
- Adequate calcium intake, preferably as dairy products, 600–1500 mg per day depending on age.
- 25-OH-vitamin D for months to years depending on cause (for infant rickets, usually treat to age 4), dose will vary but often 400–1000 units per day.
- Stoss/megadose therapy is alternative method, using 100,000–150,000 units 25-OH-vitamin D at 0, 6–12 weeks then every 3–6 months as required, with appropriate monitoring.
- 1,25-diOH-vitamin D for vitamin D resistant rickets, hypoparathyroidism, patients on anticonvulsants.

Hypercalcaemia
Background
For causes, see Table 13.6.

Clinical features
- Polyuria, polydipsia
- Vomiting, dehydration

- Failure to thrive
- Abdominal pain (constipation, renal stones, pancreatitis)
- Confusion, apathy (if severe)

Investigation
- Total and ionised calcium, phosphate
- Magnesium, albumin
- Alkaline phosphatase
- PTH level
- 25-OH-vitamin D $\pm$ 1,25-diOH-vitamin D
- Thyroid function
- Chest radiograph $\pm$ skeletal survey
- Parathyroid imaging
- Urinary calcium/creatinine ratio
- Renal ultrasound (nephrocalcinosis)
- ECG (short QT interval)

Management
Severe
- Rehydration with 0.9% saline + 5% dextrose. For infants <2 years use 0.45% saline + 5% dextrose.
- Diuretics are used in two situations:
  - Acute hypercalcaemia: frusemide is given to reduce fluid overload while the patient is aggressively rehydrated.
  - Chronic hypercalcaemia with hypercalciuria (or normocalcaemia with hypercalciuria): thiazides are given to reduce oedema and prevent nephrocalcinosis (by decreasing urinary calcium excretion).
- Bisphosphonates, particularly for increased bone resorption (e.g. immobilisation).
- Steroids for vitamin D excess (prednisolone 2 mg/kg per day, reducing).
- Low-calcium diet.
- Surgery if indicated, treatment of underlying condition.

Paediatric bone health – fragility fractures
Background
A wide variety of conditions can lead to both primary and secondary issues with skeletal development. The effects on bone health of a number of chronic conditions in paediatrics is increasingly recognized (immobility, glucocorticoid use, chronic inflammation, poor nutrition, hypogonadism, etc.). While fractures are a relatively common part of childhood, recurrent fractures, fractures with low levels of force or fractures in clinical settings mentioned above should be further investigated.

Clinical features
The following factors should be considered during a bone health assessment:

- Number/type/mechanism/management of fractures
- Ambulatory status/activity levels
- Medication usage (i.e. glucocorticoids, anticonvulsants)
- Calcium intake/vitamin D levels
- Pubertal status
- Family history of fragility fractures (timing, number, mechanism)
- Presence of features suggesting collagen defects (ligamentous laxity, blue/grey sclerae, dental issues)

Investigations
- Blood tests: calcium, phosphate, vitamin D, alkaline phosphatase, PTH, thyroid function, coeliac screen.
- Urine tests: Urine calcium, phosphate, creatinine (needs to be paired with serum to interpret).
- Plain X-rays – examine existing films looking at cortical width, general appearance/mineral content (can be difficult to judge), vertebral wedging/collapse if lateral spine X-ray performed.

- Bone density scanning – usually dual energy X-ray absorptiometry (DXA) scan, often lumbar spine, hip and/or total body. Paediatric software is required to generate age matched Z score. Remember confounders – short stature and maturational delay.

Management

- Optimization of any simple risk factors (calcium intake, vitamin D levels, activity levels, pubertal induction).
- If recurrent fragility fractures, especially vertebral changes, consider the use of intravenous bisphosphonates. These should be prescribed by a specialist with experience in paediatric bone health disorders. Dental review is required prior to commencement. Monitoring for first dose effects of acute phase reaction and hypocalcaemia.
- Modification of environment to limit fracture risk.

CHAPTER 14
Growth and puberty

Matthew Sabin
Michele O' Connell
Georgia Paxton

Slow weight gain

Slow weight gain is arbitrarily defined as being <3rd percentile for weight or dropping ≥2 percentiles. It implies failure to gain weight, with height and head circumference being initially well preserved. Slow weight gain is often called 'failure to thrive (FTT)', however this term may be distressing to parents/families, and is probably best avoided. Many children with slow weight gain do not have an organic medical cause. A good history and examination of the child, along with assessment of family growth patterns, is usually adequate to exclude significant pathology. Investigations should be limited and focused. Short stature is discussed on p. 208.

Is this weight normal or is it slow weight gain?

When assessing children's growth, it is important to recognize that being in the lower/lowest percentiles does not necessarily indicate a problem. Weight and height are distributed in the population (thus the 3rd percentile represents the lower 3% of the population). By definition, children who are growing along a percentile line (including the 3rd percentile line) have normal growth. Children who have a discrepancy between their height and weight percentiles still have normal growth if both parameters are tracking, although they will be lean, and may have a body mass index (BMI) that is low. They will appear healthy, with good muscle bulk, adequate subcutaneous fat, and normal activity and development. It is important to plot family growth parameters to get an idea of expected height (mid-parental height (MPH) – p. 209).

Birthweight percentile does not predict future weight and in the first months of life, many infants will equilibrate to their 'true' growth channels and cross percentile lines. After the first months, crossing percentile lines does usually represent slow weight gain.

Children who are lean because they are undernourished are usually apathetic and withdrawn with poor muscle bulk.

Slow weight gain can be due to any one (or combination) of the following:

- Reduced intake
- Inadequate absorption
- Increased losses – upper or lower gastrointestinal (vomiting or diarrhoea) or urine
- Increased metabolic requirements
- Poor utilisation (genetic/metabolic conditions)

Considering these aspects provides a useful framework for history, alongside assessment of familial patterns of weight gain and growth, and psychological and developmental assessment of the child (Table 14.1).

History

History is focused on intake, output and excluding organic causes of slow weight gain.

- **Intake**: breast/bottle feeding history, number and volume of feeds per day (duration of feeds if breastfeeding), breast milk supply, whether formula is made up correctly, time taken to feed, age solids commenced, age when three meals and two snacks per day achieved, composition and quantity of meals, intake of different food groups, behavioural issues/fussing around eating and mealtime routine

Paediatric Handbook, Ninth Edition. Edited by Amanda Gwee, Romi Rimer and Michael Marks.
© 2015 John Wiley & Sons, Ltd. Published 2015 by John Wiley & Sons, Ltd.

Table 14.1 Causes of slow weight gain

Non-organic	Organic
Accounts for >50% of cases of slow weight gain. Essentially caused by poor intake, often combined with reduced amount of food offered, and poor intake by the child (slow eating, fussiness, issues with mealtime routine). This is strongly affected by psychosocial factors, such as parent/child mental health issues, and food access/poverty. In some cases it may be due to child protection issues, such as neglect.	**Poor intake** • Dental caries • Tonsillar hypertrophy (if severe) **Inadequate absorption** • Post infectious diarrhoea • Gastrointestinal manifestations of allergy • Coeliac disease • Cystic fibrosis or other pancreatic insufficiency • Short bowel syndrome or other gut mucosal abnormalities **Increased losses** • Vomiting (gastro-oesophageal reflux, pyloric stenosis, other) • Diarrhoea (infection, inflammatory bowel disease, and the other causes of inadequate absorption listed above) • Excessive urine losses/sodium losses **Increased requirements** – any chronic disease or system issue (renal, cardiac, respiratory endocrine disease, hyperthyroidism, chronic infection, immunodeficiency, malignancy, CNS or neuromuscular pathology) **Poor utilisation** • Genetic or metabolic conditions. • Disorders of protein, fat or carbohydrate metabolism (including undertreated diabetes). • Micronutrient deficiencies (from any cause) may contribute to poor utilisation of intake.

- **Output**: presence and amount of vomiting (number per day, also presence of blood/bile), stool frequency and consistency (number per day, presence of mucus, blood), urine losses (wet nappies, polyuria, polydipsia). Any identified triggers to increased output (e.g. food triggers)
- **Pregnancy/birth**
- **Past history:** chronic and current illness, recurrent infections
- **Family growth:** pattern of weight gain and growth in other family members
- **Family medical/mental health issues and social situation:** medical issues, mental health issues, household situation, food access

Examination
- **Pattern of growth:** plot serial measures of weight, height and head circumference percentiles, clarify family and health situation at times where growth trajectory changed.
- **Expected growth:** plot expected MPH.
- **Assess** growth and nutritional status and perform a full physical examination (see Chapter 9, *Fluids and nutrition*). Look for signs of macronutrient deficiency (muscle bulk, subcutaneous fat stores, buttock mass) and micronutrient deficiency (skin, hair, gums, eyes, nails) and also for evidence of system-based disease. Consider additional measures of nutrition – such as anthropometry (skinfold thickness). Assess parent–child interaction and whether the child appears well cared for. Happy, outgoing children with good muscle bulk in thighs and buttocks are unlikely to have significant under nutrition.

Investigations
Avoid random tests. The history and examination should guide the direction and pace of investigation. If the cause of slow weight gain is not readily apparent after history, examination and limited investigations (e.g. FBE, urine MCS), further investigations and management should occur in consultation with a specialist. A dietitian review will help clarify intake and provide information on estimated energy requirements and whether the child is meeting these requirements.

Second line investigations may include
- Faecal microscopy, culture, viral studies, absorption markers – pH, total sugars, reducing sugars, elastase
- Screening for coeliac disease
- Renal function
- Urine electrolytes (e.g. where salt loss suspected)
- Thyroid stimulating hormone (TSH)
- Liver function
- Inflammatory markers
- Considering testing for immune dysfunction, cystic fibrosis or other causes

Management

The underlying cause will determine the management. Infants and children require admission to hospital for
- Severe under nutrition
- Failed outpatient management
- Child abuse or neglect
- Extreme parental anxiety or depression that requires time to allow a constructive patient–doctor relationship to develop

Admission may facilitate further assessment of feeding technique, parent–child interaction and allow the involvement of a multidisciplinary team.

Obesity

Obesity is increasingly prevalent among Australian children – up to 25% are now either overweight or obese. Over the last three decades, the prevalence of overweight and obesity have doubled and trebled respectively. Although prevalence rates may now be stabilizing, paediatric obesity remains a major health concern.

Childhood obesity leads to adult obesity, with an increased long-term risk of mortality and morbidity. Parent obesity appears to be one of the strongest risk factors for persistence of obesity in children; this underpins the need for family-based change for successful weight management in children and adolescents. Adolescents who are persistently overweight are highly likely to remain overweight in their young adult years, and the prevalence of overweight and obesity has been shown to increase 65% between adolescence and early adulthood (more for males than females). However, overweight/obese children who grow up to be non-obese adults have significantly reduced risks of obesity-related conditions in adult life, such as high blood pressure and Type 2 diabetes. This is a major reason to address early-onset obesity.

Complications of obesity

- Psychosocial: body dissatisfaction, depression, bullying/teasing, school avoidance and low self-esteem
- Cardiovascular: dyslipidaemia and hypertension, metabolic syndrome
- Endocrine: glucose intolerance, insulin resistance, Type 2 diabetes, accelerated linear growth and bone age, earlier onset of puberty, polycystic ovary syndrome and menstrual abnormalities, thyroid dysfunction
- Orthopaedic: Blount disease and slipped capital femoral epiphysis
- Renal: obesity-related glomerulopathy
- Respiratory: obstructive sleep apnoea ± possible links to asthma
- Gastrointestinal: non-alcoholic fatty liver disease (NAFLD)
- Dermatological: intertrigo, furunculosis and acanthosis nigricans (marker of insulin resistance)
- Neurological: Idiopathic intracranial hypertension

Aetiology

Obesity occurs because energy intake exceeds energy requirement. Our understanding of factors that influence this balance is incomplete, but important considerations are
- Lifestyle factors: increased sedentary activities (watching television, social media and computer games), reduced time in physical activities (both incidental and organized) and increased access to energy-dense foods (i.e. food with high levels of sugar and/or fat).
- Genetic factors (susceptibility genes): may contribute to the development of obesity, although given that the gene pool changes slowly, lifestyle changes are more likely to be responsible for the recent increases in obesity prevalence. Single-gene disorders (e.g. leptin deficiency) are extremely rare.

Children with exogenous (non-medical) obesity are usually of normal intellect, have had normal development, and are either of normal or relatively tall stature.

- Hormonal and metabolic factors: Endocrine causes are rare and are usually associated with growth failure.
- Syndromal causes are often recognised by the presence of a significant developmental/intellectual disability and less frequently by dysmorphic features. Clues to syndromal or endocrine causes of obesity include
  - Height <50th centile (or less than genetic potential)
  - Dysmorphic features
  - Developmental/intellectual disabilities
  - Hypogonadism

Assessment

Definition

A simple, clinically useful definition that reflects excess body fat is the BMI. However, it does not reflect body composition and thus people with significant muscle mass may have a high BMI. This is usually clinically apparent.

$$BMI\,(kg/m^2) = weight\,(kg)/height^2\,(m^2)$$

In children and adolescents, BMI changes with normal growth; BMI is high in the first 2 years of life and this drops to a nadir, before gradually increasing to normal adult levels (see Appendix 1, *Growth charts*). The rise after the nadir is termed the **adiposity rebound** and usually occurs around the age of 6 years. The timing of the adiposity rebound may be important for later risk of obesity.

Plot BMI on a BMI centile chart, now included in standard growth charts:

- Overweight is defined as a BMI between 85th and 95th centile for age and sex.
- Obesity is defined as a BMI >95th centile for age and sex.

Once obesity is diagnosed, the aim is to identify:

- Contributing factors for the individual
- Any underlying medical causes
- Individuals at high risk of associated disease
- Complications and co-morbidities

History

In most cases, a detailed personal, family, developmental and past (including perinatal) history, complemented by a thorough dietary history, activity history and a detailed physical examination, is sufficient. Consider the following:

- Features suggestive of an underlying cause, for example poor postnatal feeding and hypotonicity during infancy (Prader–Willi syndrome) and medications (e.g. long-term steroid use).
- Risk factors for co-morbidities and symptoms of obstructive sleep apnoea.
- Family history of obesity, heart disease, diabetes, hypertension, dyslipidaemia and other complications of obesity.
- Ethnicity. Children from certain ethnic backgrounds (e.g. Australian indigenous people, Pacific Islanders, Asians and Indians) have a higher tendency for weight gain and display greater levels of co-morbidity for a given level of obesity.
- An age-appropriate developmental approach is required. Parents can be the exclusive agents of change for preschool children, whereas adolescents should be seen separately from their parents for part of a consultation to explore psychosocial co-morbidities. It is important to address body image and ensure the young person has realistic, appropriate healthy weight goals.

Examination

- Plot height, weight and BMI on percentile charts.
- Document pubertal and developmental status.
- Assess the body build, posture and distribution of adiposity.
- Measure the waist circumference (at midpoint between lowest ribs and iliac crests – be sure to include any apron of abdominal fat).

- Measure the blood pressure with an appropriate-sized cuff.
- Look for acanthosis nigricans (velvet pigmentation on the neck and/or axilla).
- Look for clues to a syndromal/endocrine cause:
  - Height <50th centile (or less than genetic potential)
  - Dysmorphic features
  - Cushingoid features (including abdominal striae)
  - Developmental/intellectual disability
  - Hypogonadism

Think of other associated problems, for example look for dental caries.

Investigations
- For aetiology.
- For underlying cause, if clinically indicated, for example karyotype/microarray. Think of thyroid function.
- For complications:
  - Hyperlipidaemia – full fasting lipid profile.
  - Type 2 diabetes – formal oral glucose tolerance testing is preferred in adolescents, although fasting glucose and insulin is often sufficient in younger children.
  - Hepatic steatosis – liver function tests $\pm$ liver ultrasound scan.
  - Vitamin D.

Although the health consequences of obesity increase with increasing age- and sex-adjusted BMI, the degree of co-morbidities in obese children and adolescents is not clearly associated with the severity of obesity. It is important to take into account other factors (such as family history of diabetes, and ethnicity) in deciding whether to investigate for health problems.

Screening for complications is particularly important in children and adolescents where obesity is resistant to lifestyle change and where there are risk factors for complication. Puberty is associated with a significant reduction in insulin sensitivity in normal individuals and investigation for Type 2 diabetes maybe needed in peri-pubertal children.

Other investigations (e.g. sleep studies in significant obstructive sleep apnoea) should be performed as clinically indicated.

General approach
The goal is to diminish morbidity and mortality risk, rather than to achieve an ideal body weight. Identifying children and adolescents who are in the early stages of weight gain is an important opportunity for clinical intervention. It is much better to start early intervention to control excessive weight gain, than to provide more intensive and difficult interventions for established obesity.

The emphasis of management should be on improved fitness, health and social functioning. The primary objective is usually to maintain weight over time, so that with normal longitudinal growth, the weight falls back into the healthy weight range. In children and adolescents with severe obesity weight loss may be required.

Successful maintenance of a healthy weight is best achieved through long-term multidisciplinary family-based interventions that include behavioural change. The aim is to shift in the child's energy balance. Principles of management include:

- Professional input that is non-judgemental, encouraging and empowering. Consider not using the word 'obese', but rather 'above the child's healthiest weight'.
- Education of families about:
  - Medical complications of obesity;
  - The concept of energy balance;
  - Healthy eating and interpreting food labels (see below);
  - Appropriate physical activities (see below).
- Family-based strategies:
  - Identify the family's readiness to change – this will guide whether the goal of the consultation is to raise awareness or to explore behaviour change.
  - Explore ways to involve all family members and caregivers.

- Aim for permanent lifestyle changes, as opposed to short-term diets or exercise programmes for rapid weight loss:
  - ○ Severely energy-restricted diets are contraindicated in the majority of obese children and adolescents.
  - ○ Self-monitoring of diet and physical activities can help maintain change.
- Regular follow-up provides an opportunity to monitor health and weight over time.

Specific approaches
Physical activity
Any increase in activity is an improvement!
- Aim for 'lifestyle' exercise: using the stairs, walking to school, walking the dog.
- Involve the whole family.
- Use after-school time to get outdoors and be active.
- Decrease screen-based activities (TV, computer, electronic games).

Nutrition
Do not forget drinks!
- Water is the best drink for kids: cut out cordial, soft drink, fruit juice.
- It is better to eat fruit rather than drink fruit juice.
- Low-fat (2% fat) milk (<500 mL per day) is preferred for children >2 years of age.
- Emphasise the importance of breakfast, regular meals and healthy snacks.
- Encourage reading food labels and an awareness of the 'traps', for example 'no fat' might mean large amounts of sugar and therefore the same number of kilojoules.
- Serving sizes – does the 5-year old get served as much as mum or dad? (see Chapter 9, *Fluids and nutrition*, Daily food needs of preschoolers). Planning ahead, avoiding regular takeaway meals. Educate about satiety and hunger cues (vs. eating when bored or emotionally distressed).
- Explore mealtime routine.

Referral to a specialist
This may be indicated when there is
- A suspected pathological cause
- Complications of obesity
- Lack of progress in weight maintenance
- Severe, progressive, or early-onset obesity
- Parent or patient request
  Some specific medical therapies are used in obese adolescents:
- Metformin may be useful in reducing obesity-associated insulin resistance.
- Orlistat can be considered in those with severe or resistant obesity. They should only be prescribed from specialist centres and must be used in conjunction with an ongoing lifestyle-modification intervention.
- Gastric banding may be indicated in severe obesity. Referrals should be made from specialist paediatric weight management centres and be in accordance with guidelines published by the Royal Australasian College of Physicians – http://www.racp.edu.au/index.cfm?objectid=64DA592 F-9F31-E67 C-CDB308F5BF17A086

Short stature
Background
Stature must be assessed in the context of parental heights and the child's pubertal status. Growth velocity must be compared with age-matched peers and assessed with regard to the child's pubertal status/bone age. A number of factors affect longitudinal growth. These include familial growth patterns, nutritional status, general health, bone health/presence of a normal skeleton, GH/IGF1 axis, adrenal function, thyroid status and the actions of insulin and sex steroids.

Assessment
Stature
Measure the child and, wherever possible, both biological parents. Height should always be measured with shoes off, with the child standing upright and fully extended against a vertical surface, with a calibrated, fixed

measuring device. The head should be directly forward. Gentle pressure can be applied beneath the mastoid processes to ensure full neck extension.

The child's height and the MPH should be plotted on the appropriate centile chart.

MPH is assessed using the following equation:

$$\frac{\text{For boys: (Mother's height} + 13 \text{ cm)} + \text{(Father's height in cm)}}{2}$$
$$\frac{\text{For girls: (Father's height} - 13 \text{ cm)} + \text{(Mother's height in cm)}}{2}$$

A child's projected final height (extrapolated from their height centile and observed growth pattern) should fall within a range of MPH $\pm$ 7.5–8 cm (one standard deviation).

Questions to consider:

- Is the child short in relation to other children of the same age (i.e. below the third percentile)?
- Is the child unexpectedly short for the family?

Growth rate

Serial measurements over time are required to fully assess stature and growth. Ideally measurements should be performed by the same clinician; however, previous height measurements, if available, are also useful to help assess the pattern over time.

Calculate the height velocity and check this against a growth velocity (GV) chart. Growth velocity can only be reliably calculated from measurements taken over 6–12 months (with a minimum of 3–4 months between consecutive readings). In most children, GV tends to fluctuate and only a consistently low GV will lead to a falling-off in height percentile. Further investigation is required in a short child with a GV below the 25th percentile.

Questions to consider:

- Is the child growing slowly?
- If the child's growth really is slow, what is the reason?
- Is the child growing at the rate expected for pubertal status? A growth spurt should always accompany puberty.

Causes of short stature

Physiological

Constitutional delay of growth and puberty

- This is a common normal variant.
- Family history of delayed puberty is often present.
- Growth slows at about 2 years of age, producing a fall in the height percentile. Thereafter, growth is parallel to the 3rd percentile, but the prepubertal decline in growth is exaggerated and the onset of the pubertal growth spurt is later than average.
- Bone age is delayed; however, height for bone age is usually within the expected mid-parental range. The final height is likely to be in keeping with that of other family members.

Familial short stature

- Several adult family members are short.
- Skeletal proportions and GV are normal.
- Bone age is equivalent to the chronological age.
- Some children from short families also have constitutional delay in maturation. Parents who have suffered protein–calorie malnutrition as children may not have achieved their own genetic potential and may be on a lower percentile than their children.

Organic

Organic causes of short stature are classified in Table 14.2. Clues to the diagnosis may emerge from the history and the child's general appearance. Some serious medical conditions (e.g. chronic renal failure, coeliac disease, inflammatory bowel disease, craniopharyngioma) may present with slow growth as the only abnormal sign.

Table 14.2 Organic causes of short stature

	Examples	Clues to diagnosis
Intrauterine	Placental insufficiency; Russell–Silver syndrome	Birth length <3rd centile for gestational age
Skeletal	Bone dysplasia (e.g. achondroplasia) Spinal irradiation	Skeletal disproportion (short limbs) Low upper: lower segment ratio
Nutritional	Malabsorption (e.g. coeliac disease/short gut)	Poor weight gain ± abdominal distension
	Rickets	History of poor nutrition or limited sunlight/dark skin
	Protein–calorie malnutrition (world no.1)	Low weight-for-height (if not chronic)
Chronic illness	Renal failure, inflammatory bowel disease, JCA, CF, inborn errors of metabolism, organic or amino acidurias	Anaemia, high ESR, findings specific to associated pathology
Iatrogenic	Corticosteroid therapy	Cushingoid features
Chromosomal/ other genetic	Turner, Down, Prader–Willi, Noonan, Cornelia de Lange, Rubinstein–Taybi syndromes	Specific dysmorphic features
Endocrine	Hypothyroidism, growth hormone deficiency, Cushing syndrome/disease, pubertal delay/arrest, pseudohypoparathyroidism, Albright hereditary osteodystrophy (AHO)	Height centile < weight centile (i.e. short and plump); associated examination findings specific to diagnosis
Other	Psychosocial deprivation	Additional child protection concerns

Important clues include:
- Dysmorphic features (e.g. Turner syndrome).
- Cutaneous changes (e.g. café au lait markings – Silver–Russell syndrome, neurofibromatosis).
- Hand and wrist changes (e.g. short fourth/fifth metacarpals, narrow deep-set nails – Turner syndrome, Madelung deformity of the wrist – SHOX gene abnormality).
- Fundal changes (e.g. optic atrophy).

Measure the skeletal proportions (arm span/height and upper/lower segment ratios):
- The lower segment should be greater than half the height beyond the age of 10 years.
- The arm span should be within a few centimetres of height at all ages.

Investigations

Check the bone age initially. If the GV is <25th percentile for bone age, or the height is out of keeping with genetic potential, then further tests are indicated. The differential diagnosis will be based on history and examination findings in a given case, but the following can be considered:

- Thyroid function tests – TSH is the usual screening test, check free T4 (FT4) if central (pituitary) dysfunction is considered.
- Haemoglobin and erythrocyte sedimentation rate (ESR) (inflammatory bowel disease).
- Renal function and urine m,c,s.
- Serum calcium, phosphate and alkaline phosphatase.
- Coeliac antibodies.
- Karyotype (all short girls – lack of dysmorphism does not exclude Turner syndrome).
- Skeletal survey (if disproportionate).

If above are all normal and concerns persist, assessment of GH axis may be considered. A baseline IGF1 may be useful (needs to be interpreted in the context of bone age). Stimulated growth hormone (GH) studies are a more definitive test. Growth hormone can be assessed in response to either:

- Exercise or
- Pharmacological stimulation (e.g. glucagon stimulation used at RCH; other agents include clonidine, insulin, arginine). These should be performed at a centre with experience in carrying out the tests.

Note: Basal GH is not a useful test as due to the pulsatile nature of GH release, a low level does not define GH deficiency.

Management
Treatment of the underlying cause, for example thyroxine replacement, gluten free diet, where applicable

Growth hormone therapy
Recombinant human GH is government-controlled in Australia; it costs an average of $20 000–$30 000 per year per child. To qualify on the basis of stature, children must meet one of the following criteria:
- Growth hormone deficiency
- Turner syndrome or SHOX gene disorders
- Chronic renal disease
- Short and slow growth, defined as height below the 1st percentile and GV below the 25th percentile for bone age

Additional criteria that must be met in all cases include:
- Bone age <13.5 years for girls, or <15.5 years for boys

Exclusion criteria include diabetes mellitus (unless proven biochemical GHD and excellent diabetes control), known risk of malignancy (e.g. Down or Bloom syndrome) or active malignancy.

Children with GH deficiency or Turner syndrome respond to growth hormone with an increase in final height. For other conditions without biochemical GH deficiency, use of growth hormone will increase GV in the short term but usually does not result in significant increase in final height.

Note: These criteria differ if a child has GH deficiency following intracranial pathology or treatment including cranial radiation. Specialist assessment is required.

In Australia, the starting dose of growth hormone is 4.5–6 mg/m^2 per week divided into 6–7 doses. Incremental increases up to 7.5 mg/m^2 per week can be made if response criteria are not met. Children with Turner syndrome/SHOX haploinsufficiency can commence therapy at a higher dose (7.5–9.5 mg/m^2 per week).

Psychological support should also be offered as short children can experience teasing or bullying and are often treated as younger than their chronological age.

Useful growth resources can be found at http://www.apeg.org.au/ClinicalResourcesLinks/GrowthGrowth Charts/tabid/101/Default.aspx

Tall stature
Causes
- Familial
- Precocious puberty
- Hyperthyroidism
- Syndromes: Marfan, Klinefelter, triple X, homocystinuria and Sotos.
- Pituitary gigantism (juvenile acromegaly).

Lifestyle-related obesity is associated with increased stature in childhood, but normal adult final height.

Assessment
Height must be considered in the context of mid-parental expectation and pubertal status, for example if puberty is 2–3 years earlier than average, the child may appear to be very tall for chronological age but have a perfectly normal final height expectation for the family. Repeated height assessments are important in assessing tall stature. Review of associated symptoms may help with differential diagnosis. Examination should include
- auxology as for short stature
- assessment for dysmorphic features
- intellectual development
- pubertal staging
- thyroid status
- assessment of arachnodactyly
- cardiovascular system
- palate and joint mobility (Marfan's)

- eyes (Marfan's/homocystinuria)
- skin and visual fields (if pituitary adenoma suspected)

Investigations
Consider:

- Bone age.
- Thyroid function.
- Karyotype.
- Urine metabolic screen/antithrombin III/coagulation/lipids (homocystinuria).
- 3 hours oral glucose tolerance test assessing for failure of suppression of GH/IGF1 if acromegaly is suspected. MRI pituitary and further assessment of pituitary function are indicated if this test is consistent with GH excess.

Management
Management of any underlying disorder, for example precocious puberty. High-dose oestrogen was previously used in very tall girls, to hasten epiphyseal closure; however, long-term follow-up indicated a reduction in fertility in treated girls and so this treatment is now rarely used.

Delayed puberty
Background
The first sign of true puberty (gonadotropin-induced sex steroid production) is breast development in girls and testicular enlargement to ≥4 mL in boys. The presence of pubarche alone is not indicative of true puberty and this may precede thelarche or testicular enlargement. Accelerated growth begins at the onset of puberty in girls and at mid-puberty in boys.

Delayed puberty is defined as the absence of early pubertal changes by 13–14 years for girls and by 15 years for boys. Delayed puberty is more common in boys, and precocious puberty is more common in girls. Always investigate if girls have delayed puberty and boys have precocious puberty. There is no absolute age for diagnosis of delayed puberty; later than average and inappropriately late in a family are common reasons for referral (see Appendix 1 for pubertal stages charts/diagrams).

Causes
With normal or low serum gonadotropins

- Constitutional delay (usually familial) is the most common cause. It is associated with slow growth and a delayed bone age in an otherwise healthy child.
- Chronic illness/poor nutrition (e.g. inflammatory bowel disease, anorexia nervosa, cystic fibrosis).
- Endocrine causes:
  - Hypopituitarism (gonadotropin and possibly GH and other hormonal deficiencies).
  - Kallmann syndrome (isolated gonadotropin deficiency with anosmia).
  - Hyperprolactinaemia (prolactinoma, secondary to medication (e.g. antipsychotics), functional (e.g. postcranial irradiation)).

With elevated serum gonadotropins
This signifies primary gonadal failure, which may be due to

- A genetic abnormality associated with gonadal dysgenesis (e.g. Turner, Klinefelter and Noonan syndromes)
- Anorchia
- Secondary gonadal destruction (e.g. due to vascular damage, irradiation, infection, torsion or autoimmune disease)

Assessment

- Detailed history to assess differential diagnosis.
- Auxology – height and weight.
- MPH and target range.
- Growth velocity.
- Pubertal stage – assessed using Tanner staging system and testicular volume in boys. Chest wall adiposity can mimic the appearance of breast tissue in a prepubertal child.

Investigations
- Bone age – may be the only test required if there is a family history of late puberty
- Serum follicle-stimulating hormone (FSH), luteinising hormone (LH), testosterone or oestradiol; serum prolactin; other pituitary function tests (e.g. GH studies), as indicated by growth
- Full blood examination, ESR
- Urea, creatinine, serum proteins
- Thyroid function test
- Karyotype

Management
Referral to a specialist is advised. A 'watch and wait' strategy may be reasonable in the first instance. If induction of puberty is thought desirable (e.g. due to psychosocial distress), testosterone may be used in boys and oestradiol in girls; however, excess or early use of sex hormones for pubertal management will result in rapid advancement of bone age, epiphyseal fusion and stunting of final height in both sexes. Growth hormone therapy may also be offered to girls with Turner syndrome.

Precocious puberty
Precocious puberty is defined as the onset of pubertal changes under 8 years in girls and under 9 years in boys. For pubertal staging, see Appendix 1.

Cause
Gonadotropin dependent ('central' or 'true' precocious puberty)
- True precocious puberty is over 10 times more common in girls than boys.
- Girls are less likely to have an underlying pathological cause than boys.
- Girls with this disorder have accelerated growth, with development of breasts and often pubic hair (± menstruation if rapidly progressive).
- Boys with true precocious puberty have enlargement of both testes, as well as accelerated linear and genital growth.
- The commonest pathological cause is an intracranial lesion such as a hypothalamic hamartoma. Practically all intracranial pathologies (malformation, trauma, tumour, infection and haemorrhage) are associated with an increased prevalence of precocious puberty. After cranial irradiation, puberty occurs on average 2 years earlier in both boys and girls.
- Investigations are directed to demonstrate the premature activity in the hypothalamic–pituitary–gonadal axis and to exclude intracranial pathology.

Gonadotropin independent ('pseudo' precocious puberty)
- Congenital adrenal hyperplasia
- Adrenal, testicular or ovarian neoplasms
- Tumours that secrete non-pituitary gonadotropin such as chorionic gonadotropin (hCG)
- McCune–Albright syndrome
- Familial male precocious puberty

Assessment
History should assess for symptoms associated with:
- pubertal changes (e.g. breast tenderness, vaginal discharge/bleeding, mood swings, enlargement of penis/testes/clitoris, voice change, acne, growth acceleration)
- features suggesting the possible aetiology (headaches, visual change, previous treatment such as irradiation, etc.).
  Examination should include auxology, careful assessment of pubertal staging (including testicular volume in boys and external genitalia in girls with apparent androgen excess), blood pressure, fundi and neurological exam, skin (McCune-Albright or NF1)

Investigation of precocious puberty (both types)
- Serum FSH and LH ± LHRH stimulation test to confirm pubertal response (if basal levels not definitive).
- Gonadal steroid (testosterone or oestradiol).

- Tumour markers – αFP and βHCG where indicated.
- Bone age.
- TFTs (long-standing primary hypothyroidism can result in precocious puberty).
- If above tests indicate a central cause, consider MRI of brain and pituitary (need to specify pituitary to ensure it is adequately imaged)
  - All boys with central precocious puberty must have an MRI scan.
  - In girls with central precocious puberty, MRI is less likely to yield an intracranial organic lesion. It is not routinely done if puberty occurs at >5 years, unless there is a specific clinical indication (e.g. headache, visual change).
- Pelvic ultrasound – if adrenal tumour suspected in either sex, or in girls for ovarian cyst or tumour.
- Testicular ultrasound if indicated.

Management

The primary goal of treatment is to preserve final height (aiming for a final height in the normal adult range and as close to MPH range as possible); treatment may also alleviate psychosocial distress relating to early puberty. In some cases, the tempo of pubertal change may be such that treatment is not indicated.

Refer to a specialist who may use a luteinising hormone releasing hormone agonist (LHRH agonist). Alternative options to suppress menses (but which won't impact on final height) include medroxyprogesterone acetate or cyproterone acetate.

Conditions resembling precocious puberty

Premature thelarche

- Isolated breast development is common in girls <2 years of age (8–10%) and can be expected to regress spontaneously in most cases.
- Simple observation is usually sufficient, but if the condition is associated with rapid growth velocity, consider true oestrogen excess of any cause and investigate (as above).

Premature adrenarche

- The isolated appearance of pubic hair (usually in a girl) under the age of 8 years may occur as a normal variant, but it may also signify non-classical congenital adrenal hyperplasia.
- Appropriate investigations are bone age, basal serum dehydroepiandrosterone sulfate (DHEA-S), androstenedione, testosterone and 17-hydroxyprogesterone (17-OHP). The measurement of 17-OHP at 30 and 60 minutes after intramuscular Synacthen (synthetic adrenocorticotrophic hormone (ACTH)) is recommended to diagnose non-classical congenital adrenal hyperplasia.
  Note: Referral to a specialist is recommended.

> **USEFUL RESOURCES**
> - *Obesity guidelines at www.nhmrc.gov.au*
> - *www.apeg.org.au* – Clinical resources and links tab.
> - *http://www.rch.org.au/childgrowth/*
> - *www.iaso.org* – International Association for the Study of Obesity. Useful general information. RACP Guidelines on Bariatric Surgery in Adolescents – http://www.racp.edu.au/index.cfm?objectid=64DA592 F-9F31-E67 C-CDB308F5BF17A086.

CHAPTER 15

Bones and joints

Peter Barnett
Jane Munro
Leo Donnan
Roger Allen

Musculoskeletal symptoms and signs are common in children and adolescents and may be the presenting feature of a broad spectrum of conditions. Clinical features and laboratory findings may be relatively non-specific in orthopaedic and rheumatological conditions and it is important to look for disease patterns when evaluating the presenting complaint and conducting a systems review.

Musculoskeletal assessment

History

- Check the nature of onset – is it acute or insidious? Have there been other episodes?
- **Acute onset monoarticular arthritis associated with fever is septic until proved otherwise.**
- Check the timing of symptoms during the day – as a general guide:
  - Early morning stiffness = inflammatory.
  - Post-activity pain = mechanical.
- Check duration of illness – if >6 weeks, it is less likely to be reactive/postviral arthritis.
- Are there any intercurrent infections (respiratory, enteric or skin)? Postviral arthritis is probably the commonest cause of transient arthritis.
- Is there a history of trauma?
- Has the child been taking any medications (e.g. cefaclor)?
- What does the child, or parent, consider to be the most symptomatic site – is it in the joint, muscle, adjacent bone or a more diffuse area?
- Check for extra-articular symptoms – ensure a thorough systems review and keep the three following diagnoses in mind:
  - Systemic lupus erythematosus (SLE).
  - Acute lymphoblastic leukaemia (ALL).
  - Inflammatory bowel disease (IBD).
- Assess whether the normal physical activities or interests have been interrupted.
- Assess the functional milieu of the patient (e.g. school progress, family and peer relationships, stress experiences).
- Check the family history for other types of inflammatory arthritis, particularly the spondyloarthropathies, autoimmune disorders and pain syndromes (e.g. fibromyalgia or other models for pain behaviour).

Examination

Observe the patient as they move about the room, looking for limitations or alterations in function, and be opportunistic when examining them.

- Examine all joints, not only the site of the presenting complaint. There may be inflammation without symptoms in juvenile idiopathic arthritis (JIA).

Paediatric Handbook, Ninth Edition. Edited by Amanda Gwee, Romi Rimer and Michael Marks.
© 2015 John Wiley & Sons, Ltd. Published 2015 by John Wiley & Sons, Ltd.

- Aim to localise the site of maximal discomfort (e.g. is it the joint capsule, adjacent bone or muscle belly, tendon or ligament attachments?).
- Examine for signs of systemic diseases with an articular component and extra-articular features of JIA. In particular, examine the skin, eyes, abdomen, nails and lymph nodes.

A musculoskeletal assessment should include

- *Joints*: signs of inflammation such as swelling or tenderness, the range of movement and deformity.
- *Entheses*: bone attachment sites of ligaments/tendons (e.g. Achilles tendon).
- *Tendon sheaths* of fingers and toes (e.g. dactylitis in psoriasis).
- *Gait*: antalgic (pain) or limp, Trendelenburg sign.
- *Muscles*: tenderness, wasting or weakness, for example inability to toe or crouch walk (walking in a full-squat position).
- *Patellar tracking pattern* – does the patella move vertically on walking?
- *Shoe sole* and heel-wearing pattern.
- *Leg length* measurement.
- *Spinal flexion*, including Schober test (the measurement of the lumbosacral range should increase by at least 6 cm on maximal flexion; the starting range is between the lumbosacral junction and a point 10 cm above).
- *Growth parameters*.

The pGALS is an excellent screening tool for joint examination. See Table 15.1.

Table 15.1 The components of paediatric Gait, Arms, Legs, Spine screen (pGALS)

Screening questions
- Do you have any pain or stiffness in your joints, muscles or your back?
- Do you have any difficulty getting yourself dressed without any help?
- Do you have any difficulty going up- and downstairs?

Gait
- Observe the child walking
- 'Walk on your tip-toes/walk on your heels'

Arms
- 'Put your hands out in front of you'
- 'Turn your hands over and make a fist'
- 'Pinch your index finger and thumb together'
- 'Touch the tips of your fingers with your thumb'
- Squeeze the metacarpophalangeal joints
- 'Put your hands together/put your hands back to back'
- 'Reach up and touch the sky'
- 'Look at the ceiling'
- 'Put your hands behind your neck'

Legs
- Feel for effusion at the knee
- 'Bend and then straighten your knee' (active movement of knees and examiner feels for crepitus)
- Passive flexion (90 degrees) with internal rotation of hip

Spine
- 'Open your mouth and put three of your (child's own) fingers in your mouth'
- Lateral flexion of cervical spine – 'Try and touch your shoulder with your ear'
- Observe the spine from behind
- 'Can you bend and touch your toes?' Observe curve of the spine from side and behind

Source: Reproduced with permission from Foster HE, Kay LJ, Friswell M, Coady D, Myers A. Musculoskeletal screening examination (pGALS) for school-age children based on the adult GALS screen. *Arthritis Care Research* 2006; 55(5): 709–716. (Foster 2006. Reproduced with permission of Wiley & Sons Ltd.)

Rheumatologic conditions
Juvenile idiopathic arthritis (previously juvenile rheumatoid arthritis and juvenile chronic arthritis)
Assessment
- Age of onset <16 years of age
- Minimum duration of arthritis – 6 weeks
- **Most acute non-septic arthritis is not JIA**

Disease subtypes
- *Oligoarticular*: affects four joints or fewer:
  - Young, often antinuclear antibody (ANA)-positive females (can get asymptomatic uveitis that does not correlate with activity of arthritis – screen 3 monthly)
  - Older, typically HLA-B27-positive males (who may have an evolving spondyloarthropathy)
- *Polyarticular*: affects five joints or more; rheumatoid factor positive or negative
- *Systemic*: joint involvement plus fever, rash and lymphadenopathy
- It is useful to look for
  - Features suggestive of a spondyloarthropathy: enthesitis, sacroiliitis or acute uveitis
  - Nail pits/scalp rash (indicative of psoriasis)
  - Rash of Still disease (faint urticarial-like erythema) – mostly when febrile
  - Uveitis (especially oligo-JIA patient) by slit lamp
  - Inflammatory features, including subtle behavioural features such as withdrawal from activity, excessive irritability or sleep disruption

Investigations
There is no single diagnostic test for JIA. Imaging will be determined by site of pain and possible diagnosis.

Often useful
- Full blood examination (FBE), erythrocyte sedimentation rate (ESR) and C-reactive protein (CRP). Normal inflammatory markers do not exclude the diagnosis.
- Synovial fluid culture – if sepsis is considered.
- ANA – beware of over-interpretation as up to 20% of normal children may have a low positive ANA.

Occasionally useful
- Rheumatoid factor – in polyarticular patients, older children or if the pattern of disease appears unusual.
- HLA-B27 – if spondyloarthropathy is suspected. Remember almost 9% of the White population are positive.
- Imaging – consider plain radiograph, bone scan and ultrasound. In early arthritis, plain films usually give no more information than a careful examination. They may be useful for difficult sites such as the hip, or if there is a long history of arthritis. MRI can be occasionally useful but is not usually an appropriate initial investigation.
- Diagnostic aspirate – worthwhile if sepsis or haemarthrosis is considered, but will not necessarily differentiate between other inflammatory arthritides.
- Specific bacterial/viral studies – if the clinical picture is suggestive (e.g. ASOT, anti-DNase B, Yersinia and parvovirus serology), see Postinfectious arthritis, p. 218.

Not useful
- Serum uric acid

Management
Depends on the clinical picture of disease severity and subtype.

Principles
- Preserve joint function
- Control pain
- Manage complications

Multidisciplinary approach, including physiotherapy, occupational therapy, and psychosocial support. Physical therapy is essential to maintain joint range and function. Splinting should be considered where appropriate.

Medication
- Initially NSAIDs, for example naproxen, indomethacin, diclofenac, piroxicam or ibuprofen.
- Then usually methotrexate to minimise joint destruction.
- Other options include corticosteroids in systemic JIA and intra-articular corticosteroid injections (used early in mono- or oligoarticular arthritis). These are usually performed under GA or procedural sedation and analgesia (e.g. nitrous oxide).
- For children with severe arthritis, persistent systemic features i.e. fever and/or uveitis resistant to treatment, biological therapies using injectable TNF and cytokine blockers may be required.

Enthesitis-related arthropathies (spondyloarthropathies)
- Uncommon (more frequent in males) with onset >10 years of age
- HLA-B27 positive (80%), often raised inflammatory markers
- Intermittent episodes of enthesitis (tender at tendon insertions) and lower back pain/sacroiliitis
- Acute uveitis (usually clinically evident)
- Management: NSAIDs such as naproxen; then methotrexate or sulfasalazine

Henoch–Schönlein purpura (HSP)
A small-vessel vasculitis.

Clinical features
- Most common age of onset 2–8 years
- May present with one or more of the following manifestations:
  - Evolving crops of palpable purpura – predominantly buttocks and legs
  - Abdominal pain (occasionally malaena) may precede rash
  - Large joint migratory arthritis of variable duration and severity
  - Nephritis
  - Other (e.g. oedema dorsum of the feet and hands, acute scrotal swelling and 'bruising', fever and fatigue)
- Exclude other causes of purpura (see Chapter 17, *Dermatologic conditions*)

Investigations
- FBE (to exclude thrombocytopenia)
- Urinalysis – haematuria, proteinuria
- Renal function – urea, creatinine and urinary protein estimation

Management
- Supportive – bed rest and analgesia.
- Corticosteroids – may reduce the duration of abdominal pain, but it is uncertain if they significantly affect other features.
- Refer to a specialist if renal dysfunction, hypertension or surgical complications develop.

Kawasaki disease
See Chapter 18, *Infectious diseases and immunisation*.

Postinfectious arthritis
Acute rheumatic fever
See Chapter 18, *Infectious diseases and immunisation*.

Reactive arthritis
Poststreptococcal reactive arthritis
- Afebrile symmetrical non-migratory poly- or pauciarticular arthritis.
- Arthritis responds slowly to NSAIDs.
- Carditis may occur and form part of a spectrum with acute rheumatic fever.
- Penicillin prophylaxis if carditis is present.

Postenteric reactive arthritis
- Mainly *Salmonella*, *Shigella* and *Yersinia* (also reported with *Campylobacter and Giardia*).
- It is clinically similar to the spondyloarthropathies; that is predominantly lower limb (including sacroiliitis), enthesitis is common and positive family history (especially if HLA-B27 positive). However, it may not present with all the classic clinical features.
- Consider Crohn's disease or ulcerative colitis.
- Associated features – acute anterior uveitis and sterile pyuria.
- Treatment – NSAIDs: indomethacin 0.5–1.0 mg/kg (max. 75 mg) p.o. 8 hourly is often the most effective.

Postviral arthritis
- Many viral illnesses are associated with arthritis.
- It is uncertain in most situations whether it is the primary (infective) or secondary (reactive) event; for example Epstein–Barr virus, rubella, adenovirus, varicella (beware of septic arthritis secondary to infected skin lesion), parvovirus B19 and hepatitis B.
- A transient arthritis often follows a non-specific 'viral' illness, the confirmation of which may be difficult and unnecessary.
- Treatment: NSAIDs probably shorten the duration.

Noninflammatory causes of joint pain
Benign nocturnal limb pains ('growing pains')
- Onset at 3–7 years, often occurs in the evenings and at night.
- Well between attacks.
- Recurrent pain mainly involving the knee, calf and shin.
- No symptoms or signs of inflammation either on history or examination.
- Investigations (if carried out) are normal.
- Management involves analgesia (usually paracetamol), ibuprofen and reassurance; heat and massage/rubbing often help.

Benign hypermobility
Common, particularly in the older child/adolescent (<7 years of age all the features are normal variants).

Typical sites
- Hyperextension of the fingers parallel to the forearm
- Apposition of the thumb to the anterior forearm
- Hyperextension of the elbows, knees or both >10 degrees
- Excessive dorsiflexion of the ankles
- Hip flexion allowing the palms to be placed flat on ground

Clinical features
- Pain occurs typically in the afternoon or after exercise and occurs mostly in the lower limbs.
- The child may have features of patello-femoral dysfunction.
- The child may have transient joint effusions.
- Management: symptomatic treatment and reassurance.

Complex regional pain syndrome
See Chapter 3, *Pain management*.

Other rheumatological disorders
Maintain an index of suspicion regarding other rheumatological disorders (e.g. SLE, dermatomyositis and other connective tissue disorders).
Enquire about the following symptoms:
- Lethargy, weight loss, mouth ulcers, alopecia or frontal hair breaking.
- Recurrent fevers.
- Raynaud phenomenon, rashes or photosensitivity.
- Ophthalmological symptoms: red sore eyes, change in vision or dry eyes.

- Weakness.
- Consider investigating with: C3, C4, ANA, dsDNA, ENA, CK, LDH or LFT.

Orthopaedic conditions
Neonatal orthopaedic conditions
Developmental dysplasia of the hip

- This condition was previously known as congenital dislocation of the hip; however, not all cases are present at birth and the hips are not necessarily dislocated.
- Risk factors: breech delivery, family history, congenital anomalies (especially foot abnormalities), being first-born and female.
- Associations: oligohydramnios, caesarean section, packaging disorders, congenital anomalies (especially foot abnormalities) and swaddling.

Diagnosis
General screening

- All neonates should have a clinical examination for hip joint instability – the Ortolani and Barlow tests. The baby should be relaxed. With the knee flexed, the thumb is placed over the lesser trochanter and the middle finger over the greater trochanter. The pelvis is steadied with the other hand and the flexed thigh is abducted and adducted.
- Any clunk or jerk where a dislocation reduces allowing the hip to abduct fully, is a positive Ortolani sign.
- The demonstration of acetabular dislocation by levering the femoral head in and out of the acetabulum is a positive Barlow sign (see Fig. 15.1).

Selective screening

Infants in high-risk groups and those with an abnormal routine clinical screening examination should have an ultrasound examination of their hips.

- As clinical diagnosis can be difficult and ultrasound has diagnostic limitations, the repeated examination of children with risk factors during the first year of life is important.
- When the ossification nucleus of the femoral head develops, between 3 and 9 months, the preferred mode of imaging changes from ultrasound to plain radiograph. Generally use ultrasound up to 6 months of age and radiography thereafter.

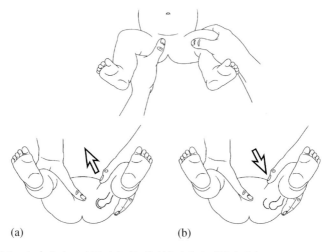

(a)   (b)

Fig. 15.1   Screening for developmental dysplasia of the hip. (a) Ortolani's sign, (b) Barlow's sign

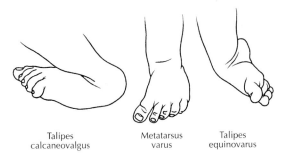

| Talipes
calcaneovalgus | Metatarsus
varus | Talipes
equinovarus |

Fig. 15.2 Congenital foot deformities

Management
The earlier the diagnosis, the easier the management.
- Most neonates can be successfully treated by abduction bracing with a Pavlik harness.
- Operative treatments, including open reduction, may be required with later diagnosis.

Swaddling
- Swaddling is a common technique used to settle infants. However, swaddling with the hips in an adducted and extended position is a risk factor for DDH.
- Parents and health professionals should be made aware of the risks associated with swaddling with the hips in extension. Safe swaddling involves the legs being wrapped loosely to allow for hip flexion and abduction. This position will assist in the proper development of the hip joint.

Club foot (congenital talipes equinovarus)
- Most infants with abnormal-looking feet are said to have 'talipes'; however, the majority have postural problems such as talipes calcaneovalgus (excessive dorsiflexion and eversion), metatarsus varus (adduction of the forefoot) or postural talipes equinovarus (see Fig. 15.2). These deformities are usually mild and mobile; that is, they correct easily and fully with the pressure of one finger. They resolve spontaneously with no treatment.
- The true club foot deformity is more severe and is often stiff. The foot is in equinus, with the hindfoot in varus and the forefoot supinated.

Management
- All require manipulation and casting.
- Soft tissue surgery is required for many.
- Bone surgery is required for a few.

Torsional and angular deformities in children
Many children are seen with normal angular or torsional variants of the lower limbs. It can be difficult to distinguish physiological variation from pathological conditions. The range of 'normality' is wide, but physiological variations can result in as much parental anxiety as pathological disorders.

Intoeing
Intoeing in childhood can be due to metatarsus varus, internal tibial torsion or medial femoral torsion. See Table 15.2 and Fig. 15.3.

Out-toeing
Infants and toddlers have restricted internal rotation at the hip because of an external rotation soft tissue contracture, not retroversion of the femur.

Infants
- Present with a 'Charlie Chaplin' posture between 3–12 months.
- The child weight-bears and walks normally.
- Resolution occurs with no treatment.

Table 15.2 Intoeing in childhood

	Metatarsus varus	Internal tibial torsion	Medial femoral torsion
Synonyms	Metatarsus adductus		Inset hips
Age at presentation	Birth	Toddler	Child
Site of problem	Foot	Tibia	Femur
Examination	Sole of foot bean shaped	Thigh–foot angle is inwards	Arc of hip rotation favours internal rotation
Management	Observe or cast	Observe and reassure	Observe, rarely surgery
When to refer if not resolved	3 months after presentation	6 months after presentation	8 years after presentation

Children
- May be due to neurologic disorder.
- Surgery may be necessary.

Bow legs (genu varum)
The vast majority are physiological. Rare causes include skeletal dysplasias, rickets and Blount disease (tibia vara).

Presentation
- Toddlers are usually bowed until 3 years of age.
- Physiological bowing is symmetrical, not excessive and improves with time.

Management
- Monitor intercondylar separation (ICS; see Figs. 15.4 and 15.5). Refer when ICS is >6 cm, is not improving or is asymmetric.

Knock knees (genu valgum)
Most children with bow legs or knock knees are normal, with <1% having an underlying problem. Rare causes are rickets and trauma.

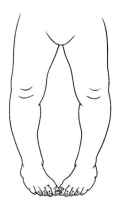

Fig. 15.3 Internal tibial torsion

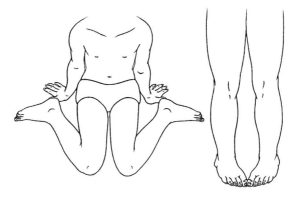

Fig. 15.4 Medial femoral torsion

Presentation
- Children are usually knock-kneed from 3–8 years.
- Physiological knock knees is symmetrical, not excessive and improves with time.

Management
- Monitor the intermalleolar separation (IMS; see Fig. 15.5).
- Refer if IMS >8 cm.

Flat feet (pes plano valgus)
This condition is painless and asymptomatic. If pain or stiffness is present, referral is needed.

Causes
- Physiological (in the vast majority): all newborns have flat feet due to fat that fills the medial longitudinal arch; 80% of children develop a medial arch by their sixth birthday. Having the child stand on their toes may reveal the 'hidden' arch.
- Tarsal coalition (in older children and adolescents only).

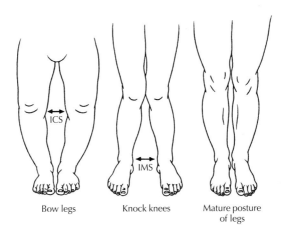

Bow legs   Knock knees   Mature posture
                                       of legs

Fig. 15.5 Postural variants in the lower limbs

Management
- No treatment is required unless symptomatic.
- The condition is unaffected by orthotics or exercises.
- Most cases resolve spontaneously.

Trauma

The management of fractures and dislocations is an integral part of the overall management of the trauma patient. Common fractures in children involve the wrist, elbow, clavicle, distal tibia, fibula and femur. Each has distinct management strategies but there are common themes.

Assessment
- Patients presenting with a suspected fracture or dislocation require a full evaluation of the fracture and exclusion of damage to other structures.
- An accurate history of the mechanism of injury will determine which structures may potentially be damaged.
- **Consider child abuse in infants with fractures (see Chapter 29, *Forensic medicine*).**

Examination
- Closed or open fracture (bone has penetrated through the skin).
- Deformity or swelling. *Note*: Acute swelling in children usually indicates a fracture.
- Neurological status distal to the injury.
- Peripheral pulses – if the blood flow to the limb is compromised, emergency orthopaedic consultation is necessary.
- Associated injuries.

Description of fractures
It is helpful to use specific, technical vocabulary to describe fractures for the purposes of documentation, and discussion with colleagues. Important features include
- *The anatomical site of the fracture*: Which bone? Which side? What part of the bone (e.g. distal, middle or proximal), for example right midshaft humerus or left distal tibia.
- *The fracture type*: that is open or closed. An open fracture has a wound which communicates with the exterior; a closed fracture has an intact soft tissue envelope.
- *The appearance of the fracture line*: for example transverse, oblique, spiral or comminuted (more than one fragment).
- Whether there is a *specific type of fracture*. Children's bones are more elastic and less brittle than adult bones. Consequently, they are more likely to bend and buckle, rather than crack or break. This results in two common patterns of fracture that are seen in children and not in adults:
  - Greenstick fractures.
  - Buckle fractures.
- *The displacement of the fracture*: for example undisplaced, angulated or displaced. Angulation is described by drawing a line along both major fragments and measuring the angle of intersection. Displacement is best described by comparing the position of the bone ends with the width of the bone at that point, for example half a diameter displaced or completely displaced.
- Fractures of the expanded ends of long bones are usually described as *metaphyseal*, and injuries to the growth plate are described according to the Salter–Harris classification (see Fig. 15.6).

  From these terms, a complete description of any fracture can be given that should be meaningful to a colleague who has not seen the radiographs. For example, a femoral shaft fracture might be described as a closed, displaced, midshaft fracture of the left femur with 30 degrees of angulation and one complete diameter of displacement.

Management
- See Table 15.3 for specific fracture information.
- The affected limb should be splinted by a board or plaster slab before radiography.
- Analgesia is required (e.g. fentanyl 0.15 µg/kg intranasally). See Chapter 3, *Pain management*.
- Anteroposterior and lateral views should be obtained of the suspected fracture site. Generally, the joint above and below should also be x-rayed.

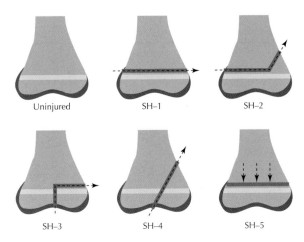

Fig. 15.6 Salter–Harris (SH) classification of growth plate injuries

- If the arm appears bent on examination, it will generally require reduction. Manipulation of the fracture needs to occur before the placement of a definitive plaster. Forearm fractures in children 5 years or older can usually be manipulated using a local anaesthetic block (e.g. Bier block, see Chapter 4, *Procedures*).
- A simple undisplaced greenstick, buckle or torus fracture can be treated in a backslab.
- Open fractures usually require operative intervention.
- Generally, any displaced or angulated fracture should be discussed with orthopaedist and may require manipulation under either local anaesthesia block or a general anaesthetic. Minor fractures of various types are discussed in the RCH Paediatric Fracture Guidelines (including their management and when to review etc.). Refer http://ww2.rch.org.au/clinicalguide/fractures
- A plaster involving the joint above and below the fracture should only be used in a diaphyseal or proximal metaphyseal fracture.
- See http://www.rch.org.au/fracture-education/management_principles/Management_Principles/ for video on closed reduction and plastering.

Home treatment after a full plaster
- Elevate the limb above the heart level for the next 24–48 hours.
- Forearm: a sling should only be worn after this period and the hand should not be below the elbow while in the sling.
- Lower limb: crutches should only be used by children over 6–7 years of age, who are coordinated enough to use them. A walking frame may be used by younger children.
- Written plaster instructions should be explained and given to parents.

Follow-up
- Patients with undisplaced greenstick or buckle fractures do not need a follow-up x-ray and can remove their backslab in 2–4 weeks. Contact sport should be avoided for a further 2–4 weeks.
- For patients who have had a manipulation of a fracture or a fracture involving both cortices of the bone, a repeat radiograph should be obtained in 1 week to ensure the correct position is maintained. Plaster should remain in place for 3–6 weeks, depending on the degree of injury and bone involved. Following the removal of the cast, the bone is still at risk of re-fracture for the next 8–12 weeks; therefore, contact sports are not recommended during this period.

Ankle injury
True sprains are common. Minor fractures of the growth plate or epiphysis should be treated like a sprain.

Table 15.3 Fractures

Site of fracture	Type	Ortho consult	Treatment	Repeat x-ray	Follow-up	Return to sport	Potential complications
Clavicle	Greenstick	No	Sling	No	No	4–6 weeks	No
	Complete	No	Sling	No	1–2 weeks	8–12 weeks	Palpable lump
Humerus – surgical neck	Greenstick/undisplaced	No	Collar and cuff	No	2–3 weeks	6–8 weeks	No
Humeral shaft	Undisplaced	Yes	Collar and cuff ± backslab	Yes	1 week	6–8 weeks	Radial nerve
Supracondylar fracture	Undisplaced/minor posterior angulation	No	Backslab to wrist	Yes	1 week	6–8 weeks	Brachial artery – check distal pulse
Lateral condyle	Undisplaced	Yes	Backslab to wrist	Yes	1 week	6–8 weeks	Displacement of fragment
Proximal radius or ulna fracture	Undisplaced	Yes	Backslab to wrist	Yes	1 week	6–8 weeks	Intra-articular fracture may require pinning
Midshaft radius and ulna	Undisplaced	Yes	Above elbow plaster	Yes	1 week	6–8 weeks	
	Greenstick angulated only	Yes	Reduction LAMP or GA	Yes	1 week	8–12 weeks	Displacement
Distal radius	Buckle, torus or undisplaced greenstick	No	Backslab wrist only	No	No	3–6 weeks	
	Angulated up to 20 degrees	No	Below elbow plaster	Yes	1 week	6–8 weeks	
	Angulated >20 degrees or displaced	Yes	Reduction LAMP or GA	Yes	1 week	8–10 weeks	
Metacarpals	Undisplaced or angulated <30 degrees	No	Backslab involving fingers	No	2 weeks	4–6 weeks	Look for rotation of finger
Phalanx	Undisplaced	No	Buddy tape	Yes (if distal fracture)	1 week	2–6 weeks (buddy tape during play)	Rotation of fracture if distal
Tibia	Undisplaced, greenstick or torus	No	Nothing or backslab	No	2–3 weeks	8–12 weeks	Toddler fracture[a]
	Spiral undisplaced	Yes	Above knee plaster	Yes	1 week	12–16 weeks	
Fibula	Undisplaced shaft or distal	No	Backslab below knee	Yes	1 week	6–8 weeks	
Metatarsal	Undisplaced or mildly displaced	No	Backslab	Yes	1 week	4–6 weeks	

[a]Toddler fracture is usually following a fall, with the child limping or nonweight-bearing, tenderness over the tibia or fibula and a normal x-ray. Treatment outlined above.

Clinical assessment

- Mechanism of injury – it is usually caused by an inversion injury to the ankle.
- Was the patient able to bear weight immediately after the injury?
- Where is the swelling most prominent?
- What is the point of maximal tenderness?

Investigation

Radiographs are required if

- Deformity is present
- Maximal tenderness occurs over the distal tibia or posterior aspect of the fibula
- The patient is unable to weight-bear at all

Management

Remember the RICE acronym:

- *Rest*: weight-bearing should occur as soon as able. If there is significant swelling and the patient is unable to weight-bear, they may benefit from immobilisation but only for a few days.
- *Ice*: should be applied for 15 minutes every 2–3 hours during the first 48 hours, then heat can be applied.
- *Compression*: should be accomplished with a firm bandage or tubigrip.
- *Elevation*: the limb should be elevated on a few pillows whenever possible to allow the swelling to subside.
- Range of motion and balance exercises should start as soon as possible followed by strength exercises (calf raises).

Pulled elbow

Pathology

- Presumed subluxation of the radial head

Clinical features

- Age: 6 months to 6 years (generally 1–3 years).
- The cause of injury is either the child's arm being forcefully pulled or related to a fall.
- There may be a crack or popping sound at the time.
- The position of arm – pronated and slightly flexed (i.e. limp by their side as if they are ignoring it).
- Examination – no tenderness or swelling noted along whole of arm. Supination of the arm causes pain.

Investigations

- If the history and/or signs are typical of a pulled elbow, no investigations are necessary.

Management

- Hold the child's hand as if to shake it and with your other hand, encircle the elbow with the thumb over the annular ligament of the radius.
- Gently apply traction and supinate the hand firmly and then flex the forearm at the elbow all the way to the shoulder. You should feel a pop as the radial head is relocated.
- The child should be moving the arm normally within 10–15 minutes. If there has been a delay in relocation, it may take longer for the child to resume using the arm.
- *Note*: If the history is not typical, there is swelling or your attempts at reduction fail, a radiograph of the elbow should be obtained to exclude a fracture.

Limp in childhood

Limp is a common presenting complaint in childhood (see Table 15.4).

Clinical assessment

Review musculoskeletal assessment, as described earlier in this chapter.

- Is the limp acute, subacute or chronic?
- Is there associated pain or fever?
- Are there other constitutional symptoms?
- Have there been previous episodes of pain or limp?
- What position is the leg held in (e.g. flexed and externally rotated)?

Table 15.4 Differential diagnosis of limp in childhood

Acute	Subacute	Chronic
Fracture	Juvenile idiopathic arthritis	Cerebral palsy
Irritable hip	Tumour/leukaemia	Developmental dysplasia of the hips
Septic arthritis	Acute or chronic SCFE	Perthes disease
Osteomyelitis		Chronic SCFE

SCFE, slipped capital femoral epiphysis.

- Does joint movement or bony pressure cause pain?
- Is there limitation of movement?

Investigations
- FBE, differential, ESR and CRP
- Plain radiograph of the joint or affected limb
- Ultrasound of hip (looking for fluid in the joint) if it is painful or tender with movement
- Bone scan

Management
This will depend on the underlying problem:
- Slipped capital femoral epiphysis (SCFE), tumours, Perthes disease or developmental dysplasia of the hip should be referred immediately to an orthopaedic surgeon.
- Toddlers' fractures may be occult and not seen on a radiograph. If the child is afebrile, then observation is appropriate.
- A bone scan should be arranged if the limp persists or symptoms worsen.

Irritable hip (transient synovitis)
The usual presentation is a child who is constitutionally well with a partial limp and difficulty walking ± a painful hip. This is a common condition which needs to be distinguished from the others listed in Table 15.4. Although it is the most common reason for limp in the preschooler, irritable hip is a diagnosis of exclusion.

Usual clinical features
- Occurs in 3–8-year olds.
- History of a recent viral illness.
- Absence of trauma.
- Child is able to walk, but with pain.
- Severity of the symptoms may vary with time.
- Child is afebrile and appears well.
- There is a mild to moderate decrease in the range of motion due to pain, particularly internal rotation.

Note: The less movement in the joint, the more likely the cause is infective.

Investigations
- These are the same as for limp (see previous; ultrasound usually demonstrates an effusion).
- Results are normal for radiographs, FBE, ESR (<20) and CRP (<8).

Note: The history, symptoms and signs of an irritable hip overlap with septic arthritis, which is a serious condition requiring urgent treatment. If there is any suspicion of bone or joint sepsis, specialist consultation is required and admission to hospital should be arranged.

Management
- Rest and simple analgesics. The more the child can rest, the quicker the recovery.
- Patients may have a relapse if they increase their activity too quickly. Occasionally, these patients need to be admitted to hospital for bed rest and observation.

Perthes disease

This is a specific hip disease of childhood. Affected children have a generalised disorder of growth with a tendency to low birthweight and delayed bone age. The pathology is avascular necrosis of the capital femoral epiphysis followed by a sequence of changes including resorption of necrotic bone, reossification and remodelling. This sequence of events is seen radiologically as density of the capital epiphysis, patchy osteolysis, new bone formation and remodelling with a variable degree of femoral head deformity.

Clinical features
- Age range: 2–12 years, but the majority present between 4 and 8 years
- Sex ratio: five males to one female, 20% bilateral
- Symptoms: pain and limp, usually for at least 1 week
- Signs: restriction of hip motion

Investigations
- X-ray.
- A bone scan is useful in the early stages before the signs are clear on radiograph.

Management principles
- Resting the hip in the early irritable phase
- Regaining motion if the hip is stiff
- Containing the hip by bracing or surgery in selected patients

Slipped capital femoral epiphysis

Can occur acutely or chronically. Early detection will prevent later morbidity.

Clinical features
- Age: this occurs in late childhood to early adolescence. Maximum incidence in girls aged 10–12 years and boys 12–14 years.
- Weight is usually >90th percentile.
- Pain in the hip or knee (often pain only in the knee).
- Limp.
- The hip appears externally rotated and shortened.
- Decreased hip movement, particularly internal rotation.
- May be bilateral (20% of cases).

Investigation
- Take an x-ray of the pelvis and a frog-leg lateral x-ray of the affected hip.

Management
- The patient should not weight-bear if this diagnosis is considered.
- Immediate transfer to hospital.
- Urgent orthopaedic referral and surgery to prevent further slipping is required. Most children can be managed with pinning.

Scoliosis

Definitions

Scoliosis is a curvature in the spine when viewed from the frontal (coronal) plane.
- A *structural scoliosis* occurs when the curvature has an element of rotation and may progress with growth.
- A *non-structural scoliosis* may be secondary to a problem outside the spine, such as unequal leg lengths or muscular spasm.

Detection

The most common type of scoliosis is adolescent **scoliosis**, affecting girls in 90% of cases. 10% of normal adolescents have a curve of 5 degrees or more, but only 2% have curves of >10 degrees. Scoliosis is also common in some developmental disorders such as Rett syndrome and complicates many conditions that affect mobility, for example spina bifida, cerebral palsy and Duchenne muscular dystrophy.

Because abnormal spinal curvatures start small and may progress with time and growth, efforts have been made to detect the condition at an early stage by school screening programmes. This is usually done by the forward bend test, in which the examiner observes the spine from behind as the subject bends forwards. Flexion of the spine usually demonstrates the deformity much more clearly because of the asymmetry of the ribs and chest wall. Very small curves are relatively common and it can be difficult to decide when a radiograph is required, which curves are likely to progress and which require brace treatment or surgery. The risk of curve progression is related to the age at presentation and the size and cause of the curve.

Management

All children with scoliosis should be referred to a paediatric orthopaedic surgeon.

- If the curvature is <20 degrees: observe.
- If the curvature is 20–40 degrees: a brace is recommended.
- If the curvature is >40 degrees: surgery is required.

USEFUL RESOURCES

- *ddheducation.com* – Clinical resource for the examination and management of hip dysplasia.
- http://ww2.rch.org.au/clinicalguide/fractures – RCH Paediatric fracture guidelines.
- **www.arc.org.uk/arthinfo/emedia.asp* – Arthritis research campaign with link to DVD on administration of pGALS.

CHAPTER 16

Head and neck conditions

James Elder
Kerrod Hallett
Elizabeth Rose
Kathy Rowe

Upper respiratory tract infections

- Background: the average child has 4–12 upper respiratory tract infections (URTIs) a year.
- Peak incidence: between 1 and 6 years.
- Risk factors: exposure to other young children (either at home, childcare or school) and passive exposure to tobacco smoke.
- Causes:
  - viruses are responsible for at least 90% of URTIs.
  - bacterial causes include Group A streptococcus and *Mycoplasma pneumoniae*.
- Local symptoms: coryza, cough, sore throat and ears aches. There may be fever, lethargy and decreased feeding. Infants and young children with a URTI may appear quite unwell. It is important to exclude serious bacterial infections in children who have severe constitutional symptoms.
- Management
  - Symptomatic if necessary.
  - Ensure adequate fluid intake.
  - Give paracetamol if the child is distressed.
  - Saline nasal drops/spray or xylometazoline nose drops (maximum duration of therapy is 48 hours) may be administered for temporary relief of nasal congestion interfering with feeding or sleep.

Note: Antihistamines are not indicated in URTIs unless coexistent allergic rhinitis is suspected. Refer to Chapter 19, *Allergy and immunology*. Antihistamines, especially sedating varieties, should be avoided in children <12–24 months of age. They can make the symptoms worse and tend to make secretions thicker.

Mouth breathing and perennial rhinitis

Mouth breathing, recurrent sore throats, stuffy nose, painful ears due to Eustachian tube dysfunction and snoring are very common in childhood and may not be obviously associated with a family history of atopy.

Management

The child with enlarged turbinates or obstructed nasal air flow may benefit from a trial of intranasal steroids for 6 weeks. If helpful, determine any seasonal variations in symptoms to better predict when topical steroids should be used.

Otitis media

This term covers a spectrum of conditions, which are characterised by the presence of fluid in the middle ear. Otitis media may be classified according to clinical presentation as either

- Acute otitis media (AOM)
- Otitis media with effusion (OME)

Paediatric Handbook, Ninth Edition. Edited by Amanda Gwee, Romi Rimer and Michael Marks.
© 2015 John Wiley & Sons, Ltd. Published 2015 by John Wiley & Sons, Ltd.

Acute otitis media

Ninety percent of children will have at least one episode before school entry with the peak prevalence being between 6 and 18 months. AOM is very often preceded by a viral URTI with 25% of AOM considered viral. The causative bacteria are usually

- *Streptococcus pneumonia* (35%)
- Non-typeable *Haemophilus influenza* (25%)
- *Moraxella catarrhalis* (15%)

This condition is characterised by both

- Middle ear effusion:
  - Otoscopic features include loss of the normal tympanic membrane translucency, loss of the light reflex with the handles of the malleus and incus not well seen and yellowish discolouration rather than the usual grey colour of the tympanic membrane. A red tympanic membrane may be due to fever or crying and by itself is not an indication of AOM.
  - Reduced tympanic membrane mobility – as assessed by pneumatic otoscopy and/or tympanometry.

and

- Clinical features of inflammation, that are either
  - Localised (e.g. ear pain); **or**
  - Generalised (e.g. fever, irritability), provided there is no other cause apparent to explain these symptoms.

Note: **Be wary of accepting AOM as the sole diagnosis in an unwell infant with a fever. There may be a coexistent serious bacterial infection. Consider a septic workup or careful observation.**

Management

Initial management

Acute symptoms resolve without antibiotics within 24 hours in most cases.

- Give adequate analgesia as required.
- Consider antibiotics:
  - Withhold in children >12 months who are only mildly unwell and immunocompetent.
  - Commence amoxicillin 15 mg/kg (max. 500 mg) p.o. 8 hourly for 5 days if the child is unwell or distress continues beyond 24–48 hours. Roxithromycin 2.5–4 mg/kg (max. 150 mg) p.o. 12 hourly for 5 days should be given instead if allergic to penicillin.

Note: Antibiotics do not reduce the incidence of recurrent AOM or OME (see below).

Follow-up

In regards to clinical inflammation:

Review in 24–48 hours. If the inflammation has not resolved, consider these possible explanations:

- Wrong diagnosis (e.g. viral URTI, serious bacterial infection).
- Failure to take the medication (antibiotics not given or vomited).
- Antibiotic resistance (switch to amoxicillin with clavulanic acid 15 mg/kg (max 500 mg) p.o. 8 hourly).
- Antibiotic reaction.
- Uncommonly, a suppurative complication of AOM may have developed (e.g. mastoiditis, facial paralysis, labyrinthitis, intracranial infection).

If the medical treatment has been unsuccessful and the child remains symptomatically unwell, refer to an otolaryngologist. Early drainage of the ear (myringotomy) with or without insertion of a tympanostomy tube may need to be considered.

In regards to the middle ear effusion:

A middle ear effusion is present for a variable period of time following AOM and may be associated with noticeable hearing loss, particularly if bilateral. A middle ear effusion will be present in approximately:

- 80% of cases at 2 weeks following AOM
- 40% at 1 month
- 20% at 2 months
- 10% at 3 months

Review at 2–3 months is recommended, particularly if symptomatic hearing loss is present.

Recurrent AOM

AOM is common in the first 3 years of life and is generally a seasonal condition with a peak incidence in winter and early spring, paralleling the incidence of viral URTI. Prevention of recurrent AOM may need to be considered during this period, depending on the frequency, severity and duration of infections. Prophylactic measures include

- Limiting exposure to viral URTI (e.g. by reducing attendance at large childcare groups)
- Reducing exposure to cigarette smoke
- Insertion of tympanostomy tubes, which should be considered particularly if infections are associated with morbidity such as persistent moderate hearing loss especially during language acquisition

Otitis media with effusion

OME usually resolves spontaneously over time. Factors contributing to persistence include recurrent URTI, recurrent AOM, poor Eustachian tube function and exposure to tobacco smoke. A persistent middle ear effusion can be associated with varying degrees of hearing loss as well as behavioural, language and educational difficulties.

Management

Medical

For symptomatic cases that persist beyond 3 months, a prolonged course of amoxicillin 15 mg/kg (max 500 mg) 8 hourly for 3 weeks will usually result in resolution. No other medical treatment has proven benefit.

Tympanostomy tubes

Tympanostomy tubes provide good short-term benefit, but their long-term value is widely debated. It does not cure the underlying Eustachian tube dysfunction responsible for OME, but temporarily removes the symptoms by providing an alternative means for middle ear ventilation. Adenoidectomy may be beneficial, particularly in children requiring recurrent tympanostomy tube insertion. The long-term impact of tympanostomy tube insertion on language, literacy and cognitive function is the subject of ongoing research.

Consider insertion of tympanostomy tubes **only** if

- middle ear effusion present for **at least 3 months** and appears likely to persist long term, **and**
- significant symptoms are present: either recurrent AOM or functionally significant hearing loss (e.g. speech delay, behavioural disturbance or poor school performance)

OME and AOM are commonly related to URTI and are therefore more common in winter and early spring. Inserting tubes towards the end of this period should be avoided, in the expectation that there may be resolution with the onset of warmer weather.

The benefits of temporary alleviation of symptoms by tympanostomy tube insertion need to be balanced against the disadvantages:

- Need for general anaesthesia and surgery.
- Tubes usually remain *in situ* for only 6–9 months (although longer-stay tubes are available) and the reinsertion rate of tubes is ~25%.
- Tympanic membrane perforation occurs at a rate of approximately 1% per year that tubes remain *in situ*. A range of other tympanic membrane and middle ear complications are associated with tubes.
- Otorrhoea occurs in up to 25% of cases. It is often associated with a URTI, and may also occur because of external contamination (e.g. swimming or bathing without ear protection).

Management of discharging ears in children with tympanostomy tubes

- Ear toilet using cotton wool
- Topical antibiotics, for example ciprofloxacin (avoid aminoglycosides)
- For refractory discharge:
  - Ear culture
  - 1.5% hydrogen peroxide ear washes
  - Refer to an otolaryngologist
  - Consider possibility of underlying immunodeficiency or cholesteatoma

Mastoiditis

This is a severe complication of AOM. Children are unwell, presenting with features of AOM associated with more severe systemic symptoms and post-auricular inflammation (ranging from cellulitis to subperiosteal abscess). Management involves referral to otolaryngologist and IV antibiotics. Unless mild, children will require insertion

Levels of hearing impairment

Hearing impairment	Decibels (dB)	Impact
No impairment	Hearing 20dB or better	Normal speech
Mild	Hearing is 26–40 dB	Difficulty hearing soft speech and in noise
Moderate	Hearing is 41–65 dB	Miss most of the conversation Reduced vocabulary Poor pronunciation
Severe	Hearing is 66–95 dB	Speech and language very limited without amplification
Profound	Hearing is 95 dB or less	Very limited speech without a cochlear implant Will need to learn sign language if no implant

of tympanostomy tubes and drainage of the subperiosteal abscess. Mastoidectomy is performed where cholesteatoma is suspected or in the presence of an additional suppurative complication.

Hearing loss

Children with impaired hearing (Tables 16.1 and 16.2) are at risk of speech and language delay, which may contribute to learning, behavioural and social problems. Hearing level is measured in decibels (dB).

Screening

All infants in Australia may have a screening hearing test (Victorian Infant Hearing Screening Program – VIHSP). Infants who have a 'refer' from either or both ears will go on to have objective, electrophysiological testing at an audiology centre. Approximately half of the babies who are referred for full testing have been found to have a hearing impairment in one or both ears.

Formal audiological testing

Hearing impairment may be conductive, sensorineural or mixed and may be unilateral or bilateral. The more severe and prolonged the hearing loss, the greater the chance of developmental impairment. However, some children may be affected by even mild levels of impairment (e.g. difficulty learning in a noisy classroom). Associated disabilities may magnify the risks of hearing impairment. Specialist referral is suggested for children with significant impairment to consider genetic testing and imaging studies.

Management options for hearing-impaired children

These will be considered by the otolaryngologist, audiologist and family. Some causes will be amenable to surgical interventions but most permanent causes of hearing impairment require optimisation of communication potential by other means. For example:

- Amplification (with hearing aids) or cochlear implant
- Sign language

Table 16.2 Commonest causes of hearing impairment in children

Conductive	Sensorineural
Recurrent AOM/OME, from middle ear effusions	Congenital: Genetic (connexins) or chromosomal Syndromic Temporal bone malformations Infections (TORCH organisms)
Chronic otitis media: Non-suppurative, for example tympanic membrane perforation Suppurative from ossicular erosion	Acquired: Prematurity Meningitis Drug-related, for example aminoglycosides cytotoxic

The impact of hearing impairment and the optimisation therapies listed above on patients and their families is significant. Family support is available through a variety of organisations, for example Hearing Australia (*www.hearing.com.au*).

Otitis externa

Clinical features

Commonly occurs due to water contamination following swimming or in children with dermatitis of the external auditory canal. It is characterised by

- Pain (often severe)
- Inflammation of the ear canal, which may include the tympanic membrane (mobility of the tympanic membrane on pneumatic otoscopy excludes otitis media)
- Pre-auricular or post-auricular tenderness

Management

- Swab for micro, culture and sensitivity.
- Ear toilet.
- Topical antibiotics combined with steroids (e.g. ciprofloxacin HC).
- An ear wick should be inserted when the ear canal is very oedematous (to maintain patency of the ear canal and allow topical antibiotics to enter the ear canal) and moistened frequently with topical antibiotics.
- Hospital admission for administration of (anti-pseudomonal) intravenous antibiotics may be necessary when ear pain is severe and not relieved by regular analgesics, or where cellulitis has extended beyond the ear canal.
- Patients with fungal otitis externa need review for ear toileting until there is no further accumulation of debris.

See Appendix 3, *Antimicrobial guidelines*.

Acute pharyngitis/tonsillitis

The combination of fever and sore throat is a common presenting problem in children. Determining the aetiology and deciding whether to treat with antibiotics can be difficult.

Background

Most sore throats are due to a viral infection (almost all in children 4 years old or less). The only clinically important bacterial pathogen is group A β-haemolytic streptococcus (GABHS), *Streptococcus pyogenes*.

- The presence of tonsillar exudate is not helpful in distinguishing viral infection from GABHS.
- GABHS is less likely if the child has associated coryza, cough, generalised lymphadenopathy or splenomegaly.
- GABHS is more likely if the child is 4 years of age or older, has tenderness and enlargement of the tonsillar cervical lymph nodes, inflammation of the tonsils and pharynx (pharyngotonsillitis), or a generalised erythematous (scarlatiniform) rash.
- Streptococcal serology (ASOT, antiDNase-B titre) can make a retrospective diagnosis but is still not always accurate.
- Penicillin reduces the duration of symptoms and the incidence of acute rheumatic fever but not of acute glomerulonephritis. Penicillin to prevent acute rheumatic fever is of questionable use as this is now rare except in some indigenous communities and developing countries.

Practical management

- Children who probably **do not** need antibiotics are those aged 4 years or younger, and/or those with associated cough or coryza, unless they are unwell enough to require hospitalisation.
- Children who **should** have treatment with penicillin include those who are Aboriginal or Torres Strait Islanders, or other Pacific Islanders, or who have a past history of rheumatic heart disease.
- Children who **might** benefit from antibiotics are those aged older than 4 years with marked pharyngotonsillitis, tender tonsillar cervical nodes, need for hospital admission for rehydration and without cough and coryza.
  - Therapy is oral phenoxymethylpenicillin 250 mg (500 mg if >10 years) 12 hourly.
  - Erythromycin 15 mg/kg (max 500 mg) 8 hourly or roxithromycin 2.5 mg/kg (max 150 mg) 12 hourly may be used for children with true penicillin allergy.

Infectious mononucleosis is a relatively common cause of acute pharyngitis in older children. The diagnosis often becomes apparent when there is no response to penicillin, other characteristic features develop (e.g. generalised lymphadenopathy, splenomegaly, mild jaundice and rashes) and the illness follows a more prolonged course. A rash commonly occurs if amoxicillin is prescribed.

Quinsy (peritonsillar abscess)
Infection can extend beyond the tonsil as cellulitis (peritonsillar cellulitis) or as a peritonsillar abscess (quinsy). In addition to features of severe tonsillitis, quinsy presents with drooling, a 'hot potato' voice, and trismus. Inflammation of the hemipalate adjacent to the tonsil is evident and an area of fluctuance (perceived as a softening) can be palpated. In the earlier cellulitic stage, the condition will settle with IV antibiotics, but where an abscess is present, drainage is necessary.

Recurrent acute pharyngitis/tonsillitis
Recurrent sore throats are a normal part of growing up for many children. Many of these children have recurrent viral pharyngitis. Many also complain of frequent sore throats associated with persistent mouth breathing due to obstructed nasal airflow.

True recurrent GABHS pharyngotonsillitis is much less common but often over-diagnosed. A variety of strategies have been used to reduce recurrences of GABHS pharyngotonsillitis. None of these is universally effective in preventing recurrent episodes and each has its own disadvantages.

- Use of another antibiotic to attempt eradication of GABHS (e.g. amoxicillin/clavulanic acid).
- Use of low-dose prophylactic penicillin.
- Treatment of culture-positive family members.
- Tonsillectomy (with or without adenoidectomy) probably works by removing a reservoir of GABHS infection. It should be considered if the pattern of infection (i.e. frequency, severity and duration of infections) is such that significant morbidity is expected to continue for a prolonged and unacceptable period of time. The presence of associated airway obstruction may influence treatment choice.

Children with suspected recurrent GABHS pharyngotonsillitis should have a throat swab taken during an acute episode to aid in treatment decisions.

Obstructive adenotonsillar hypertrophy
See Chapter 24, *Sleep problems*.

Epistaxis
This is usually due to bleeding from the anterior nasoseptal vessels, often in association with nasal crusting or nose picking. Acute bleeding usually settles with local pressure to the lower nasal septum, but occasionally the application of a cotton wool pledget soaked with a topical decongestant (e.g. ephedrine) is necessary.

Recurrent bleeding can be treated by the application of an antibiotic ointment if significant nasal crusting is present, or by cautery if enlarged blood vessels are seen (use a silver nitrate stick following the application of a topical anaesthetic and decongestant, for example co-phenylcaine spray – lignocaine (lidocaine)/phenylephrine). Epistaxis in children is very unlikely to be due to a nasal tumour or a previously undiagnosed coagulopathy.

Trauma
Nasal trauma
Treatment is required for either cosmesis or drainage of septal haematoma.

Cosmesis
A nasal deformity due to a displaced nasal fracture should be reduced within 7–10 days of injury. The presence of a bony deformity due to a nasal fracture is best determined at about 5 days following the injury, once the soft tissue swelling has resolved. The decision to reduce the nasal fracture is based on clinical grounds and radiology is unhelpful.

Septal haematoma
- This can occur after nasal trauma, regardless of whether or not there is a fracture. It invariably leads to septal abscess formation with cartilage destruction and nasal collapse.

- It presents with nasal obstruction and pain associated with a bulge of the septum that can be confirmed by palpating with an instrument (e.g. wax curette) following application of a topical anaesthetic.
- Treatment involves incision and drainage, nasal packing to prevent recurrence and anti-staphylococcal antibiotics.
- As this is the 'danger area of the face', there is also the possibility of cavernous sinus thrombosis.

Oral/oropharyngeal trauma

This may occur after a fall with a stick or similar object in the mouth and may sometimes be associated with a significant injury. Admit to hospital and evaluate if there is

- Inability to feed/swallow
- Upper airway obstruction
- Significant laceration, requiring debridement, closure or both
- Significant retropharyngeal injury (may not be obvious on oral examination)

Investigate by

- Lateral cervical spine radiograph
- Flexible nasopharyngoscopy

Consider involvement of the teeth in cases of oral trauma.

Aural trauma

Trauma to the external auditory canal is usually associated with bleeding, but is an insignificant injury and requires no treatment. The tympanic membrane can be perforated by direct trauma or a pressure wave (e.g. a slap across the ear or diving). Acute tympanic membrane perforations usually heal within weeks and do not require acute intervention. Topical antibiotics are recommended for water-related injuries. Direct trauma may rarely cause ossicular disruption, facial paralysis or inner ear damage (with complete deafness and vertigo). Follow-up at 4 weeks after injury is required to ensure perforations have healed, usually with an audiogram.

Foreign bodies

The first attempt at foreign body removal is always the easiest and should be undertaken by an experienced clinician with the appropriate instruments and good illumination. Take into account the child's developmental stage and their level of anxiety in planning this procedure. Failure of the initial removal may lead to an otherwise unnecessary general anaesthetic.

Ear

Foreign bodies in the external auditory canal are best removed with a hook-shaped instrument, which is passed behind the foreign body and then used to pull it out. Grasping instruments such as forceps invariably lead to the foreign body being displaced further medially. Suction may also be useful.

Nose

The technique for the removal of nasal foreign bodies is the same as for foreign bodies in the external auditory canal. A topical anaesthetic (e.g. co-phenylcaine) should be applied before the attempted removal, which assists with reducing pain but also provides decongestion allowing easier manipulation in the nose. The risk of inhalation of a nasal foreign body is minimal and therefore acute removal may be deferred until appropriate personnel and equipment are available. Batteries in the nose should be removed immediately, under general anaesthesia if necessary as there is a risk of septal perforation.

Fish bone in pharynx

A fish bone usually lodges in the tonsil or at the base of the tongue and therefore can be seen on oral examination and removed after the application of a topical anaesthetic. If the fish bone cannot be seen during the oral examination, a more thorough examination by nasopharyngoscopy is required. Fish bones rarely reach the oesophagus and so oesophageal evaluation is usually unnecessary. Where a fish bone is not found, despite a suggestive history, the child should be reviewed until symptoms resolve and an examination under general anaesthetic considered. Although fish bones are often radiolucent, radiology (particularly CT) may be helpful to detect the presence of complications when symptoms persist.

Oesophagus

The vast majority of swallowed foreign bodies pass without difficulty. If a foreign body becomes lodged in the oesophagus, it usually does so in the upper oesophagus, at the level of the cricopharyngeus. Lower oesophageal foreign bodies may suggest the presence of underlying oesophageal pathology (e.g. stricture).

Radiographs (including neck, chest and abdomen) should be taken if there are symptoms suggestive of oesophageal impaction (e.g. drooling and dysphagia), or if long, thin objects or button batteries have been swallowed. Oesophageal foreign bodies may be seen in the coronal plane, whereas tracheal lodgement is seen in the sagittal plane. Radiolucent foreign bodies may be imaged by barium swallow. If an object is impacted in the oesophagus, endoscopic removal is required.

If a swallowed object reaches the stomach, it will almost always pass without incident. Some objects, however, may cause problems:

- Long, thin objects (e.g. hairpins and locker keys) may impact at the duodenojejunal flexure.
- Button batteries may release alkali, causing local necrosis and perforation. Their removal is a matter of urgency.
- Multiple magnets may cause necrosis of the bowel, and should be removed as soon as possible.

Neck masses

Causes

Infectious/inflammatory (reactive) lymphadenopathy (most common): Usually results from a URTI and most resolve in 6 weeks.

Congenital: Thyroglossal duct cysts are in the midline, usually near the hyoid bone and thyroid cartilage. Branchial cysts are in the lateral neck. These may become apparent after a cold with increase in size and pain from an abscess. Branchial cleft cyst (usually second) presents as a painless enlarging neck mass anterior to the sternomastoid muscle, or with infection after a URTI.

Neoplastic (rare): Majority are lymphomas but may be from sarcomas, thyroid gland.

Diagnosis

A reasonable differential diagnosis can usually be made based on history and examination findings including clinical history (congenital or acquired, presence or absence of fever and tenderness), location (midline or lateral) and imaging characteristics (cystic versus solid).

Management

If it is likely to be an inflamed lymph node, either observe for 6 weeks or treat with a course of antibiotics. At 6 weeks if it is unchanged or enlarged, consider investigation:

- FBE and film, LFT including LDH and serology for CMV, EBV, toxoplasmosis, Bartonella and Quantiferon Gold.
- Ultrasound if concerns about possible abscess, typical or atypical mycobacterium, rapidly enlarging painless mass larger than 2 cm, or if mass has not resolved by 3 months.
- Consider referral to infectious diseases physician and/or otolaryngology if an abscess, possible malignancy or likely congenital neck mass.

Dental conditions

Dental development

Primary dentition

Teeth start to form from the 5th week *in utero* and may continue until the late teens or early twenties. The first teeth to erupt are usually the lower central primary incisors at around 7 months of age. Table 16.3 summarises the eruption dates for primary teeth. **An infant who shows no sign of any primary teeth by the age of 18 months should be referred to a paediatric dentist.**

Table 16.3 Eruption sequence of primary dentition (months after birth)

Central incisors	Lateral incisors	Canines	First molars	Second molars
6–12	9–16	16–23	13–19	23–33

Table 16.4 Eruption sequence of permanent dentition (years of age)

Central incisor	Lateral incisor	Canine	First premolar	Second premolar	First molar	Second molar	Third molar Wisdom
6–8	7–8.	9–13	10–12	10–13	6–7.0	11–13	17+

By the age of 3 years, most children will have a complete primary dentition consisting of 20 teeth (8 incisors, 4 canines, 8 molars). In most cases, all primary or deciduous teeth are ultimately replaced, but some individuals are missing permanent teeth and primary teeth may be retained into adulthood.

Permanent dentition

At around the age of 6 years, the primary incisors become mobile and fall out. This will continue for the next 6 years. The permanent dentition begins to develop, starting with the eruption of the lower first permanent incisors and molars (Table 16.4). Permanent teeth are much larger than the primary predecessors and often look more yellow or cream in colour. The period that follows, referred to as the mixed dentition phase, is highly variable. Some second primary molar teeth are replaced by the second premolars as late as 14 years of age.

The simultaneous presence of primary and permanent teeth in the same site during the mixed dentition stage is common (known as the ugly duckling stage) and is not a cause for concern.

Dental caries

Dental caries (or tooth decay) remains one of the most common childhood diseases. In Australia, just over 50% of 5-year olds and 55% of 12-year olds are decay free. Unfortunately, 80% of the decay burden is experienced by approximately 20% of children. Of these, 10–15% children have multiple decayed teeth requiring urgent surgical care. It is therefore important to identify children at high decay risk early (before 2 years of age) and specifically target them for prevention (Table 16.5).

Dental decay can occur as soon as teeth erupt. Early childhood caries (ECC) is a particular form of dental decay that is seen in infants as young as 18 months of age. It affects >6% of Australian infants and has a characteristic appearance in which the upper front teeth are affected on their labial (or lip) surfaces. The cariogenic bacteria causing ECC are transmitted from primary caregiver to child, and decay is closely associated with infant feeding habits such as bottle feeding with sweetened liquids and putting the child to sleep with a bottle.

Prevention

The prevention of dental decay should start as soon as the first tooth erupts. There are four aspects to preventing decay:

Diet

- Minimise the total amount and frequency of intake of sugary foods and drinks.
- Limit sugary snacks to mealtimes with other noncariogenic solid and liquid foods and when salivary flow is optimal.

Table 16.5 Dental caries: common risk factors assessable by medical practitioners

Risk factor	Influence
Sugar exposure	Infant feeding habits are very important with frequency of exposure being most relevant. High risk associated with prolonged on-demand night-time feeds and daytime grazing patterns
Family oral health history	Poor parental oral health places child at risk of decay as cariogenic bacteria are transmitted from the primary caregiver
Fluoride exposure	Exposure to fluoridated water source and the regular use of fluoridated toothpaste are two key factors that reduce caries risk
Social and family practices	Low socio-economic status, indigenous and immigrant groups have higher levels of dental caries
Medical illness	Medically compromised children are more at risk of dental decay and are less likely to receive appropriate treatment

- Minimise intake of drinks with high acidity (e.g. carbonated, fruit and sports drinks), as they cause erosion of the enamel tooth surface.
- Increase water intake.
- Encourage drinking from feeder cup from the age of 12 months.
- Avoid demand bottle-feeding at night-time and nursing during the night after 18 months.

Oral hygiene
- Tooth cleaning should commence following the eruption of the first tooth with a wet flannel.
- Start brushing with a soft children's toothbrush with a small head and a thin smear of paediatric fluoride toothpaste (400 ppm fluoride) at 18 months.
- Parents should supervise toothbrushing until around 8–10 years of age (when they can tie shoelaces).
- Use a soft toothbrush for children with a pea-sized amount of adult fluoride toothpaste (1000 ppm fluoride) after 6 years of age.
- Flossing should start once the child is proficient at toothbrushing.

Fluoride and amorphous calcium phosphate (ACP or tooth mousse)
- Fluoride enhances the ability of teeth to resist enamel demineralisation caused by sugar-related acids.
- Apart from systemic water fluoridation, the most common source of fluoride is toothpaste applied twice daily to the tooth surface.
- The preventive effect is dose dependant (400, 1000 and 5000 ppm) and dental prescription is now based on perceived caries risk.
- ACP applied topically after toothbrushing can enhance enamel remineralisation.
- Fluoride supplements in the form of tablets or drops should no longer be used in fluoridated communities (NHMRC guideline, 2006).

Regular dental check-ups
- A child should see a dental professional within 6 months of the eruption of the first tooth.
- The first visit is a 'well baby' visit and aimed at providing 'anticipatory guidance'.
- Children should have a dental check-up at least annually or sooner if risk is high.
- Developmental problems such as malocclusion should be identified early for interceptive treatment.

Dental emergencies
Toothache
- Assess level and nature of pain, for example sharp intermittent pain on eating or in response to hot/cold (pulpitis) or spontaneous dull pain (apical periodontitis) at night.
- Provide analgesia (paracetamol should be adequate in most cases).
- Refer to dentist for assessment and treatment of the affected tooth.

Dental abscess
Presentation
- History of spontaneous dull (usually constant) pain, particularly at night.
- Swelling or sinus evident intraorally near the diseased or carious tooth.
- Red swollen face, commonly unilateral and often spreading up under the orbit or under the mandible is consistent with facial cellulitis of dental origin.
- Limited mouth opening and difficulty swallowing.
- Elevated temperature, enlarged lymph nodes and a generally unwell child.
- Teeth tender to palpation on side of the swelling.

Investigations
- An orthopantomogram (OPG) will often show dental pathology, usually dental caries and pulpal pathology.

Management
- Consider oral amoxicillin for early infection.
- Admit to hospital if red swollen face, fever and generally unwell.
  - IV antibiotics (amoxicillin and metronidazole in the first instance).
  - IV fluids if dehydrated.

Table 16.6 Dental trauma – primary dentition

Injury	Management
No tooth displacement	Non-urgent referral to dentist for review
Intrusion – tooth upwards and inwards	Needs dental review within 24 hours to accurately locate the tooth. Likely that extraction will be required
Luxation – tooth palatal or sideways	Needs dental review within 12 hours
Avulsion – knocked out completely	**Do not** replant primary teeth

- Extraction of the tooth or intra canal drainage of the abscess is almost always indicated.
- Occasionally, additional soft tissue drainage is required; however, dental abscesses in young children usually manifest with cellulitis rather than a collection of frank pus.

Dental trauma

Traumatic injuries to the facial region can affect the teeth, soft tissues and jaw bones. **In all cases of dental trauma, lift the lips and look in the mouth!**

Primary teeth
Consider:
- How did the injury occur?
- Were there any other facial injuries?
- Time of the injury?
- Where are the teeth or fragments of teeth?
- How much of the tooth is broken off or how far is the tooth displaced?
- Can the patient bite their teeth together or does the displaced tooth get in the way?
- Are there associated soft tissue (mucosal) injuries?

Never replant a lost primary tooth. Injury (particularly intrusion) to a primary incisor can damage the permanent successor; therefore, dental review for all suspected intrusion injuries is important (Table 16.6).

Permanent teeth
Whenever possible, an OPG is useful as it allows a full examination of the jaws, temporomandibular joints and teeth (Table 16.7). A chest radiograph is useful if the tooth or fragments cannot be located. Many injuries can be managed under local anaesthesia, depending on the cooperation of the child and the presence of associated soft tissue or other bony injuries.

Locate all teeth or tooth fragments because
- Most permanent teeth and tooth fragments can be replaced or re-cemented.
- 'Missing' teeth may have been intruded (pushed in) rather than knocked out.
- Associated mucosal injuries may require suturing by the dentist.
- An avulsed permanent tooth is a genuine emergency and should be triaged as such. Try to replant the tooth or keep the tooth stored in milk until the dentist arrives. The longer the tooth is out of the mouth, the worse the prognosis.
- The long-term psychosocial and economical impact on a young person of losing a front tooth should not be underestimated. Appropriate emergency management can make a significant difference to the prognosis of any injured tooth.

Mucosal lacerations
- Check carefully intraorally for degloving injuries (where the gum tissue around the teeth is stripped away from the underlying bone). Unless the lips are retracted, this injury is easily missed. These injuries need suturing under general anaesthesia.
- Many superficial tongue and intraoral lip lacerations do not need suturing and heal well when left.
- Extraoral lacerations, particularly those crossing the vermilion border on to the skin, should be referred to a plastic surgeon.

Table 16.7 Dental trauma – permanent dentition

Injury	Management
Fractures	
<1/3 crown	Non-urgent referral to dentist
>1/3 crown	Locate fragments, store in milk Needs dental review within 24 hours Some fragments can be reattached to broken teeth
Mobile but not displaced	Soft diet and analgesia
Displacements	Needs dental review within 12 hours May need dental splint
Intrusions (tooth upwards and inwards)	Locate teeth, using radiographs Tooth may re-erupt or require surgical/orthodontic repositioning Use gentle finger pressure to reposition teeth, if in doubt leave alone
Luxations (tooth pushed out/inwards or sideways)	Loose splinting can be achieved using tin foil until patient sees dentist Urgent referral to dentist
Avulsions[a] (knocked out completely)	Urgent referral to dentist Replace tooth in socket if possible If not, store in milk at all times

[a] An avulsed permanent tooth is a genuine dental emergency.

Fractures to the jaw bones
- Whenever a jaw fracture is suspected, a maxillofacial surgeon should be called. If teeth are also obviously displaced or lost, a paediatric dentist should also be called.
- An OPG and a lateral skull examination and/or a variety of occipitomental/anteroposterior radiographic views can be useful in inspecting the facial complex for fractures.
- Tetanus prophylaxis should be considered in any compound fractures opening to mouth or skin, and IV antibiotics commenced.

Bleeding from the mouth
- Rinse the mouth with cold water or saline and remove any debris, blood, tissue etc. from the teeth and gums.
- Identify the source of bleeding – usually an extraction socket.
- If the child has been bleeding for some time, assess haemodynamic status.
- Bleeding socket:
  - Compress the sides of the socket together using finger pressure.
  - If the child is cooperative, place a slightly damp gauze pack over the socket and have the child bite down on to it for 20 minutes. Parents may be asked to assist. Do not pack anything into socket.
  - Refer to dentist for further treatment if the bleeding has not stopped after 20 minutes.

Eye conditions
Important principles
- Eye examination:
  - Always test and record vision as the first part of any eye examination.
  - In infants, observe following and other visual behaviour and listen to the parents' impressions of their child's vision.
- Instilling eye drops:
  - Do not use local steroid drops unless corneal ulceration has been excluded by fluorescein staining. Only use steroids for short periods (2 days or less), unless an ophthalmologist directs otherwise.
  - Instilling eye drops/ointment in a young child: carer sits on the floor with legs extended; lay child between carer's legs with child's arms under the carer's thighs and the child's feet near the carer's feet. This leaves

the child's head secured and the carer with both hands free to hold open the child's eyelids and instill eye medication.
- Padding eyes:
  - Never pad a discharging eye.
  - Pad an eye or keep the child indoors if local anaesthetic has been instilled, until the effect of the local anaesthetic has worn off (10–20 minutes).
- Referral to an ophthalmologist:
  - Transient malalignment of the eyes is common up to 6 months of age. However, a child with a transient squint after 6 months or a constant squint at any age should be referred promptly to an ophthalmologist. True squints rarely improve spontaneously.
  - All children with a white red reflex or white masses in the retina must be referred immediately to an ophthalmologist to exclude retinoblastoma.
  - In cases of photophobia or watery eyes with no significant discharge in the first year of life, consider congenital glaucoma.

Trauma

Trauma to the eye can take many forms. Physical trauma to the eye and surrounding structures may be blunt or sharp. Trauma can also result from radiation (thermal and electromagnetic) and chemical agents.

Foreign bodies

Foreign bodies on the surface present with a painful, watery eye. If a foreign body or corneal ulcer is suspected, instill one drop of local anaesthetic to ease the pain and facilitate examination. Suitable local anaesthetics are proxymetacaine 0.5%, amethocaine 0.5 or 1%, or benoxinate 0.4%. *Do not use local anaesthetics for the continuing treatment of ocular pain under any circumstance.*

Conjunctival foreign bodies are common and often found on the posterior surface of the upper lid. Therefore, eversion of the lid is essential. To evert an eyelid: ask the patient to look down, then with a cotton bud resting on the eyelid at the level of the top of the tarsal plate, gently push down on the cotton bud while grasping the eyelashes with the other hand and rotating the lid margin in an upward direction.

Most foreign bodies are easily removed with a moist cotton wool swab. If they are embedded and/or difficult to remove, refer the child to an ophthalmologist. Beware of an iris naevus (small pigmented lesion on the iris that can be mistaken for a corneal foreign body) or iris prolapse through a perforating injury of the cornea mimicking a corneal foreign body.

Intraocular foreign bodies are generally the result of high-velocity fragments. Suspect them if the history involves an explosion, metal(s) striking on metal, or any other situation that involves high-speed objects (e.g. power tools or a lawn mower). If the history is at all suggestive, even in the absence of local signs, radiography of the orbit (AP and lateral) is necessary. If an intraocular foreign body is demonstrated or suspected, immediate referral to an ophthalmologist is mandatory.

Eyelid injuries

All eyelid lacerations except the most minor should be repaired under general anaesthesia. Refer to an ophthalmologist if lacerations involve the lid margin or the medial aspect of the eyelids (canalicular injury is likely).

Hyphaema (blood in the anterior chamber)

This is the result of blunt trauma to the eye and all cases require referral to an ophthalmologist. The potential complications include other eye injuries, secondary haemorrhage and vision loss. Minor hyphaemas can be managed as an outpatient. More significant hyphaemas require admission and bed rest.

Fracture of the orbital bones

A blowout fracture through the wall of the orbit is suspected if ≥ 1 of the following three cardinal signs are present:

- Restricted movement of the eye, particularly in a vertical plane, with double vision
- Infra-orbital nerve anaesthesia
- Enophthalmos – this may be difficult to assess initially because of eyelid haematoma

Diagnosis is usually clinical. Refer to an ophthalmologist before organising a CT scan. A CT scan is used to demonstrate the fracture of the orbital wall and entrapped orbital tissue (the classic sign is a teardrop 'polyp' hanging from the roof of the maxillary antrum).

Penetrating injury (including intraocular foreign body)

This should always be considered in patients with lacerations involving the eyelids, particularly after motor vehicle accidents. Clinical clues include distortion of the pupil, shallowed anterior chamber, prolapse of the iris through the cornea, or presence of pigmented tissue over the sclera. If suspected, protect the eye with a cone or shield that does not place pressure on the eyelids or eye and admit. Prevent vomiting with an antiemetic, as this may cause extrusion of eye contents. Refer to an ophthalmologist immediately.

Chemical burns

Irrigate the eye with saline or water copiously for 15 minutes using an IV giving set under local anaesthesia. Continue this until the fluid is neutral on pH testing. Refer all chemical burns to an ophthalmologist.

Thermal burns

The ocular surface is rarely involved. Check for ulceration with fluorescein staining. Butesin picrate ointment is suitable for use on lid burns. Secondary lid swelling may result in corneal exposure and the exposed cornea should be protected with ocular lubricants until the swelling subsides.

Non-accidental injury

The presence of retinal haemorrhages in cases of unexplained head injury raises the possibility of non-accidental injury. An appropriate investigation of the circumstances of the injury should be initiated. The retinal haemorrhages must be assessed by an ophthalmologist (refer to Chapter 29, *Forensic medicine*).

Acute red eye

Common causes of the acute red eye are conjunctivitis, corneal ulceration, corneal or conjunctival foreign bodies (see above). Less common causes are preseptal and orbital cellulitis. Table 16.8 gives a brief outline of the presenting features of red, sticky and watery eyes, which have a large number of causes and whose clinical presentations may overlap.

Conjunctivitis

Aetiology

- Bacterial: generally pus is present
- Viral: generally there is watery discharge
- Allergic: history of atopy and 'itchy eyes'

Neonatal conjunctivitis (ophthalmia neonatorum)

Neisseria gonorrhoea

- *Clinical.* Presents within a few days of birth with acute, severe, purulent discharge associated with marked conjunctival and lid oedema ('pus under pressure').
- *Diagnosis.* Urgent Gram stain for Gram-negative intracellular diplococci and direct culture to appropriate culture media.
- *Treatment.* **This is an ocular emergency because of the risk of corneal perforation.** Admit and give IV ceftriaxone for 7 days. Penicillin (same duration) is an alternative if the organism is known to be susceptible. In all cases, local measures such as ocular lavage and topical antibiotics (chloramphenicol) may be helpful.
- Investigate and treat the mother and partner.

Chlamydia

- *Clinical.* Usually occurs at 10–14 days of age. Fails to respond to routine topical antibiotics. If left untreated, there is a risk of pneumonitis.
- *Diagnosis.* Giemsa stain of conjunctival scraping for intranuclear inclusions. Also antibodies in tears and immunofluorescent stains of conjunctival scrapes. Use a *Chlamydia* kit, ensuring conjunctival cells are collected.

Table 16.8 The causes of red, watery and sticky eyes

Problem	Pain	Itch	Epiphora	Discharge	Erythema	Photophobia	Reduced eye movements	Other
Neonatal conjunctivitis (ophthalmia neonatorum)	+++		++	+++	++–+++			
Congenital nasolacrimal duct obstruction			+–++	+–+++				
Infantile glaucoma			++		+	++		Enlarged and cloudy cornea
Viral conjunctivitis	++		++	+	++–++			
Bacterial conjunctivitis	++–+++		++	+++	++–+++			
Allergic conjunctivitis		++–+++	++–+++	Stringy	+			
Chemical conjunctivitis	+++		+++	+	++–+++			
Corneal abrasion	+++		++	Variable				
Foreign body	+++		++	Variable				Variable fluorescein staining
Preseptal cellulitis	++		+	Variable	+++ Swelling of eyelids			Conjunctiva not inflamed
Orbital cellulitis	+++		+	Variable	+++ Swelling of eyelids		+–+++	Eye is often inflamed and proptosed

- *Treatment.* Erythromycin 12.5 mg/kg oral q.i.d. for 14 days or azithromycin 20 mg/kg oral daily for 3 days. Eye toilet.
- Investigate and treat the mother and partner.

Other bacteria

- Other causes of conjunctivitis are *Staphylococcus, Streptococcus* or diphtheroids. Culture and treat with chloramphenicol eye drops/ointment. A rapid clinical response is anticipated.
- Occasionally, *Neisseria meningitidis* can cause conjunctivitis and should be treated as for invasive infection (see Chapter 18, *Infectious diseases and immunisation*).

Blocked nasolacrimal duct

Presents with mucopurulent discharge with a watery eye. On waking the discharge is worse and conjunctiva is not inflamed (see Watering eyes, p. 247).

Conjunctivitis in older children

Viral

- This condition usually clears spontaneously.
- If it is unclear whether the infection is viral or bacterial, chloramphenicol eye drops may be given.

Bacterial

- *Severe:* chloramphenicol eye drops: 2 hourly by day and ointment at night
- *Less severe:* chloramphenicol eye drops or ointment three times a day

Herpes simplex conjunctivitis

- Suspect if the child has eyelid vesicles.
- Check for corneal ulceration and treat with 4 hourly acyclovir ointment if ulceration is present.
- Refer to an ophthalmologist.

Allergic

- In mild cases, use an astringent (phenylephrine 0.12% or naphazoline 0.1%).
- In moderate cases, use a topical antihistamine (antazoline 0.5%).
- In severe cases, refer to an ophthalmologist. Topical steroid or sodium cromoglicate should only be given under the supervision of an ophthalmologist.

Corneal ulceration

Ulceration causes pain, photophobia, lacrimation and blepharospasm. It is diagnosed by eye examination. For causes and management, see Table 16.9.

Periorbital and orbital cellulitis

Both periorbital and orbital cellulitis present with erythematous, swollen lids in a febrile child. Orbital cellulitis is differentiated by the presence of proptosis and ophthalmoplegia. Hence, the lids **must** be separated (a Desmarres lid retractor may be used) to enable a thorough examination.

Table 16.9 Causes and management of corneal ulceration

Cause	Appearance of ulcer (with fluorescein staining)	Management
Trauma (with or without a foreign body)	Scratch – linear Subtarsal foreign body – round or vertically linear	Chloramphenicol ointment (1%) and pad if possible Review in 24 hours. If not healed in 48 hours, refer to an ophthalmologist When ulcer has healed, continue chloramphenicol ointment twice daily for 1 week
Herpes simplex (dendritic ulcer)	Dendritic (occasionally 'geographic' if late presentation)	Aciclovir eye ointment (1 cm inside the lower conjunctival sac) five times a day for 14 days and refer to an ophthalmologist

Periorbital (preseptal) cellulitis

Periorbital (preseptal) cellulitis refers to infection in the soft tissues of the eyelids. This may arise from purulent conjunctivitis, dacryocystitis, or entry via local trauma or insect bite.

Distinguish this from a *periorbital allergic reaction*. A well child, who has eyelid swelling with minimal or no erythema, fever, tenderness nor local warmth, may simply have an allergic reaction to an allergen that has been blown or rubbed into the eye, or be secondary to an insect bite. In this case, no specific radiological imaging is required. An oral antihistamine may be used. The child should be reviewed if the swelling does not settle in the next 24 hours or if signs of inflammation develop.

Recommended antibiotics
- Mild – amoxycillin/clavulanate
- Moderate – IV flucloxacillin
- Severe or <5 years and unimmunised – ceftriaxone and flucloxacillin

Failure to respond in 24–48 hours may indicate orbital cellulitis or underlying sinus disease.

Orbital (septal) cellulitis

Orbital (septal) cellulitis occurs when infection is present around and behind the globe of the eye and is usually due to spread from sinus infection (especially the ethmoid sinuses). It usually occurs in children >2 years. **Orbital cellulitis is a medical emergency and should be treated with the same level of urgency as meningitis or a brain abscess**. The potential for loss of vision and suppurative intracranial complications is significant.

Orbital cellulitis is differentiated from periorbital cellulitis by the presence of
- Chemosis
- Proptosis
- Ophthalmoplegia
- Systemic symptoms

If the features of orbital cellulitis are present, a CT scan is required to determine if the sinusitis is complicated by abscess formation. This is most commonly a subperiosteal abscess on the medial wall of the orbit adjacent to the ethmoid sinus (displacement of the medial rectus muscle is often an indication of abscess formation). An abscess will often require surgical drainage. If no abscess is present, treatment is by IV antibiotics alone; however, CT scanning may need to be repeated if there is clinical deterioration, or if there is lack of improvement with medical treatment.

Management is with IV flucloxacillin and ceftriaxone (See Appendix 3, *Antimicrobial guidelines*). Urgent ENT and ophthalmology consultation are also required in suspected orbital cellulitis.

Watering eyes

Watery eyes are common in children and are the result of either poor tear drainage or overproduction. The latter is usually the result of eye irritation and causes include foreign bodies (see p. 243), corneal ulcer (see p. 246), conjunctivitis (see p. 246) and infantile glaucoma (see p. 249).

Nasolacrimal duct obstruction is the most common cause of watery eyes and discharge that persist after the first 2 weeks of life. The discharge is worse on waking and the conjunctiva is not inflamed. It usually resolves spontaneously, due to an opening of the lower end of the nasolacrimal duct. Local eye cleaning is usually the only treatment indicated. If the eye is red and inflamed, topical framycetin sulfate eye drops may be given (avoid repeated courses of chloramphenicol). Secondary irritation of the skin can be minimized by protecting it with an application of soft white paraffin ointment after discharge is cleaned off. If the discharge and watering have not settled by 12 months of age, refer to an ophthalmologist for probing under general anaesthetic.

Strabismus or squint (turned eye)

Refer all children with squint or suspected squint to an ophthalmologist. This will allow early detection (and possibly prevention) of amblyopia and detection of any underlying pathology such as retinoblastoma or cataract. Urgent referral to an ophthalmologist is required if
- The red reflex is abnormal (very dull or white); or
- There is limitation of eye movement on one or both eyes.

A child does not 'grow out of' a squint. However, in the first few months of life, babies may have an intermittent squint, especially when feeding. A child of any age with a constant large-angle squint or a child over

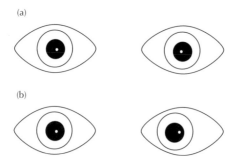

Fig. 16.1 Corneal light reflex. Shine a light at the child's eyes and observe the reflection. (a) Eyes are straight and the corneal light reflex is symmetrical. (*Note*: It is displaced slightly to the nasal side of the centre in each eye.) (b) Left convergent strabismus. The reflection from the deviated eye is displaced laterally

6 months with any squint (constant or intermittent) should be referred to an ophthalmologist. All children with a first-degree relative with a squint should be seen by an ophthalmologist at about 3–3.5 years of age, even if there is no squint, as they may have a refractive error alone.

A pseudostrabismus (pseudosquint) is due to a broad nasal bridge or epicanthic folds, or both. This results in the appearance of a squint, but corneal light reflexes are central and there is no movement on cover testing (see Figs. 16.1 and 16.2). Only make the diagnosis of pseudostrabismus if absolutely certain. Refer doubtful cases to an ophthalmologist.

Eyelid lumps and ptosis

- *Styes* are acute bacterial infections of an eyelash follicle. They occur at the eyelid margin and are red and tender. Removing the lash directly related to the stye will often result in discharge of pus and hasten its resolution. Local antibiotics are sometimes indicated. Systemic antibiotics are rarely needed.
- A *chalazion* is an obstructed tarsal (or meibomian) gland. These glands are situated within the substance of the eyelid and thus a chalazion will present as a lump within the eyelid. There may be no associated symptoms. Redness associated with a chalazion is usually the result of sterile inflammation due to leakage of the contents, rather than a bacterial infection. Thus local or systemic antibiotics seldom influence the natural

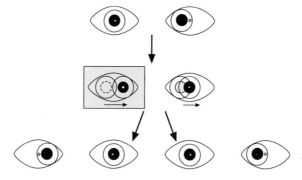

Fig. 16.2 The cover test. The child's attention is attracted with a toy. The eye that appears not to be deviating is covered. The uncovered eye is then observed for movement. If there is a convergent squint, the eye will move outwards (top and middle). The uncovered eye should also be observed when the cover is removed from the fellow eye. In an alternating squint there will be no movement of the uncovered eye and the previously covered eye will now be deviated (bottom left). In non-alternating or constant squint (vision is usually reduced in the deviating eye), there will be a rapid return to the original situation (bottom right). If no movement is detected, the test should be repeated but cover the other eye first

history of these lesions. Warm compresses may hasten resolution. If the chalazion is persistent (>6 months), large or causes discomfort, incision and drainage under general anaesthesia may be indicated.

- *Ptosis* is a droopy or lowered upper eyelid. In children, it is usually the result of a minor and isolated anomaly in the development of the levator muscle. It may be unilateral or bilateral, and is sometimes inherited in a dominant manner. If the lowered eyelid obstructs the pupil in a young child, visual loss will occur secondary to amblyopia. Urgent referral to an ophthalmologist is appropriate in such cases. Referral is also indicated if there are associated pupil abnormalities. In more minor degrees of ptosis, surgical intervention is for cosmesis and is less urgent.

Rare but important eye conditions
Iritis
Acute iritis is very rare in children and presents with an acute red eye similar to the symptoms for a corneal ulcer. The pupil is small and does not react well to light. Consider iritis in children with juvenile chronic arthritis (JCA). This form of iritis is chronic and painless. Refer to an ophthalmologist.

Infantile glaucoma
The presenting features are
- A hazy cornea
- An enlarged cornea
- Watery eyes
- Photophobia

This is a rare condition, but early recognition is vital. Prompt surgery offers a chance of cure and preservation of vision. All infants with suspected glaucoma require urgent referral to an ophthalmologist for assessment and treatment.

Congenital cataracts
Congenital cataracts are rare, but early detection and removal with subsequent optical correction (contact lenses or spectacles) offers a good chance of visual preservation. All newborn infants should have their red reflexes examined before discharge from hospital. Check the red reflexes and fundi in any infant with poor visual performance (fixation and following). Nystagmus is a late sign of congenital cataracts. A unilateral cataract will often present as a squint. Any child suspected of having a congenital cataract must be referred urgently.

Retinoblastoma
This is a rare childhood cancer of the retina and presents with a white pupil (cat's eye reflex), squint, poor vision or a family history of the tumour. Prompt recognition is vital to maximise the possibility of preserving vision. Untreated this is a fatal disorder. If suspected, refer urgently to an ophthalmologist.

USEFUL RESOURCES
- *www.hearing.com.au* – Hearing Australia.
- *www.entnet.org* – American Academy of Otolaryngology and Head and Neck Surgeons. Links to websites and case scenario teaching.
- *www.tracheostomy.com* – Aaron's tracheostomy page. An excellent site regarding tracheostomy management, run by an American parent and nurse.
- Spencer AJ. The use of fluorides in Australia: guidelines. *Australian Dental Journal* 2006; 51(2): 195–199.
- www.dentaltraumaguide.org/
- *cim.ucdavis.edu/eyes/version1/eyesim.htm* – A brilliant simulation program addressing eye movements and associated defects in muscles or cranial nerves.
- *www.aapos.org/* – American Association for Pediatric Ophthalmology and Strabismus™. Covers information on most major topics in paediatric ophthalmology (search section entitled "Eye terms & conditions").

CHAPTER 17

Dermatologic conditions

Rod Phillips
David Orchard

The key to accurate diagnosis and hence to appropriate management of skin disorders in children is a careful history and astute observation of rashes, particularly focusing on their appearance, site and pattern of development. During the examination, consider a few key questions (see also Fig. 17.1).

- Are there any vesicles, that is fluid-filled lesions? Finding these greatly narrows the range of possible diagnoses. Small circular erosions may be the only signs of an underlying vesicular process.
- Is the rash raised (papular) or flat (macular)?
- Is the rash red? Redness is from haemoglobin. Most red rashes blanch, that is the redness disappears with pressure. If not, the haemoglobin is outside the blood vessels (purpura).
- Is the rash scaly? If so, the epidermis may be broken (eczematous) to give weeping, crusting or bleeding, or it may be intact (papulosquamous).

Vesiculobullous rashes

Vesicles are usually caused by infections (herpes simplex virus (HSV), varicella zoster virus (VZV), enterovirus, tinea, scabies or impetigo) or contact dermatitis. Also, consider drug reactions and erythema multiforme. Larger blisters may be from staphylococcal infections, tinea, Stevens–Johnson syndrome, arthropod bites, contact dermatitis, burns or trauma.

Impetigo (school sores)
Cause
Staphylococcus aureus or *Streptococcus pyogenes* (impetigo but not bullous lesions), or both.

Clinical features
- Presents as areas of ooze and honey-coloured crusts on the face, trunk or limbs. Occasionally, the primary lesions are bullous but because the blisters are very superficial and break easily, one mostly only sees the 'peeling' edge of the blister.
- Lesions are rounded and well demarcated and are most often grouped and asymmetrical but may be solitary and widespread.
- Their onset and spread may be rapid or occur over days.
- In more chronic cases, there may be central healing with peripheral spread to give annular lesions.

Management
- Bathe off crusts.
- Apply topical mupirocin 2% ointment 8 hourly if localised, or cephalexin 25 mg/kg (max. 500 mg) orally, 12 hourly if severe or extensive.
- Isolate the child from other children or from sick adults unless all lesions are covered or treated.
- Treat any underlying condition such as scabies (a common cause of widespread impetigo).
- Treat coexistent eczema with topical corticosteroids.

Staphylococcal scalded skin syndrome
Clinical features
- Usually seen in younger children.

Paediatric Handbook, Ninth Edition. Edited by Amanda Gwee, Romi Rimer and Michael Marks.
© 2015 John Wiley & Sons, Ltd. Published 2015 by John Wiley & Sons, Ltd.

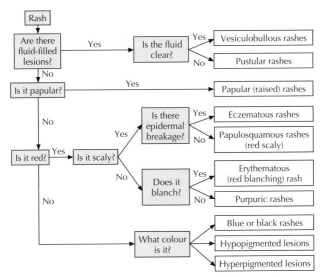

Vesiculobullous rashes
- Impetigo (school sores)
- Eczema herpeticum
- Erythema multiforme
- Single blisters
- Stevens–Johnson syndrome/toxic epidermal necrolysis

Pustular rashes
- Acne

Papular (raised) rashes
- Scabies
- Urticaria/serum sickness
- Papular urticaria
- Keratosis pilaris
- Papular acrodermatitis
- Molluscum
- Warts

Eczematous rashes
- Atopic eczema

Red scaly rashes (papulosquamous)
- Seborrhoeic dermatitis
- Psoriasis
- Tinea corporis
- Pityriasis rosea

Red blanching rashes (erythematous)
- Fever and exanthem
- Erythema infectiosum

Red blanching rashes (erythematous)
- Roseola infantum
- Kawasaki disease

Purpuric rashes
- Enteroviral infection
- Septicaemia
- Leukaemia
- Henoch–Schoenlein purpura
- Child abuse
- Idiopathic thrombocytopenic purpura (ITP)
- Trauma and vasomotor straining

Blue or black rashes
- Vascular malformations
- Haemangiomas
- Mongolian spots

Hypopigmented lesions
- Tinea versicolor
- Pityriasis alba
- Vitiligo
- Post-inflammatory hypo- and hyperpigmentation

Hyperpigmented lesions
- Congenital pigmented naevi
- Acquired pigmented naevi

Fig. 17.1 Classification of skin disorders in children

- Mediated by an epidermolytic toxin released from an often insignificant staphylococcal focus (e.g. eyes, nose or skin).
- Fever and tender erythematous skin are early features.
- Exudation and crusting develops, especially around the mouth.
- Wrinkling, flaccid bullae and exfoliation of the skin are seen – Nikolsky sign ('normal' skin separates if rubbed).
- Blisters are very superficial and heal without scarring.

Management

- Flucloxacillin 50 mg/kg (max. 2 g) IV 6 hourly if there is any evidence of sepsis or systemic involvement.
- Look for a focus of infection. Drain foci of pus if present.
- Monitor temperature, fluids and electrolytes if large areas are involved. Increased fluids will aid renal excretion of toxin.
- Handle skin carefully and use an emollient ointment.

Erythema multiforme

Clinical features

- Occurs at any age.
- Lesions are usually symmetric and appear most commonly on the hands, feet and often the face. They can be found anywhere, including mucous membranes.
- Typical target lesions have an inner zone of epidermal injury (purpura, necrosis or vesicle), an outer zone of erythema and sometimes a middle zone of pale oedema. They are not migratory.
- Most cases are caused by herpes simplex, some by other infections. Drugs are an uncommon cause.

Management

- Fluid maintenance.
- Apply emollient ointment to the lips, if needed.
- If the condition is recurrent, it is highly likely to be related to HSV. Prophylactic aciclovir should be considered if recurrences are frequent and affecting the quality of life.

Stevens–Johnson syndrome/toxic epidermal necrolysis

Clinical features

Stevens–Johnson syndrome and toxic epidermal necrolysis are believed by many to be variants of the same condition.

- They are characterised by widespread blisters on an erythematous or purpuric macular background, often with extensive mucous membrane haemorrhagic crusting.
- There may be tender erythematous areas with a positive Nikolsky sign ('normal' skin separates if rubbed).
- Conjunctivitis, corneal ulceration and blindness can occur. Some degree of permanent scarring around the conjunctivae is common even if eye symptoms are not severe.
- Anogenital lesions can lead to urinary retention.
- Fever, myalgia, arthralgia and other organ involvement can occur.
- Drugs, usually commenced a few weeks earlier, are the most common cause, occasionally *Mycoplasma*.

Management

- Cease any drug that may be the cause.
- Monitor temperature, fluids and electrolytes.
- Fluid maintenance.
- Apply emollient ointment to the skin, lips and anogenital areas – this may be required many times a day. Careful attention to emollients and/or dressing of the glans and undersurface of the foreskin may prevent secondary scarring, adhesions and phimosis. For eroded areas, dressings with or without silver impregnation as per burns therapy is appropriate.
- A regular eye examination with a specialist review for topical steroid drops if any eye involvement is noted.
- Good pain management is essential. Occasional or regular brief inhalational general anaesthetics may be necessary to facilitate dressings, eye care, etc., which **must** not be compromised.
- IV gamma globulin is seen by many as standard therapy for cases threatening to become severe.
- Cyclosporin (5–6 mg/kg per day for a few days, then taper to 3–5 mg/kg per day for 2–3 weeks) commenced at diagnosis may prevent worsening. Immunosuppression is controversial (beware sepsis).

Note: Stevens–Johnson syndrome is not severe erythema multiforme (EM). They are distinct conditions with different aetiologies. Permanent sequelae are rarely seen in severe EM and concurrent drug use is unlikely to be the cause. Skin lesion morphology is the best discriminating factor. Classic target lesions are not seen in Stevens–Johnson syndrome. Mucous membrane involvement can be seen in both conditions but is usually localised in EM, often confluent in Stevens–Johnson syndrome.

Eczema herpeticum

Clinical features

- HSV infection in children with eczema is common, but many cases are misdiagnosed as either an exacerbation of the eczema or bacterial infection.
- Grouped vesicles may be prominent, but more often vesicles are rudimentary or absent and the infection presents as a group of shallow 2–4 mm ulcers on an inflamed base.
- The infected area may not be painful or itchy and does not respond to standard eczema therapy.
- If untreated, resolution usually occurs in 1–4 weeks, but dissemination may occur.
- Recurrences may occur at different sites.

Management

- Collect epithelial cells from the base and roof of the vesicles for herpes immunofluorescence and culture.
- Local disease in an otherwise well child requires regular observation but does not need antiviral therapy.
- A child with fever or multiple sites of cutaneous herpes infection may need admission to hospital and treatment with IV aciclovir.
- Milder cases demonstrating progression or facial involvement can be managed with oral aciclovir.
- Eye involvement requires aciclovir and urgent review by an ophthalmologist.
- The underlying eczema can be treated with moisturisers, topical steroids and wet dressings. Topical corticosteroids can be used during the active infection phase.

Eczema coxsackium

Some coxsackie viruses (usually type A6) can give a widespread vesicular eruption with prominence around mouth, hands and feet in otherwise well children. Previous areas of eczema may be involved. Differentiate from eczema herpeticum by the sudden symmetrical onset. Swab for both HSV and enterovirus if unsure.

Single blisters

When a child presents with a single blister as an isolated finding, consider impetigo, tinea, mastocytoma, insect bite, cigarette burn, friction or spider bite.

Pustular rashes

Consider acne, folliculitis, scabies, perioral dermatitis, acute generalised exanthematous pustulosis and rarely psoriasis.

Acne

Clinical features

- Undertreated acne is a cause of significant morbidity in adolescents and may be a factor in teenage suicide.
- Mainly affects the forehead and face but can involve other sebaceous areas (neck, shoulders, upper trunk).
- Early lesions include blackheads, whiteheads and papules. In more severe cases, there may be pustules or inflammatory cysts that can lead to permanent scarring.
- Consider underlying endocrine disorders if acne begins before puberty.

Management

- Acne is treatable. No person with acne should just be told it is an inevitable part of adolescence. Effective acne therapies are now available and should be used to control the disease.
- For mild disease, use topical benzoyl peroxide 2.5–5%. Other topical agents include antibiotics (clindamycin, erythromycin or tetracycline), isotretinoin (not in pregnancy) or azelaic acid. These can be used singly or in combination. Improvement occurs over 1–2 months, not within days. All of these topical agents have side effects with which practitioners must be familiar.
- Treatment of moderate acne often involves the addition of oral antibiotic therapy (e.g. tetracycline 500 mg twice daily, erythromycin 500 mg twice daily, doxycycline 50–200 mg per day) for 3–6 months.
- Oral hormone therapy can help female patients.

    If antibiotics and topical treatment have not resulted in considerable improvement within 3 months, oral isotretinoin is indicated. Provided pregnancy is avoided, this is safe and highly effective. Isotretinoin is also indicated if there is scarring, cyst formation or significant depression. Treatment of severe acne with isotretinoin may decrease the risk of suicide. Assessment and treatment of any depression is required.

Papular (raised) rashes

If the child is itchy, consider scabies, urticaria, serum sickness, papular urticaria or molluscum. If not, consider urticaria, molluscum, warts, melanocytic naevi, keratosis pilaris and papular acrodermatitis. For vascular swellings, consider pyogenic granuloma.

Scabies

Clinical features

- An intensely itchy papular eruption develops 2–6 weeks after first exposure to the *Sarcoptes scabiei* mite or 1–4 days after subsequent reinfestation.
- The characteristic lesion is the burrow that is several millimetres in length. Burrows are best seen on the hands, especially between the fingers, and on the feet. Early burrows may be vesicular.
- A clue to the diagnosis of scabies is the distribution of papules and pruritus.
- Involvement of the palms, soles, axilla, umbilicus, groin and genitalia is common and the head is usually spared.
- Excoriations and secondary impetigo may be present.
- There is currently a worldwide pandemic of this contagious disease affecting both adults and children.

Management

- Treatment is expensive and upsetting. If diagnosis is unclear, confirm by scraping to find a mite, or refer before treating.
- Use permethrin 5% cream. An alternative for pregnant women or neonates is sulfur 2% in yellow soft paraffin.
- Oral ivermectin at the stat dose of 200 mcg/kg is effective and can be used particularly for more widespread or institutional breakouts.

Note: The following are **not recommended:** lindane 1% (contraindicated in infants or women who are pregnant or breastfeeding) or benzyl benzoate 25% (too irritating for children and ineffective).

- Treat all family members and any other people who have close skin contact with the affected individuals.
- Apply to dry skin (not after a bath) from the neck down to all skin surfaces. For infants, apply to the scalp as well (not face). Use mittens if necessary to prevent finger sucking.
- Leave the cream on for at least 8 hours.
- Wash the cream off. Wash clothing, pyjamas and bed linen at this time.
- The itch takes a week or two to settle and can be treated with potent topical steroids.
- Reinfestation is common. The family should notify all social contacts (e.g. crèche, school or close friends) to ensure that all those infected receive treatment.

Urticaria/serum sickness

See also Chapter 19, *Allergy and immunology*.

Clinical features

- Characterised by the rapid appearance and disappearance of multiple raised red wheals on any part of the body.
- Individual lesions are often itchy and clear within 1 day.
- There may be central clearing to give ring lesions (these are not the so-called target lesions of EM that persist for several days).
- The child is usually well.
- Urticarial episodes usually resolve over days or weeks and rarely last longer than 6 months.
- In most cases of short duration, the trigger is either a transient viral infection, allergic reaction or cannot be determined.
- Some children develop fever and arthralgias in association with urticarial lesions that are more fixed and may bruise or be tender (serum sickness). In Australia, serum sickness is usually idiopathic or following a course of cefaclor.

Management

- Urticaria may be the first sign of anaphylaxis. If there is associated angio-oedema (prominent subcutaneous swelling) or wheeze, continued observation and appropriate treatment is required (see Chapter 1, *Medical emergencies*, p. 5).

- Investigation is usually not required. The trigger is usually a previous viral illness.
- Ask about medications, new foods and environmental allergens. Consider food allergy testing only if urticaria starts suddenly, on the lips and face and within 1 hour of a newly introduced food.
- Treat the itch with oral antihistamine (see Chapter 19, *Allergy and immunology*). Oral prednisolone (1 mg/kg per day, max 50 mg) for 2–5 days is beneficial in serum sickness and is warranted in urticaria when pruritus is severe.
- Urticaria can become chronic, and in the vast majority of cases, no underlying ongoing trigger is found. Consider mast cell degranulating drugs, foods, animals, parasitic infections, heat, cold and physical pressure. Consider investigating with a throat swab (for streptococcal carriage), full blood examination (for eosinophilia and anaemia), antinuclear antibodies, urine culture for bacteriuria, nocturnal check for threadworms and a possible challenge with any suspected agent. Adding cimetidine (10 mg/kg (max 200 mg) p.o. 6 hourly) to the antihistamine may help.
- If individual lesions last >2 days or are tender or purpuric, consider investigation for cutaneous vasculitis.

Papular urticaria

Clinical features

- This is a clinical hypersensitivity to insect bites.
- New bites appear as groups of small red papules, usually in warmer weather.
- Older bites appear as 1–5 mm papules, sometimes with surface scale or crust, or with surrounding urticaria.
- Vesicles or pustules may form.
- Individual lesions may resolve in a week or last for months and may repeatedly flare up after fresh bites elsewhere.
- The itch is often intense and secondary ulceration or infection is common.

Management

- Prevent bites (e.g. adequate clothing, modifying behaviour that leads to exposure, occasional repellent and the treatment of pets and house for fleas if necessary).
- Treat the itch with an agent such as aluminium sulfate 20% (Stingose), liquor picis carbonis 2% in calamine lotion, potent steroid ointment or antihistamines (see Chapter 19, *Allergy and immunology*). Protective dressings (e.g. Duoderm) can speed the healing of lesions.
- Treat secondary infection with topical mupirocin ointment 2% or oral antibiotics.

Keratosis pilaris

Clinical features

- This is a rough, somewhat spiky papular rash on the upper outer arms, thighs, cheeks or all three areas, with variable erythema.
- It is common at all ages and most often present in one or both parents to some degree.

Management

- Reassure the patient. Therapy is only needed for cosmetic appearance. Soap avoidance and moisturisers can improve the feel. Steroids do not help.
- Older children may get some benefit from topical keratolytics (e.g. Dermadrate, Calmurid).
- Older children with troublesome facial redness can be treated with vascular laser.

Papular acrodermatitis

Clinical features

- Characterised by the acute onset of monomorphic red or skin-coloured papules mainly on the arms, legs and face.
- It is usually asymptomatic.
- It can be caused by coxsackie virus, echovirus, mycoplasma, EBV, adenovirus and others.

Management

- Reassure and advise that clearing can take several weeks

Molluscum

Clinical features

- Uncomplicated molluscum lesions are easily recognised as firm, pearly, dome-shaped papules with central umbilication.
- Presentation to a doctor is often prompted by the development of eczema in surrounding skin. In such cases, recognition can be difficult as eczematous changes can obliterate the primary lesions. A careful history of the initial lesions is usually diagnostic.

Management

Education – molluscum is caused by a virus and is very common. A child may develop a few, or a great many lesions and individual lesions may last for months. Complete resolution will not happen until an immune response develops, which may take from 3 months to 3 years.

Children with molluscum should not share towels but should not be restricted in their activities.

The treatment depends on the age of the child, the location of the lesions and any secondary changes. Things to note include

- Treatment of the surrounding eczema may be all that is required.
- Uncomplicated lesions not causing problems and not spreading can be left alone.
- Isolated or troublesome lesions (e.g. on the face) can be physically treated. One method is gentle cryotherapy.
- Rarely, children warrant curettage under topical anaesthesia. This is well tolerated and usually curative but can potentially scar. Alternatively, the stimulation of an immune response can be attempted with cantharidin, aluminium acetate solution (Burow solution 1:30) for large areas, or benzoyl peroxide 5% daily to small areas and covered with the adhesive part of a dressing.
- Inflamed lesions do not require antibiotic treatment, but if true cellulitis or abscess formation occurs, treat with antibiotics and/or drainage.

Warts

Many serotypes of the papilloma virus can cause warts. Different serotypes have a predilection for different areas of the skin. No treatment is necessary unless the warts are causing a problem to the child (e.g. social embarrassment, or pain from a plantar wart). Avoid painful procedures unless chosen by older children. Resistant warts on the limbs often respond to contact sensitisation (e.g. Diphenylcyclopropenone (DCP) 0.1% cream after sensitisation with 2% solution). DCP use requires caution, supervision and possible dose adjustment, as there is a wide variation in individual responses.

- *Ordinary warts:* if tolerated by the child, paring every 2–3 days with a razor blade or nail file will remove the surface horn. Apply a proprietary keratolytic agent that contains salicylic or lactic acid, or both, each day or two as directed.
- *Plantar warts:* these can be painful and can appear flat. Pare as for ordinary warts. Apply a proprietary keratolytic agent that contains salicylic or lactic acid, or both, each day or two. Alternatively, place a small pad of cotton wool soaked in 3% formalin in a saucer on the floor. Rest the wart-affected sole on the pad/saucer for 30 minutes each night. Cryotherapy and surgery are often ineffective and can lead to painful keloid scarring.
- *Plane (flat) warts:* these are smooth, flat or slightly elevated, skin-coloured or pigmented lesions. They may occur in lines or coalesce to form plaque-like lesions. If treatment is needed for plane warts on the hands, apply a formalin solution as for ordinary warts. Lesions on the face are often subtle and may not need treatment. Topical retinoid creams can reduce the size of the warts whilst waiting for immune response but can be irritating for some.
- *Anogenital warts:* these are soft, fleshy warts that occur at the mucocutaneous junctions, especially around the anus. They may be isolated flesh-coloured nodules or may coalesce into large cauliflower-like masses. Management options include awaiting resolution, imiquimod, curettage and diathermy and carbon dioxide laser.

Note: by itself, the presence of genital warts in a young child is not an indication for mandatory reporting to government protective services, as transmission is usually by normal close parent–child contact.

Eczematous rashes

Consider atopic eczema, allergic contact dermatitis, irritant contact dermatitis, photosensitivity eruptions, molluscum, tinea corporis and scabies.

Atopic eczema

See also Chapter 19, *Allergy and immunology*, p. 309.

Clinical features

- Eczema usually begins in infancy.
- It commonly involves the face and often the trunk and limbs as well.
- In older children, the rash may be widespread or may be localised to flexures.
- Erythema, weeping, excoriation and rarely vesicles may be seen in acute lesions. Chronic lesions may show scale and lichenification. In some children, the lesions are more clearly defined, thickened discoid areas that may intermittently be itchy.
- There is usually a cyclical pattern of improvement and exacerbation.
- Weeping and yellow-crusted areas that do not respond to therapy may indicate secondary bacterial or herpetic infection.

Management

- *Education:* parents need to know the triggers and that treatments are effective in controlling the disease.
- *Avoid irritants* which may worsen eczema: soaps, bubble baths, prickly clothing, seams and labels on clothing, car seat covers, sand, carpets, overheating or contact with pets. Smooth cotton clothing is preferred.
- *Keep the skin moist:* use a moisturiser such as paraffin ointment (50:50 white soft paraffin/liquid paraffin) as often as several times a day if necessary.
- *Treat inflammation:* in mild or moderate cases, steroid creams can be used intermittently with good effect. Hydrocortisone 1% is usually adequate. If not, moderate potency (e.g. betamethasone valerate 0.02%) or potent (e.g. mometasone 0.1% or methylprednisolone 0.1%) ointment can be used for exacerbations in areas other than the face or nappy area. Oral steroids are rarely indicated in eczema. For chronic eczema on the limbs, zinc and tar combinations are alternatives to steroids.
- *Control itch:* advise parents to avoid saying 'Stop scratching' all the time, and to distract the child instead. Avoid overheating, particularly at night. Wet bandaging is very helpful if warranted. Antihistamines are often unhelpful but may be tried if the itch is not controlled by other measures (see Chapter 19, *Allergy and immunology*).
- *Treat infection:* take cultures and treat with simple wet dressings and oral antibiotics (e.g. erythromycin, cephalexin or flucloxacillin). Consider if herpes simplex is present. For recurrent bacterial infection, use antiseptic wash or 15-minute soak in salt/bleach baths (for each 30 litres of bath water add 30 mL of standard household bleach – about 4% hypochlorite – and one cup of ordinary sodium chloride, for example pool salt).
- Diet: a normal diet is usually indicated. If a child has immediate urticarial reactions to a particular food, that food should be avoided. Food allergy is more likely to be relevant in a child less than 12 months of age with widespread eczema. Environmental and food allergens may contribute to the exacerbation of symptoms in some patients. Allergen avoidance in these children may be of some benefit. In difficult cases, consider a more formal allergy assessment.
- Hospitalisation: if a child is missing school because of eczema, they should generally be in hospital for intensive treatment or seen urgently in a specialist clinic for consideration of oral immunosuppressive agents.

Red scaly rashes (papulosquamous)

Consider seborrhoeic dermatitis, psoriasis, tinea corporis, pityriasis rosea, pityriasis versicolor and atopic eczema. Ichthyosis vulgaris is a common cause of generalised scale without itch or redness.

Seborrhoeic dermatitis

Clinical features

- This condition presents in the first months of life, partly due to the activity of commensal yeasts.

- Red or yellow/brown scaly areas will commonly affect the scalp and forehead (The 'seborrhoeic' rash in infants affecting areas without sebaceous glands (e.g. axillae, napkin area) is probably best considered as a form of psoriasis.) The folds behind the ears and around the neck, axillae, groin and gluteal clefts are also affected.
- Resolution by the age of 4 months is usual.

Management
- Paraffin or olive oil applied to scalp to loosen scale.
- Imidazole creams with hydrocortisone 1% cream or with a mixture of salicylic acid (1%) and sulfur (1%) ointment, twice daily.
- Anti-yeast shampoos (e.g. selenium sulfide – Selsun) can be helpful. Use carefully to avoid irritation or toxicity.

Psoriasis
Clinical features
- Can occur at any age.
- Lesions begin as small red papules that develop into circular, sharply demarcated erythematous patches with prominent silvery scale.
- Common presentations include plaques on extensor surfaces, generalised guttate (small) lesions, red scaly scalp lesions or moist red anogenital rashes. Itch can be a variable feature. Nail changes are often seen in childhood.

Management
The treatment depends on the site and extent of disease and the age of the child. Adolescents are less tolerant of tar creams.
- Treat isolated skin plaques with either topical steroids (e.g. intermittent mometasone with clinical monitoring) or tar-based creams (e.g. liquor picis carbonis 3%, salicylic acid 2% in sorbolene cream). Generally avoid tars on the face, flexures and genitalia.
- Use hydrocortisone 1% ointment on the face and anogenital region. Topical steroids are not used for large areas in childhood psoriasis because of the possible development of rebound pustular disease.
- Thick scalp plaques can be softened overnight with a similar tar cream and removed with a tar shampoo.
- Topical calcipotriol can be used in conjunction with steroid creams or as a combination cream (Daivobet).
- Widespread psoriasis may need treatment with one or more of etretinate, methotrexate, cyclosporin or ultraviolet therapy, all of which are effective. Biologic therapies have recently become available for severe childhood psoriasis.

Tinea corporis
Clinical features
- The typical lesion is a slow-growing erythematous ring with a clear or scaly centre; however, tinea corporis can present in a wide variety of ways, particularly if previously treated with steroid ointments. It can be pustular, vesicular or bullous, or spread to many sites within days.
- Tinea should be considered in any red scaly rash where the diagnosis is unclear.

Management
- If in doubt about the diagnosis, confirm by scraping the scale for microscopy and culture.
- Lesions are treated with terbinafine cream (twice daily for 1 week) or an imidazole cream (e.g. clotrimazole, miconazole or econazole 2–4 times daily, for 4 weeks).
- Oral griseofulvin (20 mg/kg per day in divided doses) is required for tinea capitis or for widespread lesions.

Pityriasis rosea
Clinical features
- The condition is common between the ages of 1 and 10 years.
- Initially, a pink scaly patch appears, followed a few days later by many pink/red scaly oval macules mainly on the trunk.
- It is usually asymptomatic but can be itchy.

Management
- Reassure the patient. The condition can persist for weeks.

Red blanching rashes (erythematous)

Macular erythematous lesions are most commonly caused by viral infections (e.g. coxsackie, echovirus, Epstein–Barr virus, adenovirus, parainfluenza, influenza, parvovirus B19, human herpes virus 6, rubella and measles) or drug reactions. Consider also septicaemia, scarlet fever, Kawasaki disease (see Chapter 18, *Infectious diseases and immunisation*) and *Mycoplasma* infection.

Fever and exanthem

The onset of fever and exanthem is usually due to a viral illness, often enterovirus. Some infections have specific clinical features that aid diagnosis; for example measles and erythema infectiosum. However, in most instances, a diagnosis cannot be made with certainty. To manage such a child, consider

- Is the child sick? Is the child lethargic, cold peripherally or young? Consider meningococcal disease, other bacterial sepsis and Kawasaki disease. Investigate and treat.
- Are they taking any medication? Consider ceasing medication.
- Are there other people at risk? If relatives are immunosuppressed or pregnant, consider serology, stool viral culture and advising the at risk person to consult their doctor.
- Is the rash papular? Consider papular acrodermatitis.

  If the answer to all the above is 'no', reassurance and review is probably appropriate.

Erythema infectiosum and Kawasaki disease

See Chapter 18, *Infectious diseases and immunisation*.

Roseola infantum

This condition is seen most days in paediatric emergency departments. Typically, an infant has had a high fever for 2–4 days and has often been put on antibiotics. The fever then goes but a widespread erythematous rash appears. The family needs reassurance that the rash is not a drug reaction. See Chapter 18, *Infectious diseases and immunisation*, p. 276.

Purpuric rashes

Consider viral infections, meningococcal sepsis, platelet disorders, vasculitis, drug reactions and trauma.

Septicaemia

Suspect septicaemia (usually meningococcal) in a child with recent onset of fever and lethargy. Skin lesions may be erythematous macules progressing to extensive purple purpura. Even if there is doubt, take blood cultures, give antibiotics and arrange admission (see also Chapter 1, *Medical emergencies*).

Enteroviral infection

Scattered petechiae are common in children who have fever from enteroviral infections. These children are usually well. If in doubt, or if the child appears unwell, investigate (full blood examination, blood cultures) and consider treatment for septicaemia. See Approach to the febrile child, Chapter 18, *Infectious diseases and immunisation*, p. 266.

Leukaemia

Suspect leukaemia in a child with generalised petechiae or purpura in the absence of trauma. Look for tiredness or pallor. Obtain an urgent full blood examination (see Chapter 12, *Haematologic conditions and oncology*).

Henoch–Schönlein purpura

See detailed summary including Investigations and management in Chapter 15, *Bones and joints*.

Non-itchy, painless macules, papules or urticarial lesions with purpuric centres occur in a symmetrical distribution mainly on the buttocks and ankles, occasionally on the legs, arms and elsewhere. There may be associated abdominal pain, arthralgia, arthritis or haematuria. Renal involvement leading to chronic renal failure is rare, but can occur irrespective of the severity of the rash and other symptoms and may be delayed until weeks or months after the onset of the illness.

Idiopathic thrombocytopenic purpura

See also Chapter 12, *Haematologic condition and oncology*, p. 169.

Bruises, petechiae or purpuric lesions appear over a period of days or weeks, mainly in sites of frequent mild trauma. The child is otherwise well. Full blood examination will show a low platelet count.

Child abuse

See Chapter 29, *Forensic medicine.*

Twisting, compression, pinching and hitting can all cause petechial or purpuric lesions. Look for bruises of bizarre shapes and different ages, evidence of bony fractures and an abnormal affect.

Trauma and vasomotor straining

In some ethnic groups, it is common to treat a febrile or unwell child by rubbing or suctioning the skin with a variety of implements. This produces bizarre circular and linear patterns of petechiae that can alarm the unwary.

Petechiae can appear around the head and neck in normal children after coughing or vomiting. Restraining a small child for a procedure such as a lumbar puncture or venepuncture can also lead to the development of petechiae on the upper body.

Blue or black rashes

Consider vascular malformations, haemangiomas, Mongolian spots, blue naevi and melanoma.

Vascular malformations

- These can be blue, red, purple or skin coloured. They are developmental defects and do not resolve.
- Such malformations can involve capillaries (e.g. port wine stain), veins, arteries (e.g. arteriovenous malformation) and lymphatics (e.g. cystic hygroma).
- Small vascular malformations may not cause any problems and do not require treatment.
- Extensive malformations can be associated with pain, soft tissue or bony hypertrophy, bone erosion, haemorrhage, thrombosis, infection and platelet trapping. Troublesome or large lesions may benefit from anticoagulation, oral sirolimus, surgery or sclerotherapy. A multidisciplinary approach using expertise from surgical, paediatric, dermatological and radiological fields is helpful.

Haemangiomas

Clinical features

- Superficial haemangiomas begin as macular erythematous lesions in the first weeks of life and become soft, partly compressible, sharply defined, red or purple swellings that can occur anywhere on the body.
- Deeper haemangiomas may appear as blue or skin-coloured swellings.
- Most haemangiomas are not present at birth; they grow for several months and resolve fully over several years.

Management

Parents need reassurance about the inherently benign nature of these lesions. Most haemangiomas are best left alone and allowed to involute spontaneously. In some sites, however, haemangiomas can rapidly lead to problems such as permanent disfigurement, ulceration, blindness, destruction of cartilage, respiratory obstruction or death.

Urgent assessment by an experienced clinician is needed if any developing haemangioma

- Is ulcerating and/or potentially disfiguring
- Is on the eyelid or adjacent to the globe of the eye
- Deforms structures such as the lip, ear cartilage or nasal cartilage
- Begins as an extensive macule that grows thicker, especially if on the face
- Is associated with stridor

If treatment is warranted, topical timolol (for smaller flat lesions) or oral propranolol (e.g. wean dose upwards to 2 mg/kg per day) is usually effective at stopping growth and accelerating shrinking. Oral prednisolone (3 mg/kg per day weaning over 6 weeks) can be used if propranolol is contraindicated. Vascular laser, surgery or gamma interferon may be used in certain circumstances.

Hypopigmented lesions

In hypopigmented lesions, look for a fine scale. If it is scaly, consider pityriasis versicolor or pityriasis alba. If it is not scaly, consider pityriasis versicolor, post-inflammatory loss of pigment, halo naevi or vitiligo.

Pityriasis versicolor

- This is common in adolescents and is caused by an increased activity of commensal yeasts.

- Multiple oval macules, usually covered with fine scale, appear on the trunk or upper arms. The lesions may appear paler or darker than the surrounding skin.
- Treatment with anti-yeast shampoos is effective. For example, apply selenium sulfide 2% (Selsun shampoo). Leave on for 5–10 minutes, rinse and treat weekly for 4 weeks and then monthly. The pigmentation takes weeks to resolve and relapses are common without ongoing maintenance.

Pityriasis alba

This condition is common in prepubertal children and represents post-inflammatory hypopigmentation secondary to mild eczema. Single or multiple, poorly demarcated hypopigmented 1–2 cm macules are seen on the face or upper body. Lesions are not itchy but often have a fine scale. Most families only need reassurance. If needed, treat with hydrocortisone 1% to active lesions and educate regarding skin care for eczema. Resolution of the discolouration takes months.

Vitiligo

This condition is characterised by sharply demarcated, often symmetrical areas of complete pigment loss. Eventual repigmentation in childhood vitiligo is common and is helped by topical steroids. Some children develop extensive areas of vitiligo that do not respond for treatment.

Post-inflammatory pigmentation changes

This condition occurs particularly in dark-skinned people. Many inflammatory skin disorders may leave diffuse, hypo- or hyperpigmented macules after healing. No treatment makes much difference. Most lesions resolve over months or years.

Hyperpigmented lesions

If they are flat, consider junctional melanocytic naevi, café-au-lait spots, naevus spilus, pityriasis versicolor and post-inflammatory hyperpigmentation. If raised, consider compound melanocytic naevi, Spitz naevi and warts.

Congenital pigmented naevi

Congenital melanocytic naevi that cover large areas or are likely to cause significant cosmetic concern need very early assessment by a skin specialist and plastic surgeon, preferably in the first week of life, for diagnosis, surgery, laser treatment and/or long-term follow up. Small congenital melanocytic naevi have no increased risk for the development of melanoma over other moles.

Acquired pigmented naevi

During childhood, most children develop multiple pigmented lesions, which may be freckles, lentigines, naevus spilus, acquired melanocytic naevi or very rarely, melanoma.

Immune-suppressed children and those who have had chemotherapy are at greater risk of skin malignancy.

Anogenital rashes

Most anogenital rashes seen in infants who wear nappies are primarily caused by reaction with urine or faeces (irritant napkin dermatitis). Soaps, detergents and secondary yeast infection may contribute. In older children, threadworms (*Enterobius vermicularis*) are a common cause of an itchy anogenital rash. Look for the worms at night and treat with mebendazole 50 mg (<10 kg), 100 mg (>10 kg) (not in pregnancy or <6 months) or pyrantel 10 mg/kg (max 500 mg) oral stat. A repeat dose 2 weeks later helps reduce the high rate of reinfestation.

Consider also less common causes such as malabsorption syndromes (diarrhoea, erosive dermatitis and failure to thrive), zinc deficiency (a sharply defined anogenital rash with associated perioral, hand and foot 'eczema'), Langerhans' cell histiocytosis, psoriasis and Crohn's disease.

Irritant napkin dermatitis

Clinical features

- This is the most common cause of napkin dermatitis in infants.
- Typically presents as confluent erythema that typically, but not always, spares the groin folds. Variant presentations include multiple erosions and ulcers, scaly or glazed erythema and satellite lesions at the periphery.
- Satellite lesions are suggestive of *Candida* infection.

Management

- Keep the area clean and dry. Leave the nappy off whenever possible.
- Gel-based disposable nappies or a non-wettable under-napkin can be helpful. Cloth nappies should be thoroughly washed and rinsed.
- Use topical zinc cream or paste for mild eruptions.
- Add hydrocortisone 1% cream if inflamed. Do not use stronger steroids.
- Consider mupirocin 2% cream if not settling. Antifungal therapy is often not needed, even if *Candida* is present.

Candida napkin dermatitis

This occurs secondary to irritant napkin dermatitis and antibiotic use. Swab to confirm and treat the underlying cause as above and use topical imidazole cream.

Perianal streptococcal dermatitis

Streptococcus pyogenes infection.

Clinical features

- A localised, well-demarcated erythema that covers a circular area of 1–2 cm radius around the anus.
- Tenderness and painful defecation are typical.
- If not treated, it may persist for months.
- May have fissures and constipation.

Management

- Take perianal and throat cultures to confirm the presence of *Streptococcus pyogenes*.
- Apply paraffin ointment three times daily to the perianal area for symptomatic relief. Treat with oral antibiotics (phenoxymethylpenicillin 15 mg/kg (max. 500 mg) 6 hourly) for a minimum of 2 weeks. Several weeks of therapy may be required. Intramuscular penicillin can be used if there are concerns about compliance.
- Keep stools soft with oral liquid paraffin for several weeks.

Lichen sclerosis

This condition presents as an area of atrophy with white shiny skin, purpura or telangiectasia in the perivulvar region of girls aged 3 years or older. It may be itchy. Cases have been misdiagnosed as sexual abuse. Management is with moisturisers and courses of potent steroid ointment. Even after treatment, unrecognised scarring and atrophy can occur. Long term follow-up is required.

Hair problems

Consider alopecia areata, traumatic alopecia, tinea capitis, kerion and head lice.

Alopecia areata

Clinical features

- Typically one or more oval patches of hair loss develop over a few days. Some hairs may remain within the patches but usually there is complete alopecia in the affected areas. Occasionally, the hair loss is diffuse.
- The scalp appears normal and does not show scaling, erythema or scarring.
- Most cases in childhood resolve spontaneously but progression to total scalp or body hair loss or recurrent alopecia can occur.
- Regrowth can occur decades later.

Management

- For isolated small patches present for weeks without further progression, no treatment is needed.
- For recent or progressive hair loss, treatment with intralesional steroids for a few weeks is beneficial. In difficult cases, other therapies including contact sensitisation, irritant agents and pulsed corticosteroids need to be considered.

Traumatic alopecia

Clinical features

- This condition is usually caused by rubbing (as on the occiput of many babies), cosmetic practices (e.g. tight braiding) or hair tugging as a habit (trichotillomania). Trichotillomania may be largely nocturnal and parents are often unaware of it.
- The affected areas are usually angular and on the anterior or lateral scalp.
- The areas contain hairs of different lengths and are never completely bald, unlike alopecia areata.

Management

- Recognition of the problem and a careful explanation to the family is often sufficient.
- Trichotillomania in younger children does not usually indicate that significant psychological problems are present. It is a habit similar to thumb sucking or nail biting, and a low-key approach similar to that used in those conditions is appropriate.

Tinea capitis

Clinical features

- In Australia, tinea capitis is usually caused by *Microsporum canis* contracted from cats or dogs.
- It is characterised by patches of hair loss with some short, lustreless, bent hairs a few millimetres in length.
- Redness and scaling are present in the patch. Hair loss without any of these features is not likely to be fungal.

Management

- Confirm the diagnosis, if possible, by greenish fluorescence of the hair shafts with Wood light (not present with some fungi) or by microscopy and culture of hair and scale.
- Treatment usually comprises griseofulvin orally 15–20 mg/kg (max. 1 g) daily for 4–6 weeks or until non-fluorescent. Pulse therapy (1 week treatment, 3 weeks off, then repeat) with terbinafine or itraconazole is also effective.
- Children may attend school provided that they are being treated.

Kerion (inflammatory ringworm)

This represents an inflammatory scarring immune response to tinea. It is an erythematous, tender, boggy swelling that discharges pus from multiple points. The swellings appear fluctuant but skin incision should be avoided. Treatment is with oral antifungals, often with antibiotics for secondary infection, and a brief course of oral steroids to suppress the immune response. Other inflammatory granulomas can mimic kerions.

Head lice

Clinical features

- Infestation of the scalp with *Pediculus capitis* is associated with itching.
- Eggs (nits) can be seen attached to the hairs just above the scalp surface.
- Epidemics of head lice regularly sweep through primary schools in all areas.

Management

- Suitable treatments include pyrethrin 0.165% (e.g. Pyrifoam), maldison 0.5% and permethrin 1% (e.g. Nix and Lyclear cream rinse), although resistance to all of these therapies has been reported.
- Wash the hair with soap and water. Thoroughly moisten the hair with the treatment and leave for 10 minutes. Rinse well and comb out with a fine-toothed comb. Reapply 1 week later to kill any eggs that have subsequently hatched.
- Reinfestation is common. A regular physical inspection, use of conditioner and combing of the hair are as important as chemical treatment.
- Children should continue to attend school whilst treatment is being undertaken.
- In very difficult cases, consideration to oral Bactrim for 2 weeks or single dose oral ivermectin should be given.

Nail problems

Congenitally abnormal nails are usually atrophic and can be the presenting feature of rare inherited conditions such as ectodermal dysplasias, dyskeratosis congenita, pachyonychia congenita, congenital malalignment of the great toenails and the nail–patella syndrome.

Acquired nail disease is usually a result of fungal infection, psoriasis, ingrown toenails or 20-nail dystrophy. It may also be seen in association with diseases such as alopecia areata and lichen planus. Nail biting and picking can lead to marked deformity of involved nails.

Tinea unguium (onychomycosis)

Clinical features

- Dermatophyte infection may affect one or more nails.
- White or yellow patches develop at the distal and lateral nail edges. The rest of the nail may become dis-coloured, friable and deformed with accumulation of subungual debris.
- Tinea is often also present on the adjacent skin, particularly in between the toes.

Management

- Always confirm the diagnosis by microscopy and culture of nail clippings.
- Oral terbinafine is the therapy of choice, taken daily for 12 weeks (<20 kg 62.5 mg, 20–40 kg 125 mg, >40 kg 250 mg).

USEFUL RESOURCES
- *www.dermnet.org.nz* – An excellent website with online courses (including pictures, investigations and management) and patient information.

CHAPTER 18

Infectious diseases and immunisation

Nigel Curtis
Mike Starr
Tom Connell
Nigel Crawford

Infectious Disease
Rational antibiotic prescribing

- Unnecessary antibiotic use for viral illnesses contributes to the increasing problem of antibiotic resistance. Most respiratory tract infections in children, including tonsillitis and otitis media, are self-limiting and do not require antibiotic therapy. If the diagnosis is unclear, it is preferable to repeat the clinical evaluation rather than use empiric antibiotic therapy 'just in case'.
- Antibiotics do not prevent secondary bacterial infection in viral illnesses.
- The use of antibiotics may make it more difficult to establish a definitive diagnosis and make rational decisions about management.
- Empiric antibiotic therapy (i.e. not based on specific aetiological diagnosis) should only be prescribed when a *serious* bacterial infection is suspected (e.g. meningitis).
- Empiric therapy should be based on the likely cause, local antibiotic resistance patterns and individual host factors (e.g. immunocompromise) in accordance with local guidelines.
- For mild infections use the safest and best-tolerated antibiotic with the narrowest spectrum against the most likely pathogens (e.g. trimethoprim for urinary tract infection).
- For serious infections use broad-spectrum antibiotics until the pathogen and its antibiotic susceptibility is available (e.g. cefotaxime/ceftriaxone for meningitis).
- Theoretical benefits of new antibiotics based on *in vitro* data do not necessarily translate into greater efficacy. Newer antibiotics often do not offer any advantages. They are usually more expensive with potentially more side effects and, if broad spectrum, have a greater likelihood of leading to resistance.

Antibiotic resistance

Although many bacteria are still susceptible to long-established treatments, antibiotic resistance is an increasing problem worldwide. Examples of particular clinical concern include

- Penicillin (and cephalosporin) resistant *Streptococcus pneumoniae* (PRP)
- Methicillin (multidrug) resistant *Staphylococcus aureus* (MRSA)
- Community-acquired non-multi-resistant MRSA (CA-MRSA)
- Glycopeptide (vancomycin and teicoplanin) intermediate-resistant *S. aureus* (GISA)
- Vancomycin-resistant *Enterococcus* (VRE)
- Multidrug-resistant (MDR) and extensively drug-resistant (XDR) *Mycobacterium tuberculosis*
- Bacteria that produce inducible beta-lactamases (IBL) which are always present in bacteria of the 'ESCHAPPM' group comprising *Enterobacter* spp., *Serratia marscesens*, *Citrobacter freundii*, *Hafnia* spp., *Aeromonas* spp., *Providencia* spp., *Proteus vulgaris* and *Morganella morganii*
- Bacteria that produce extended-spectrum β-lactamases (ESBL), for example some *E. coli* and *Klebsiella* spp. which are associated with cephalosporin (and often gentamicin resistance)

Paediatric Handbook, Ninth Edition. Edited by Amanda Gwee, Romi Rimer and Michael Marks.
© 2015 John Wiley & Sons, Ltd. Published 2015 by John Wiley & Sons, Ltd.

- MDR *Salmonella* spp.
- Macrolide-resistant *Streptococcus pyogenes*

Infections with resistant organisms should be considered in patients who have had prolonged hospitalisation, known exposure to, or prior colonisation with resistant organisms, or failed response to initial empiric antibiotic therapy. Specialist consultation is strongly advised in managing infections caused by resistant organisms.

Approach to the febrile child

- Fever is the most common presenting symptom in children in the primary care setting.
- Definition: generally considered to be present if core temperature (rectal or tympanic) is >38.0°C. Axillary and oral temperatures may underestimate body temperature by 0.5°C or more.
- Measuring temperature
  - Babies <3 months: use rectal thermometer (tympanic is not as accurate).
  - Immunocompromised patients: best to use oral or axillary.
- Although tympanic thermometers provide some advantages over other thermometers (ease of use, rapid results and convenience), several studies have found that they are not as accurate for the detection of fever, particularly in infants <3 months of age. Rectal (neonates), oral and axillary (immunocompromised patients) temperatures are preferable for accurate measurement of temperature.
- Self-limiting viral infections are the most common cause of fever in children. However, the challenge to the clinician is to identify those children with a more serious cause. Fever in children may be classified into three groups:
  - Fever with localising signs.
  - Fever without focus.
  - Fever (or pyrexia) of unknown origin.

Fever with localising signs

A careful history and examination will identify the source of infection in most patients. These children should be managed according to their source of infection and its severity.

Fever without focus

In a small number of children presenting with fever, no focus is found. Most will have a viral infection, but a more serious illness such as a urinary tract infection (5–8%), occult bacteraemia (<1%) or meningitis may be present. Infants (<12 months old) have a higher risk of occult bacteraemia.

Most children who present with fever and no identifiable focus do not appear unwell. History should include systems review and details about immunisation status, infectious contacts, travel, diet and contact with animals. Physical examination should pay particular attention to

- General appearance: the level of activity and social interaction; peripheral perfusion and colour.
- Vital signs: pulse, respiratory rate, blood pressure and oxygen saturation.
- Possible clues to source: full fontanelle, neck stiffness, photophobia; respiratory distress (tachypnoea; grunting; nasal flare; intercostal and subcostal retraction), abnormal chest signs; rhinitis; pharyngitis; otitis or mastoiditis; lymphadenopathy; abdominal distension, tenderness or masses; hepatosplenomegaly; bone and joint tenderness or swelling; skin rashes, petechiae or purpura, or skin infection.
- **Always consider Kawasaki disease in any child with a fever that persists for more than a few days**. It is the only rare cause of persistent fever that requires urgent treatment.

Patients with unexplained fever with a higher likelihood for serious infection include the following patients or conditions:

- Neonates and infants <3 months of age.
- Children <6 months of age (higher chance of UTI).
- Children <12 months of age with febrile convulsion, or any children with prolonged febrile convulsion (>10 minutes), consider lumbar puncture to exclude meningitis.
- Immunocompromised patients (e.g. congenital immunodeficiency, human immunodeficiency virus (HIV) infection, neutropenia, patients on cytotoxic drugs, immunosuppression or steroids).
- Asplenic children (congenital, post-splenectomy or functional, e.g. sickle cell disease).
- Patients who have received prior antibiotics.

Table 18.1 Management of fever without focus

Age	Investigations	Management
<1 month	FBE; blood, urine and CSF cultures; CXR	Admit Empiric IV benzylpenicillin and gentamicin, *plus* cefotaxime if meningitis is suspected (see Antimicrobial guidelines)
1–3 months	As above (CXR may be omitted if no respiratory symptoms or signs present)	If WCC 5–15 × 10⁹/L with other investigations normal: discharge and review within 12 hours, or sooner if deterioration occurs If child is unwell, or any results are abnormal: admit and consider empiric antibiotics (see Antimicrobial guidelines)
3 months to 3 years *and well*	Consider urine culture (mandatory if <6 months)	If <6 months and UTI is suspected from dipstick urine testing: admit for IV benzylpenicillin and gentamicin (see Antimicrobial guidelines) Otherwise: discharge and review within 24 hours, or sooner if deterioration occurs
3 months to 3 years *and unwell*	FBE; blood, urine and CSF cultures; CXR if respiratory symptoms or signs present	Admit and start empiric antibiotics: • if CSF normal: IV flucloxacillin and gentamicin • if CSF abnormal or unavailable: IV cefotaxime (see Antimicrobial guidelines)

Fever = rectal temperature >38°C (>38.9°C over 3 months of age).
FBE, full blood examination, including film; CSF, cerebrospinal fluid; WCC, white cell count; CXR, chest x-ray.
Urine specimens should be obtained by suprapubic aspiration or catheter drainage. Bag specimens are useless in this context.
Lumbar puncture should not be performed in a child with impaired conscious state or focal neurological signs (see Chapter 1, *Medical emergencies*; Chapter 3, *Procedures*).
Ceftriaxone can be substituted for cefotaxime (see Antimicrobial guidelines).

• Children with indwelling lines/devices (e.g. central venous lines, arterial catheters, ventriculoperitoneal shunt, intercostal drain, cardiac devices).
• Sickle cell disease, cystic fibrosis or structural cardiac defects (e.g. endocarditis).
• Children who appear toxic and unwell (e.g. altered conscious state, decreased peripheral perfusion (check central capillary refill) or purpuric rash).

These children require admission to hospital, culture of blood, urine and cerebrospinal fluid (CSF) (full septic screen) and a chest x-ray if indicated. Antibiotic therapy should be based on the patient's clinical illness, local epidemiology and likely antibiotic susceptibility (see Antimicrobial guidelines).

In the absence of these risk factors, a febrile child >6 months of age without a focus of infection who appears well does not require laboratory testing or treatment, although a urine microscopy and culture may be appropriate.

There is no evidence that empiric oral or parenteral antibiotics prevent focal infections from occult bacter-aemia; instead, they may cause delayed diagnosis, potential drug side effects, additional costs and the development of antibiotic resistance. The child should have a careful clinical assessment, scheduled early review and parental education. See Table 18.1 and Box 18.1.

Occult bacteraemia

Infants with bacteraemia may clear the bacteria spontaneously. This is particularly likely for pneumococcal bacteraemia. A common clinical scenario is children who have had a blood culture taken during fever that grows *S. pneumoniae,* but who are well and afebrile without having received any antibiotics by the time the culture result is available. In this situation children have generally cleared the organism, and do not require further investigation or treatment, although parents should be asked to bring their children back for immediate review if they develop further fever within the following 7 days. Refer for specialist advice if uncertain.

Other pathogens causing occult bacteraemia should be treated with appropriate antibiotics.

Box 18.1 **Advice for parents about fever**

When caring for your child:

- Make the child comfortable, for example dress in light clothing.
- Give small, frequent drinks of clear fluid, for example water or diluted juice.
- Fever does not necessarily require treatment with medication. Finding the cause and treating the cause is often more important.
- Paracetamol may be given if the child is irritable, miserable or appears to be in pain (15 mg/kg p.o. 4 hourly when required, to a maximum of 90 mg/kg per day).
- Giving paracetamol has **not** been shown to prevent febrile convulsions.
- Do not continue giving regular paracetamol for more than 48 hours without having the child assessed by a doctor.
- Avoid aspirin and other non-steroidal anti-inflammatory drugs (NSAIDs):
  - Aspirin because of risk of Reye's syndrome.
  - NSAIDs because of potential association with invasive staphylococcal and streptococcal disease (including necrotising fasciitis).

Parents should be advised to seek immediate medical attention if there is no improvement in 48 hours or at any time if their child

- Looks 'sick': pale, lethargic and weak.
- Has severe headache, neck stiffness or complains of light hurting their eyes.
- Has breathing difficulties.
- Refuses to drink anything.
- Has persistent vomiting.
- Shows signs of drowsiness.
- Has a non-blanching petechial/purpuric rash.

Partially treated bacterial infection

Patients presenting with fever who have received prior antibiotics should be assessed carefully. Although the child may still have a viral illness, partial treatment with antibiotics may mask the typical clinical presentation of a serious bacterial infection, such as meningitis. A full septic screen should be considered, even if the child looks well. For this reason, neonates should almost never be treated with oral antibiotics in the community.

Pyrexia (fever) of unknown origin

Pyrexia of unknown origin (PUO) is defined as prolonged fever (usually defined as ≥2 weeks or longer) where history, examination and initial investigations have failed to reveal a cause. In general, PUO in children is more likely to be due to chronic, non-infectious conditions, such as juvenile chronic arthritis and other collagen vascular diseases, inflammatory bowel disease or malignancy. Infectious causes include systemic viral syndromes (such as infectious mononucleosis), upper or lower respiratory infections (e.g. sinusitis), urinary tract infection, CNS infection, bone infection, TB, abscess (e.g. parameningeal, intra-abdominal), endocarditis and enteric infections (e.g. typhoid fever). The term PUO is often *incorrectly* applied to patients who have frequent recurrent viral infections.

Febrile neutropenia

See Chapter 12, *Haematological conditions and oncology*, p. 179.

Common bacterial infections

Group A streptococcus

Group A β-haemolytic streptococci (GABHS or *S. pyogenes*) cause a variety of diseases including pharyngo-tonsillitis (see Chapter 24, *Ear, nose and throat conditions*), impetigo, cellulitis, scarlet fever, otitis media, streptococcal toxic shock syndrome, necrotising fasciitis, glomerulonephritis and rheumatic fever. Group A streptococcal pharyngitis is extremely uncommon in children <5 years of age. *S. pyogenes* is currently always sensitive to penicillin.

Scarlet fever

- Transmission: droplet, direct contact.
- Incubation period: 2–5 days.
- Infectious period: 10–21 days (24–48 hours, if adequate treatment).

Clinical features

- Prodrome: sudden-onset high fever, vomiting, malaise, headache and abdominal pain.
- Rash: appears early during prodrome, blanching, diffuse, erythematous, involving torso and skin folds.
- Associated features: circumoral pallor, strawberry tongue (initially white, then red day 4–5), pharyngotonsillitis and tender cervical/submaxillary nodes.

Complications

Otitis media, retropharyngeal abscess, quinsy, rheumatic fever, glomerulonephritis and rarely meningitis.

Diagnosis

Culture of throat swab may confirm clinical impression.

Treatment

- Phenoxymethylpenicillin (penicillin V) 250 mg p.o. (<10 years), 500 mg p.o. (>10 years) 12 hourly for 10 days.
- Control of case: exclude from school until treated for 24 hours.

Differential diagnosis

Kawasaki disease, streptococcal or staphylococcal toxic shock syndrome, viral infection.

Acute rheumatic fever

- Incubation period: 7–28 days after group A streptococcal infection.

Clinical features

Specific criteria for diagnosis can be found at www.rhdaustralia.org.au. Carditis, polyarthritis and chorea are major manifestations.

Complications

Increased risk of recurrent disease; particularly for first 5 years after an attack. Heart valve damage may be permanent, especially after severe or recurrent disease, leading to rheumatic heart disease.

Diagnosis

Clinical features and culture/serology. Echocardiography may be useful in detecting subclinical lesions or typical rheumatic valvular involvement.

Treatment

- Admission to hospital.
- Oral phenoxymethylpenicillin (penicillin V): or a single IM injection of benzathine penicillin G. Use oral erythromycin if allergic to penicillin.
- Aspirin.
- Corticosteroids are often used when carditis with cardiac failure is present, although there is no definitive evidence that they improve long-term outcome.
- For severe chorea, haloperidol, sodium valproate/carbamazepine or other major tranquilisers have been used with limited success.

Follow-up

Secondary prophylaxis is essential to prevent subsequent group A streptococcal infections, which may cause recurrences. Daily phenoxymethylpenicillin (penicillin V), or 4-weekly IM benzathine penicillin G. Long-term clinical and echocardiographic follow-up is essential.

Post-infectious glomerulonephritis

See Chapter 10, *Genitourinary conditions*.

S. pneumoniae

S. pneumoniae (pneumococcus) is a Gram-positive coccus that causes a wide variety of infections including severe, invasive disease (e.g. meningitis, septicaemia, septic arthritis, peritonitis), or mild, often self-limited, invasive disease (occult bacteraemia), pneumonia, otitis media and sinusitis.

Transmission: droplet

Epidemiology

This is changing as a result of the routine use of conjugate pneumococcal vaccine (7-valent and more recently 10-valent and 13-valent vaccines).

The 13-valent conjugate pneumococcal vaccine (13PCV, Prevenar 13®) has been part of the routine immunisation schedule in Australia since 2011. It is given at 2, 4 and 6 months of age. A fourth dose in the second year of life is recommended for children at high risk of invasive pneumococcal disease (IPD), including those with hyposplenism.

The 23-valent polysaccharide vaccine provides protection against a broader range of serotypes but is not immunogenic in children <18–24 months of age and protection is not long-lasting (2–3 years). The vaccine is routinely recommended in risk groups such as Aboriginal children, children with respiratory or cardiac comorbidities, hyposplenia or certain immunodeficiencies.

In trials, the vaccine provided ~70% protection against IPD (meningitis, septicaemia), ~50% protection against radiographically proven pneumonia, and <5% protection against otitis media caused by *S. pneumoniae*. However, IPD remains high in Aboriginal children due to the high proportion of disease caused by non-vaccine serotypes. The incidence of IPD in central Australian Aboriginal children prior to the introduction of vaccine was among the highest in the world (~1000–2000 per 100,000 aged <5 years).

Despite the decreasing incidence of pneumococcal disease, *S. pneumoniae* remains the most common cause of pneumonia, otitis media and meningitis in children. There also remains concern about the possibility of a rise in disease caused by non-vaccine serotypes (serotype replacement).

Clinical features

The most common presentations of *S. pneumonia* infection are pneumonia and otitis media, followed by septicaemia and meningitis. Soft tissue, bone and joint infections are less common manifestations.

Diagnosis

Meningitis, septicaemia or other sterile site infection is confirmed by culture/Gram stain of appropriate specimen. In pneumococcal pneumonia, a blood culture is positive in only ~10–20% of cases. Polymerase chain reaction (PCR) based testing of blood and CSF is available and may be useful when antibiotics have been started prior to the collection of specimens. Pneumococcal urinary antigen has poor specificity due to pharyngeal carriage of pneumococcus being common.

Treatment

Penicillin or amoxicillin is the drug of choice, except in CNS infection with penicillin non-susceptible pneumococci (PNSP).

- If non-CNS infection with PNSP, treat with high-dose penicillin (benzylpenicillin 60 mg/kg (max. 2 g) IV 4–6 hourly for invasive disease including pneumonia, or amoxicillin 30–40 mg/kg (500 mg) p.o. 8 hourly for otitis media or sinusitis).
- If CNS infection with cefotaxime/ceftriaxone-non-susceptible (or intermediate susceptible) pneumococci, use vancomycin plus rifampicin or, for PNSP with cefotaxime MIC ≤2.0 mcg/mL, use high-dose cefotaxime (300 mg/kg per day)/ceftriaxone (100 mg/kg per day) as an alternative (see Bacterial meningitis, p. 286). Duration of treatment is 10 days for meningitis and usually 5–7 days for other infections.

Neisseria meningitidis

N. meningitidis (meningococcus) is a Gram-negative diplococcus that mainly causes meningitis and/or septicaemia. Less commonly, it may cause other infections including conjunctivitis, septic arthritis, pharyngitis, pneumonia and occult bacteraemia. For recommendations specific to meningitis see Bacterial meningitis, p. 286.

- Transmission: droplet.
- Incubation period: hours to 3 days.
- Infectious period: as long as carried – may be months. Most are virulent within days of acquisition.

Epidemiology

- Peak age groups: <2 years and 15–24 years.
- Most common serogroups in Australia: B (in young children) and C (in adolescents).
- Incidence of group C meningococcal infection has fallen rapidly since the introduction of routine conjugate group C vaccine.

- Even with antibiotic treatment, the overall case fatality in invasive disease has been reported as 5% for group B and 14% for group C infection.

Clinical features
- Meningitis – see below, p. 286.
- Septicaemia: often non-specific prodrome suggestive of viral illness, followed by rapid progression with any or all of the following: fever, rash (classically purpuric or petechial, but can be less specific), malaise, myalgia, arthralgia, vomiting, headache, reduced conscious state.
- Chronic meningococcaemia occurs rarely (consider terminal complement deficiency), and may be associated with progressive purpuric rash.

Diagnosis
Diagnosis is initially based on clinical features, with confirmation by culture of blood and/or CSF, preferably collected before first dose of antibiotics. Under no circumstances should treatment be delayed while awaiting collection of clinical samples. Additional tests may include skin scrapings of purpuric skin lesions for Gram stain and culture and PCR on blood or CSF.

Treatment
- Manage shock appropriately (see Chapter 1, *Medical emergencies*).
- Administer IV antibiotics (cefotaxime 50 mg/kg per dose (max. 2 g) 6 hourly, or ceftriaxone 50 mg/kg (max. 1 g) IV 12 hourly or if unavailable, benzylpenicillin 60 mg/kg (max. 2 g) IV 4–6 hourly).
- Change to IV benzylpenicillin when meninogococcus is isolated.
- Duration of antibiotics is usually 5–7 days.
- All cases should be notified immediately to statutory health authorities.
- Steroids
  ○ Meningococcaemia: Consider corticosteroids (hydrocortisone 1 mg/kg IV 6 hourly) in severe cases.
  ○ Meningitis: (Children >4 weeks old) give dexamethasone 0.15 mg/kg IV 6 hourly for 4 days.
- Immunoglobulin 0.5 g/kg IV over 4 hours may be considered in those requiring ICU.

Clearance antibiotics for contacts of patients with meningococcal infection
Contacts should receive prophylaxis (see Table 18.2). Patients with invasive disease who have received only penicillin should also receive treatment to eradicate carriage.

Meningococcal vaccines
Meningococcal group C conjugate vaccine is effective in all age groups and given as part of the routine NIP schedule to all Australian children at 12 months of age. Children at higher risk should be offered two doses of conjugate vaccine from 2 months of age with a third dose in the second year of life. Recently, 4-valent meningococcal conjugate vaccines (A, C W135 and Y) have become available and are recommended for travellers (e.g. to African 'meningitis belt' or attending the Haj) and for controlling outbreaks. They are also used in patients with asplenia.

Staphylococcus aureus
S. aureus is a Gram-positive coccus that causes a wide variety of invasive and non-invasive disease.

Epidemiology
S. aureus is present in the nose of about one-third of individuals. Both hospital- and community-acquired multi-resistant *S. aureus* (MRSA) have emerged as a significant public health problem.

Clinical features
S. aureus causes a variety of diseases including impetigo, boils and abscesses, cellulitis (including periorbital cellulitis), osteomyelitis, septic arthritis, endocarditis, pneumonia, food poisoning, bacteraemia, septicaemia, toxic shock syndrome and scalded skin syndrome in younger children. Staphylococcal infection may be accompanied by significant systemic symptoms (e.g. myalgia) in addition to localising features.

Diagnosis
- Sterile site infection is confirmed by appropriate culture/Gram stain.

Table 18.2 Prophylaxis regimens for contacts of meningitis cases

Organism	Antibiotic	Those requiring prophylaxis
Haemophilus influenzae type b	Rifampicin 20 mg/kg (max. 600 mg) p.o. daily for 4 days *Infants <1 month of age:* Rifampicin 10 mg/kg p.o. daily for 4 days *Pregnancy/contraindication to rifampicin:* Ceftriaxone 250 mg IM daily for 2 days	Index case and all household contacts if household includes other children <4 years of age who are not fully immunised. Index case and all household contacts in households with any infants <12 months of age, regardless of immunisation status. Index case and all household contacts in households with a child 1–5 years of age who is inadequately immunised. Index case and all room contacts, including staff, in a childcare group if index case attends >18 hours per week and any contacts <2 years of age who are inadequately immunised. **AND** children who are not up to date with Hib should be immunised.
N. meningitidis	Rifampicin 10 mg/kg (max. 600 mg) p.o. 2 hourly for 2 days *Infants <1 month of age:* Rifampicin 5 mg/kg p.o. 12 hourly for 2 days *Pregnancy/contraindication to rifampicin:* Ceftriaxone 250 mg (>12 years) or 125 mg (<12 years) IM as a single dose or Ciprofloxacin 500 mg (>12 y) or 250 mg (6–11 y) p.o. as a single dose	Index case (if treated only with penicillin) and all intimate household or day care contacts who have been exposed to index case within 10 days of onset. Any person who gave mouth-to-mouth resuscitation to the index case
S. pneumoniae	Nil	No increased risk to contacts

It is important that rifampicin is given early to both the index case and contacts, especially for *N. meningitidis* disease, because of the rapidity with which secondary cases may develop.
As prophylaxis is not infallible, any febrile household contact should seek urgent medical attention.
Nasopharyngeal carriage of Hib is not eradicated by a single injection of ceftriaxone.
Rifampicin interferes with the metabolism of several medications, including the oral contraceptive pill (alternative contraception should be instituted), anticonvulsants, warfarin and chloramphenicol.
Rifampicin colours body fluids red, for example urine, saliva, tears (soft contact lenses may be damaged), sweat.

- Patients with *S. aureus* bacteraemia should undergo careful clinical examination to identify any focal infection.

Treatment
- Surgical drainage is often necessary for abscesses and other foci of infection.
- Anti-staphylococcal antibiotics include flucloxacillin, cephalexin, cephazolin and clindamycin.
- MRSA is resistant to all penicillin and cephalosporin antibiotics.
  - Community-acquired MRSA is often sensitive to a wide range of antibiotics including clindamycin, co-trimoxazole, ciprofloxacin, vancomycin, teicoplanin, rifampicin and fusidic acid. (*Note*: ciprofloxacin, rifampicin or fusidic acid should never be used alone for *S. aureus,* as resistance develops rapidly.)
  - Hospital-acquired MRSA is often only sensitive to vancomycin and teicoplanin. Although vancomycin may be necessary to treat some MRSA infections, it is not as effective as flucloxacillin for the treatment of susceptible isolates.
- *S. aureus* bacteraemia needs prolonged (up to 14 days) treatment to prevent recurrence.

Mycoplasma pneumoniae

- Transmission: droplet.
- Incubation period: 1–4 weeks.
- Infectious period: unknown, likely to be many months; typically infects all members of a family over a period of weeks/months although most are asymptomatic.
- Epidemiology: all ages.

Clinical features

- Pneumonia: malaise, fever, headache, non-productive cough for 3–4 weeks (may become productive); 10% have rash (usually maculopapular); bronchitis, pharyngitis, otitis media; chest x-ray may demonstrate unilateral lobar or bilateral diffuse changes.
- CNS manifestations (uncommon; likely post-infectious): aseptic meningitis, meningoencephalitis, encephalitis, polyradiculitis/Guillain–Barré syndrome, acute cerebellar ataxia, cranial nerve neuropathy, transverse myelitis, acute disseminated encephalomyelitis (ADEM) and choreoathetosis.

Diagnosis

- Serology: Not useful in acute setting. Infection can be diagnosed by fourfold rise in IgG over 2–4 weeks; IgM alone has very poor specificity in children as positive results occur in ∼30% of healthy preschoolers.
- PCR of respiratory specimens: Recent studies show asymptomatic well children are as likely as symptomatic children to have a positive respiratory such suggesting current diagnostic tests can not distinguish between asymptomatic carriage and symptomatic infection.

Treatment

- Roxithromycin 2.5–4 mg/kg (max. 150 mg) p.o. 12 hourly for 10 days or Azithromycin 10 mg/kg (max. 500 mg) p.o. daily for 5 days, although the role of antibiotics is uncertain.
- Despite definitive evidence, macrolides (e.g. IV azithromycin) are recommended in cases with suspected CNS disease.

Viral infections

Cytomegalovirus

Cytomegalovirus (CMV) is a ubiquitous herpes virus. It persists in latent form after primary infection and reactivation can occur years later, particularly with immunosuppression. The acquisition of primary CMV infection in early pregnancy may affect the unborn infant and lead to congenital CMV infection.

Transmission

- *Horizontal*: salivary contamination or sexual transmission; blood transfusion/organ transplantation.
- *Vertical*: transplacental, intrapartum via passage through infected genital tract and postnatal via ingestion of CMV-positive breast milk.

Incubation period

Unknown; symptoms usually develop between 9 and 60 days after primary infection. Infection may manifest 3 weeks to 3 months after blood transfusion and 4 weeks to 4 months after bone marrow and other transplants.

Clinical features

The presentation varies with age and immune status of child; asymptomatic infection is common. Symptomatic presentations include CMV mononucleosis, cervical lymphadenopathy, hepatosplenomegaly in children, fever in adults. Note: clinical signs of CMV infection are similar to graft rejection in transplant patients. Both events peak 30–90 days after transplantation. Infants with congenital CMV may be asymptomatic (majority) or have clinical signs including low birth weight, microcephaly, rash (petechial), jaundice, hepatosplenomegaly (see below). Auditory brainstem evoked responses may show sensorineural hearing loss.

Diagnosis

Identification of the virus by culture or PCR of urine or saliva in the first 3 weeks of life is diagnostic of congenital disease. After this period, positive results may represent postnatally acquired infection. PCR of stored dried blood spots taken for the neonatal screening test may aid the diagnosis in infants suspected after 3 weeks of life to have congenital CMV (e.g. infants identified with sensorineural hearing loss that were asymptomatic at birth).

Distinguishing past infection from active infection can be difficult. Viral culture or PCR of urine, saliva and even blood may be misleading as CMV can be excreted intermittently for life after primary infection, especially in immunocompromised patients. Leucocyte antigenaemia assay (degree of antigenaemia) correlates with the severity of CMV disease and may assist in predicting disease and monitoring progression in immunocompromised patients. Serial quantitative PCR may also be helpful.

Complications

- Encephalitis, myocarditis, pneumonia, haemolytic anaemia, thrombocytopenia are rare manifestations.
- Primary CMV infection has been described in conjunction with Guillain–Barré syndrome and other peripheral neuropathies.
- Pneumonia, retinitis, hepatitis and colitis in immunocompromised patients.
- Congenital infection: >90% infants appear normal at birth. CNS sequelae occur in 10–20% (mainly sensorineural hearing loss); 5% of infants with congenital CMV present early with petechiae, hepatosplenomegaly, microcephaly and thrombocytopenia – this group have high rates of neurological sequelae.

Treatment

- Ganciclovir or valacyclovir for active CMV disease in the immunocompromised. CMV hyper immune globulin is also sometimes used in these patients.
- Ganciclovir therapy should be considered in any neonate with symptomatic congenital CMV to reduce the risk of hearing loss and other neurological sequelae. Specialist advice is recommended.

Enterovirus (non-polio)

Coxsackie A, B and echoviruses are important causes of childhood infections, especially in the summer months. These include a wide range of clinical presentations, including non-specific febrile illness; pharyngitis; herpangina; hand, foot and mouth disease; gastroenteritis; aseptic meningitis; encephalitis; myocarditis; pericarditis and several forms of viral exanthem (maculopapular, vesicular, petechial). Infection in agammaglobulinaemic patients can cause severe or persistent meningoencephalitis. In neonates, enteroviral infection may be difficult to distinguish from bacterial sepsis.

Hand, foot and mouth disease

- Cause: coxsackie A virus (usually A16).
- Transmission: direct contact/droplet.
- Incubation period: 3–6 days.
- Infectious period: until blisters have gone.

Clinical features

Vesicles on cheeks, gums, sides of the tongue; papulovesicular lesions of palms, fingers, toes, soles, buttocks, genitals, limbs (may look haemorrhagic); sore throat; fever and anorexia.

Diagnosis

Tests are usually unnecessary as the clinical picture is sufficient for diagnosis.

Control of case

Exclusion is not indicated and is impractical as virus is excreted in stool for weeks.

Treatment

Symptomatic

Epstein–Barr virus (infectious mononucleosis)

- Incubation period: 30–50 days.
- Infectious period: unknown, viral excretion from oropharynx for months.

Clinical features

Fever, malaise, exudative tonsillopharyngitis, generalised lymphadenopathy and hepatosplenomegaly. The acute phase lasts 2–4 weeks and convalescence may take weeks to months. It may be associated with hepatitis or CNS involvement. In immunocompromised (particularly transplant) patients, it may be associated with the development of lymphoproliferative disease.

Diagnosis

Atypical lymphocytes in the peripheral blood. The Monospot test (blood) for heterophile antibodies identifies 90% of cases in older children and adults, but has poor sensitivity in children less than 4–5 years of age. Serology is the gold standard. PCR of blood or tissue may be helpful to detect lymphoproliferative disease in immunocompromised patients (i.e. transplant patients).

Complications

- Upper airway obstruction
- Dehydration from poor oral intake (uncommon)
- Chronic fatigue syndrome (uncommon)

Treatment

Prednisolone 1–2 mg/kg (max. 50 mg) or dexamethasone 0.6 mg/kg p.o. daily may be considered in patients who are hospitalised for airway obstruction. Patients with splenomegaly should be advised to avoid contact sports to prevent splenic rupture. Amoxicillin and ampicillin cause florid rash in up to 90% of children with EBV infection.

Herpes simplex virus

Manifestations of herpes simplex virus (HSV) infection include skin and mucous membrane involvement, gingivostomatitis (mainly HSV-1), genital herpes (mainly HSV-2), eczema herpeticum (see Chapter 23, *Dermatologic conditions*), herpetic whitlow and eye involvement. Although rare, HSV encephalitis is an important treatable condition that should be considered in patients that present with fever and focal neurological signs or seizures. Pneumonia and disseminated infection may occur in immunocompromised patients. Congenital infection also occurs. Infection can be primary (e.g. gingivostomatitis) or from a reactivation of the latent virus (e.g. cold sores).

Primary herpes gingivostomatitis

- Transmission: droplet, direct contact
- Incubation period: 2–14 days
- Infectious period: indeterminate; virus can be excreted for at least 1 week, occasionally months. It is shed intermittently with or without symptoms (including cold sores) for years afterwards

Clinical features

Fever, irritability, cervical lymphadenopathy, halitosis, diffuse erythema and ulceration within the oral cavity (buccal mucosa, palate, gingiva and tongue) and mucocutaneous junction. Lesions typically take between 7 and 14 days to heal.

Diagnosis

Immunofluorescence or culture of vesicular scrapings used to be standard testing, but more recently, PCR-based testing of vesicular fluid is used to establish a rapid diagnosis.

Complications

Poor oral intake; autoinoculation resulting in herpetic whitlow, keratitis or genital herpes; eczema herpeticum; dissemination (particularly in immunocompromised).

Treatment

Symptomatic relief with topical anaesthesia (e.g. 1–2% lignocaine (lidocaine) gel, xylocaine viscous), analgesia (paracetamol), fluids and a soft diet. Aciclovir, valaciclovir or famciclovir should be considered in immunocompromised patients. Antiviral medications can also be used to prevent recurrent HSV in certain patients.

HSV in pregnancy

Primary infection during the first 20 weeks of gestation is associated with an increased risk of spontaneous abortion, stillbirth and congenital disease. Beyond 20 weeks, premature labour and growth retardation are more common. Primary infection after 34 weeks is associated with high rates of neonatal HSV disease.

Neonatal HSV

Transmission

- Intrapartum (70%–85%): perinatal acquisition from maternal genital tract; usually presents day 5–19.

- Postnatal (10%): usually presents day 5–19.
- Intrauterine (5%): transplacental; usually presents within 48 hours of birth.

Transmission is 10 times more likely to occur with primary infection than with recurrent infection. Both primary and recurrent infection may be asymptomatic in women – more than 70% of women who give birth to infants with neonatal HSV infection give no history of genital HSV in themselves or their partners. The risk of HSV infection in a baby of an asymptomatic woman with a history of recurrent genital herpes is <3%.

Clinical features
Neonatal infection presents in three ways:
- Localised skin, eye and/or mouth (SEM) disease (20%)
  - Onset 7–14 days.
  - Neurological involvement in 30% or more.
  - Death is rare.
- CNS disease (30%)
  - Onset 14–21 days in the form of encephalitis or a more disseminated disease.
  - Mortality is 15%.
  - Fifty to sixty per cent of survivors have psychomotor retardation, with or without microcephaly, spasticity, blindness, etc.
- Disseminated disease (25%)
  - Onset 5–10 days.
  - Involves any organ but primarily liver and adrenals; encephalitis occurs in 70% or more of patients. Presentation includes irritability, seizures, respiratory distress, jaundice, coagulopathy, shock and characteristic vesicular rash. About 20% of babies never have skin lesions.
  - Mortality is 50–60% and neurological sequelae in 40%, even with appropriate treatment.

Diagnosis
Viral isolation from neonatal vesicular fluid, mouth or conjunctival swabs, stool, urine, leucocytes and maternal genital tract swabs. Serology is not always helpful, as maternal IgG (which crosses the placenta) confounds interpretation in the neonate and IgM may not be produced until 2 weeks after the onset of illness. Detection of viral DNA by PCR (in blood or CSF) is helpful. Changes on EEG (PLEDs) and MRI may provide supporting evidence of HSV infection.

Complications
The overall mortality (following treatment) is 15–20% and 40–50% of infants have some neurological impairment.

Treatment
Aciclovir 20 mg/kg IV 8 hourly (see Appendix 3, *Antimicrobial guidelines*) for at least 14 days (SEM disease) or 21 days (CNS or disseminated disease). Recent evidence supports the use of aciclovir suppressive treatment for 6 months in infants with disseminated disease (with the greatest benefit in infants with CNS involvement) with improved developmental outcomes compared to placebo.

Prevention
20% of babies born to women with primary HSV will be infected, even if delivered by Caesarean section. Some experts recommend aciclovir prophylaxis in pregnant women with a history of recurrent HSV (from 35 weeks gestation) in an effort to prevent congenital infection.

HSV encephalitis
See Encephalitis, Chapter 11, *Neurologic conditions*, p. 151.

Human herpes virus 6 (roseola infantum)
Ninety-five per cent of children are infected with human herpes virus 6 (HHV-6) by the age of 2 years. Up to 30% will present with clinical features of roseola. HHV-7 has also been shown to be the cause in a small number of children. HHV-6 infection may also present as an acute febrile illness without a rash.
- Transmission: direct contact/droplet (asymptomatically shed).
- Incubation period: 9–10 days.
- Infectious period: unknown (greatest during period of the rash).

Clinical features

Fever with occipital lymphadenopathy; then rapid defervescence corresponding with appearance of a red, maculopapular rash over trunk and arms lasting 1–2 days.

Note: Many children are started on antibiotics for the fever and then misdiagnosed as having a drug reaction when the rash appears.

Diagnosis

Serology and PCR are available and may be helpful in some settings (immunocompromised patients) but usually do not alter management.

Complications

Febrile convulsions (HHV-6 is thought to be the cause of up to one-third of febrile convulsions in children <2 years of age), aseptic meningitis, encephalitis (rare), hepatitis. HHV-6 can cause severe disease in immunocompromised patients including meningoencephalitis, bone marrow failure, hepatitis and severe colitis.

Treatment

Symptomatic in immunocompetent children. In immunocompromised patients, several antiviral medications are available and specialist advice is recommended.

Influenza virus

- Cause: influenza A or B virus.
- Transmission: direct contact/droplet.
- Incubation period: 1–4 days.
- Infectious period: 3–7 days after onset of symptoms. Longer in immunocompromised patients.

Epidemiology

Continuous genetic reassortment of influenza A viruses can lead to epidemics; the degree of cross-immunity from previously circulating strains and vaccines determines whether epidemics occur. Large-scale epidemics (pandemics) occur when there is no protection from previous exposure. Although the virus may cause disease at any time, seasonal epidemics occur during winter.

Clinical features

Variable. May be asymptomatic. Severity of illness is dependent on partial immunity from previous exposure to related influenza viruses and vaccines. Commonly presents with fever and rigors; respiratory symptoms including coryza, pharyngitis, cough, pneumonia, wheeze or croup; headache, myalgia, fatigue. Vomiting and diarrhoea are less common.

Complications

Important complications include bacterial superinfection causing pneumonia (especially *S. aureus*), otitis media or sinusitis; neurological (encephalitis, meningitis, encephalopathy); myositis and cardiomyopathy. Death occurs in ~1% of hospitalised children.

Diagnosis

- Rapid diagnosis by immunofluorescence or PCR on respiratory specimens (nasal swab or NPA) may allow for early treatment.
- Viral culture is also important for epidemiology.

Control of case

Exclude from school until symptoms have resolved.

Treatment

- Neuraminidase inhibitors (zanamavir, oseltamivir) reduce the severity and length of illness by up to 36 hours if started within 48 hours, but earlier initiation is associated with the best outcome. **Routine treatment of influenza in immunocompetent patients is not recommended**.
- Neuraminidase inhibitors (oseltamivir ≥1 year of age, zanamavir ≥7 years of age) should be considered in children with laboratory-confirmed influenza, who are severely unwell, immunocompromised or who have chronic medical conditions.

Prevention

Vaccines can be used to prevent influenza in children.

- Trivalent inactivated intramuscular vaccine is ~65% protective against influenza and prevents ~30% of influenza-like illnesses, but efficacy varies from year to year. Annual vaccination with vaccine containing the most recent strains is necessary to provide continued protection. Two doses at least one month apart are recommended for children ≤9 years receiving influenza vaccine for the first time.
- Live attenuated vaccine is more effective (~79% protective) but is not yet available in Australia.

Neuraminidase inhibitors may be used to prevent influenza in children at risk of complications.

Measles virus (rubeola)

Measles is now uncommon as a result of widespread measles immunisation. However, outbreaks continue to occur in most parts of the world.

- Transmission: droplet, direct contact.
- Incubation period: 7–18 days (usually 14 days) to the appearance of a rash.
- Infectious period: 1–2 days before the onset of symptoms to 4 days after the onset of the rash. Measles is highly infectious.

Clinical features

- Prodrome: fever, conjunctivitis, coryza, cough and Koplik spots (white spots on a bright red buccal mucosa).
- Rash: appears 3–4 days later; erythematous and blotchy; starts at hairline and moves down the body, then becomes confluent; lasts 4–7 days; may desquamate in the second week.

Diagnosis

Serology (IgM is usually detectable 1–2 days after onset of rash, and almost always 4 days after), immunofluorescence and culture or PCR on nasopharyngeal aspirate.

Complications

Otitis media (25%), pneumonia (4%), encephalitis (1 in 2000), subacute sclerosing panencephalitis (SSPE) (1 in 25,000).

Treatment

Predominantly symptomatic, observing for any complications. Vitamin A should be considered for young infants with severe measles, immunocompromised patients and patients with vitamin A deficiency.

Control of case

Exclude from school for at least 5 days from the appearance of the rash.

Contacts

- Measles, mumps, rubella (MMR) vaccine should be given within 72 hours of exposure, to unimmunised children >9 months of age (another dose should be given at 12 months of age or 4 weeks after the first dose, whichever is later).
- If MMR is contraindicated, or if >72 hours since exposure, normal human immunoglobulin (NHIG) should be given IM within 7 days (see Chapter 29, *Haematologic conditions and oncology*).
- NHIG should be given to exposed pregnant women who have had only 1 dose of MMR.
- Exclude from school for 2 weeks if unimmunised.

Parvovirus B19 (erythema infectiosum, slapped cheek disease, fifth disease)

- Transmission: droplet, direct contact.
- Incubation period: 4–21 days.
- Infectious period: highly infectious until rash appears (50% of adults are immune).

Clinical features

Non-specific prodrome with a fever in 15–30%. The rash has three stages:

- Slapped cheek appearance (1–3 days).
- Maculopapular rash: on proximal extensor surfaces, flexor surfaces and trunk; fades over next few days, then central clearing, forming a reticular pattern (after 7 days).
- Reticular rash: reappears with heat, cold and friction (weeks/months).

Diagnosis

Mainly clinical. PCR on blood and serology may be helpful, but are rarely required.

Complications

Arthritis; aplastic crisis in children with chronic haemolytic anaemia; bone marrow suppression; foetal hydrops in newborns.

Treatment

Predominantly symptomatic. Blood transfusions may be required in certain patient groups (severe haemolytic anaemia, in utero hydrops).

Control of case

School exclusion is inappropriate as the patient is no longer infectious once the rash appears.

Contacts

Pregnant contacts should seek advice regarding the unlikely possibility of intrauterine infection as treatment of foetal infection may prevent sequelae (i.e. hydrops).

Rubella virus

- Transmission: droplet, direct contact.
- Incubation period: 14–21 days.
- Infectious period: 5 days before to 7 days after rash.

Clinical features

- Twenty-five to fifty per cent have no symptoms.
- Prodrome: (1–5 days) low-grade fever, malaise, headache, coryza, conjunctivitis (more common in adults), postauricular/occipital/posterior triangle lymphadenopathy precedes rash by 5–10 days.
- Rash: small, fine, discrete pink maculopapules; starts on face and spreads to chest and upper arms, abdomen and thighs, all within 24 hours.

Diagnosis

Serology. PCR on urine or throat swab may be helpful but a negative result does not exclude infection.

Complications

Congenital rubella syndrome: ~50% of infants will be affected if their mother is infected during first trimester; 10–20% have single congenital defect if infection occurs at 16–40 weeks. Clinical manifestations include deafness, neurological abnormalities, cataracts, retinopathy, tooth defects and growth retardation.

Control of case

Exclude from school for at least 5 days from the onset of the rash.

Contacts

Check serology if pregnant. Immunoglobulin given after exposure in early pregnancy may not prevent infection or viraemia, but may modify risk of abnormalities in the baby.

Varicella zoster virus (chickenpox, shingles)

- Transmission: Droplet from respiratory secretions or direct contact with vesicle fluid from skin lesions. Highly contagious.
- Incubation period: 10–21 days. Shorter incubation in immunocompromised patients. Prior administration of Zoster immune globulin (ZIG) may prolong incubation to 28 days.
- Infectious period: 1–2 days before appearance of the rash until skin lesions fully crusted.

Clinical features

Fever, irritability, anorexia and lymphadenopathy. A pruritic rash develops over the next 3–5 days, which progresses from maculopapular to vesicular, followed by crusting within 5–10 days. Lesions appear in crops with a central distribution. May affect scalp, face, trunk, mouth, conjunctivae and extremities.

Diagnosis

Clinical diagnosis is usually sufficient. PCR of vesicular fluid has largely replaced immunofluorescence and culture. Varicella serology may also be helpful to support diagnosis.

Complications

Although varicella is usually a mild infection in children, complications occur in ∼1% of cases. These include secondary bacterial infection of skin lesions (most commonly group A streptococcus or *S. aureus*); bacterial pneumonia; neurological complications (cerebellitis, transverse myelitis, Guillain–Barré syndrome) and, rarely, dissemination (pneumonitis, hepatitis, encephalitis), particularly in patients with abnormal T-cell immunity.

Herpes zoster (shingles), resulting from a reactivation of the latent virus, is more common in children who have had chickenpox in infancy or who have been exposed *in utero*. Post-herpetic neuralgia as a complication of herpes zoster is less common in children than in adults.

Treatment

- Aciclovir, famciclovir or valaciclovir in patients with impaired T-cell immunity. Antiviral treatment is **not** indicated in the immunocompetent child.
- Antibiotics for secondary bacterial skin infection (e.g. flucloxacillin).
- **Aspirin is contraindicated because of the association with Reye's syndrome.**
- Other NSAIDs (including ibuprofen) should be avoided because of possible increased risk of invasive group A streptococcal disease.
- Paracetamol can be used.

Prevention

ZIG should be administered within 96 hours of exposure but may have some efficacy up to 10 days following exposure (dose is based on weight: 600 IU for >30 kg, 400 IU for 11–30 kg and 200 IU for 0–10 kg). ZIG is indicated for the following patients in contact with varicella (or direct contact with shingles):

- Immunocompromised children (e.g. HIV, immunosuppressive therapy – including high-dose steroids; prednisolone 2 mg/kg or more per day – and patients with transplants, lymphoma, leukaemia or severe combined immune deficiency).
- Newborn infants whose mothers develop varicella from 7 or fewer days before delivery to 2 days after delivery.
- Infants under 28 days of age if mother has no history of chickenpox or is seronegative.
- Hospitalised premature infants with no maternal history of varicella.
- Hospitalised premature infants <28 weeks gestation or <1000 g, regardless of maternal history or varicella.

Varicella vaccine

Live attenuated varicella vaccine is available as a monovalent vaccine and from July 2013 will be available in Australia as a quadrivalent vaccine combined with the MMR vaccine.

Infectious diarrhoea

See also Chapter 8, *Gastrointestinal conditions*, p. 90.

Infectious diarrhoea continues to cause significant morbidity in children from developed and developing countries. Aside from rotavirus, other important pathogens include norovirus, enteric adenoviruses, astroviruses, *Salmonella* spp., *Campylobacter jejuni*, *Giardia intestinalis (lamblia)*, *Cryptosporidium parvum*, enteropathogenic (and other) *Escherichia coli*, *Shigella* spp. and *Yersinia enterocolitica* and *Clostridium* spp.

- Children <5 years of age with rotavirus-positive gastroenteritis are unlikely to have another pathogen isolated from their faeces.
- It is unusual to find a protozoal parasite in the setting of acute diarrhoea.
- Repeat stool examination and culture are not helpful except in patients with chronic diarrhoea, suspected *Salmonella* carriage or suspected parasitic infection.
- Most bacterial causes of diarrhoea are self-limiting and do not usually require antibiotic therapy. Antibiotics should be considered for the immunocompromised and neonates and in those with persistent symptoms.
- Nosocomial infection is common. Hence, adequate infection control measures established by the hospital are essential in preventing spread.

Rotavirus

- *Incubation period*: illness usually begins from 12 hours to 4 days after exposure.
- *Infectious period*: most children shed the virus in the stools for up to 10 days; however, about one-third of patients with severe primary rotavirus infection continue shedding for >21 days.

Clinical features

Prior to the introduction of routine vaccine, this was the major cause (>50%) of diarrhoea in children <5 years of age admitted with acute gastroenteritis, and a common cause of nosocomial infection. Annual peak period of infection occurs in the winter–spring period. Symptoms generally resolve within 7 days. Commonly presents with

- Vomiting (may precede diarrhoea)
- Diarrhoea
- Respiratory symptoms
- Fever in the first few days

Complications
Dehydration, electrolyte imbalance and acidosis.

Diagnosis
Enzyme immunoassay (EIA) and latex agglutination assay can confirm the diagnosis but are not necessary as results rarely influence management.

Treatment
Supportive, with particular attention to hydration.

Vaccine
Two safe and efficacious rotavirus vaccines are available. There is reasonable evidence that intussusception is not associated with these new vaccines (a concern with previous vaccines) (see Chapter 9, *Immunisation*).

Adenovirus diarrhoea

Similar clinical presentation to rotavirus, but there is no seasonality. Infection is more common under 12 months of age. Diarrhoea and vomiting may persist for longer and high fever is less common. May be associated with prolonged diarrhoea and other manifestations in immunocompromised children.

Salmonella (non-typhi) gastroenteritis

- Transmission: faecal–oral route from person to person or animal to person; ingestion of contaminated or improperly cooked foods.
- Incubation period: 6–72 hours.

Clinical features

Non-typhoidal salmonella (NTS) may be associated with a broad spectrum of clinical features including asymptomatic carriage, gastroenteritis (cramping abdominal pain and loose stools), bacteraemia and focal infections (e.g. bone and joint). Age-specific attack rates are highest in children <5 years of age (peak at <1 year of age) and the elderly. Invasive infections and mortality are more common in infants, the elderly and those with underlying diseases (e.g. sickle cell, HIV, immunocompromise)

Diagnosis

NTS may be cultured from stool, blood or other clinical specimens. Serology and PCR are also available.

Treatment

Antibiotic treatment is not usually indicated for uncomplicated gastroenteritis (symptoms usually resolve within 7 days) as it may prolong excretion. Antibiotic treatment is indicated for bacteraemia, systemic involvement or infection in infants <3 months of age, patients with underlying disease (e.g. immunocompromised) and the elderly. The choice and duration of treatment depends on the clinical manifestation and antibiotic susceptibility.

Campylobacter jejuni

Transmission

Ingestion of contaminated food or water or undercooked poultry.

Clinical features
More common in children >5 years of age. Causes diarrhoea with visible or occult blood, abdominal pain, malaise and fever.

Diagnosis
Isolation of *Campylobacter* spp. from culture of stool is diagnostic. Serology is also available but not routinely recommended.

Treatment
Antibiotic treatment is not usually necessary (symptoms improve in 60–70% within 7 days), except in special circumstances where the elimination of the carrier state is important, such as infection in food handlers.

Giardia intestinalis (lamblia)
Transmission
The major reservoir and means of spread is contaminated water and to a lesser extent, food. Person-to-person spread may occur and the infective dose is low in humans. Giardia is the most common parasite identified in stool specimens from children, it is more common in children (and staff) in childcare centres and returned travellers.

Clinical features
There is a broad spectrum of clinical manifestations, but the most common are diarrhoea (usually persistent and non-bloody), abdominal distension, flatulence, abdominal cramps and weight loss/failure to thrive.

Diagnosis
Confirmed by microscopy of fresh or preserved stool specimens. These do not usually contain blood, mucus or leucocytes. Repeat specimens (up to three) may be necessary over a week to increase the chance of detection. Stool antigen tests and PCR are also available but are not routinely recommended.

Treatment
Metronidazole 30 mg/kg (max. 2 g) PO daily for 3 days **or** tinidazole 50 mg/kg (max. 2 g) p.o. as a single dose.

Dientamoeba fragilis
Transmission
This parasite is thought to be transmitted with the eggs of *Enterobius vermicularis* (pinworm).

Clinical features
Symptoms include acute or chronic diarrhoea and abdominal pain, although many infected children are asymptomatic. May be associated with eosinophilia (up to 50% of children).

Diagnosis
Confirmed by microscopy of a permanently stained smear of a fresh stool sample. Up to three stool specimens collected on alternate days may be necessary to increase the chance of detection.

Treatment
May be treated with metronidazole (dose as above) although treatment is unnecessary in asymptomatic patients where the organism is found incidentally.

Escherichia coli
There are at least five categories of diarrhoea-producing *E. coli*:
- Enterohaemorrhagic *E. coli* (EHEC): haemolytic uraemic syndrome (HUS), haemorrhagic colitis.
- Enteropathogenic *E. coli* (EPEC): watery diarrhoea in children <2 years of age in developing countries.
- Enterotoxigenic *E. coli* (ETEC): the major cause of traveller's diarrhoea (usually self-limiting).
- Enteroinvasive *E. coli* (EIEC): usually watery diarrhoea, but may cause dysentery.
- Enteroaggregative *E. coli* (EAEC): chronic diarrhoea in infants and young children.

Antibiotic treatment is not usually indicated for diarrhoea caused by *E. coli* and may be associated with increased rates of HUS in EHEC infection.

Clostridium difficile

Transmission
Acquired from the environment or by faecal–oral transmission from a colonised host. Up to 50% of healthy neonates and infants <2 years of age are colonised (usually asymptomatic), compared to 5% of children >2 years of age.

Clinical features
Rare cause of diarrhoea in infants <12 months of age, but can cause diarrhoea in older children. Pseudomembranous colitis usually occurs only in patients on antibiotics (particularly penicillins, clindamycin and cephalosporins).

Diagnosis
Stool culture is the most sensitive test. Stool cytotoxin, EIA and PCR tests are also available.

Treatment
- Cessation of antibiotics, **and**
- Oral metronidazole 7.5 mg/kg (max. 400 mg) p.o. 8 hourly for 10 days, **and**
- Consider probiotics – *Saccharomyces* spp. (baker's or brewer's yeast) or *Lactobacillus* spp.

Failure of treatment or relapse (in ~25%) may be due to reinfection, non-compliance, continued antibiotic use, or, rarely, a metronidazole-resistant organism. Options in this context include repeat metronidazole, oral vancomycin (not IV) or probiotics.

E. vermicularis (threadworm, pinworm)
Pinworm is the most common worm infection in Australia. The highest rate of infection occurs in school-age children.

Transmission
Eggs survive for up to 2 weeks on clothing, bedding or other objects and can remain under the fingernails. Reinfection by autoinfection is common. Infection often occurs in more than one family member.

Incubation period
At least 1–2 months from the ingestion of eggs until the adult female migrates to the perianal region to deposit eggs.

Infectious period
Eggs are infective within a few hours of being deposited on the perianal skin.

Clinical features
Causes pruritus ani and vulvae and occasionally can cause perineal pain in females.

Diagnosis
Visualisation of worms in the perianal region (at night) or microscopy of eggs collected on sticky tape briefly applied to perianal skin in the morning.

Treatment
Mebendazole 50 mg (<10 kg), 100 mg (>10 kg) p.o. (not in pregnancy or in those <6 months of age) or pyrantel 10 mg/kg (max. 750 mg) PO as a single dose, followed by a second dose 2 weeks later. All family members should be treated. Wash bedding in hot water, avoid sharing towels, and cut fingernails.

Hepatitis viruses
See also Chapter 8, *Gastrointestinal conditions*, p. 101.

Hepatitis A
Hepatitis A virus (HAV) is the most common viral hepatitis; it is particularly prevalent in developing countries.
- Transmission: faecal–oral route.
- Incubation period: mean of 4 weeks (2–7 weeks).
- Infectious period: viral shedding lasts 1–3 weeks; the highest viral load in stool occurs 1–2 weeks before the onset of illness, corresponding to the highest risk of transmission; lowest risk after onset of jaundice.

Clinical features

Either asymptomatic or associated with an acute self-limited illness in children: mild, non-specific symptoms without jaundice in infants and preschoolers; fever, malaise, jaundice, anorexia and nausea in older children and adults. The presence of dark urine may precede the onset of jaundice.

Complications

Relapse (unusual), fulminant hepatitis (rare). Hepatitis A does not cause chronic liver disease.

Diagnosis

Serology for HAV-specific IgM and IgG. Abnormal liver function tests usually normalise within 4 weeks.

Treatment

Supportive

Control of case

Children should be excluded from childcare or school for 7 days from the onset of illness, although the virus is excreted for many weeks.

Prevention

Inactivated HAV vaccine is recommended for travellers to endemic areas and patients with chronic liver disease (e.g. hepatitis B or C infection) or transfusion-dependent illness. Several monovalent HAV vaccines are available as well as HAV-containing combination vaccines.

Hepatitis B

Hepatitis B virus (HBV) infection is endemic in Africa and south Asia. The prevalence of HBV and carriage rates vary in different parts of the world. The carriage rate is about 0.2% in Australians of European origin, and >10% in some indigenous and migrant populations. Rates are highest in those born in Asian, sub-Saharan Africa or Mediterranean countries. Immunisation against hepatitis B is part of the Australian Immunisation Schedule, and is a priority in non-immune children and adolescents (and adults) in high-prevalence subgroups and household contacts of people with hepatitis B.

- Transmission: blood or body fluids that are hepatitis B surface antigen (HBsAg) positive. Vertical transmission can occur in infants born to HBsAg-positive mothers; there is a high risk of horizontal transmission in the first years of life. Transmission may also occur through needle-stick injury in a health care setting.

Incubation period: 7 weeks–6 months

- Infectious period: from several weeks before the onset until documented clearance of virus.
- Incubation period: 7 weeks–6 months.
- Infectious period: from several weeks before the onset until documented clearance of virus.

Clinical features

Symptomatic acute hepatitis (jaundice, anorexia, malaise and nausea) in adults; usually asymptomatic in young children, particularly in those with vertically acquired infection.

Diagnosis

Test for

- HBsAg (active disease or (if detectable for >6 months) chronic carrier).
- HBsAb (protective immunity due either to past infection or immunisation). HBsAb >10 IU/L indicates adequate immunity.
- HBcAb (past or present HBV infection).
- Children who are HBsAg positive need further tests (LFTs, HBcAb, HBeAg, HBeAb, and HBV PCR (increased infectivity and risk of sequelae).and a screen for hepatitis A, delta and C, and HIV (immunise against hepatitis A if needed). Hepatitis B is a notifiable disease.
- STI screening may be needed depending on age and history.

Treatment

There is no specific therapy for HBV; α-interferon and nucleoside analogues may resolve chronic infection but are less effective for infection acquired during childhood. Hepatitis A vaccination is recommended. All acute cases of hepatitis with clinical illness need immediate discussion with a specialist and children with hepatitis B infection and abnormal liver function tests require specialist review. All patients with chronic hepatitis B should have

- Explanation/education/counselling about:
  - Blood spills and infection risk
  - Not sharing toothbrushes (or razors where relevant)
  - The need to notify other treating doctors when starting medications, and to commence hepatotoxic drugs cautiously – particularly anti-TB therapy
  - Avoiding excess alcohol consumption
  - Using barrier contraception and sexual health in adolescents
  - The need to screen household contacts for hepatitis B and vaccinate those who are non-immune (and check post-immunisation serology to confirm immunity)

  Other management depends on serology, LFTs and clinical status. The primary goal of therapeutic management in the individual is to eliminate or suppress hepatitis B.

Complications

Fulminant hepatitis is rare. Chronic HBV infection results in chronic hepatitis. Cirrhosis occurs in up to one-third of affected individuals and these individuals have an increased risk of hepatocellular carcinoma. Chronic infection is most likely to occur after exposure in early life: 70–90% of infants infected at birth develop chronic HBV (particularly if the mother is HBeAg positive), in contrast to only 5% of adults who acquire hepatitis B infection. Chronic HBV infection is associated with 25% mortality from hepatocellular carcinoma or liver disease; lifelong follow-up is indicated. People who clear the infection generally have no long-term effects.

Prevention

- In Australia, recombinant HBV vaccine is currently recommended for all infants from birth, as well as those at high risk of hepatitis B. Infants born to HBsAg-positive mothers should be given HBV-specific immunoglobulin in addition to HBV vaccination. They should be tested at 12–18 months with HBsAg and HBsAb.
- See needle-stick injuries (p. 294) for management of exposure to infected blood or body fluid.

Hepatitis C

Hepatitis C virus (HCV) causes acute and chronic hepatitis. The carriage rate is ∼0.3% in apparently healthy new blood donors in Australia, but this probably underestimates the prevalence in the population, which may be around 1%.

Transmission

Parenteral exposure to HCV-infected blood and blood products; vertical transmission occurs in ∼6% of HCV-positive mothers (higher if the mother is co-infected with HIV). Avoid use of foetal scalp electrodes; breast-feeding is not contraindicated but should be avoided if the mother has bleeding or cracked nipples; sexual transmission is rare.

- Incubation period: 6–7 weeks (range 2 weeks to 6 months).
- Clinical features: mild, insidious hepatitis; usually asymptomatic in children.
- Diagnosis: current or past infection is detected by serology (anti-HCV antibodies); current infection is confirmed by PCR for HCV RNA.

Treatment

- Patients must be screened for chronic hepatitis, cirrhosis and hepatocellular carcinoma.
- Optimal treatment regimens are under investigation and include interferon alpha and ribavarin. The probability of a response to treatment is related to the viral genotype.
- Hepatitis A and B vaccination is recommended and provide advice on avoiding transmission (see hepatitis B above).

Complications

Persistent infection in >85% (most children with chronic infection are asymptomatic); 65–70% develop chronic hepatitis, 20% develop cirrhosis. Uncommonly, hepatocellular carcinoma may develop in the absence of chronic hepatitis.

Hepatitis E

Hepatitis E virus (HEV) is an uncommon cause of hepatitis, which occurs predominantly in tropical countries, especially in parts of India. Cases have been reported in travellers returning from these regions. HEV is transmitted by the faecal oral route and the clinical features are similar to HAV infection.

Bacterial meningitis

Bacterial meningitis is a medical emergency.

Clinical features

- Infants: often non-specific, for example fever, lethargy, irritability, high-pitched crying or vomiting.
- Older children: headache, vomiting, drowsiness, photophobia and neck stiffness may be present. Kernig sign (inability to extend the knee when the leg is flexed at the hip) and Brudzinski sign (bending the head forward produces flexion of the legs) may be positive.

Diagnosis

Diagnosis is confirmed by examination of the CSF. Lumbar puncture (LP) may be contraindicated in certain situations (see Chapter 4, *Procedures*). If LP is deferred or reveals no organism, identification of the pathogen may still be possible through

- Blood cultures – often positive where clinical signs of meningitis are present.
- PCR on blood or CSF for *N. meningitidis*, *S. pneumoniae* and consider TB.
- Skin scraping or aspirate of purpuric lesions for Gram stain, PCR or (less likely) culture.
- Throat swab.

Interpretation of CSF findings

CSF findings should always be interpreted in the light of the clinical setting (see Table 18.3).

Cell count

- **Perform microscopy without delay**. Cell lysis begins shortly after collection: neutrophils may decrease by up to one-third after 1 hour and by half after 3 hours (lymphocytes may decrease by ~10% after 2 hours).
- Macroscopic appearance of CSF may be misleading: $200–500 \times 10^6$/L cells are required before CSF appears cloudy to the naked eye.
- In early bacterial meningitis there may be no increase in the CSF cell count.

Table 18.3 Classical cerebrospinal fluid (CSF) findings

	Neutrophils ($\times 10^6$/L)	Lymphocytes ($\times 10^6$/L)	Protein (g/L)	Glucose (CSF:blood ratio)
Normal (>1 month of age)	0	≤5	<0.4	≥0.6 (or ≥2.5 mmol/L)
Normal term neonate	Higher than for older infant/child	<20–30	Higher than for older infant/child usually <1	Lower than for older infant/child
Bacterial meningitis	100–10,000 (but counts may be normal)	Usually <100	>1.0 (but protein may be normal)	<0.4 (but glucose may be normal)
Viral meningitis	Usually <100	10–1000 (but counts may be normal)	0.4–1 (but protein may be normal)	Usually normal
TB meningitis	Usually <100	50–1000 (but counts may be normal)	1–5 (but protein may be normal)	<0.3 (but glucose may be normal)
Encephalitis	Usually <100		0.4–1 (but protein may be normal)	Usually normal
Brain abscess	Usually 5–100		>1 (but protein may be normal)	Usually normal

- CSF contaminated by blood can be difficult to interpret. There is no reliable rule to correct for red blood cells (RBCs) in CSF, although a ratio of one white blood cell to 500–700 RBCs is sometimes used. Similarly, 0.01 g/L protein for every 1000 RBCs may be allowable. It is safer to be cautious and interpret the white cell count of CSF as if it has *not* been contaminated with blood.
- Even in bacterial meningitis, the CSF cell count may remain normal in up to 4% of young infants and up to 17% of neonates.
- Presence of neutrophils in the CSF should always raise concern (except in neonates, see Table 18.3).
- In early viral (typically enteroviral) meningitis, the CSF findings can mimic bacterial meningitis with a neutrophil predominance. This usually shifts to a lymphocytic picture after 6–8 hours.
- In bacterial meningitis there can be a shift to a lymphocyte predominance after 48 hours of therapy.
- *Listeria* infection is associated with a lower neutrophil rise than other causes of bacterial meningitis.
- Gram stain may be negative in up to 60% of cases of bacterial meningitis even without prior antibiotics.
- Antibiotics usually prevent the culture of bacteria from the CSF, but they do not significantly alter the CSF cell count or biochemistry in samples taken early. In 'partially treated meningitis' the CSF should be interpreted like any other CSF.
- Seizures do *not* cause an increased CSF cell count.
- In neonates, interpretation of CSF may be difficult. Normal values for CSF cell counts and biochemistry differ from those of older infants (typically they have higher cell count and protein and lower glucose, particularly in premature neonates) (see Table 18.3).

Biochemistry
- CSF protein is normal in about 40% of school-age children with bacterial meningitis.
- CSF glucose is normal in about 50% of school-age children with bacterial meningitis.
- CSF glucose may be decreased in mumps meningitis and lymphocytic choriomeningitis, as well as in bacterial and TB meningitis.

Adjunctive steroid treatment of meningitis
- Adjunctive steroid therapy should be given at the time of LP if there is strong clinical suspicion of bacterial meningitis in children >4 weeks old, as this can reduce the risk of hearing loss.
- Antibiotics should *not* be delayed by any more than 30 minutes to administer steroids.
  - Initial dose: dexamethasone 0.15 mg/kg IV ideally given 15 minutes before, but up to 1 hour after, the first dose of antibiotics.
  - Ongoing dose: dexamethasone 0.15 mg/kg IV 6 hourly should be continued for 4 days (unless bacterial meningitis has been excluded).

Antibiotic treatment of meningitis
Antibiotics must be given immediately after the collection of appropriate cultures, but should not be delayed if an LP is deferred. Antibiotics should only be rationalised when *final* CSF or blood culture results are available.

Age >2 months
The incidence of bacterial meningitis has fallen dramatically since the introduction of conjugated *Haemophilus influenzae* type b (Hib) vaccine. The major pathogens are now *S. pneumoniae* and *N. meningitidis*.

Penicillin (and cephalosporin) resistant pneumococci (PRP) are an increasing problem worldwide. Local patterns of resistance determine treatment.
- Initial therapy
  - cefotaxime 50 mg/kg (max. 2 g) IV 6 hourly or 50 mg/kg (max.1 g) IV 12 hourly.
  - In areas with a significantly high incidence of PRP, or when PRP are suspected, vancomycin 15 mg/kg (max. 500 mg) IV 6 hourly should be added to a third generation cephalosporin as empiric therapy (particularly if CSF Gram stain shows Gram positive cocci).
- Continued therapy: give IV antibiotics for a total of
  - 7 days for *N. meningitidis*.
  - 10 days for *S. pneumoniae*.
  - 7–10 days for Hib.
- For sensitive *S. pneumoniae* or *N. meningitidis*: benzylpenicillin 60 mg/kg (max. 2 g) IV 4 hourly, or amoxicillin 50 mg/kg (max. 2 g) IV 4 hourly, or continue with cefotaxime.

- If there is prolonged or secondary fever, or where sensitivity testing indicates the pneumococcal isolate has reduced susceptibility to third-generation cephalosporins, LP should be repeated to detect treatment failure, and CT brain should be considered, looking for abscess or empyema.

Age <2 months

The most common organisms are neonatal pathogens (e.g. group B streptococcus (GBS), *E. coli* and other enteric Gram negatives, and *Listeria monocytogenes*), or the same pathogens commonly detected in older children (e.g. *S. pneumoniae, N. meningitidis*, Hib).

- Initial therapy: IV benzylpenicillin and cefotaxime (see Appendix 3, *Antimicrobial guidelines*).
- Continued therapy: treatment is adjusted according to culture and sensitivity results. Gentamicin is used for its synergistic action with penicillin for the treatment of GBS and *Listeria* meningitis. Therapy should be continued for
  - 2–3 weeks for GBS and *Listeria* meningitis
  - At least 3 weeks for Gram negative meningitis.

Meningitis associated with shunts, neurosurgery, head trauma and CSF leak

In addition to common pathogens causing meningitis, meningitis associated with neurosurgery, trauma or CSF leak can also be caused by *S. aureus*, coagulase negative staphylococci and (especially with a ventriculoperitoneal shunt *in situ*) Gram negative bacilli including *Pseudomonas aeruginosa* or anaerobes.

- Initial therapy: vancomycin 15 mg/kg (max. 500 mg) IV 6 hourly **plus**:
  - (with ventriculoperitoneal shunt) ceftazidime 50 mg/kg (max. 2 g) IV 8 hourly
  - (without ventriculoperitoneal shunt) cefotaxime 50 mg/kg (max. 2 g) IV 6 hourly

Antibiotic prophylaxis for contacts of meningitis cases

See Table 18.2.

General measures

Requirement for intensive care

Admission to ICU should be discussed with a specialist in the following circumstances:

- Age <2 years
- Coma
- Cardiovascular compromise
- Intractable seizures
- Hyponatraemia

Fluid management

Careful fluid management is important in the treatment of meningitis as many children develop the syndrome of 'inappropriately' increased antidiuretic hormone secretion. The degree of fluid restriction varies with each patient according to their clinical state. Hypovolaemia should be corrected with 10 mL/kg of normal saline and repeated as required. A patient who is not in shock who has a normal serum sodium, should initially be given 50% maintenance fluid requirements. If the serum sodium is <135 mmol/L give 25–50% of maintenance requirements. Serum sodium should be measured every 6–12 hours for the first 48 hours and the total fluid intake adjusted accordingly.

Observations

Neurological observations and blood pressure should be recorded every 15 minutes for the first 2 hours and then at intervals determined by the child's conscious state. Head circumference should be monitored daily in infants. Weight is measured daily or more frequently if required.

Seizures

Hypoglycaemia, electrolyte imbalance (especially hyponatraemia) and raised intracranial pressure should be excluded before attributing seizures to the underlying infection or febrile convulsion. Control of seizures is vital and specialist consultation is advised.

Analgesia

Ensure adequate analgesia; children in the recovery phase may have significant headache.

Fever persisting for >7 days

May be due to nosocomial infection, subdural effusion or other foci of suppuration. Uncommon causes include inadequately treated meningitis, a parameningeal focus or drug related fever.

Outcome/follow-up

All patients require a hearing assessment 6–8 weeks after discharge, or sooner if hearing loss is suspected. More than one-fourth of the survivors have mild disabilities that adversely affect school performance and behaviour. Consequently, all children surviving bacterial meningitis should be regularly reviewed during their early school years. Less common sequelae include epilepsy, visual impairment and cerebral palsy.

Prevention

Many cases of meningitis are now preventable. All parents should be encouraged to have their children fully immunised.

Other CNS infections
Viral meningitis

Common pathogens: enterovirus (coxsackie and echoviruses) and HHV-6 (see p. 276).

Clinical presentation: can mimic bacterial meningitis.

Diagnosis: enterovirus may be isolated from throat swabs and stool or PCR in CSF.

Natural History: most cases are self-limiting.

Treatment: support except in immunocompromised patients where IV immunoglobulin and antiviral may be used (specialist advice is recommended).

Tuberculous meningitis

Tuberculous meningitis is uncommon in Australia, although it should be considered in children from countries where TB is more common. TB meningitis often presents in an insidious manner and can be difficult to recognise without a high index of suspicion. Large volumes of CSF are required (at least 10 mL) for diagnosis by microscopy and culture of mycobacteria, or mycobacterial PCR (which is not necessarily more sensitive). Treatment with combination antituberculous medications plus steroids should be started early and specialist advice is recommended.

Encephalitis

Most common pathogens: HSV-1 or 2, EBV, VZV, enterovirus, adenovirus, influenza virus or *M. pneumoniae*.

Clinical presentation: usually presents with one or more of fever, headache, vomiting, change of behaviour, drowsiness, convulsions (particularly focal), focal neurological deficits and signs of raised intracranial pressure. Focal seizures and neurological signs are more typical of herpes encephalitis but clinical presentation, especially early in the disease, is not specific to a particular pathogen.

Diagnosis: CSF findings are non-specific (see Table 18.3). CT or MRI of the brain and EEG may be more helpful.

Treatment: any child with encephalitis of an uncertain cause should be started on IV aciclovir (see Appendix 3, *Antimicrobial guidelines*). If the patient does not regain consciousness over a short period of time, IV aciclovir should be continued until

- An alternative diagnosis is reached; **or**
- Herpes encephalitis is excluded by
  - Absence of typical clinical features.
  - Normal serial MRI scans.
  - Normal serial EEG.
  - Negative PCR for HSV on CSF obtained >72 hours into the illness (this may necessitate a repeat LP).

Macrolides (e.g. azithromycin) are sometimes used in encephalitis due to *M. pneumoniae* but their benefit is uncertain.

Brain abscess

Brain abscess classically presents with fever, headache and focal neurological deficit. Although rare, early recognition is important because most cases are readily treated and delayed diagnosis can lead to complications. Diagnosis is by brain CT or MRI. Neurosurgical intervention for diagnosis (aspiration for microscopy and culture) and management is usually necessary. Empiric treatment to cover the likely aetiological pathogens is flucloxacillin 50 mg/kg (max. 2 g) IV 4 hourly, cefotaxime 50 mg/kg (max. 2 g) IV 6 hourly **and** metronidazole 15 mg/kg (max. 1 g) IV stat, then 7.5 mg/kg (max. 500 mg) IV 8 hourly (see Antimicrobial guidelines). Treatment is usually continued for up to 6 weeks. Specialist advice is recommended.

Kawasaki disease

Kawasaki disease (KD) is a systemic vasculitis that predominantly affects children under 5 years of age. Although the specific causal agent remains unknown, it is believed that KD is initiated by an infectious agent, although it is not transmitted from person to person. Early recognition and treatment are essential to reduce the risk of life-threatening complications.

Diagnosis

Diagnosis is often delayed because the features are similar to many viral exanthems. The features of KD can occur sequentially and may not all be present at the same time. The diagnostic criteria for KD are

- Fever for 5 days or more; **plus**
- Four of the following five features:
  ○ Polymorphous rash.
  ○ Bilateral (non-purulent) conjunctivitis.
  ○ Mucous membrane changes; for example reddened or dry cracked lips, strawberry tongue, or a diffuse redness of oral or pharyngeal mucosa.
  ○ Peripheral changes; for example erythema of the palms or soles, oedema of the hands or feet and desquamation *in convalescence*, particularly involving skin of hands, feet or perineal region.
  ○ Cervical lymphadenopathy (>15 mm in diameter, usually unilateral, single, non-purulent and painful).
- Exclusion of diseases with a similar presentation: staphylococcal infection (e.g. scalded skin syndrome and toxic shock syndrome), streptococcal infection (e.g. scarlet fever and toxic shock-like syndrome, but not just isolation from throat), measles, adenovirus and other viral exanthems, leptospirosis, rickettsial disease, Stevens–Johnson syndrome, drug reaction and juvenile chronic arthritis.

Although irritability is not considered one of the diagnostic criteria, children with KD are frequently inconsolable and their fever is resistant to antipyretics.

Clinical vigilance is needed to recognise patients with 'incomplete' or 'atypical' KD. These patients do not fulfil the formal diagnostic criteria, but are still at risk of developing coronary artery complications (see below). Other relatively common features of KD include arthritis, diarrhoea and vomiting, coryza and cough, and hydropic gallbladder.

Investigations

Laboratory features may include neutrophilia, raised erythrocyte sedimentation rate and C-reactive protein, mild normochromic, normocytic anaemia, raised transaminases, hypoalbuminaemia and marked thrombocytosis in the second week of the illness.

Complications

Up to 30% of untreated children develop coronary artery dilation or aneurysm formation. This can occur up to 6–8 weeks after the onset of the illness. Echocardiography should therefore be done at least twice: at presentation and if negative, again at 6–8 weeks to exclude coronary artery involvement. Coronary artery aneurysms can be associated with early ischaemic heart disease.

Management

Management includes early (preferably within the first 10 days of the illness) administration of IVIG (single dose of 2 g/kg IV over 10 hours) and aspirin (3–5 mg/kg p.o. once a day (antiplatelet dose) for at least 6–8 weeks; maximum dose 150 mg). There is no evidence that using high (anti-inflammatory) dose aspirin decreases the risk of aneurysm development over and above that prevented by IVIG. However, some guidelines suggest using high dose aspirin (10 mg/kg p.o. 8 hourly) until defervescence. Paracetamol can be used for symptomatic relief. Recent trials have evaluated the use of steroids in addition to IVIG early in the course of the illness. Although results were encouraging, further trials are needed before any change to current recommendations can be made.

A repeat dose of IVIG (2 g/kg) should be given to patients who fail to defervesce within 24 hours after finishing the first dose. Refractory cases with continuing fever and other signs of inflammation after IVIG need specialist advice for further treatment that may include high-dose steroids (e.g. methylprednisolone 30 mg/kg IV).

Treatment with IVIG is highly effective in preventing coronary artery complications. Treatment should still be undertaken in patients presenting after 10 days of illness if they have evidence of ongoing inflammation (fever, raised acute phase markers).

Cervical lymphadenitis

This is usually caused by an infection or inflammation of the lymph nodes. Malignancy is much less common.

Infectious causes

Acute bilateral lymphadenitis

- Viral upper respiratory tract infections.
- Systemic viral infections (e.g. EBV and CMV: may have generalised lymphadenopathy and hepatosplenomegaly).
- Kawasaki disease: may present initially as cervical lymphadenitis alone (see p. 414 above).

Acute unilateral lymphadenitis

- Group A streptococcus or *S. aureus*: 40–80% of acute unilateral lymphadenitis; occurs at 1–4 years of age; fever, tenderness, overlying erythema; may be associated with cellulitis.
- Anaerobic bacteria: older children with dental caries or periodontal disease.
- GBS may have overlying cellulitis (neonates).

Subacute/chronic unilateral lymphadenitis

- *Bartonella henselae* (cat-scratch disease): occurs about 2 weeks after a scratch or lick from a kitten or dog, usually involves axillary nodes, tender nodes; there may be a papule at infection site.
- *Mycobacterium avium complex* (MAC – formerly known as MAIS): patient usually 1–4 years of age, afebrile, systemically well and not immunocompromised; node usually unilateral, slightly fluctuant, non-tender, sometimes tethered to underlying structures and with violaceous hue to overlying skin.
- *Toxoplasma gondii*: systemic features (fatigue, myalgia), there may be generalised lymphadenopathy.
- *M. tuberculosis*: usually a contact history or relevant history of migration; affects older children; systemic symptoms (e.g. fever, malaise, weight loss), non-tender nodes.
- HIV.

Management

Acute bilateral lymphadenitis without other signs (e.g. pallor, bruising or hepatosplenomegaly) is usually viral and does not need specific treatment or investigation. Acute unilateral lymphadenitis with a fluctuant node may require incision and drainage (contra-indicated in suspected TB as may result in sinus formation). Otherwise, acute unilateral lymphadenitis is treated with oral flucloxacillin 25 mg/kg (max. 500 mg) p.o. 6 hourly for 10 days (see Appendix 3, *Antimicrobial guidelines*), with review in 48 hours. If the child is unwell with large tender nodes, admission to hospital for IV antibiotics may be required.

Cellulitis
Clinical features

- An infection of cutaneous and subcutaneous tissue characterised by erythema, warmth, oedema and tenderness.
- Predisposing factors include a break in the skin (e.g. insect bite, trauma) or a pre-existing skin lesion.
- May be associated with regional lymphadenopathy, fever, chills and malaise.
- It may be associated with deeper involvement including necrotising fasciitis (usually extremely painful), osteomyelitis, septic arthritis, or features of toxin-mediated illness (diffuse erythema, conjunctival injection and systemic features).
- Usually caused by *S. pyogenes* or *S. aureus*.
- Hib is uncommon but should be considered in unimmunised children aged <5 years. In this setting, cellulitis is often accompanied by bacteraemia or meningitis, or both.

Diagnosis

Cultures of blood, skin aspirate or skin biopsy are positive in about 25% of cases.

Management
- Flucloxacillin 25 mg/kg (max. 500 mg) p.o. 6 hourly.
- Parenteral therapy is needed if there is fever, rapid progression, lymphangitis or lymphadenitis. Non-immunised children <5 years with facial cellulitis should be treated with cefotaxime 50 mg/kg (max. 2 g) IV 6 hourly or ceftriaxone 50 mg/kg (max. 1 g) IV 12 hourly, **and** flucloxacillin 50 mg/kg (max. 2 g) IV 6 hourly. Seek specialist advice if toxin-mediated disease is suspected.

Toxin-mediated disease
Gram-positive bacteria (group A β-haemolytic streptococci and *S. aureus*) can cause disease as a result of production of protein (superantigen) toxins.

Clinical features
Fever, erythematous rash, diarrhoea, conjunctivitis, reddened mucous membranes, strawberry tongue and prolonged capillary refill time. A range of clinical presentations may be seen. At the most severe end of the spectrum, capillary leak leads to hypotension, shock and multi-organ failure (toxic shock syndrome).

Diagnosis
Early diagnosis depends on recognition of clinical features. A blood culture may be positive in ~30% of children with group A β-haemolytic streptococcus but is positive in <5% of children with *S. aureus* toxic shock.

Management
- Remove any possible focus of infection (including retained tampon if present).
- Appropriate fluid management and intensive care as needed.
- Antibiotics should include an anti-staphylococcal agent (e.g. flucloxacillin 50 mg/kg (max. 2 g) IV 4 hourly, see Antimicrobial guidelines). Treatment should also include clindamycin (to inhibit bacterial toxin and host cytokine production) and IV immunoglobulin (2 g/kg) (as an immunomodulatory agent).

Mycobacterium tuberculosis
Epidemiology
Up to one-third of the world's population is infected with *M. tuberculosis*. The majority will remain well and not go on to develop tuberculosis (TB) disease.

Transmission
Human-to-human transmission through infected droplets. Children are less infectious compared to adults as generally they have paucibacillary disease and do not develop cavitary TB. A new presentation of TB disease in a child should lead to a search for the index (adult) case.

Infectiousness
Related to burden of disease. Smear-positive individuals are highly infectious. Only cases with pulmonary TB can transmit the organism to others.

Risk factors for progression to TB disease
These include
- Age <3 years;
- Immunosuppression (e.g. HIV infection or immune-modulating medications);
- Malnutrition;
- Low body weight; and
- Migration within 5 years from a high TB prevalence area (recently infected).

Clinical features
Infection with *M. tuberculosis* is associated with a wide variety of clinical presentations from asymptomatic latent TB infection (LTBI) to invasive TB disease.
- Pulmonary TB disease: chronic cough, weight loss and night sweats or non-specific signs and symptoms including fatigue.
- Extra-pulmonary TB disease: enlarged cervical or axillary lymph nodes that are characteristically painless, although symptoms will reflect the site of infection.

- Infants and children with TB meningitis may present with lethargy, decreased feeds, headache, photophobia, neck stiffness, focal seizures or coma.

Diagnosis

The diagnosis of LTBI relies on detection of an immune response to *M. tuberculosis* using either the tuberculin skin test (TST) or an interferon gamma release assay (IGRA) blood test. Asymptomatic children with normal examination and chest radiograph who have either a positive TST and/or IGRA have LTBI. Although more specific than the TST, an IGRA is not recommended as the sole test for identifying children with LTBI as false negative results occur in this age group. For children with symptoms suggestive of TB disease, appropriate clinical specimens (sputum/gastric aspirates/lymph node/CSF) should be sent for culture (gold standard) but it can take up to 6 weeks for the organism to grow in the laboratory. Culture of *M. tuberculosis* allows for drug susceptibility testing to guide treatment and identify MDR TB. New molecular assays (e.g. PCR, *GeneXpert*) can detect *M. tuberculosis* DNA within 2 hours in appropriate clinical specimens.

Treatment

- LTBI: Preventive therapy is either isoniazid for 6 months or a combination of isoniazid and rifampicin for 3 months.
- TB disease: at least 6 months of treatment with several TB medications. Specialist advice should be sought.

Screening

Refugee and asylum seeker children and adolescents (as well as adults) should have testing for LTBI or TB disease using a TST as part of post-arrival refugee health screening. Ideally, TB screening should also be completed in any child migrating from a country with a high prevalence of TB.

Prevention

Bacillus Calmette–Guérin (BCG) vaccine is highly effective in preventing the severe forms of TB (e.g. disseminated or military TB, and TB meningitis) that affect infants and young children. BCG immunisation is recommended for infants and children (particularly those aged <5 years) travelling to high TB incidence countries and also for Aboriginal and Torres Strait Islander neonates living in certain regions.

HIV infection and AIDS

Cause

Acquired immunodeficiency syndrome (AIDS) is caused by HIV.

Transmission

Blood and body fluids. Perinatal (vertical) transmission is the most common mechanism of paediatric HIV infection. Without treatment, HIV-infected mothers will pass infection to the neonate in up to 30% of cases. Horizontal transmission is the main means of transmission in adolescents and adults (see below).

Incubation period

It is important to distinguish between infection with HIV, which may be asymptomatic during a variable latent period and the progressive immunological derangement that leads to AIDS. Perinatally infected infants may be asymptomatic for months or years.

Risk groups

- Infants of mothers who are known to be HIV positive or who are members of a high-risk group (e.g. sex workers, IV drug users and those with bisexual partners).
- Intravenous drug users (HIV prevalence 1–17%).
- Men who have sex with men (HIV prevalence 5–10%).
- Sexual contacts (including sexually abused children) of individuals with HIV.
- Transfusion recipients, particularly patients with congenital bleeding disorders who received blood products before 1985.
- Individuals from countries with a high prevalence of HIV infection.

Clinical features

Clinical presentations of HIV infection include prolonged fever, failure to thrive or weight loss, generalised lymphadenopathy, hepatosplenomegaly, parotitis, chronic or recurrent diarrhoea, recurrent otitis, chronic candidiasis and chronic eczematous rash.

The indicator diseases for the diagnosis of AIDS in children include candidiasis, lymphoid interstitial pneumonitis, recurrent episodes of serious bacterial infection, opportunistic infection (e.g. *Pneumocystis carinii* pneumonia and disseminated *Mycobacterium avium complex* disease), CMV retinitis, cerebral toxoplasmosis, progressive neurological disease and malignancy (e.g. primary brain lymphoma).

Diagnosis

Patients ($\pm$ their families) require counselling and informed consent before testing for HIV. Specific antibody detection is a sensitive indicator of HIV infection in adults and children, but passively transferred maternal antibodies may persist for up to 18 to 21 months in infants. Prior to 18 months, HIV ultrasensitive viral load (PCR) can detect actively replicating HIV infection. The disease is monitored using a combination of absolute CD4+ T-cell count and quantification of HIV RNA (viral load). Patients may also have lymphopaenia, abnormal T-cell subsets and hypergammaglobulinaemia.

Management

A multidisciplinary approach by a specialised team is required to manage the unique needs of these patients and their families. Medical management of HIV-positive patients includes

- Antiretroviral drugs (highly active antiretroviral treatment, HAART). All infants diagnosed in the first year of life require treatment to prevent complications. Beyond the first year of life, decisions regarding treatment are based on a combination of clinical features and blood test results (CD4 count and HIV viral load).
- Prevention of opportunistic and other infections (immunisation (live vaccines may be contraindicated) and prophylactic antimicrobials (e.g. trimethoprim-sulphamethoxazole)).
- The early diagnosis and aggressive management of opportunistic infections.
- Cases of sexual assault need specialist advice for consideration of post-exposure prophylaxis.

Control

Antiretroviral therapy given to the HIV-infected woman during pregnancy and delivery, and to the newborn, complete avoidance of breastfeeding (where formula is available and safe) and with other measures can decrease the rate of transmission to the child from 25–35% to <1%. Antenatal testing of pregnant women to detect HIV infection is therefore critical. Antiretroviral therapy and other interventions (e.g. immunisation, *Pneumocystis* prophylaxis) can have a significant impact on disease progression.

Needle-stick injuries

Community-acquired needle-stick injuries

The risk of seroconversion to HIV, HBV or HCV from a community-acquired needle-stick injury is very low. Exposed individuals should be reassured. Immunity to hepatitis B should be confirmed, and if incomplete, hepatitis B vaccine should be given. Unless the injury is considered to be particularly high risk, no further management is required at the time. Follow-up should be arranged for counselling and serology. Tetanus toxoid $\pm$ immunoglobulin should be considered.

Occupational needle-stick injuries

Standard precautions

It is recommended that all health care workers are aware of their hepatitis B immune status and are appropriately vaccinated.

- All sharp objects and body fluids should be considered as potentially contaminated.
- Avoid contact with blood and other body fluids by
  - Using protective barriers (e.g. gloves) if contact is likely.
  - Immediately cleaning up accidental spills.

  Managing needle-stick injury or exposure to blood/blood-stained body fluid
- Squeeze the puncture wound.
- Wash blood off the skin with soap and water.
- Rinse blood from the eyes and mouth with running water.

Table 18.4 Evaluation of needle-stick injury sources

High risk of HIV and HBV	High risk of HCV
Unsafe sex, particularly with multiple (or homosexual) partners Intravenous drug users (IVDU) (particularly if they share equipment) and their sexual partners • Family members of an infected person • Individuals from communities with high HIV prevalence	Recipients of blood products prior to 1985 IVDU past or current (particularly if they share equipment)

- Document the date and time of exposure, details of incident, names of the source and exposed individuals.
- Inform source individual of exposure.
- Assess the risk of HIV, HBV and HCV in the source individual (see below).
- If indicated, test known source for HBV surface antigen (HBsAg), HCV antibody (anti-HCV Ab) and antibodies to HIV-1 and HIV-2 (HIV Abs). Obtain consent from the source individual.
- Even if the source individual is not infected with a blood-borne pathogen, storage of a serum specimen from the exposed person is recommended.
- Follow-up should be arranged for counselling (of the exposed person).
- Give HBV-specific immunoglobulin ± HBV vaccine if appropriate (see Tables 18.4 and 18.5).
- HIV post-exposure prophylaxis is only required if source is HIV Ab positive, or if the source is unknown and HIV is considered likely.

Assessing risk

A significant exposure is considered to have occurred if there has been

- An injection of blood/body fluid (particularly if >1 mL).
- A skin-penetrating injury with a sharp that is contaminated with blood/body fluid.
- A laceration from a contaminated instrument.
- A direct inoculation in the laboratory with contaminated material.
- A contaminated wound or skin lesion.
- Mucous membrane/conjunctival contact with blood/body fluid.

Table 18.5 Management of needle-stick injury

Exposure	Virus	Bloods to take from the exposed individual	Bloods to take from the source individual	What to give the exposed individual
High-risk	Hepatitis B	Anti-HBsAb (urgent)	HBsAg (urgent)	HBV immune: Nil HBV non-immune: Source HBsAg positive/unknown HBV immunoglobulin (within 48 hours)[a] + HBV vaccine Source HBsAg negative HBV vaccine
	Hepatitis C	ALT + hold serum	Anti-HCV Ab (urgent)	Nil
	HIV	Hold serum	HIV Ab (urgent)	HIV prophylaxis[b] if source is HIV positive and/or risk of transmission is significant
Low-risk	All viruses	Anti-HBsAb (if unsure of immunity)Hold serum	HBsAg	HBV immune: Nil H BV non-immune: HBV vaccine

[a] HBV immunoglobulin should be given as soon as possible, but can be deferred for 48 hours, while awaiting results of serology to confirm affected individual's immunity (when checking whether a vaccinated individual has maintained immunity or whether the individual is immune from previous infection).
[b] Urgent expert advice should be sought.

The incidence of HBV, HCV and HIV in Victorian IV drug users is 1.8, 10.7 and 0.2 per 100 person-years, respectively. The estimated risk of virus transmission from an occupational needle-stick injury from a *known positive donor* (e.g. in Victoria) is

- HBV: 6–30%
- HCV: 0–7%
- HIV: ~0.4%

Note: These figures are for needle-stick injury from a positive source. When the source is unknown, the actual risk of infection for the affected individual depends on the probability of infection in the source population.

Immunisation

Immunisation is one of the most cost-effective public health measures. They prevent clinical manifestations of disease or substantially reduce severity. In Australia, vaccinations for children <7 years are captured in the Australian Childhood Immunisation Register (ACIR). Immunisations are also detailed in the childhood health book and whilst vaccination is not compulsory in Australia, immunisation status must be detailed at childcare and school entry. Modern vaccines are safe and effective. As a disease becomes less common through a successful immunisation programme, the occurrence and perception of side effects assume greater relative importance. Health care providers may need to explain the risks of the diseases themselves and inform parents clearly that disease complications far outweigh the potential vaccine side effects. With explanation, the vast majority of parents feel comfortable about immunising their children.

Health professionals have a responsibility to know the immunisation status of patients in their care and to offer due or overdue vaccinations. Use every health care visit as an opportunity and minimise missed opportunities to vaccinate. The ACIR can be used to check vaccination status for children up to 7 years of age (1800 653 809). The Australian Commonwealth Government website (*www.immunise.health.gov.au*) also has extensive information including the latest Australian Immunisation Schedule, parent fact sheets and *The Australian Immunisation Handbook* (10th edition, 2013); downloadable at http://www.health.gov.au/internet/immunise/publishing.nsf/Content/Handbook10-home. The Melbourne Vaccine Education Centre (http://www.mvec.vic.edu.au/) also has local up-to-date resources, including an Immunisation Schedule App.

Current Australian standard vaccination schedule.

Current vaccines, their abbreviations and available forms with trade names are indicated in Table 18.6.

Although vaccine antigens to be given are the same throughout Australia, the schedule differs slightly in different by state, depending on the vaccine(s) purchased. The Australian schedule, at 1 July 2013, is shown in Table 18.7. Schedules applicable to other states are available in *The Australian Immunisation Handbook* (10th edition) or via state health departments.

Additional vaccine requirements

- Some preterm infants require additional hepatitis B and pneumococcal vaccines (see Fig. 18.1).
- Influenza vaccine can be administered to any infant ≥6 months. It is funded for all children and adolescents with special risk conditions. The dose varies by age (see Table 18.8).

Catch-up doses

When infants and children have missed scheduled vaccine doses, a 'catch-up' schedule should be recommended. Sometimes the catch-up schedule is relatively simple to devise, for example the 2- and 4-month vaccines can be given 1 month apart, hence a late 2-month vaccine given at 3 months can be followed by the routine 4-month vaccines just 1 month later. Catch-up schedules for newly arrived immigrants can be complex; see Chapter 27, *Immigrant health* and the RCH website. Comprehensive catch-up doses according to the overdue vaccine are detailed in the Victorian Department Health Immunisation section website at http://www.health.vic.gov.au/immunisation/quick-guide-catch-up.htm.

Contraindications to vaccination

There are few complete contraindications. Anaphylaxis to a vaccine or one of its constituents is considered a contraindication and requires allergy specialist assessment. Immunosuppression is generally a contraindication to live vaccines such as BCG, varicella and measles, mumps, rubella (MMR) vaccines.

The RCH immunisation service

The RCH Immunisation Service assists doctors, immunisation providers and parents through its telephone service (03 9345 6599) and weekly outpatient clinics for discussion of individual cases. There is a drop-in centre

Table 18.6 Current immunisation schedule vaccines, their abbreviations and available forms with trade names (alphabetical)

Disease	Vaccine	Available products
Diphtheria, tetanus, pertussis, hepatitis B, *Haemophilus influenzae* type B, polio	DTPa-hepB-Hib-IPV	Infanrix-hexa
Diphtheria, tetanus, pertussis, polio	DTPa-IPVdTpa-IPV	Infanrix-IPV, Boostrix-IPV
Diphtheria, tetanus, pertussis	dTpa	Boostrix, Adacel
Diphtheria, tetanus	dT	ADT Vaccine
Haemophilus influenzae type B	Hib (PRP-T)	Hiberix
Haemophilus influenzae type B – meningococcal C	Hib (PRP-T)-meningoccal C conjugate vaccine	Menitorix
Hepatitis B	hepB	Engerix-B, H-B VaxII
Human papillomavirus	HPV 4-valent vaccine HPV 2-valent vaccine	Gardasil Cervarix
Influenza	Trivalent influenza vaccine	Agrippal, Fluvax[a], Fluarix, Influvac, Vaxigrip
Measles, mumps, rubella	MMR	MMR II, Priorix
Measles, mumps, rubella, varicella	MMR–VZV	ProQuad, Priorix-Tetra
Meningococcal C disease	Meningococcal C conjugate vaccine (MCCV)	Meningitec, Menjugate, Neis-VacC
Meningococcal disease A, C, W, Y	4-valent Meningococcal conjugate vaccine	Menveo, Menactra
Poliomyelitis	IPV	IPOL
Rotavirus	Rotavirus vaccine	Rotarix, RotaTeq
Varicella	VZV	Varilrix, Varivax

[a]bioCSL Fluvax not licensed for children <5 years of age; not recommended <10 years.

at the hospital (open business hours) to assist in the provision of opportunistic immunisations for inpatients and outpatients. More information available on the RCH Immunisation service website (http://www.rch.org.au/immunisation/).

Vaccines in the Australian schedule – further information
Pertussis vaccines: childhood
There is limited clinical protection against pertussis following the initial vaccine (see Table 18.7). However, this fully killed combination vaccine is highly effective once the three-dose primary course is completed. A childhood pertussis booster is recommended at 3.5–4 years of age and again in adolescents.

Pertussis vaccines: adults
Although the pertussis vaccine is highly effective, it does not provide lifelong immunity against disease. Adults can contract pertussis 5–10 years after their most recent pertussis vaccine and spread it to infants, causing serious illness. Target immunisation of adults is important as they have been shown to be the major source of the disease in the community. The vaccine should be considered for parents, close household contacts and childcare workers who are in contact with infants <6 months of age. Further data is required to determine the timing of repeat boosters in adults to maintain adequate immunity.

Hepatitis B vaccine
Neonatal and infant schedule
This inactivated vaccine is recommended to be given within 7 days of birth. Infants born to mothers who are positive for hepatitis B surface antigen should receive passive protection with 100 IU hepatitis B immunoglobulin

Table 18.7 Australian immunisation schedule (from 1st January 2015)

Birth	hepB	—		
2 months (can be administered from 6 weeks of age)	DTPa-hepB-IPV-Hib	Rotavirus[a]	13vPneumococcal	
4 months	DTPa-hepB-IPV-Hib	Rotavirus	13vPneumococcal	
6 months[b]	DTPa-hepB-IPV-Hib	Rotavirus (RotaTeq only)	13vPneumococcal	
12 months	Hib -MenC[c]			MMR
18 months				MMR–Varicella[d]
3.5–4 years	DTPa-IPV			
School year 7	dTap[e]	HPV[f]3 doses		(Varicella[g])

[a]RotaTeq, 2 mL at 2, 4 and 6 months of age. Rotarix, 1 mL at 2 and 4 months only. Minimum interval between doses is 4 weeks. Oral rotavirus vaccine is not recommended beyond the following age limits: RotaTeq first dose by 12 weeks of age and third dose by 32 weeks of age, Rotarix first dose by 14 weeks of age and second dose by 24 weeks of age.

[b]Influenza vaccine can be given to infants ≥6 months. Children in special risk groups are highly recommended annual influenza vaccine. (see Table 9.4).

[c]Meningococcal C conjugate vaccine can be given <1 year but is not funded (2–6 months, 3 doses; 6–12 months, 2 doses min. 2 months apart, with final booster ≥12 months).

[d]Varicella vaccine is funded for infants aged 18 months, administered as combined MMR-V vaccine. This is the second dose of MMR, separated by minimum of 4 weeks.

[e]dTap is administered in Year 7 as part of the secondary school program, a catch-up for Years 8–10 will be undertaken in 2015.

[f]HPV vaccine is funded for males and females aged 12–13 years. Three doses spaced 0, 2 and 6 months.

[g]Catch-up varicella vaccine is given to students in Year 7 (single dose) who have not had chickenpox or varicella vaccine.

(0.5 mL) preferably within 12 hours of birth. Their active hepatitis B vaccination should be commenced at the same time. Three further doses of hepatitis B vaccine are required for all infants (see Table 9.2).

Preterm infants
Preterm babies do not mount as strong an antibody response to hepatitis B-containing vaccines, so those born at <32 weeks gestation or <2000 g should have a 'booster' given at 12 months of age (see Figure 18.1).

Pneumococcal vaccines
Background
S. pneumoniae is an important cause of bacterial infections in children. IPD includes meningitis, septicaemia and pneumonia. *S. pneumonia* is also a cause of otitis media. A 7-valent killed conjugate pneumococcal vaccine (PCV7) was licensed for use in Australia in December 2000 and replaced by an extended 13-valent (PCV13) vaccine in 2011. It is highly effective against IPD caused by the 13 vaccine serotypes. The vaccine is safe and effective in children, with the primary doses administered in early infancy due to the high morbidity and mortality in children <2 years of age.

Extra recommended free vaccines for babies born:
- **<28 weeks gestation**: Pneumococcal conjugate vaccine and hepatitis B vaccine at 12 months and pneumococcal polysaccharide vaccine at 4 years
- **<32 weeks gestation and/or**
- **<2000g** birth weight: Hepatitis B at 12 months of age
- **underlying medical condition**: Influenza vaccine annually, pneumococcal conjugate vaccine at 12 months and pneumococcal polysaccharide vaccine at 4 years

Figure 18.1 Additional vaccines required for premature infants

Table 18.8 Influenza vaccine dosing guidelines by age

Age	Dose	Number of doses in the first year the vaccine is received	Number of doses in subsequent years
<6 months	Not recommended (poor immune response)	–	–
6 months to <3 years	0.25 mL	2 4 weeks apart	1
3 years–9 years	0.5 mL	2 4 weeks apart	1
≥10 years	0.5 mL	1	1

Schedule

Conjugate pneumococcal vaccine is given routinely at 2, 4 and 6 months of age. A booster (fourth dose) of PCV13 is recommended at 1 year of age for children with special risk medical conditions (e.g. preterm <28 weeks, cystic fibrosis, cardiac disease, nephrotic syndrome, haematological malignancies). These children are at higher risk of IPD. A full list of the children recommended additional doses of pneumococcal vaccine is available in *The Australian Immunisation Handbook* (10th edition). These children are also recommended to have a 23-valent-polysaccharide pneumococcal vaccine at 4–5 years of age.

Aboriginal and Torres Strait Islander children in Northern Territory and Central Australia are given an additional PCV13 at 12–18 months of age and a booster of the 23-valent-polysaccharide pneumococcal vaccine (23vPPV) between 18 and 24 months. The recommendations for indigenous children living in other areas of Australia vary; refer to *The Australian Immunisation Handbook* (10th edition) for details.

Meningococcal vaccines

Background

There are at least 13 meningococcal serogroups. Group B is currently the most common in Australia. A vaccine against MenB has recently been licensed in Australia (Bexsero® Novartis), but is not currently part of the National Immunisation Program schedule.

Conjugate C vaccine

Meningococcal serogroup C was the main cause of disease in the late 1990s to early 2000s and has dramatically decreased following the protein-conjugated group C vaccine introduction in 2003. All three brands of meningococcal vaccine (see Table 18.6) are safe and effective at preventing group C meningococcal disease at all ages. The killed conjugate vaccine does provide long-term immunity.

Who should be vaccinated?

A single MenC vaccine is given routinely to all 1-year olds. Whilst meningococcal C disease is rare under the age of 1 year, families can choose to purchase the vaccine for infants from 6 weeks of age. Infant doses at 2 and 4 months or 2, 4 and 6 months still require the booster dose at 1 year of age to provide lasting immunity. Newly arrived refugees should receive a catch-up meningococcal C vaccine. See Chapter 27, *Immigrant health* for further details on this group of patients.

4-valent Meningococcal conjugate vaccines

Two vaccines are also now available with broader serogroup coverage, the 4-valent A, C, Y and W135 meningococcal conjugate vaccines (Menactra, Menveo). They are not on the routine national immunisation program, but are recommended for children and adults at higher risk of encapsulated bacteria such as asplenia, HIV and complement deficiency (see Immunisation Handbook).

MMR vaccine

Two doses of live-attenuated MMR vaccine are given to improve seroconversion and long-term protection. The two doses were previously given at 12 months and 4 years, but since July 2013 it has been given at 12 months and 18 months of age.

Egg allergy
The MMR vaccine is safe for children with egg allergy, even in those with past anaphylaxis, as the vaccine is produced in chicken fibroblast cell cultures, not eggs.

Does MMR vaccine cause inflammatory bowel disease or autistic spectrum disorder?
There is **no** link between MMR vaccination and inflammatory bowel disease or autistic spectrum disorder. Families with further concerns about this topic should discuss them with a specialist.

Co-administration with other vaccines
The MMR vaccine can be given on the same day as the varicella vaccine, at a separate site. If MMR is not given on the same day as the varicella vaccine, they should be spaced at least 4 weeks apart. MMR-V is recommended to be the second dose of MMR vaccine, administered at 18-months of age.

Post-exposure prophylaxis
The MMR vaccine can be administered to susceptible contacts >9 months of age within 72 hours of exposure to measles as post-exposure prophylaxis. NHIG can be given within 7 days of contact as an alternative for subjects with contraindications to MMR such as immunosuppression.

Previous proven measles, mumps or rubella
Children require protection from all components of MMR. Monovalent measles vaccine is not available in Australia. As vaccination of children who have been previously infected with any of the three components of this vaccine is not dangerous, MMR should be given to all children.

Varicella vaccine
Background
Chickenpox disease used to be considered a childhood rite of passage. Many children are hospitalised and a few die each year in Australia from chickenpox. The most common complication is secondary bacterial infection of varicella skin lesions, but more severe sequelae include pneumonitis and encephalitis.

One or two doses for infants
Varicella vaccine is a live attenuated vaccine, highly effective against severe varicella disease. When a single dose is used the chance of mild breakthrough cases is about 7% in the next 10 years. USA introduced a two-dose schedule in 2006 to reduce the rate of breakthrough varicella from 7% to 2%. Australia currently only funds a single dose, but a second dose can be considered and bought privately (a minimum of 4 weeks between doses).

Who should be given varicella vaccine?
- According to the 2013 schedule, a single varicella vaccine at 18 months of age is recommended for all immunocompetent children who do not have a definite history of varicella. Families can purchase this dose earlier if required. It was included on the routine schedule in 2005, so a dose is also currently recommended for children in Year 7 at school if they did not receive the vaccine in infancy. The vaccine is not required if they have had confirmed chickenpox infection, although it is safe to give if uncertain.
- Individuals ≥14 years of age without a definite history of chickenpox and those with serologically proven non-immunity are recommended two doses, at least 4 weeks apart.
- Varicella vaccine should be spaced at least 4 weeks apart from the MMR if it is not given on the same day.
- It is highly recommended for non-immune health care workers and family members who are in contact with immunosuppressed subjects.
- Health care workers with a negative or uncertain history of varicella should have serology and vaccinated if negative. Checking serology after vaccination is not routinely necessary.
- Non-immune women immediately postpartum or women planning a pregnancy should be given two doses of varicella vaccine ≥4 weeks apart and should not become pregnant for 1 month after a varicella vaccine dose.
  Note: Approximately 40% of adults who do not think they have had chickenpox are found to be immune on serology and do not need vaccination. However, there is no known harm giving the vaccine to immune subjects.

Varicella vaccine rash
Rash and/or fever can occur in 2–5% of vaccinees during a period of 5 days to 3 weeks after the vaccine. This can occur over the injection site or be generalised and the appearance is either maculopapular or vesicular.

Although rare, varicella vaccine virus can be spread from vesicular rash lesions. If vaccinees develop a rash they should avoid contact with immunocompromised persons for the duration of the rash. If a health care worker develops a vesicular rash following the vaccine, they should be reassigned to duties that do not require patient contact or placed on sick leave for the duration of the rash (not for 4–6 weeks as the product information states). The duration of the rash is likely to be <1 week. Florid vesicular rash after the vaccine is highly suspicious of wild-type varicella.

Post-exposure prophylaxis

Varicella vaccine is effective in preventing varicella in those already exposed if used within 3–5 days, with earlier administration preferable. It is not 100% effective but, as with pre-exposure vaccination, if breakthrough varicella occurs it is usually milder. Post-exposure varicella vaccine can be considered in children >9 months of age, with a second dose still recommended at the routine 18 months of age.

Oral rotavirus vaccine

Background

Rotavirus is the leading cause of severe childhood gastroenteritis in children <5 years. There are at least four main serotypes. Infection with any two of the natural strains provides broad protection to most children. There are two oral live attenuated vaccines licensed: Rotarix (two doses) and RotaTeq (three doses).

At what age should oral rotavirus vaccine be given?

The oral rotavirus vaccine should be given at the same time as the routine 2- and 4-month immunisations. If the three-dose vaccine (RotaTeq) is used, the third dose should be given with the 6-month immunisations. The rotavirus vaccines have been associated with a very small increased risk of intussusception (two additional cases of intussusception among every 100,000 infants vaccinated, or fourteen additional cases per year in infants in Australia). They are, therefore, recommended for use in children within the specified age ranges: RotaTeq, first dose by 12 weeks and third dose by 32 weeks. For Rotarix, first dose is recommended by 14 weeks and second dose by 24 weeks. The vaccine is not licensed or funded for use beyond these age limits and hence infants late for the routine immunisation doses may miss out on a rotavirus vaccine dose. Knowledge of this should encourage parents and immunisation providers to have the 2-, 4- and 6-month immunisations on time. Preterm and hospitalised infants can have the oral rotavirus vaccine.

Who can't have oral rotavirus vaccine?

There are some groups of infants for whom this live attenuated vaccine is **contraindicated**:

- Infants with severe combined immunodeficiency (SCID).
- Previous history of intussusception or a congenital abnormality that may predispose to intussusception.
- Anaphylaxis following a previous dose of either rotavirus vaccine.

Human papillomavirus vaccine

Background

Human papillomavirus (HPV) is responsible for most cervical carcinoma in females, as well as anogenital warts in both sexes. There are multiple types with approximately 70% cervical carcinoma caused by types 16 and 18. HPV types 6 and 11 are responsible for 90% of genital warts. Two killed vaccines are licensed in Australia, derived from inactive virus-like particles. Gardasil contains types 6, 11, 16, and 18, and Cervarix contains types 16 and 18.

Who should be vaccinated?

The funded Australian HPV vaccine program is with the 4-valent HPV vaccine (Gardasil) and since 2013, has been recommended for both sexes. The female HPV program commenced in 2007 and has already had an impact on cervical cancer screening programs and the incidence of anogenital warts. The vaccine is administered as part of the secondary school program or at the local doctor at age 12–13 years. The 2-year catch-up program for males aged 14–15 years was completed in December 2014. The HPV vaccination is most effective when it is given before exposure to HPV. Even if young people have already begun to have sexual contact, the HPV vaccine will provide excellent protection against types an individual may not have been exposed to. The three doses are administered over a 6-month period at 0, 2 and 6 months. There is no need to recommence the schedule if there is a delay between doses.

Influenza vaccine

Who should have annual influenza vaccine?

All children and adolescents >6 months of age can have the annual influenza vaccine. It is funded for all children with medical special risk conditions that predispose them to an increased risk of influenza-related complications. This includes children with chronic illnesses requiring regular medical follow-up, such as chronic suppurative lung disease (e.g. cystic fibrosis), congenital cardiac disease and those receiving immunosuppressive therapy (e.g. childhood cancer). Health care workers and family members of those at increased risk of severe influenza disease are highly recommended to be vaccinated to reduce risk of transmission to at-risk individuals.

Vaccine dose varies according to age

The dose requirements vary by age and are detailed in Table 18.8. In children 9-years and under, two doses are recommended in the first year that an annual influenza vaccine is received. Children and adolescents on immunosuppression should also have two doses (a minimum 4 weeks apart) if there has been a strain change from the last influenza season.

Other influenza vaccine facts

The majority of influenza vaccines are inactivated and currently contain three strains (two Type A and one Type B influenza). It has been found that children with a non-anaphylaxis egg allergy can safely receive the influenza vaccine. Children with egg anaphylaxis should discuss the vaccine with a paediatric allergist or vaccine safety service.

Influenza vaccine can be administered concurrently with most childhood vaccinations. Due to a small possible increase in febrile convulsions, it can be separated from pneumococcal conjugate vaccines (e.g. Prevenar 13) by 3 days. Influenza vaccination is carried out during a season where it is common to have regular intercurrent illness. Symptoms post vaccine may be due to the killed vaccine dose or may be due to a coincidental intercurrent illness.

Vaccine administration

- Cold chain: never use a vaccine if there is any doubt about its safe cold chain storage. Vaccines should be kept in a refrigerator reserved for vaccine/medicine storage at 2–8°C and never frozen.
- Prevent immunisation errors: always check about a vaccine dose, route of administration and potential side effects before prescribing. If in doubt check with a pharmacist or the RCH Immunisation Service.
- Post-vaccine observation: Recipients of any vaccine should remain in the vicinity of medical care for approximately 15 minutes. Although anaphylaxis is very rare, it can occur with any vaccine and should be treated with adrenaline urgently; refer to Chapter 1, *Medical emergencies*, p. 5.

Common misconceptions for missing vaccinations

Children may be under-immunised for their age when health professionals miss opportunities to vaccinate, when parents forget appointments or when parents actively oppose vaccination (only 1–2%). Some common misconceptions about vaccination include

- Natural infection is the best way to achieve immunity.
- Vaccination weakens the immune system or is too much for the immune system to handle.
- 'Homeopathic immunisation' is safer and more effective.

It is essential to address parental concern, to emphasise the well-established risks associated with not vaccinating their child and to provide reassurance about vaccine safety. The back cover of *The Australian Immunisation Handbook* has an invaluable table for immunisation providers and parents comparing the effects of vaccines and diseases. This table compares the range and rate of disease effects, and the range and rate of vaccine side effects. This table also appears on the back of the parent-checklist sheet that is given to each family when their child is having a vaccine. Table 18.9 details false contraindications to vaccines.

Adverse events associated with vaccinations

All vaccines are medications and all medications have side effects. For each individual vaccine there are a known list of fairly common relatively minor symptoms and an important small list of significant major side effects. It is helpful for families to understand the risks and benefits of immunisations to feel comfortable and confident with their decision to vaccinate their young child.

Table 18.9 False contraindications to vaccination

Usually, children **should** still be vaccinated, even if they

- Have a cold, or low-grade fever (<38.5°C).
- Have a family history of any reactions following vaccination.
- Have a family history of convulsions.
- Have a history of pertussis-like illness, measles, rubella or mumps infection.
- Are premature (vaccination should not be postponed as immunisations are recommended at actual **not** corrected age).
- Have a stable neurological condition such as cerebral palsy or Down syndrome.
- Have been in contact with an infectious disease.
- Have asthma, eczema, or hay fever.
- Are on antibiotics.
- Are on locally acting (inhaled or low-dose topical) steroids.
- Have a pregnant mother.
- Are being breastfed.
- Have had recent or imminent surgery.
- Are of low weight but otherwise healthy.

Source: Adapted from *The Australian Immunisation Handbook*, 10th edition. (2013) National Health and Medical Research Council (Australia), and Department of Health and Ageing (Canberra). Reproduced with permission of Commonwealth of Australia.

The vast majority of adverse events experienced after the scheduled vaccinations are minor (e.g. fever, local redness, swelling or tenderness) and do not contraindicate further doses of the vaccine. Parents who have questions regarding potential adverse events should discuss these with their vaccine provider.

SAEFVIC: surveillance of adverse events following vaccinations in the community

When symptoms occur in the hours or days after a vaccination, they may be directly due to the vaccine or totally unrelated and coincidental in nature. Adverse events following immunisations (AEFI) should never be dismissed and often require individual assessment to provide accurate advice for the family about the actual adverse event and about options for further doses of the same vaccine. Maintaining confidence in immunisations following an adverse event is very important. Notifying significant or unexpected adverse events is also very important to assist with safety monitoring of vaccines used in Australia.

SAEFVIC is on the RCH campus based in the Murdoch Children's Research Institute and is funded by the Department of Health. This surveillance service provides telephone advice, outpatient clinic appointments and immunisation under supervision following significant adverse events. SAEFVIC reports AEFI to the national Therapeutic Goods Administration. Notifications of vaccine adverse events can be made online: www.saefvic.org.au, phone 1300 882 924 (option 1), fax (03) 9345 4163 or by email (saefvic@mcri.edu.au).

Immunisation guidelines for special groups

Vaccines in the setting of immunosuppression

Live vaccines (e.g. varicella vaccine, MMR, BCG) are generally not recommended for immunosuppressed individuals. The MMR vaccine can be given to some children with HIV but the safety of this should be assessed in each case in discussion with their treating physician.

- Children who have recently received high-dose oral steroid therapy (prednisolone 2 mg/kg per day for >1 week, or 1 mg/kg per day for >1 month)
  - Delay live vaccine administration until at least 1 month after therapy has stopped.
  - The use of inhaled steroids is not a contraindication to vaccination with either live or inactivated vaccines.
- Children who have recently received immunoglobulin products
  - Varicella vaccine should be delayed for 5 months in children who have received zoster immunoglobulin.
  - Delay MMR and varicella for 9–11 months if immunoglobulin has recently been given to avoid reduced effectiveness of the vaccine(s).
- Children who have received bone marrow transplants
  - Require booster doses or complete revaccination, depending on their serological and clinical status, as per guidelines in the *Australian Immunisation Handbook* (10th edition).

- Children who receive cancer chemotherapy
  - Require booster doses 6 months after completion of therapy.
  - Inactivated vaccines (such as pertussis), modified toxins (such as diphtheria and tetanus vaccines) and subunit vaccines (such as Hib and hepatitis B vaccines) can be safely given to children receiving immuno-suppressive therapy, but may produce a diminished serum immune response and additional doses are recommended.
  - Influenza vaccine is an important safe vaccine for children with immunosuppression, even though it may not work optimally because of the reduced immune function.

Functional or anatomical asplenia

- All children post-splenectomy should receive pneumococcal and meningococcal vaccinations in addition to the vaccinations of the standard schedule, as well as annual influenza vaccine.
- In cases of elective splenectomy, the vaccinations should ideally be given at least 2 weeks before the operation.
- A detailed immunisation protocol for children with asplenia is available from the Melbourne Vaccine Education Centre website.

For further details of immunisation in immunosuppressed special risk children refer to *The Australian Immunisation Handbook* (10th edition).

Household contacts of children with immune deficiency

Siblings and close contacts of immunosuppressed children are recommended to ensure vaccination status is up-to-date for MMR, varicella and pertussis (whooping cough). Annual influenza vaccines are also recommended for household contacts. Immunisation will ensure that they have less chance of infecting their immunosuppressed siblings.

Vaccination of newly arrived immigrants to Australia

See Chapter 10, *Immigrant child health*, and the RCH Immigrant Health Resources (*www.rch.org.au/ immigranthealth/resources.cfm?doc_id=10813*).

Acknowledgements

We thank Dr. Josh Wolf for his contribution to the previous version of this chapter.

Thanks to Associate Professor Jim Buttery and Dr. Jenny Royle for their contribution to previous drafts of the 'Immunisation' section of the RCH Handbook.

USEFUL RESOURCES

- *http://www.mvec.vic.edu.au/* – The Melbourne Vaccine Education Centre is a resource developed by RCH and provides up-to-date immunisation information for healthcare professionals, parents and the public.
- *http://www.health.vic.gov.au/ideas/bluebook/* – Australian national information on infectious diseases and their control, from the Department of Human Services. Has detailed information on most infections.
- *http://www.cdc.gov* – The US Centers for Disease Control and Prevention has an enormous array of information on infectious diseases and travel medicine.
- http://www.rch.org.au/genmed/clinical_resources/RCH_Immunisation_Service/ – RCH immunisation resources
- *www.saefvic.org.au* – SAEFVIC Victorian vaccine safety service.
- *http://www.health.vic.gov.au/immunisation* – Victorian Department Health Immunisation Section.
- *www.ncirs.usyd.edu.au* – National Centre for Immunisation Research and Surveillance of Vaccine Preventable Diseases website includes fact sheets related to specific vaccines, vaccine-preventable diseases and vaccine safety.
- *www.immunise.health.gov.au* – Immunise Australia Program website where *The Australian Immunisation Handbook* (10th edition, 2008) is downloadable. Also contains useful fact sheets and links to State and Territory Health Department websites.

CHAPTER 19

Allergy and immunology

Ralf Heine
Joanne Smart
Dean Tey

Allergic diseases affect up to 40% of children in the community, including food allergy, eczema, asthma, allergic rhinoconjunctivitis, and allergies to insect stings or drugs.

Definitions
- Allergy is an objective, reproducible reaction mediated via the body's immune system, initiated by exposure to a defined stimulus at a dose tolerated by normal persons.
- Sensitisation is defined by the production of IgE antibodies against an antigen, as detected either via a skin prick test (SPT) or serum-specific IgE (sIgE).
- Atopy is the genetic tendency to develop sensitisation in response to ordinary exposure to allergens, and subsequently develop typical symptoms of food allergy, eczema, asthma and allergic rhinitis.

Diagnostic methods
Skin prick testing

- Detect evidence of IgE-sensitisation *in vivo*
- Highly sensitive, inexpensive, simple and rapid.
- Can be performed from early infancy; albeit with lower sensitivity in those under 2 years of age.
- SPT is typically performed by using a single-, dual- or multi-point device to introduce the allergen extract into the epidermis (on the back or forearm). Wheal diameter is measured 15 minutes later. Histamine and saline are used as positive and negative controls.
- False-negative SPT can occur after antihistamine use (within 4–5 days), or after recent anaphylaxis (within 6 weeks due to mast cell tachyphylaxis). False-positive SPT results may occur with dermatographism.

Serum-specific IgE antibodies (sIgE)

- Useful in the primary care setting as initial investigation to confirm a suspected, **single** allergy (e.g. confirmation of IgE-mediated food allergy to cow's milk, egg or peanut; or assessment for house dust mite, pet dander or pollen sensitisation in asthma or allergic rhinitis).
- Also useful alternative to SPTs if there is dermatographism, widespread skin disease, or if antihistamines cannot be discontinued.
- They have reduced sensitivity, are more expensive and have a slower turnaround time.
- Measurement of sIgE to food allergen panels/mixes is **not** recommended.

Interpretation of SPT and sIgE

- A positive SPT or sIgE in the setting of a recent immediate allergic reaction is diagnostic of IgE-mediated allergy.
- A positive SPT or sIgE in the absence of a clinical reaction is not diagnostic (sensitisation only, but not allergic disease).
- The size/level of positive SPT and sIgE results correlates with the probability of IgE-mediated allergy but does not predict the severity of allergic reactions or risk of anaphylaxis.

Paediatric Handbook, Ninth Edition. Edited by Amanda Gwee, Romi Rimer and Michael Marks.
© 2015 John Wiley & Sons, Ltd. Published 2015 by John Wiley & Sons, Ltd.

- Where SPT or sIgE results are equivocal, an *in vivo* challenge is required to assess the true allergic status (e.g. food challenges).

In-vivo challenges

- *In vivo* challenges are the gold standard for the diagnosis of food allergy and antibiotic reactions.
- Performed if SPT or sIgE result is equivocal or to determine if previously diagnosed food allergy has resolved.
- Due to the risk of anaphylaxis, food challenges should only be performed by experienced specialists in centres with facilities for resuscitation.
- Increasing quantities of an allergen are administered until either a threshold dose is tolerated, or objective signs of an allergic reaction are observed in the patient.
- The diagnosis of delayed, non-IgE-mediated reaction to foods requires a sequence of food elimination (generally for 2–4 weeks) and subsequent food challenge in a supervised setting (at home or in hospital, depending on clinical scenario).

Food allergy

- The prevalence of food allergies and infantile eczema has increased dramatically over the past decades.
- A population-based study in Melbourne in 2007 found that more than 10% of 12-month-old infants suffer from challenge-proven IgE-mediated food allergies (egg 9%, peanut 3%).
- Infants with IgE-mediated food allergy often present with eczema in the first year of life.
- While some IgE-mediated food allergies (cow's milk, soy and wheat) may resolve during childhood, peanut, tree nuts, fish and shellfish allergy often persist into adult life.
- Non-IgE-mediated food allergies present in the first years of life, mainly with chronic manifestations of the gastrointestinal tract or skin (atopic dermatitis).
- Population prevalence of non-IgE-mediated food allergy in infancy is not known but may be as high as 10%.

Terminology

- Food hypersensitivity is an objective, reproducible reaction initiated by exposure to a defined food allergen (Fig. 19.1).
- Food hypersensitivity reactions may be either mediated through the immune system (allergy) or not (intolerance e.g. lactose intolerance).

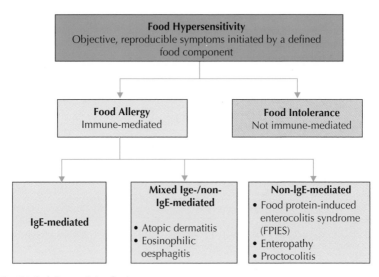

Fig. 19.1 Food allergy terminology flowchart

- Food allergies can be further classified as IgE-mediated, non-IgE-mediated, or mixed IgE- and non-IgE-mediated.

Clinical presentation

IgE-mediated reactions to food

- Occur within 30–60 minutes of food ingestion.
- Symptoms include oral tingling, lip swelling, urticaria, facial angioedema, vomiting and acute diarrhoea.
- More severe reactions (anaphylaxis) involve the respiratory tract (stridor, wheezing, hoarse voice persistent coughing, chest tightness) and/or the cardiovascular system (hypotension, collapse).

Non-IgE-mediated reactions to food

- Delayed onset 24–48 hours after food ingestion (exception FPIES).
- Relatively common in the first year of life (gastrointestinal or cutaneous).
- A **small** proportion of infantile eczema is triggered by non-IgE-mediated food allergy.
- Cow's milk, soy and wheat are the most common trigger foods for non-IgE-mediated reactions.
- Gastrointestinal symptoms in infants include frequent regurgitation/vomiting, chronic diarrhoea, rectal bleeding, unsettled behaviour and abdominal pain.
- Feeding difficulties and food refusal are common in infants with non-IgE food allergy and may cause poor weight gain or failure to thrive.
- Natural history is generally good, with development of tolerance in most cases by 18–24 months of age.

There are three main clinical syndromes of non-IgE-mediated gastrointestinal food allergy:

1. Food-protein-induced proctocolitis
   - Most common cause of rectal bleeding in early infancy.
   - Presents in the first months of life with mild rectal bleeding, increased mucus and low-grade diarrhoea (occurs in breastfed and formula-fed infants).
   - Infants otherwise well and thriving.
2. Food-protein-induced enterocolitis syndrome (FPIES)
   - Delayed-onset forceful and repeated vomiting (may become bilious) >2 hours after ingestion of offending food allergen.
   - Typically occurs after first ingestion of formula (cow's milk, soy) or solid foods (rice, oats, chicken).
   - Rarely occurs in exclusively breastfed infants.
   - Infants present with pallor and lethargy, but have no fever or cutaneous manifestations.
   - About 20% of infants with FPIES develop severe dehydration and hypovolaemic shock.
   - Diarrhoea may persist for 24 hours, occasionally containing blood.
   - Reactions may be mistaken for gastroenteritis, sepsis or intestinal obstruction.
3. Food-protein-induced enteropathy
   - Clinical picture similar to that of coeliac disease.
   - Usually occurs in formula-fed infants (cow's milk or soy), or after early introduction of intact cow's milk.
   - Infants present with irritability, persistent diarrhoea, vomiting (in two-thirds of cases) and poor weight gain/growth failure.
   - Signs of secondary lactose malabsorption, including abdominal bloating and perianal excoriation, may be present.

Mixed IgE-mediated/non-IgE-mediated food allergy

- Patients with eczema or eosinophilic oesophagitis (EoE) (see below) often have evidence of IgE-mediated food allergy and non-IgE-mediated food allergy.

Investigation

- Take detailed history
  - Symptoms of reaction, including features of anaphylaxis, type/dose of food ingested, timing of reaction after ingestion, prior and subsequent exposures, and treatment required.
  - Explore early birth and feeding details, including birth mode, duration of breast feeding, formula use, timing of introduction of solid foods, growth details (refer to percentile charts).
  - Document co-existing atopic diseases, including other food allergies, and the presence and severity of eczema, asthma and allergic rhinitis.

- IgE-mediated food allergy
  - Diagnosis relies on clinical history of typical immediate reaction **plus** demonstration of IgE antibodies by either SPT or specific serum IgE antibodies (ImmunoCAP®).
  - If the history is uncertain or diagnosis not supported by demonstration of sIgE, specialist referral is warranted where further evaluation by formal food challenge in hospital may be considered.
- Non-IgE-mediated food allergy
  - No specific *in vitro* test for non-IgE-mediated food allergy is available.
  - SPT or ImmunoCAP® is negative.
  - Diagnosis requires demonstration of symptom resolution after food elimination (within 2–4 weeks), followed by relapse of symptoms after reintroduction of offending food.
  - Some patients require additional investigations to exclude other diagnoses, such as such sigmoidoscopy and biopsy (when presenting with atypical rectal bleeding) and HLADQ2/DQ8 testing, gastroscopy and biopsy (when presenting with enteropathy).

Management

- Strict elimination of the offending food allergen(s) from the diet. This requires parental education and attention to reading of ingredient labels.

Cow's milk allergy

In infants with CMA, all cow's milk-based products should be eliminated.

- In breastfed infants, a maternal dairy-free diet may be effective (see below).
- In formula-fed infants, a soy-based formula can be used in infants from age 6 months (if the infant is not also allergic to soy). Calcium-fortified soy milk can be used from age 12 months.

In infants with soy allergy, an *extensively hydrolysed formula* should be used.

- About 10% of infants will not tolerate an extensively hydrolysed formula (due to residual allergenicity) and require an *amino acid based formula* (i.e. elemental formula).
- Use of amino acid based formula is generally reserved for infants with complex or severe manifestations of food allergy, including cow's milk anaphylaxis, multiple (non-IgE-mediated) food allergy, or children with eosinophillic oesophagitis (EoE).
- Partially hydrolysed formula is not suitable for the treatment of CMA (but may have a role in allergy prevention).

Maternal elimination diets

- Food allergens may transfer from the maternal diet into breast milk and may cause allergic reactions in the infant. The clinical relevance can be determined via a maternal elimination-reintroduction diet over a 2–4 week period.
- Maternal elimination of specific food proteins may be effective in a range of food allergic conditions, including infantile eczema and gastrointestinal food allergy (food-protein-induced proctocolitis).
- The maternal elimination diet needs to be closely supervised by a dietitian, and maternal micronutrient/vitamin supplementation is generally required (NB maternal RDI for calcium 1200 mg daily).

Treatment of IgE-mediated food allergy

- Patients should be provided with a written management plan for accidental allergen exposure (available from *www.allergy.org.au*).
- The Australasian Society of Clinical Allergy and Immunology (ASCIA) guidelines recommend provision of an adrenaline autoinjector (Epipen® or Anapen®) when there has been a history of anaphylaxis and suggests consideration of prescription in patients with limited access to emergency medical care, have co-morbid asthma, have a nut or insect sting allergy, or are in the adolescent age group.
  - Dose for adrenaline autoinjector
    - Child >20 kg: 300 mcg single dose.
    - Child 10–20 kg: 150 mcg single dose.
    - Child <10 kg: not usually recommended.
  - Note: this is different to current product information dosage guidelines, where both the Epipen and Anapen 300 mcg is recommended for children >30 kg.
- Patients should be monitored with repeat SPT and/or sIgE to monitor for possible development of tolerance to determine the need for ongoing avoidance or for the need to perform food challenges.

Eosinophilic oesophagitis

- Recently recognised eosinophilic gastrointestinal disorder affecting the oesophagus.
- Defined by histological evidence of at least 15 eosinophils per high power field on oesophageal histology, plus symptoms attributable to upper gastrointestinal dysfunction.
- Associated with other atopic disorders (asthma, eczema, allergic rhinitis).
- Occurs in any age group, with a strong male preponderance.
- Infants/young children often present with reflux-like symptoms/regurgitation, food refusal, feeding difficulties and persistent unsettled behaviour.
- In older children and adolescents, swallowing difficulties and increasing dysphagia (food bolus obstruction) are characteristic symptoms.
- The diagnosis of EoE always requires a gastroscopy with oesophageal biopsies (from upper and lower oesophagus).
- A repeat biopsy after a trial of a proton pump inhibitor for 4–8 weeks is also required to delineate EoE against so-called 'proton pump inhibitor-responsive oesophageal eosinophilia'.
- Children with EoE often respond to elimination diets. Amino acid-based (elemental diet) is effective in over 90% of patients but poorly tolerated in the long term. Targeted elimination diets (based on SPT) are effective in about 60–70% of children. Empirical elimination diets eliminate the most common food allergens in EoE (cow's milk, egg, wheat and soy). The diet is gradually liberalised, as tolerated, based on repeat gastroscopy after food challenges.
- Older children with EoE may require topical corticosteroids (swallowed fluticasone aerosol or viscous budesonide).
- Natural history of EoE is not well documented, but generally follows a chronic relapsing course.
- In patients with long-standing uncontrolled EoE, narrowing of the oesophageal lumen or strictures can develop (may require endoscopic food disimpaction or balloon dilatation of oesophageal strictures).

Atopic dermatitis (eczema)

See also Chapter 17, *Dermatologic conditions*, p. 258.

- Eczema is often the first allergic manifestation in infants and young children.
- Eczema is the result of a complex interaction between skin barrier dysfunction and environmental triggers, such as irritants, allergens and microbial infections.
- Moderate-to-severe eczema in the first year of life is strongly associated with IgE-mediated food allergy.
- *Staphylococcus aureus* – colonisation is common in patients with moderate-to-severe eczema, even in the absence of overt infection.
- Acute staphylococcal infections should be treated with appropriate oral antibiotics.
- Staphylococcal reduction measures may reduce severity of eczema. Measures include daily bathing, avoidance of 'double dipping' into moisturiser tubs and regular dilute bleach baths (12 mL of household bleach in 10 L of water).
- House dust mite can be a trigger in eczema and measures to reduce exposure may be advised in selected patients.
- SPT and measurement of sIgE have a poor positive predictive value in determining offending foods that may be exacerbating eczema. Screening SPT or sIgE (in the absence of immediate reaction to the food(s) in question) is **not** recommended.
- An elimination diet should only be considered after optimisation of topical therapies (moisturising and topical corticosteroid creams) and anti-staphylococcal measures have been implemented. Elimination diets should be supervised by an allergy specialist. Dietary restriction is generally not recommended for children with mild atopic dermatitis.

Allergic rhinitis and conjunctivitis

- Presents with paroxysmal sneezing, itching, congestion and rhinorrhoea (caused by sensitivity to environmental allergens).
- Commonly unrecognised and may impact significantly on quality of life and school performance.
- Traditional classification into *perennial* (throughout the year), *seasonal* (for example, during summer and spring) or *triggered by a specific allergen* (e.g. cats or horses).

- Recent classification uses *persistent* (symptoms for >4 days a week **and** >4 weeks a year) or *intermittent* (symptoms <4 days a week or <4 weeks a year), and as *mild, moderate* or *severe*. Both classification systems may be used in combination.
- Diagnosis requires the demonstration of an allergic basis for symptoms.
- Other causes of rhinitis should be considered: non-allergic rhinitis with eosinophilia syndrome, infective rhinitis, vasomotor rhinitis, hormonal rhinitis or rhinitis medicamentosa (rhinitis induced by excessive use of topical decongestants).

Perennial allergic rhinitis

- Can occur at any age.
- More common than seasonal rhinitis in preschool and primary school children.
- Sneezing and congestion are prominent especially on waking in the morning. There may be significant nasal obstruction and snoring at night.
- House dust mite is the major allergen involved but concurrent sensitivity to pollens is also common.
- Patients with allergic rhinitis and significant nasal obstruction are at risk of obstructive sleep apnoea.

Seasonal allergic rhinitis

- More frequent in teenagers and young adults.
- Seasonal sneezing, itching and rhinorrhoea are prominent. Nasal symptoms are frequently associated with symptoms of itchy, red and watery eyes.
- Symptoms occur in the relevant pollen season.
- In general, trees pollinate in early spring, grasses in the late spring and summer and weeds in the summer and autumn, although there is some overlap. Rye grass is the commonest provoking antigen in Australia, but multiple sensitivities to tree, grass and weed pollens are also observed.

Examination

- Assess the nasal mucosa and nasal airflow (no assessment is complete until the nose is examined).
- Pale, oedematous mucosa and swollen turbinates indicate ongoing rhinitis. In seasonal rhinitis, examination may be normal outside pollen season.

Management

- Second-generation antihistamines (loratadine, desloratadine, cetirizine, levocetirizine) are minimally sedating and can be used as first-line therapy for mild intermittent rhinitis. They are also useful for control of breakthrough rhinitis while on a nasal topical corticosteroid or can be taken prophylactically before an anticipated exposure (e.g. to cats). Terfenadine and astemizole should be avoided as they may cause cardiac arrhythmia when taken with other medications.
- Topical corticosteroid nasal sprays are the treatment of choice for both allergic and non-allergic rhinitis. They are indicated for moderate–severe or persistent symptoms. Continuous use of prescription-strength nasal corticosteroid sprays (refer Table 19.1) are safe and do not suppress the hypothalamic–pituitary–adrenal axis. Local side effects such as epistaxis and irritation can be avoided by directing patients to look down and to aim the nozzle laterally towards the ears.
- The initial course of treatment should be for 2–3 months and patients should be informed that improvements may not be apparent until 3–4 weeks. In seasonal rhinitis, commence treatment 1 month prior to the relevant pollen season and continue over the symptomatic period.
- Allergen avoidance measures may be of benefit to selected patients. Dust mite reduction involves washing bedding in hot water weekly, removing soft toys and soft furnishings from the bed, vacuuming carpet and damp-dusting hard surfaces (including hard flooring) weekly and using allergen-impermeable covers for the mattress, pillow and doona or duvet. Avoidance of grass pollens is challenging and may include closing the house and car windows, having a shower after being outdoors and switching the car's air conditioning to recirculate.
- Immunotherapy involves the systemic administration of house dust mite and/or grass pollen allergen extracts to achieve clinical tolerance and may be considered for patients with refractory disease despite optimal pharmacotherapy. Immunotherapy has traditionally been administered via the subcutaneous injection route, initially with weekly injections at increasing doses until the target dose is achieved (updosing phase), followed by monthly injections for approximately 3 years (maintenance phase). Sublingual immunotherapy involves daily administration of the allergen extract at home with a similar time commitment of 3 years. This route

Table 19.1 Nasal corticosteroids

Nasal corticosteroid spray (generic)	Dose (mcg)	Age indicated for use in seasonal rhinitis	Age indicated for use in perennial rhinitis
Over the counter			
Rhinocort hayfever (budesonide)	32	≥12 year old	≥18 year old
Beconase allergy and hayfever 12 hours (beclomethasone)	50	≥12 year old	≥12 year old
Beconase allergy and hayfever 24 hours (fluticasone propionate)	50	≥12 year old	≥12 year old
Nasonex (mometasone)	50	≥3 year old	≥3 year old
Prescription-only			
Avamys (fluticasone dipropionate) – Dymista (azelastine hydrochloride and fluticasone propionate) – Dose (mcg) = 125/50 – Age indicated for seasonal rhinitis: ≥12 year old – Age indicated for perennial rhinitis: ≥12 year old	27.5	≥2 year old	≥2 year old
Rhinocort (budesonide)	64	≥6 year old	Adults
Omnaris (ciclesonide)	50	≥6 year old	≥12 year old

of administration is widely used in Europe and increasingly used as an alternative to traditional injection immunotherapy in Australia.

Allergic conjunctivitis

Allergic conjunctivitis is commonly associated with allergic rhinitis.

- Occasionally eye symptoms occur in isolation.
- Red, watery, itchy eyes.
- May be persistent or intermittent.

Management

- Eye toilette with normal saline to flush out allergen, cool compresses.
- Oral antihistamine is usually adequate.
- Topical antihistamine eye drops (e.g. Patanol), and combination antihistamine/mast cell stabilisers eye drops (e.g. Zaditen) may be of added benefit.
- Occasionally symptoms may be severe and warrant topical corticosteroid therapy, but this should only be prescribed with caution and in consultation with an allergy specialist or ophthalmologist.

Asthma

See also Chapter 7, *Respiratory conditions*, p. 74.

- Allergic factors may contribute to the symptoms of asthma, particularly in cases of chronic asthma requiring ongoing corticosteroid therapy.
- The major allergens implicated are the indoor inhalants (house dust mite, cat and dog dander). Pollens may also contribute to seasonal exacerbations of asthma, especially if the patient also suffers from seasonal allergic rhinitis. Moulds may trigger asthma symptoms in arid climates.
- Untreated allergic rhinitis can exacerbate asthma and treatment of co-existent allergic rhinitis is likely to benefit asthma control.
- Food does not generally induce asthma symptoms in isolation. They may cause asthma symptoms as part of an immediate allergic reaction (i.e. anaphylaxis) when urticaria is usually also observed.

- In some patients with chronic asthma, NSAIDs (e.g. aspirin) and the preservative metabisulfite can provoke an acute exacerbation. Confirmation of this requires specialist consultation.

Urticaria and angio-oedema

- Urticarial rashes (hives) are characterised by papular, pruritic patches of erythema and oedema.
- Angioedema frequently accompanies urticaria and involves painful, rather than pruritic, swelling in areas of low tension, such as the eyelids, lips and scrotum.
- Hereditary angioedema should be considered in patients who present with isolated angioedema without urticaria (see below).
- Urticaria and angioedema are further classified as either acute (<6 weeks' duration) or chronic (>6 weeks' duration).

Acute urticaria and angioedema

- Acute urticarial reactions to foods generally subside within 24 hours.
- Persistence or recurrence of urticarial rashes for several days is generally not due to food allergy. In the vast majority of these cases, no precipitating factor is identified. Some cases follow an intercurrent viral infection.
- A careful history should be obtained to determine possible exposure to drugs (especially antibiotics) or foods that may have induced an immediate allergic reaction.

Chronic urticaria and angioedema

- Can persist or occur intermittently for months or years.
- The possibility of a physical urticaria (e.g. heat, cold, exercise, cholinergic) should be considered.
- In protracted cases, the possibility of an underlying connective tissue or autoimmune disorder should be considered. In these cases, there are usually other features, including arthritis or vasculitis.
- Chronic urticaria is rarely caused by specific allergic factors and therefore investigation with SPT and sIgE is not helpful.

Treatment

- Second-generation antihistamines are the mainstay of therapy, with cetirizine being particularly effective (for doses see Table 19.2). If patients do not respond to standard dose antihistamines, increase to 2–3× the usual daily dose.
- In resistant cases, refer to a specialist to consider additional therapy with an H_2 antihistamine (ranitidine), or combined H_1 and H_2 antihistamine (doxepin) and/or montelukast.
- Dietary manipulation is not helpful in the vast majority of children.

Hereditary angio-oedema

- Rare autosomal dominant condition in which C1 esterase inhibitor levels are reduced (HAE type I), poorly functional (HAE type II) or normal (HAE type III), resulting in uninhibited activation of the complement, kinin and fibrinolytic cascade.
- This results in recurrent episodes of angio-oedema involving limbs, upper respiratory or gastrointestinal tract. Hence patients present with
  - Angio-oedema **without** pruritus or urticaria.
  - Abdominal pain ± nausea/vomiting (due to intestinal oedema).
  - Laryngeal oedema.
- Diagnosed by the finding of low C1 esterase inhibitor level or function. C4 level is also low during episodes of angio-oedema.

Management

Refer to the Clinical Practice Guideline at *www.rch.org.au/clinical guide* (C1 Esterase Inhibitor Deficiency) and Australasian Society of Clinical Immunology and Allergy (ASCIA) position paper on HAE (www.allergy.org.au).

- Adrenaline, antihistamines and corticosteroids have **no** role in the management.
- Tranexamic acid may be considered in mild episodes to shorten the duration of symptoms.
- Severe angio-oedema episodes can be fatal. Intravenous C1 esterase inhibitor concentrate (Berinert (CSL) or Cinryze (ViroPharma)) should be administered. Icatibant (Firazyr®) is a bradykinin 2 receptor antagonist now

Table 19.2 H₁ antihistamines

Antihistamine type	Common brand name	Doses
Second-generation antihistamines (less-sedating)		
Loratadine	Claratyne (10 mg tablet, 1 mg/mL suspension)	1–2 years: 2.5 mg daily 3–6 years: 5 mg daily >6 years and adults: 30 mg daily
Desloratadine	Aerius (5 mg tablet, 0.5 mg/mL suspension)	6–11 months: 1 mg daily 1–5 years: 1.25 mg daily 6–11 years: 2.5 mg daily ≥12 years and adults: 5 mg daily
Fexofenadine	Telfast (30 mg, 60 mg, 120 mg, 180 mg tablets, 6 mg/mL suspension)	6–23 months: 15 mg b.i.d 2–11 years: 30 mg b.i.d ≥12 years: 120–180 mg daily
Cetirizine	Zyrtec (10 mg tablet, 1 mg/mL suspension, 10 mg/mL drops = 0.5 mg/drop)	2–12 years: • 8–14 kg: 2 mg b.i.d • 14–18 kg: 2.5 mg b.i.d • 18–22 kg: 3 mg b.i.d • 22–26 kg: 3.5 mg b.i.d • 26–30 kg: 4 mg b.i.d • >30 kg: 5 mg b.i.d Adults: 10 mg daily
Levocetirizine	Xyzal (5 mg tablet)	≥12 years and adults: 5 mg daily
First-generation antihistamines (sedating)		
Trimeprazine	Vallergan (1.5 mg/mL suspension) Vallergan Forte (6 mg/mL syrup) Vallergan tablets (10 mg)	Urticaria • ≥2 years: 2.5–5 mg t.d.s or q.i.d • Adults: 10 mg t.d.s or q.i.d (max 100 mg per day) Sedation (eczema) • 3–6 years: 15–60 mg per day • 7–12 years: 60–90 mg per day
Promethazine	Phenergan	Sedation (give 1–2 hours prior to procedure) • 2–12 years: 0.5–1 mg/kg • 12–18 years: 25–75 mg once daily Allergy • 2–12 years: 0.125 mg/kg/dose t.d.s and 0.5 mg/kg nocte • 12–18 years: 10–25 mg 2 or 3 times daily

listed on the Pharmaceutical Benefits Scheme for emergency treatment of acute angioedema in patients with known HAE, and can in suitable circumstances be self-administered at home.
• Children undergoing surgery: preoperative discussions with the anaesthetist, immunologist and intensive care unit are recommended. Depending on the procedure Danazol for 5 days before and 2 days following surgery may be considered. For any procedure requiring intubation, or for tooth extraction, C1 INH concentrate should be given 1–6 hours before the procedure with further doses readily available if needed.

Antibiotic allergy and adverse drug reactions
• Self-reported antibiotic allergy is common, however, formal evaluation is important as the majority of patients can tolerate the medication.
• The most common reported reactions are to the penicillin family.

- Patients with skin-test confirmed penicillin allergy have a 3% chance of reacting to first- and second-generation cephalosporins (third-generation cephalosporins usually tolerated).

History

- Take a careful history, including details of the reaction, severity and its timing in relation to drug dose; prior and subsequent drug exposure; concurrent illness; and other concurrent new food or drug ingestion.
- Check for features of anaphylaxis (cardiovascular and/or respiratory involvement), mucocutaneous involvement (Stevens–Johnson syndrome) or signs of toxic epidermal necrolysis.

Investigation and management

- No reliable *in vitro* or *in vivo* tests for drug allergy are available.
- SPT and sIgE tests for drug allergy have low sensitivity and the majority of patients will require intradermal testing to the penicillin metabolites (major and minor determinants) and amoxicillin (for side chain reactions).
- In the majority of cases, intradermal test results are negative or equivocal, and patients can undergo inpatient oral drug challenge to confirm or exclude allergy.
- In the majority of patients with suspected multiple antibiotic allergies, a challenge to a single antibiotic is done (which is considered appropriate for future treatment).

Insect sting allergy

- Insect sting reactions in Australia commonly occur to honey bees, European wasps and jack jumper ants (Tasmania and regional Victoria).
- Majority of patients present with transient local reactions, while a minority with large, localised or systemic allergic reactions.

Large localised reactions

- Occur in 5–15% of patients.
- Consists of local angioedema and erythema at the sting site, peaking in size at 24–48 hours post-sting, and lasting 1 week or more.
- The risk of a future systemic allergic reaction is 10% and patients can be reassured that no further assessment is indicated.
- Management is symptomatic and includes use of an ice pack, simple analgesia, a second generation antihistamine and a single dose of oral steroid (if significant spreading angio-oedema).
- Antibiotics are rarely required despite extensive swelling.

Systemic allergic reactions

- Occurs in <1% of children and 3% of adults.
- Rapid onset of gastrointestinal, respiratory and/or cardiovascular symptoms.
- The risk of a future systemic allergic reaction is 40–70%.
- Investigate with either SPT, intradermal testing and/or sIgE to confirm sensitisation to the suspected insect.
- Baseline mast cell tryptase is performed to exclude mastocytosis, as patients with this condition are at increased risk of insect sting anaphylaxis.
- Management consists of general sting precautions and provision of an adrenaline autoinjector.
- Specialist referral for venom immunotherapy (VIT) in all patients with insect sting anaphylaxis).

Venom immunotherapy

- VIT commences with an *updosing phase*, where increasing doses of venom are administered via subcutaneous injections until the maintenance dose is achieved over a period of months (traditional protocol), weeks (modified-rush protocol), 2–3 days (rush protocol) or a single day (ultra-rush protocol).
- Because of the risk of anaphylaxis during the updosing phase, these injections are typically administered in a tertiary hospital.
- Patients then undergo a 5-year *maintenance phase* where the injections are provided monthly by their general practitioner.
- After 5 years of VIT, patients have a 10% risk of a systemic allergic reaction.

Latex allergy

- Latex products contain two types of compounds that may cause reactions: chemical additives that cause dermatitis and natural proteins that induce immediate allergic reactions.

- Most reactions to latex in the hospital setting involve disposable gloves.
- Common latex products used in the community include balloons, baby-bottle teats and dummies, elastic bands and condoms.

Irritant dermatitis
- Irritant dermatitis is the most common problem with the use of latex gloves. This is a non-allergic skin rash characterised by erythema, dryness, scaling and cracking.
- Caused by sweating and irritation from the glove or its powder, or by irritation as a result of frequent washing with soap and detergents.

Immediate allergy to latex
- IgE-mediated allergic reactions to latex proteins are serious and potentially life threatening.
- Reactions may occur after contact with latex or the inhalation of airborne powder particles containing latex proteins.
- Sensitisation may occur following direct exposure of mucosal surfaces to latex (e.g. catheterisation).
- Some patients experience cross-reactivity between latex and certain foods (e.g. avocado, kiwi fruit and banana).
- SPTs and/or sIgE testing are useful in confirming suspected allergy.

Contact dermatitis
- Delayed hypersensitivity (Type IV) to chemical additives is used in the processing of latex.
- Reactions are limited to the site of contact (e.g. back of hands from glove exposure).
- Patients with irritant and contact dermatitis are at an increased risk of developing immediate hypersensitivity to latex and exposure to latex should be minimized.

Management
- Patients at high risk for latex sensitivity should be referred to a paediatric allergist/immunologist for further evaluation.
- Patients who have a confirmed latex allergy (either immediate or delayed) should undertake strict latex avoidance including implementation of latex-free precautions during surgery.

Immunodeficiency disorders
When to suspect immunodeficiency
Infections are common in immunocompetent children who average 5–10 viral upper respiratory tract infections per year in the first few years of life (frequently more if the child attends childcare or has older siblings). Recurrent viral infections in a well, thriving child do not suggest immunodeficiency. Immune deficiency should be suspected when there is a history of severe, recurrent or unusual infections particularly when more than one anatomical site is affected.
- Recurrent/chronic bacterial infections or more than one severe pyogenic infection may indicate antibody deficiency.
- Severe or disseminated viral infections, persistent mucocutaneous candidiasis, chronic infectious diarrhoea and/or failure to thrive (FTT) in infants suggest a severe T-cell deficiency. These children should be investigated for severe combined immune deficiency (SCID). The most important warning signs for SCID are FTT, the need for IV antibiotic therapy and a known family history.
- SCID should be managed as a paediatric emergency with urgent referral to an immunologist for further evaluation, management and bone marrow transplant. Immediate isolation in an infection free environment (barrier nursing ideally in a positive pressure ventilation room) should be initiated.
- Beware the infant with persisting lymphopaenia even in the absence of a history of significant infections. Any infant with a reduced lymphocyte count should have their FBE repeated to ensure normalization of previously low lymphocyte counts.
- The presence of autoimmune cytopaenias, together with recurrent sinopulmonary infections, raises the possibility of less severe forms of combined immune deficiency.
- Recurrent pyogenic infections affecting lymph nodes, skin, lung and bones suggest a neutrophil defect.
- Recurrent or severe meningococcal disease suggests a late component complement deficiency.
- Early component complement deficiencies may present with clinical features that are similar to antibody defects or with autoimmune disease.

Investigations if immunodeficiency is suspected

Table 19.3 Primary immunodeficiency workup

Immune defect	Clinical	Pathogens			Investigations
		Bacteria	Viruses	Fungi/parasites	
T cell	FTT	Sepsis	CMV, EBV Severe varicella Resp and GIT	Candida PJP	FBE (NB. Lymphopaenia) IgG, IgA, IgM Lymphocyte markers
B cell	Sinopulmonary suppuration	Strep, Staph H. influenza	Enteroviral encephalitis	Severe giardiasis	FBE IgG, IgA, IgM Specific antibody responses
Neutrophils	Abscess suppuration granuloma	Staphylococcus Pseudomonas Catalase +ve	NA	Candida Aspergillus Nocardia	FBE Neutrophil function
Complement	Sepsis meningitis	Neisseria Strep,	NA	NA	C3, C4 CH100, AH50

Basic immunodeficiency screen

- Investigations should be guided by the clinical presentation (see Table 19.3).
- An FBE with differential and immunoglobulin levels (IgG, IgA and IgM) will identify the vast majority of treatable primary immunodeficiencies (e.g. agammaglobulinaemia, common variable immune deficiency, selective IgA deficiency and SCID). IgG subclass levels should **not** be done as part of a basic immunological screen, as isolated IgG subclass deficiency is of uncertain clinical significance.
- Note that immunoglobulin levels vary with age and are lower in infancy and early childhood. It is therefore important that the relevant age-related reference ranges are used (see Table 19.4). In the first months of life

Table 19.4 Immunoglobulin normal ranges (5th to 95th percentile)

Age	IgG (g/L)	IgA (g/L)	IgM (g/L)
0–1 month	2.5–12.0	<0.07–0.94	0.19–1.93
1–2 months	2.5–12.0	<0.07–1.31	0.19–1.93
2–3 months	2.5–12.0	<0.07–1.31	0.21–1.92
3–4 months	2.86–16.8	<0.07–1.31	0.21–1.92
4–12 months	2.86–16.8	0.1–1.29	0.21–1.92
1–2 years	2.86–16.8	0.19–1.75	0.43–1.63
2–3 years	3.41–19.6	0.22–2.20	0.43–1.63
3–4 years	3.41–19.6	0.48–3.45	0.43–1.63
4–5 years	5.28–21.9	0.61–3.45	0.48–2.26
5–6 years	5.28–21.9	0.43–2.53	0.48–2.26
6–7 years	5.28–21.9	0.41–2.97	0.48–2.26
7–10 years	5.28–21.9	0.51–2.97	0.48–2.26
10–13 years	5.28–21.9	0.44–3.95	0.48–2.26
13–19 years	5.28–21.9	0.44–4.41	0.48–2.26

Source: Davis ML, Austin C, Messmer BL, Nichols WK, Bonin AP, Bennett MJ. IFCC-standardised pediatric reference intervals for 10 serum proteins using the Beckman Array 360 system. Clinical Biochemistry. 1996; 29(5): 489–492. (South 2012. Reproduced with permission of Elsevier.)

IgG levels reflect maternally acquired IgG and a normal IgG at this time does not exclude a severe antibody deficiency disorder.

- If these tests are normal and the clinical suspicion of immune deficiency persists, referral to a clinical immunologist for further evaluation is indicated.

Specific antibody responses

- Should be considered when there is evidence of persistent or recurrent suppurative upper and/or lower respiratory tract infection and hypogammaglobulinaemia has been excluded.
- Can be evaluated by examination of specific antibody production pre-immunization and 4 weeks post immunization with the unconjugated pneumococcal vaccine, Pneumovax R.
- In general, regular gammaglobulin therapy is only indicated for severe recurrent infections despite appropriate antibiotic therapy when a specific antibody defect has been identified.

T-lymphocyte numbers and function

- Consider a chest x-ray to look for absent thymic shadow when a T-lymphocyte defect is suspected.
- Lymphocyte markers for T cells (CD3, total T cells; CD4, T Helper cells, CD8, Cytotoxic T cells), B cells (CD19), and NK cells (CD56) should be evaluated where a significant PID is suspected.
- Naïve T cell (CD45RA+) evaluation is a useful test where a severe T cell defect is suspected.
- Specialised T-lymphocyte function tests are used to help in the diagnosis of SCID and Di George syndrome (absent thymus, hypocalcaemia and cardiovascular anomalies). Referral to an immunologist is indicated if these conditions are suspected.

Neutrophil function tests

- Specific defects of neutrophil function (e.g. chronic granulomatous disease and leucocyte adhesion deficiency 1) are very rare. They are almost always associated with gingivitis and careful examination of the mouth is important when considering abnormalities of neutrophil function.
- Markedly elevated circulating neutrophil counts and delayed separation of the umbilical cord (>4 weeks) suggest the possibility of a leucocyte adhesion deficiency.
- Suspected cases of defective neutrophil function should be referred to an immunologist for further evaluation.

Complement studies

- Deficiencies of complement are rare.
- Should be suspected in patients presenting with overwhelming sepsis, severe complicated pneumonia or severe meningitis.
- The best screening test for congenital deficiency is a CH50, which measures the function of the classical complement pathway and AH50 which measures the function of the alternative complement pathway.

Evaluation of haemophagocytic lymphohistiocytosis

Haemophagocytic lymphohistiocytosis (HLH) is a rare life-threatening disease of severe hyperinflammation caused by uncontrolled proliferation of activated lymphocytes and macrophages secreting high amounts of inflammatory cytokines. It frequently manifests in patients with predisposing genetic defects, but can occur secondary to various infectious, malignant, and autoimmune triggers in patients without a known genetic predisposition. Impaired secretion of perforin is a key feature in several genetic forms of the disease, but not required for disease pathogenesis.

Diagnostic criteria for HLH

Molecular diagnosis consistent with HLH or five out of eight following criteria:

1. Fever
2. Splenomegaly
3. Cytopenias in two out of three cell lines (haemoglobin <9 mg/dL (<10 mg/dL in infants <4 weeks old), platelets <100,000/μL, neutrophils <1000/μL)
4. Hypertriglyceridemia (fasting triglycerides ≥265 mg/dL) and/or hypofibrinogenemia (fibrinogen ≤1.5 g/L)
5. Haemophagocytosis in bone marrow, spleen, lymph nodes, or liver
6. Ferritin >500 ng/mL
7. Soluble CD25 >2400 U/mL
8. Decreased or absent natural killer cell cytotoxicity

Increasingly atypical variants presenting with signs of chronic immunodeficiency are being recognised.

HLH is an immunologic emergency requiring an aggressive chemotherapy regimen to achieve disease control. Despite progress in diagnostics and therapy, mortality of patients with severe HLH is still above 40%.

HIV tests

HIV infection is rare in the Australian population. HIV testing should be considered in the setting of recurrent, severe or unusual infections, particularly if there is hypergammaglobulinaemia. Testing requires informed consent and appropriate counselling. This specialised immune function testing is best undertaken in consultation with a clinical immunologist. See also Chapter 18, *Infectious diseases and immunisation*.

Immunodeficiency treatment
Immunisation
See also Chapter 18, *Infectious diseases and immunisation*.
- As a general rule, all live viral vaccines should be avoided in immunodeficiency unless advised by a specialist.
- Patients with a T-cell defect and their immediate family should receive the killed injectable polio (Salk) vaccine, not live oral polio vaccine. This is now the standard form of polio vaccine in Australia.
- In certain circumstances, measles immunisation may be given to patients with a T-cell defect (e.g. Di George syndrome or paediatric HIV infection) as the risks of wild-type measles infection are considerable, but adverse reactions to the vaccine are largely theoretical.
- In cases of antibody deficiency, T-cell deficiency and combined immunodeficiency, immunisation with killed vaccines will not promote a significant antibody response.
- If the patient is on immunoglobulin replacement therapy (IRT), passively acquired antibody will prevent viral infections such as measles and chickenpox. See also Chapter 18, *Infectious diseases and immunisation*.
- Patients of any age with asplenia should be immunised with Hib, pneumococcal and meningococcal vaccines.

Immunoglobulin replacement therapy
- IRT (400–600 mg/kg IV monthly or subcutaneously in divided dosage administered at home weekly) is given when a significant deficiency of antibody production is demonstrated in a patient with clinically significant infections (usually sinopulmonary).
- In hypogammaglobulinaemia, IRT is generally lifelong.
- In patients with a severe combined immunodeficiency, IRT may be discontinued once normal B-cell function can be demonstrated following bone marrow transplantation.

Antibiotics
- As IRT does not provide significant levels of IgA antibody (the mucosal surface antibody), aggressive treatment of respiratory infections in patients with antibody deficiency is important in order to prevent bronchiectasis and permanent damage to the lungs.
- In severe cases or those with end organ damage (e.g. bronchiectasis), long-term prophylactic antibiotics are used to prevent recurrent severe sinopulmonary infections.
- Antibiotic prophylaxis with cotrimoxazole 2.5/12.5 mg/kg (max. 80/400) p.o. b.d. 3 days per week is indicated in patients with T-cell or combined immune deficiency to prevent infection with pneumocystis.

Use of blood products
- If it is suspected or known that the patient has a significant T-cell deficiency, blood products that contain cells (e.g. whole blood, packed red cells or platelets) should be irradiated to prevent graft versus host disease.
- In infants with SCID or any significant T-cell deficiency, attempts should be made to provide cytomegalovirus (CMV) antibody-negative blood, as CMV infection can be a significant problem in such patients. If this is not possible, the blood product should be filtered to remove contaminating white blood cells as it is delivered to the patient.

Immunological assessment and monitoring in patients receiving rituximab
- Rituximab is a monoclonal antibody that binds the CD20 molecule on B cells resulting in depletion of precursor, naïve and memory B cells. It is a therapy that is being increasingly used to treat a number of autoimmune and inflammatory conditions. Prior to initiation of rituximab therapy, assessment of B cell numbers and IgG, IgA and IgM levels is recommended.

- Following a single infusion of rituximab, B cell regeneration can take months to years and in some patients may never occur. This can result in a secondary antibody deficiency disorder.

Haematopoietic stem cell transplantation (HSCT)

- HSCT is the definitive treatment for SCID. It may also be useful for the treatment of other immune deficiencies (e.g. chronic granulomatous disease, hyper IgM syndrome).
- HSCT sources include bone marrow, cord blood or peripheral blood stem cells. Donors may be HLA matched related donors or unrelated donors from cord cell banks and bone marrow donor registries nationally and internationally.
- The cure rate can be 80–90% if the transplant is from a matched sibling or a parent.
- Survival is about 50% if the transplant is only partially matched and from an unrelated donor.

USEFUL RESOURCES
- *www.allergy.org.au* – The Australian Society of Clinical Allergy and Immunology. Contains excellent information for patients and health care professionals. Includes anaphylaxis action plans.
- *www.primaryimmune.org* – Immune Deficiency Foundation. Patient organisation website containing excellent handouts for primary immune deficiencies.
- *www.esid.org* – European Society for Immunodeficiencies. Contains a useful clinical section which details diagnostic criteria of various primary immunodeficiencies.

CHAPTER 20

Genetics and metabolics

David Amor
Joy Lee

Modes of inheritance (see Table 20.1)

Approach to the diagnosis of genetic syndromes
Important features on history
In addition to pregnancy, birth, neonatal and developmental histories, the following should be included:

- Family history: birth defects, miscarriage, neonatal death, consanguinity. Draw a family tree including minimum of three generations.
- Organ defects (e.g. congenital heart disease, renal malformations) and medical problems, for example seizures.
- Growth history.
- Hearing and vision.
- Evidence of progression of symptoms or developmental regression.
- Behavioural problems: autistic features, self-harm, aggression, sleep disturbance.

Important features on examination
- Growth parameters (height, weight, head circumference), relative proportions.
- Dysmorphic features. Describe overall impression and specifically note head shape, ears, eyes, nose, philtrum, mouth, lips, tongue, palate, dentition, chin, chest wall.
- Hands and feet. Describe fingers and toes (number, size, shape). Note palmar and plantar creases, nails.
- Skin abnormalities. Note birth marks, pigmentary abnormalities, neurocutaneous stigmata, skin texture, hair.
- Nervous system. Note gait, muscle tone (hypotonia, spasticity), reflexes, behaviour.
- Abdomen. Note hepatosplenomegaly, male genitalia.
- Skeleton. Note scoliosis, joint mobility.
- Consider patient photographs, which can aid in diagnosis.

Investigations
- Chromosome analysis.
  - Chromosome microarray (CMA) has now replaced microscope chromosome analysis and fluorescence *in situ* hybridisation testing for nearly all paediatric indications. CMA detects pathogenic abnormalities in approximately 15% of children with cognitive impairment, autism spectrum disorders or multiple congenital abnormalities; however because of its high resolution CMA also detects abnormalities of unknown significance, abnormalities with incomplete penetrance, and incidental findings.
- Fragile X testing should be undertaken in all males and females with cognitive impairment.
- Metabolic tests are especially important in the setting of a history of regression or progression of symptoms, seizures, hepatosplenomegaly, periodicity of symptoms, or microcephaly.
- Specific genetic tests are helpful to confirm the diagnosis of many single gene disorders; however, sequencing of single genes remains expensive.
- Next-generation sequencing is a new technology that allows the simultaneous and cost-effective testing of large numbers of individual genes or even the whole genome. A number of disease-specific next-generation

Paediatric Handbook, Ninth Edition. Edited by Amanda Gwee, Romi Rimer and Michael Marks.
© 2015 John Wiley & Sons, Ltd. Published 2015 by John Wiley & Sons, Ltd.

Table 20.1 Modes of inheritance

Inheritance	Mechanism	Main features	Examples
Autosomal dominant	A mutation in one copy of a gene (located on an autosome) is sufficient to cause disease	<ul><li>No difference whether you are male or female</li><li>A 50% chance that a child will inherit the gene mutation from a parent with it</li><li>There may be incomplete *penetrance*, variable *expressivity*</li><li>A single affected person in a family may have a *de novo* mutation</li></ul>	Marfan syndrome Neurofibromatosis Tuberous sclerosis Achondroplasia
Autosomal recessive	Mutations in both copies of a gene (located on an autosome) are necessary to cause disease	<ul><li>No difference whether you are male or female</li><li>Both parents must carry gene mutations in the same gene for their children to be at risk</li><li>If both parents carry the mutation each child has a 25% chance of inheriting the disease</li></ul>	Cystic fibrosis Thalassaemia Spinal muscular atrophy Phenylketonuria
X-linked	The disease gene is located on the X chromosome *X-linked recessive:* female carriers show no phenotype *X-linked dominant:* female carriers show a phenotype	<ul><li>Affected males linked by unaffected/mildly affected females</li><li>*Transmission from female carrier:* 50% of sons will be affected; 50% of daughters will be carriers</li><li>*Transmission from affected males:* 100% of daughters will be carriers; no sons will be affected</li></ul>	Duchenne muscular dystrophy Fragile X syndrome Haemophilia A G6PD deficiency
Polygenic	Multiple genes play an additive role in the development of a disease	<ul><li>These conditions cluster in families but do not follow predictable inheritance patterns</li><li>Environmental factors often contribute to disease development</li></ul>	Autism Hypertension Type 2 diabetes Schizophrenia
Mitochondrial	Mutations in the *mitochondrial* genome follow matrilineal inheritance	<ul><li>Affected mothers pass on the mutation to all children</li><li>Males cannot pass on the disorder</li><li>Variable expressivity is common</li></ul>	Leber hereditary optic neuropathy

sequencing gene panels are now available. An alternative approach is to sequence the 'exome', comprising the parts of the genome that code for protein.

- Brain imaging by MRI should be undertaken when developmental delay is associated with microcephaly, macrocephaly, seizures, focal neurological signs, or developmental regression.
- Skeletal survey should be considered in the setting of short stature, disproportionate growth, bone malformations or fractures associated with minimal trauma.
- Consider genetics consultation for the following reasons:
  - To provide an accurate diagnosis
  - To help understand aetiology
  - To guide investigations
  - To advise about prognosis
  - To guide management and possible therapeutic interventions
  - To discuss recurrence risk in a future pregnancy
  - To discuss options for prenatal diagnosis

  Common genetic syndromes (see Tables 20.2 and 20.3)

Metabolic conditions

Metabolic disorders, whilst individually rare, collectively represent an important cause of paediatric morbidity and mortality. The majority of metabolic disorders are inherited in an autosomal recessive manner. The clinical presentation can be easily confused with common acquired conditions. A high index of suspicion is therefore important.

Approach to the diagnosis of a metabolic disorder

Important features on history

In addition to pregnancy, birth, neonatal and developmental histories, the following should be included:

- Maternal history – for example HELLP syndrome (foetus may have a fatty acid oxidation disorder), diet and nutritional status (vegetarian/vegan diet causing low carnitine or B12 levels)
- Family history – consanguinity, ethnicity, Sudden Infant Death Syndrome (SIDS), unexplained deaths
- Dietary – aversions, food intake in relation to onset of symptoms
- Review of organ systems
- Progression of symptoms, developmental regression, diurnal patterns, recurrent unexplained symptoms (vomiting, ataxia, respiratory symptoms), presence of precipitating factors (infection, prolonged fasting, surgery, or certain medications), unusual smell and urine colour, for example black urine in alkaptonuria

Clinical Presentation (signs and symptoms)

Metabolic disorders can present for the first time at any age. The presentation may be non-specific and there is often variability in presentations, even within families. A review of organ systems is important since most metabolic disorders involve more than one organ system. The pattern of abnormalities and degree of organ involvement may suggest a specific metabolic disorder. Common clinical presentations of some metabolic disorders are shown in Table 20.4.

Laboratory investigations

Metabolites indicative of a metabolic diagnosis are best detected at the time of the acute presentation and may normalise between events. Therefore, blood and urine samples collected **at the time of presentation** are most valuable. Proper collection and handling of these samples is important. However, collection of samples should not delay management of patients in critical situations.

The first line metabolic investigations include

- Blood – acid base, glucose, lactate, ammonia, plasma amino acids (AA), Guthrie card acylcarnitine (do not put in a plastic specimen bag). See http://ww2.rch.org.au/specimen/ for specimen collection handbook.
- Urine – smell, pH, glucose, ketones, urine-reducing substances, amino acids, organic acids and glycosaminoglycans screen.
- Ancillary – FBE, LFT, U&E, CK, uric acid, cholesterol, triglycerides.

  Note: collect and freeze extra urine and plasma samples.

  Interpretation of some of these tests is shown in Table 20.5.

Table 20.2 Common genetic syndromes

	Clinical features	Key management points	Genetics
Down syndrome	Hypotonia, small ears, upslanting palpebral fissures, flat facial profile, brachycephaly, congenital heart disease (40–50%), intellectual disability, hypothyroidism (20–40%), acute leukaemia (2%), dementia in fifth to sixth decade	Early developmental intervention and educational support. Regular paediatric follow-up and surveillance for complications See Table 20.3	Additional chromosome 21, usually sporadic. Two per cent result from Robertsonian translocation of which 50% are familial. Mosaic Down syndrome accounts for another 2% of cases and typically has a less severe phenotype
Trisomy 18	Growth retardation, dysmorphism (prominent occiput, simple ears, overlapping fingers, rocker bottom feet, short sternum), congenital heart disease (>90%), short life expectancy, profound disability in survivors	Supportive care	Additional chromosome 18, usually sporadic.
Trisomy 13	Growth retardation, holoprosencephaly, scalp defects, cleft lip/palate, congenital heart disease, polydactyly, short life expectancy, profound disability in survivors	Supportive care	Additional chromosome 13, usually sporadic
Klinefelter syndrome	Infertility, small testes, testosterone insufficiency, tall stature, learning difficulties in some	Testosterone replacement from around 10 years. Monitor development and behaviour. Assisted reproduction	Karyotype 47,XXY. Sporadic
Fragile X syndrome	Moderate intellectual disability in males and mild intellectual disability in females. Males may have a characteristic appearance (large head, long face, prominent forehead and chin, protruding ears), joint laxity, and large testes after puberty. Features of autism spectrum disorder are common.	Early developmental intervention and educational support.	Expansion of CGG trinucleotide repeat in FMR1 gene on the X chromosome. Fragile X full mutation is >200 repeats
Noonan syndrome	Early feeding difficulties, short stature, pulmonary stenosis (20–50%), hypertrophic cardiomyopathy (20–30%), variable developmental delay, webbed neck, sternum abnormality, cryptorchidism, characteristic facies.	Treat cardiovascular complications. Early developmental intervention and educational support.	Heterozygous mutation (de novo or inherited) in one of several genes including PTPN11, SOS1
Velocardiofacial syndrome (22q11.2 deletion syndrome)	Highly variable, but include learning difficulties (70%), congenital heart disease (75%), cleft palate (10%), major abnormal immune dysfunction (1%), neonatal hypocalcaemia (60%), subtle dysmorphism (short palpebral fissures, prominent nasal bridge, rounded ears)	Early developmental intervention and educational support. Surveillance for complications	Microdeletion at chromosome 22q11.2. Usually de novo but 7% inherited from a parent who may be mildly affected

(continued)

Table 20.2 (Continued)

	Clinical features	Key management points	Genetics
Williams syndrome	Feeding difficulties in infancy, supravalvular aortic stenosis, distinctive facies, mild intellectual disability with unique personality characteristics, hypercalcaemia	Early developmental intervention and educational support. Surveillance for complications	Microdeletion at chromosome 7q11.2 (de novo)
Prader–Willi syndrome	Severe hypotonia and feeding difficulties in infancy, followed by excessive eating and development of morbid obesity (unless eating is controlled). Variable cognitive impairment and obsessive-compulsive characteristics, hypogonadism, incomplete pubertal development, short stature	Strict supervision of daily food intake. Early developmental intervention and educational support.	Microdeletion at chromosome 15q11.2-q13 (de novo on paternal chromosome) or maternal UPD of chromosome 15
Angelman syndrome	Intellectual disability, severe speech impairment, gait ataxia, microcephaly, seizures, frequent laughing, smiling, and excitability	Early developmental intervention and educational support	Microdeletion at chromosome 15q11.2-q13 (de novo on maternal chromosome) or paternal UPD of chromosome 15 or mutation in the gene UBE3 A
Beckwith–Wiedemann syndrome	Macrosomia, macroglossia, embryonal tumours (Wilms tumour, hepatoblastoma, neuroblastoma, and rhabdomyosarcoma), omphalocele, neonatal hypoglycaemia, ear creases/pits, hemihyperplasia	Tumour surveillance: abdominal ultrasound every 3 months until age 8 years. Serum alpha fetoprotein every 3 months until age 4 years.	Abnormal imprinting or UPD of chromosome 11p.
Achondroplasia	Short limbs, large head, frontal bossing and midface retrusion. Normal intelligence	Regular surveillance for complications, including craniocervical junction compression, obstructive sleep apnoea, middle ear dysfunction, bowed legs	Heterozygous mutation (de novo or inherited) in FGFR3 gene
Neurofibromatosis type 1 (NF1)	Multiple café au lait spots, axillary and inguinal freckling, multiple cutaneous neurofibromas, iris Lisch nodules, learning difficulties (50%)	Regular surveillance for complications including plexiform neurofibromas, optic nerve gliomas, central nervous system gliomas, malignant peripheral nerve sheath tumours, scoliosis	Heterozygous mutation (de novo or inherited) in NF1 gene
Marfan syndrome	Skeletal manifestation: long limbs, scoliosis, sternum deformity, joint laxity. Eye manifestations: lens dislocation (60%) and myopia. Cardiovascular manifestations: dilatation of the aorta, predisposition for aortic rupture, mitral valve and tricuspid valve prolapsed.	Surveillance for eye and cardiac manifestations. Medication to reduce haemodynamic stress on aortic wall (e.g. beta blockers). Surgical repair of aorta when maximum diameter reaches ~5 cm. Avoid contact sports	Heterozygous mutation (de novo or inherited) in FBN1 gene

Table 20.3 Routine screening for children with Down syndrome at different ages

	Prenatal	Birth to 1 month	1 month to 1 year	1–5 years	5–13 years	13–21 years
Counselling regarding prenatal diagnosis results						
Plan for delivery						
Referral to geneticist						
Physical exam for evidence of trisomy 21 with particular attention to cardiac, gastrointestinal and ophthalmologic examinations						
Chromosomal analysis to confirm diagnosis						
Offer genetic counselling – discuss risk of recurrence of Down syndrome						
ECG		Prior to discharge after birth				
Echocardiogram done by a *paediatric* cardiologist Note that serious cardiac disease can be missed on physical examination						
Radiographic swallowing assessment if marked hypotonia, poor feeding, possible aspiration						
Newborn hearing screen and follow-up						
Audiology and ENT assessment			6 and 12 months		Annual	
History and examination for duodenal or anorectal atresia						
If constipated, evaluate dietary intake. Consider hypotonia, hypothyroidism, GI anomalies, Hirschsprung's disease			Any visit			

(continued)

Table 20.3 *(Continued)*

	Prenatal	Birth to 1 month	1 month to 1 year	1–5 years	5–13 years	13–21 years
Full blood examination				Annual		
TSH (may be part of newborn screening)	As part of newborn screen		6 and 12 months		Annual	
Discuss atlanto-axial instability with parents and monitor for evidence of myelopathy. See http://www.dsmig.org.uk/library/articles/CSI%20revision%20final%202012.pdf				Any visit		
Assess for symptoms of obstructive sleep apnoea and consider polysomnography				Any visit		
Ophthalmology assessment			Annually		Every 2 years	Every 3 years
If congenital heart disease, monitor for signs and symptoms of congestive heart failure			All visits			
Screen for symptoms of coeliac disease					Annual	
Assess developmental progress. Early referral to Early Childhood Intervention Services				All visits		
Assess behavioural issues						
Establish optimal dietary and physical exercise patterns						
Discuss physical and psychosocial changes though puberty, need for gynaecologic care in the pubescent female, sexual development and behaviours						
Facilitate transition: guardianship, financial planning, behavioural problems, school placement, vocational training, independence with self-care						

Table 20.4   Clinical features suggestive of a metabolic disease

Age	Clinical symptoms and signs	Possible diagnosis
Neonatal to infancy	Acute encephalopathy[a] Vomiting, feeding refusal Lethargy or irritability Changes in respiration Hypo/hypertonia, seizures Altered conscious state	Aminoacidopathies, For example maple syrup urine disease (MSUD) Organic acidurias (OA) Urea cycle disorders (UCD) Fatty acid oxidation disorders (FAOD) Mitochondrial disorders
	Liver dysfunction, prolonged cholestatic jaundice, hepatomegaly, hypoglycaemia, +/− kidney dysfunction	Galactosaemia Tyrosinaemia I Hereditary fructose intolerance Glycogen storage disorders (GSD) Certain FAOD Disorders in ketogenesis Bile acid defects Mitochondrial disorders
	Seizures as a predominant feature	Pyridoxine responsive seizures Pyridoxal 5 phosphate responsive seizures Glucose transporter defect I Biotinidase deficiency Nonketotic hyperglycinaemia
Early to late childhood	Psychomotor delay, regression, seizures Behavioural problems, learning difficulties Psychiatric symptoms, ataxia Stroke-like episodes, movement disorder	Aminoacidopathies, for example classic homocystinuria Organic acidurias (OA) Urea cycle disorders (UCD) Lysosomal storage disorders, for example mucopolysaccharidosis Disorders of creatine metabolism Disorders of purine and pyrimidine X-linked adrenoleukodystrophy Mitochondrial disorders Congenital disorders of glycosylation
	Cardiac (conduction defects cardiomyopathy) +/− rhabdomyolysis, muscle pain	Certain GSD, for example GSD III or GSD V Pompe disease Certain FAOD Mitochondrial disorders
	Dysmorphism, progressive symptoms +/− other systems: hepatomegaly, splenomegaly, cherry red spot, obstructive sleep apnoea, hair, skin and skeletal changes	Biosynthetic defects, for example Smith–Lemli–Opitz Peroxisomal disorders Lysosomal storage disorders, for example mucopolysaccharidosis

[a]Can present at ANY AGE and usually precipitated by infections, prolonged fasting, large protein meal or changes in diet.

Second tier of metabolic investigations include **(always discuss with a metabolic physician)**
- Paired blood/CSF for glucose, AA, lactate, pyruvate (lumbar puncture should be done in fasting state and blood should be collected first to avoid stress-related hyperglycaemia)
- CSF neurotransmitters
- Serum transferrin isoforms; Biotinidase testing; Galactoscreen
- Lysosomal enzymes testing; Very long chain fatty acids and phytanic acid
- Urine for: bile acids, creatine and guanidinoacetic acid, purines and pyrimidines

Table 20.5 Interpretation of results

Metabolic condition	Glucose	Lactate	Metabolic acidosis	Ammonia	Anion gap[b]	Urine ketones
Mitochondrial disorder	N	Usually very high	Usually present	N	May be increased	Negative
MSUD	Low or N	N	Variably present	N	May be increased	Positive
OA	Low or N	May be high	Very acidotic	May be high	Usually increased	Positive
FAOD	Low or N	May be high	Variably present	May be high	May be increased	Negative or low[a]
UCD	N	N	No	Very high	N	Negative

N, normal.

[a] Inappropriately low.

[b] Calculate by using Na- (Chloride + Bicarbonate). Normal <16 mmol/L.

Management of metabolic disorders (always discuss with a metabolic physician)

Treatment principles

- In the acute setting, stop the intake of potentially toxic compounds (e.g. protein, galactose, fructose).
- Avoid catabolism, which can lead to further accumulation of toxic metabolites, by providing sufficient calories in the form of glucose and fat. Do not use more than 5% dextrose for suspected mitochondrial disorders to prevent exacerbation of lactic acidosis.
- Increase the disposal of toxic metabolites by giving certain medications. Haemofiltration in severe cases, for example rapid neurological deterioration.
- Enhance enzymatic activity by providing vitamins and cofactors.

Management should also include proper hydration, antibiotic cover as needed, and avoidance of certain medications (e.g. phenylalanine containing for PKU; valproic acid for urea cycle disorders, fatty acid oxidation disorders and mitochondrial disorders).

Expanded newborn screening by tandem mass spectrometry

The sample is collected on day 2 or 3 of life. There are more than 20 metabolic conditions included on the screen (e.g. aminoacidopathies, fatty acid oxidation disorders and organic acidurias). This is a screening test, not a diagnostic test. Further follow-up and confirmatory testing are required. Newborn screen does not detect all disorders reliably and will miss certain disorders (e.g. certain urea cycle disorders, Tyrosinaemia I). Screening for galactosaemia is not included in Victoria.

Post-mortem samples

Urgent tissue collection after death for suspected metabolic disease [This is not a replacement for full autopsy which should be requested if the diagnosis is unclear.]:

- Collect samples as soon as possible after death, preferably within 2 hours.
- Note the time between death and freezing or collection of the samples.
- Obtain blood, urine, CSF and bile samples, if possible for further metabolic analysis. A vitreous humour specimen should be obtained if urine is unavailable.
- Collect blood on Guthrie cards (1–2) for biochemical testing and source of DNA.
- Obtain a skin biopsy for fibroblast culture. One piece of full-thickness skin (2–3 mm surface diameter) in a tissue culture medium bottle, or a viral medium bottle or sterile container with normal saline without preservatives. Store in a refrigerator at 4°C. *Do not freeze this sample.*
- Tissue biopsies for enzyme testing should be placed in aluminium foil or Parafilm®, frozen immediately (on dry ice) and put in screw-cap tubes. Store in a freezer at −70°C. Note the time of sampling.
- Tissue biopsies for light microscopy should be placed in a formalin bottle. Store at room temperature.

- Tissue biopsies for electron microscopy should be cut down to small pieces (1–2 mm in diameter) and placed in a glutaraldehyde bottle. Store in a refrigerator at 4°C. *Do not freeze this sample.*
- Muscle samples are preferably from the quadriceps. If the parents object to the two incisions (the muscle and liver), suggest a right upper quadrant incision to take samples from the liver, rectus muscle and skin biopsy.
- Blood for DNA tests: 10 mL of EDTA blood (no mixing beads or separating gel) can be sent at room temperature if they are expected in the laboratory within 24 hours or store in a refrigerator at 4°C until sent to the molecular laboratory.

Acknowledgements

I would like to acknowledge Associate Prof. Avihu Boneh as previous author and Dr. Heidi Peters for reviewing the section and for her suggestions.

USEFUL RESOURCES
- Paediatric Pharmacopoeia 13th edition
- RCH Specimen Collection Handbook
- Victorian Clinical Genetics Service (VCGS) Website: Metabolic Screening, Tests and Collection
- Genereviews and Emedicine websites

CHAPTER 21

Neonatal conditions

Rod Hunt

Routine care

The vast majority of deliveries are uncomplicated and do not require medical intervention.

The first minutes

Establishing breathing

The major stimuli to start breathing include cooling of the face and physical stimulation as well as hypoxia and acidosis. Babies usually start breathing within seconds of birth. If the baby is not breathing, drying with a towel is a very effective stimulus.

Heat loss after birth

Evaporative cooling occurs very quickly after birth. It is minimised by drying and wrapping the baby in warm towels. A well, term infant will be kept warm by being swaddled and cuddled by the mother. Early contact helps with establishing bonding and breastfeeding. The baby's rectal temperature should stabilise around 37°C (+/−0.3°C) by 1 hour of age. If a baby becomes cold, he/she may need controlled warming under a radiant heater or in an incubator and should be assessed for illness. Both hypothermia and hyperthermia should be avoided and when present, may be the first signs of being unwell.

The umbilical cord

This is clamped and cut cleanly close to the skin just after birth. The cut end and the base of the cord must be kept clean and dry. Bathing with clean water is usually all that is required. Antiseptic solution, such as chlorhexidine in alcohol, may be applied daily until the cord stump drops off. The plastic clamp can be removed after 2 days. Failure of the cord to detach after 7 days may indicate leukocyte adhesion deficiency.

The first hours

Once the infant's temperature is stable, he/she can be washed with soap and water. There is no hurry to do this. Record the heart rate, colour, respiratory rate and effort, at intervals depending on the infant's condition. Often the baby will be alert and breastfeeds should be started at these times.

Vitamin K

All infants, regardless of size, maturity, or health status, should receive vitamin K mixed micelles (Konakion) 0.1 mL intramuscularly. This eradicates haemorrhagic disease of the newborn. An increased incidence of both early and late haemorrhagic disease of the newborn occurs in breastfed infants who have received either an oral or inadequate IM dose, or no prophylactic vitamin K. Parents who insist on their infant having oral vitamin K must be given instructions that it must be given for 3 doses at 2-weekly intervals from birth.

The first day

After an initial period of alertness a healthy newborn will often sleep for long periods and may not be too demanding with feeds. However, the infant must

- Suck and swallow easily: if he/she does not, consider unrecognised prematurity, a congenital abnormality, hypoglycaemia or infection.
- Pass urine: this often occurs at birth without being noticed. If a boy does not pass urine in the first 24 hours, consider posterior urethral valves.
- Pass meconium within the first 48 hours: if not, consider bowel obstruction or Hirschsprung disease.

Paediatric Handbook, Ninth Edition. Edited by Amanda Gwee, Romi Rimer and Michael Marks.
© 2015 John Wiley & Sons, Ltd. Published 2015 by John Wiley & Sons, Ltd.

The first examination

The purpose of this examination is to detect congenital abnormalities, reassure the parents and to discuss their concerns. Most major abnormalities will have been seen on antenatal ultrasound, but not all.

- Observation: before disturbing the baby observe the posture, behaviour, general appearance, colour and well-being.
- Chest: while the baby is quiet examine the heart sounds, rate, presence of femoral pulses and the pulse characteristics. Many babies have a very soft murmur in the first few days. If it sounds pathological, is associated with other signs or persists, then refer to a cardiologist. Normal babies breathe so shallowly when they are sleeping that it can be difficult to see. Tachypnoea, recession and laboured breathing are the most important signs of respiratory distress. In babies the depth of each breath can be very variable.
- Head and neck: look for scalp defects; fractures; haematomas; lacerations; eye size, anatomy and red reflex; neck cysts, lumps or fistulae; cleft palate; tongue size and shape; ear position, shape, size and tags or fistulae and facial symmetry when crying. A cephalohaematoma is a soft boggy swelling over one bone (usually the parietal) due to blood under the periosteum. It needs no treatment. **Beware of a generalised boggy swelling all over the scalp in a shocked baby**. This may be a subgaleal haemorrhage and is a neonatal emergency as babies can bleed profusely into them.
- Abdomen: feel for masses (liver, spleen, kidneys, bladder and ovaries), distension and tenderness. Examine the genitalia, anus and inguinal and umbilical region for herniae. The umbilicus should be clean and dry. The liver is often just palpable or percussible in normal babies.
- Limbs: examine for abnormal fingers, hands, toes and feet; posture of the hands and feet; and the flexibility of the joints.
- Hips: carefully examine for congenital dislocation by observation and specific manoeuvres. (See Chapter 15, *Bones and joints*, p. 220.)
- Measurement: naked weight, length and head circumference should be recorded and plotted on the growth chart in the baby's record book.

The first week

- Feeding: will be established during this time. After an initial phase of waking frequently until lactation is established, the breastfed baby should establish a regular cycle of waking for feeds, followed mostly by sleeping. However even in the first week of life, some babies will stay awake after some feeds. Some babies will sleep for 4 hours; others will wake frequently for small feeds. After an initial weight loss of up to 10%, over the first few days, the baby's weight should stabilise and then increase towards the end of the first week.
- Stools: change over the first 4–5 days from black sticky meconium, to dark-green, yellow–green and finally to loose yellow once full breastfeeding is established. The frequency of bowel actions varies, but is usually once per feed after feeding is established.
- Urine: production is usually low in the first few days, but increases after feeding has been established, with a urinary frequency of usually at least once per feed.
- Jaundice: occurs in more than 50% of babies after the first 24 hours of age, see p. 335.
- Metabolic screening: is performed on the third day for cystic fibrosis, hypothyroidism, phenylketonuria, and other metabolic conditions from a heel prick. Results are available approximately 1 week after sampling. Negative (normal) results are not notified, but the laboratory will contact the baby's doctor regarding the management of children with positive (abnormal) results and advise on appropriate management. This usually involves an immediate referral to a tertiary paediatric hospital for further testing and treatment.

The first month

The baby should be weighed weekly to ensure adequate nutrition. The results must be recorded and plotted on growth charts. Weight gain for term babies vary from 150 to 250 g per week.

Maternal concerns about the baby usually relate to crying, not sleeping enough, not gaining weight, rashes or poor feeding (see Chapter 9, *Fluids and nutrition*; Chapter 24, *Sleep problems*; and Chapter 25, *Behaviour and mental health*) (Fig. 21.1).

- Ventilation is provided by positive pressure ventilation delivered with bag and mask, or Neopuff.
- Resuscitation should be with air rather than oxygen as this reduces perinatal mortality. If despite effective ventilation there is no increase in heart rate, or if oxygenation remains unacceptable, use of a higher

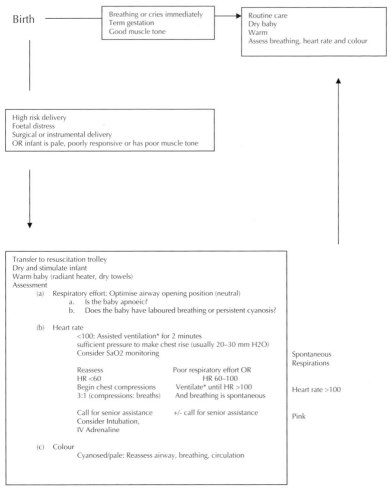

Birth ——— Breathing or cries immediately
Term gestation
Good muscle tone

→ Routine care
Dry baby
Warm
Assess breathing, heart rate and colour

High risk delivery
Foetal distress
Surgical or instrumental delivery
OR infant is pale, poorly responsive or has poor muscle tone

Transfer to resuscitation trolley
Dry and stimulate infant
Warm baby (radiant heater, dry towels)
Assessment
   (a) Respiratory effort: Optimise airway opening position (neutral)
      a.   Is the baby apnoeic?
      b.   Does the baby have laboured breathing or persistent cyanosis?

   (b) Heart rate
        <100: Assisted ventilation* for 2 minutes
        sufficient pressure to make chest rise (usually 20–30 mm H2O)
        Consider SaO2 monitoring

Reassess	Poor respiratory effort OR
HR <60	HR 60–100
Begin chest compressions	Ventilate* until HR >100
3:1 (compressions: breaths)	And breathing is spontaneous
Call for senior assistance	+/- call for senior assistance
Consider Intubation,	
IV Adrenaline	

   (c) Colour
        Cyanosed/pale: Reassess airway, breathing, circulation

Spontaneous Respirations

Heart rate >100

Pink

*Using bag and mask

Fig. 21.1 Neonatal resuscitation. Diagram adapted from the ILCOR Guidelines, Part 11, October 2010.

concentration of oxygen should be considered. It should be noted that 'normal' oxygen saturations in the preterm infant are as low as 40% for the first 4 minutes of life, with those in the term infant ranging from 60% at 1 minute, to 90% at 5 minutes, without intervention with supplemental oxygen.

- The most common cause for failure of resuscitation is inadequate ventilation. This may be due to a poor seal at the facemask or inadequate pressure. Sometimes pressures up to 30–40 cm H_2O are required for the first few breaths.
- A baby who does not respond and has a slow heart rate (<60 beats/min) needs cardiac massage and may need infusions of volume (normal saline or blood) and intravenous adrenaline to improve cardiac output

Table 21.1 Endotracheal tubes

Weight	ETT size	Tie at lips
<1000 g	2.5 mm	6.5–7.0 cm
1000–2000 g	3.0 mm	7–8 cm
2000–3000 g	3.0/3.5 mm	8–9 cm
>3000 g	3.5/4.0 mm	>9 cm

depending on the underlying problem. Chest compressions should be provided in association with adequate inflating breaths in a ratio of 3:1.

- In general, admission to a neonatal intensive care unit is required if spontaneous ventilation is not established by 5 minutes of age (Table 21.1).
- The Apgar score is used to assess the condition of the baby at 1, 5 and occasionally 10 minutes of age. The total score ranges from 0 to 10. A score between 7 and 10 indicates the infant is well. A score between 4 and 7 indicates the baby needs assistance. A score between 0 and 3 indicates severe cardiorespiratory depression (Table 21.2).
- Naloxone is rarely required. It should only be given if a mother has received narcotics within 2 hours of delivery. When using Naloxone, be aware that the effect can wear off quickly and the baby may then develop apnoea, the most serious sign of narcotic overdose. Do not use Naloxone if there is a possibility of maternal narcotic abuse (risk of fulminant withdrawal in the baby).

Variations from normal

When the baby is fully examined, normal variants or minor problems are often noted. If they are obvious to the doctor, most will be obvious to the parents who often need explanation and reassurance.

Skin

- Naevus flammeus (stork-bite): dilated capillaries, on the nape of the neck and on the bridge of the nose, eyelids and adjacent forehead. They fade over 6–12 months.
- Milia: small white blocked sebaceous glands on the nose. They disappear over the first month.
- Miliaria: there are two types – 'crystallina' and 'rubra'. Miliaria crystallina are beads of sweat trapped under the epidermis and are most prominent on the forehead in babies who are overheated. Miliaria rubra, also called 'heat rash', usually appear after a few weeks of age, fluctuate over 2–3 weeks and then disappear. They are related to an increasing activity of the sweat glands. They are prominent on the face, in babies who are overheated.
- Erythema toxicum (toxic erythema or urticaria of the newborn): these are red 'urticarial' spots over the baby's trunk that peak at 2–3 days of age and generally resolve by the first week of life, but occasionally runs a fluctuating course over a few weeks. It is harmless and of unknown cause. New lesions have a broad

Table 21.2 The Apgar score

Sign	0 (absent)	1 (present but depressed)	2 (normal)
Heart rate	Absent	<100	>100
Respiratory effort	Absent	Slow, irregular	Good, crying
Muscle tone	Limp	Some flexion	Active
Response to stimulation	No response	Grimace	Cry
Colour	Pale, blue	Centrally pink, blue periphery	Pink

Source: Practice Parameter: Management of Hyperbilirubinemia in the Healthy Term Newborn. Provisional Committee on Quality Improvement and Subcommittee on Hyperbilirubinemia, Pediatrics 1994, 94: 558–565. PCQI 1994. Reproduced with permission of American Academy of Pediatrics.

erythematous base up to 2–3 cm diameter with a 1–2 mm papule or pustule. The diagnosis can be made with confidence on clinical appearance alone. The differential diagnosis is staphylococcal skin infection, which is persistent and purulent. An examination of the fluid reveals neutrophils and Gram-positive cocci in infection, or eosinophils and no organisms in erythema toxicum.

- 'Mongolian' blue spot: this results in areas of increased melanin deposition over the lower back and sacrum. It can be extensive and is sometimes mistaken for bruising. It is present in most babies born to dark-skinned parents and gradually lightens over a few years, as the rest of the skin becomes more pigmented.
- Dry skin: babies who are post-term have a thicker epidermis and hence drier-looking skin after birth. This may occasionally crack and bleed around the hands and feet during the first few days. Emollients will help. Otherwise the dry skin should be allowed to peel off naturally, which may take up to 1–2 months.

Deformities

- Moulding: the skull moulds to enable the head to be delivered. This changes to a normal shape over the first few days. In addition there may be postural deformities of the face, skull and limbs that are related to the baby's position in the uterus. These gradually improve after birth, but sometimes they do not disappear completely – very few people are symmetrical, especially in their face.
- Positional talipes: The foot is deformed from being compressed in the uterus and is quite common. To determine whether this is pathological, test the range of movements of the foot. A normal foot can be flexed and extended so that the angle with the shin is less than or more than 90°. The forefoot should be mobile. A fixed deformity should be referred to a paediatric orthopaedic surgeon for management (see Orthopaedic Chapter)

Other

- Puffy eyelids/scalp oedema: the newborn infant has excess body fluid at birth. Fluid accumulates easily in the eyelids and after lying on one side, the lower eye may be more swollen. Scalp oedema is common in the first few hours after a normal birth and can persist for several days. This needs further investigation if it persists, or is generalised.
- Bruising/petechiae/subconjunctival haemorrhages: the part of the baby that was presenting during delivery is commonly bruised. If the cord was wrapped tightly around the neck, the baby may have petechial haemorrhages on the face and head (traumatic cyanosis). Subconjunctival haemorrhages occur in up to 25% of babies delivered normally and do not adversely affect vision. They may persist for up to 2 weeks and must not be confused with postnatal trauma. Bruising is common after forceps deliveries, particularly over bony prominences, but disappears over the first week of life. Less commonly after forceps deliveries, firm nodules may be noted in the subcutaneous tissue over similar sites. This is subcutaneous fat necrosis and resolves spontaneously over the first month of life.
- Sucking blisters: these are common on the lips, particularly the upper lip and need no treatment.
- Epstein's pearls: these are small white cysts on the hard palate in the midline. They are benign and disappear in the first weeks after birth.
- Breast hyperplasia: a breast bud is palpable in most term babies, regardless of gender. The breasts may become enlarged during the first week and milk may be observed. They should be left alone and the swelling will subside over several months. However, a breast that is swollen, hot, red and tender may be infected.

Common minor problems

- Hiccups: these occur frequently after a feed. They are not caused by inadequate burping and are harmless.
- Snuffles: these occur in about one-third of normal babies in the few weeks after birth. Despite the noise, the baby is otherwise well and is able to feed normally. The problem diminishes with time as the baby's feeding becomes more efficient and the nasal passages enlarge. It is only important if it interferes with the baby's ability to suck.
- Vomiting: small vomits are harmless. The serious signs are vomit that is bile-stained (grass green), blood-stained, projectile, persistent or associated with frequent choking or failure to thrive. Bile-stained vomiting must be referred to a tertiary paediatric centre for an upper barium study.
- Bleeding umbilical cord: small amounts of bleeding occur rarely as the cord is separating and require no treatment. More profuse bleeding may indicate a bleeding disorder.

- Umbilical hernia: this is present in approximately 25% of babies and resolves in almost all. Consider surgical referral if present beyond 2 years.
- Vaginal skin tag: a small tag of vaginal skin commonly protrudes between the labia in newborn girls. It is benign and disappears as the labia enlarge.
- Vaginal discharge: a small amount of vaginal mucus is universal. In some it can be blood-stained during the first week as the endometrium involutes.
- Red urine: a red-orange discoloration of the napkin when the urine is concentrated (common in the first few days of life) may be mistaken for blood, but is usually due to urates.
- Clicky hips: some ligamentous clicking is common in all large joints, including the hips. It can be considered normal in the absence of any abnormal movement of the femoral head, restriction of hip movement, strong family history, or breech presentation. However, if there is any doubt, hip ultrasound is indicated.

Jaundice

Jaundice is common in the newborn period and is almost always caused by unconjugated hyperbilirubinemia. The clinical importance of jaundice depends on the time at which it is observed and the gestational age of the baby. Jaundice needs to be taken seriously; if the bilirubin level is too high (>340 µmol/L) brain damage (kernicterus) may occur.

The first 24 hours

- Jaundice in the first 24 hours is abnormal. The infant must be admitted to a special care nursery and investigated urgently.
- It is mostly caused by haemolysis, usually ABO or rhesus incompatibility between mother and foetus. Severe haemolysis leads to a rapid rise in serum bilirubin over a few hours.
- The following investigations are required urgently: the mother and baby's blood group, the baby's serum bilirubin (total and unconjugated), direct Coombs' test, haemoglobin, white cell count, and platelets. The mother's red cell antibodies may need to be tested.
- Further investigations are needed if there is no haemolysis, or conjugated hyperbilirubinemia is present.
- Phototherapy should be commenced if the bilirubin level is >150 µmol/L in the first 24 hours in a term infant.
- An immediate exchange transfusion may be required if the jaundice is due to rhesus incompatibility and the infant is anaemic (Hb <110 g/L). This primarily corrects the anaemia and removes antibodies. Further exchange transfusions may be required to control the jaundice.
- Frequent monitoring of bilirubin levels is essential as rapid changes may occur. The results should be plotted on a chart and an 'action level' for exchange transfusion established so that mistakes are not made.

Days 2–7

Jaundice is considered to be 'physiological' if the following criteria are satisfied:

- The jaundice appeared on day 2–4.
- The baby is not premature.
- The baby is well (afebrile, feeding well and alert).
- The baby is passing normal-coloured stools and urine.
- There are no other abnormalities.
- Bilirubin levels are not above treatment threshold.

About a one-third of term babies become visibly jaundiced by 2–4 days of age. Jaundice is visible once serum bilirubin is above 85–120 µmol/L. In physiological jaundice, serum bilirubin rarely exceeds 220 µmol/L. If the unconjugated bilirubin is >220 µmol/L, other causes, including infection, should be considered.

Well, term infants with no haemolysis are at minimal risk of kernicterus. Infants whom are at higher risk of kernicterus are

- Unwell infants (particularly those exposed to hypoxic insults)
- Infants with haemolysis
- Preterm infants

These infants should have treatment started at lower bilirubin levels (Tables 21.3, 21.4 and 21.5).

Table 21.3 Management of non-pathologic jaundice in healthy term infants

	Serum bilirubin (μmol)			
Age (hours)	Consider phototherapy	Phototherapy	Exchange transfusion if intensive phototherapy fails	Exchange transfusion and intensive phototherapy
<24[a]	–	–	–	–
25–48	>170	>260	>340	>430
49–72	>260	>310	>430	>510
>72	>290	>340	>430	>510

Source: Practice Parameter: Management of Hyperbilirubinemia in the Healthy Term Newborn. Provisional Committee on Quality Improvement and Subcommittee on Hyperbilirubinemia, Pediatrics 1994, 94: 558–565. PCQI 1994. Reproduced with permission of American Academy of Pediatrics.
In cases of pathologic jaundice, these guidelines are modifi ed and treatment is typically more aggressive.
[a] Pathologic jaundice is clinical jaundice at less than 24 h of age, and/or bilirubin rising at greater than 8.5 μmol/L/h, and/or true haemolysis.

Prolonged jaundice (>14 days)

In a well infant, prolonged neonatal jaundice is usually secondary to breastfeeding and is benign. A serum bilirubin should be checked to determine whether hyperbilirubinaemia is conjugated or unconjugated.

- Unconjugated bilirubinemia: hypothyroidism, infection or red cell enzyme abnormalities should be considered.
  - A sudden onset of jaundice at this age is suggestive of haemolysis caused by a red blood cell enzyme abnormality, most frequently glucose-6-phosphate dehydrogenase (G6PD) deficiency. Urgent admission to hospital is indicated.
- Conjugated bilirubinemia (>25% total or >25 μmol/L): is uncommon and always pathological. Consider biliary atresia (the stools are acholic – grey colour), neonatal hepatitis, a choledochal cyst obstructing the bile duct, galactosaemia or parenteral nutrition.

If the above are excluded and the baby is well and breastfeeding, the likely diagnosis is breast milk jaundice. This occurs in approximately 10% of breastfed infants, is not associated with kernicterus and does not need any treatment. Reassurance that breastfeeding should continue is very important. Prolonged jaundice (after the first few days of life) can usually be managed as an outpatient, but may require readmission for investigation or treatment.

Respiratory distress

Most major causes of respiratory distress will present within the first hours of life. The signs are
- Increased work of breathing (recession of the lower chest wall and upper abdomen).

Table 21.4 Management of jaundice in preterm infants: guidelines for phototherapy

	Serum bilirubin (μmol)		
Age (hours)	<1500	Weight (g)1500–2000	>2000
<24	>70	>70	>85
24–48	>85	>120	>140
49–72	>120	>155	>200
>72	>140	>170	>240

Source: Practice Parameter: Management of Hyperbilirubinemia in the Healthy Term Newborn. Provisional Committee on Quality Improvement and Subcommittee on Hyperbilirubinemia, Pediatrics 1994, 94: 558–565. PCQI 1994. Reproduced with permission of American Academy of Pediatrics.

Table 21.5 Management of jaundice in preterm infants: guidelines for exchange transfusion

Age (hours)	Serum bilirubin (μmol)		
	<1500	Weight (g)1500–2000	>2000
<24	>170–255	>255	>270–310
24–48	>170–255	>270	>290–320
49–72	>255	>290	>310–340

For high-risk premature infants: use lower end of range and weight, next lower weight category, and next lower age category in that order.
Premature LGA infants: use average birthweight for gestational age.
These 3 tables and guidlines can be found at www.rch.org.au/nets/handbook

- Rapid breathing (>60 breaths per minute).
- Expiratory grunt.
- Central cyanosis.

Babies need to be considered for level 3 neonatal intensive care if they require >40% oxygen to maintain saturations >88% (usually measured by pulse oximetry).

Common pulmonary diseases

Respiratory distress syndrome (RDS) or hyaline membrane disease

- RDS is primarily caused by deficiency of surfactant, immaturity of lung structure and delayed fluid clearance; hence the lungs do not expand easily or evenly. The incidence increases with decreasing gestation. It usually affects babies <30 weeks' gestation, but it can occur in term babies, especially those delivered by elective Caesarean section.
- Respiratory distress (O_2 requirement, work of breathing) typically increases over 12–24 hours before improvement is seen. Rapid deterioration may occur leading to respiratory failure (rising arterial CO_2 level).
- The diagnosis is made by clinical features and chest x-ray, which has a generalised fine reticulogranular (ground glass) appearance with air bronchograms.
- Respiratory support with oxygen, assisted ventilation (CPAP, IPPV) and surfactant therapy may be required.

Transient tachypnoea of the newborn or 'wet lung syndrome'

- This is caused by delayed clearance of foetal lung fluid and commonly occurs in babies born near term by elective Caesarean section. It presents as mild respiratory distress and lasts for up to 1 to 2 days.
- It is diagnosed by chest x-ray, which demonstrates coarse streaking of lung fields with fluid in the fissures. The baby is usually not very ill, needing <30% oxygen.

Bacterial infections

- Group B β-haemolytic streptococcus (GBS) is the most common and serious cause of pneumonia and septicaemia in the newborn. It is acquired around the time of birth from a colonised mother. Other organisms, including *Escherichia coli*, can also cause pneumonia.
- Pneumonia presents early with severe and progressive respiratory failure. If not treated immediately there is rapid progression to collapse and death.
- Later infections can present with lethargy, temperature instability, poor feeding, respiratory difficulty, apnoea or poor perfusion.
- The chest x-ray of GBS infection is similar to severe RDS and is not diagnostic.
- Because of the rapid and severe nature of GBS septicaemia, all babies with early onset respiratory failure must be treated with penicillin and gentamicin until the cause is confirmed.

Meconium aspiration syndrome

- Hypoxia before delivery may cause the baby to gasp *in utero* and inhale meconium. This causes respiratory difficulty. It is associated with pulmonary hypertension and right-to-left shunting.

- The chest x-ray shows hyperinflation and patchy consolidation (pneumothorax and pneumomediastinum may follow) or a diffuse hazy appearance.
- Oxygen is the mainstay of therapy, but other respiratory support (CPAP or ventilation) may be required. Antibiotics are given to counter infection.

Pneumothorax

- May occur spontaneously at birth, or secondary to other lung disease. It is a serious cause of respiratory distress and vital to be recognised and treated early.
- The diagnosis is by chest x-ray. Transillumination using a cold light source can be useful.
- The main treatment is an intercostal catheter with an underwater drain at low negative pressure.
- Asymptomatic pneumothorax usually needs no treatment.

Tension pneumothorax

- This is a medical emergency.
- If a baby is deteriorating rapidly despite full resuscitation this diagnosis should be considered particularly if there is poor air entry on auscultation to one or both sides of the chest. There may be no time for a chest x-ray.
- In the event of severe deterioration perform needle aspiration of the chest using a 25-gauge scalp vein needle attached via a three-way tap to a 10 mL syringe. The needle is inserted into the second or third intercostal space in the midclavicular line. Aspirate the chest with the 10 mL syringe.
- This manoeuvre may be life-saving and is followed by insertion of an intercostal catheter.

Upper airway obstruction

- Nasal: may be due to an upper respiratory tract infection, choanal atresia (obstruction to the back of the nose) or traumatic deviated nasal septum. It presents with difficulty in breathing or feeding. Suspect choanal atresia/stenosis when the baby's condition improves with opening the mouth. Choanal atresia is diagnosed when a 10-French suction tube cannot be passed from the nose to the nasopharynx.
- Oral: macroglossia may be associated with Beckwith–Wiedemann syndrome or hypothyroidism. Micrognathia may result in a tongue that obstructs the pharynx. Pierre Robin sequence is an association of mandibular hypoplasia (micrognathia), cleft palate and upper airways obstruction caused by the tongue falling back into the cleft palate. The severity of the upper airways obstruction can vary from mild to severe. There is usually a soft inspiratory stridor associated with subcostal and intercostal indrawing of variable severity. Babies with mild upper airways obstruction feed reasonably well, gain weight and usually need no intervention other than prone posturing. However, babies who feed poorly, vomit and fail to thrive usually have significant airways obstruction. These babies often adopt an extensor posture in an attempt to relieve their obstruction. Presentation at 2–4 weeks of age with these features is not uncommon. Insertion of a nasopharyngeal tube is necessary to relieve airway obstruction. Babies needing prolonged treatment with a nasopharyngeal tube respond well to mandibular distraction surgery. Tracheostomy is rarely needed.
- Larynx: laryngomalacia, subglottic stenosis, laryngeal inflammation or occasionally vocal cord palsy, present with inspiratory stridor and suprasternal and lower chest indrawing.
- Trachea: tracheal obstruction presents with an inspiratory and expiratory wheeze and lower chest indrawing. It may be due tracheomalacia or a vascular ring.

Non-pulmonary causes of respiratory difficulty
Cardiac
- Left-to-right shunts or left-sided obstructions cause pulmonary oedema.
Pulmonary hypertension
- Presents with an increased oxygen requirement and little respiratory difficulty.
- Chest x-ray often reveals clear lung fields.

Management of respiratory diseases
Before birth
- If possible, anticipate high-risk babies and transfer to a hospital with a level 3 nursery for delivery and neonatal care.

- Betamethasone given to mothers with threatened preterm labour reduces the severity of hyaline membrane disease (HMD), halves the mortality and incidence of brain haemorrhages and improves long-term outcome.

General care
- Observation, usually in an incubator.
- Temperature control is essential – aim for a rectal temperature of 37°C (+/−0.3°C) or axillary temperature range 36.8°C (+/−0.3°C).
- Measure blood glucose, electrolytes, full blood count and CRP.
- Take a blood culture (but not an LP in the acute stage).
- Avoid enteral feeds initially as they worsen respiratory distress via splinting the diaphragm.
- Give IV fluids.
- Treat with benzylpenicillin and gentamicin until blood cultures are negative.

Respiratory care
- A chest x-ray provides the diagnosis in most cases.
- Monitor cardiorespiratory and blood gas measurements.
- Arterial pH should be maintained at 7.35–7.45.
- Arterial Pco_2 should be 40–60 mmHg.
- Arterial Po_2 – a low PO_2 means the baby is hypoxic. If the pH is also low, the baby may have a metabolic acidosis and a higher level of inspired oxygen is required. If this does not improve oxygenation, suspect cyanotic heart disease as a cause (see Chapter 6, *Cardiac conditions*).
- Arterial bicarbonate should be 22–26 mmol/L. A low level is due to a metabolic acidosis. The pH will also be low unless the baby has compensated by blowing off CO_2.
- Base excess should be between +3 and −3. If low it indicates a metabolic acidosis. A level of −5 is usually tolerated in small babies without out a significant change in pH.

Note: if arterial blood gases cannot be obtained, sample the capillary blood. This is simple and rapid to perform, providing some information about acid–base status and CO_2 levels to guide further therapy, while tertiary assistance is sought.

- In ventilated babies with RDS, especially those <30 weeks' gestation, surfactant should be given via the endotracheal tube as early as possible.
- The inspired oxygen requirement is initially determined using a pulse oximeter. Aim for an oxygen saturation of 88–95%.
- Arterial blood gases should be measured in babies needing >30% oxygen. Aim for a P_aO_2 level between 50 and 80 mmHg.
- Nasal continuous positive airway pressure (CPAP) is effective for treating RDS or apnoea. It should be used early for any baby who is grunting or showing increased respiratory effort (starting at 7 cm H_2O).
- The decision to ventilate a baby is made on the following criteria:
  - Apnoea not responding to simple treatment.
  - Unsatisfactory arterial blood gases: pH <7.25 with a PCO_2 >60 mmHg, or inspired oxygen >60% despite treatment with CPAP (up to 10 cm H_2O).

Hypoglycaemia
This is defined as a true blood glucose of <2.5 mmol/L. 'Dextrostix' or 'BM stix' are only useful for screening purposes. If these suggest hypoglycaemia, a true blood glucose must be measured.

Blood glucose should be measured before 1 hour of age for infants with the following conditions: infants of diabetic mothers, infants weighing <10th centile, prematurity, large for gestational age, shock, seizures and infants receiving intravenous infusions.

Clinical features
The infant may be asymptomatic, or may have apathy, hypotonia, poor feeding, temperature instability, apnoea, jitteriness or convulsions.

Management

Asymptomatic infants with a true blood glucose of 1.5–2.5 mmol/L: give early, frequent small milk feeds at 90 mL/kg per day. If no response occurs within 2 hours, give IV 10% dextrose.

- If the blood glucose is <1.5 mmol/L intravenous dextrose should be given. A bolus of 10% dextrose, 2 mL/kg, should be followed by an infusion providing 5–10 mg/kg/min of glucose. The response to therapy should be monitored by frequent blood glucose measurements.
- To calculate an infusion of 10 mg/kg/min
  - A fluid bag of 10% dextrose = 10 g/100 mL = 0.1 g/mL = 100 mg/mL of dextrose.
  - Hence, 10 mg/kg/min = 0.1 mL/kg/min of 10% dextrose infusion.
- If the blood glucose is <1 mmol/L and it is difficult to insert an intravenous line, give 0.3 units/kg of glucagon IM pending successful insertion of the line, or transfer to a higher level of care.
- Further investigation and treatment is necessary if the glucose requirement is 10 mg/kg/min or greater (see Chapter 20, *Genetics and metabolics*).

Neonatal infection

Infection is one of the most common preventable causes of neonatal mortality and morbidity. Infection may be acquired from the mother before or at birth (early onset) or postnatally from the environment by droplet spread or handling (late onset). The most frequently encountered bacteria are

Early onset (within the first week of life): GBS, *E. coli* and Listeria monocytogenes.

Late onset (between week 1 and 4 of life): Coagulase-negative staphylococci, *Staphylococcus aureus*, GBS, *Klebsiella* spp. and *Pseudomonas* spp.

The most serious viral infection is herpes simplex virus (HSV), although other viruses, especially respiratory syncytial virus (RSV), can cause problems in neonatal nurseries, or soon after discharge home in ex-premature infants. There are occasional outbreaks of enteroviral infections in the community causing significant illness in babies.

Clinical features

The early symptoms and signs may be minimal, however, if ignored rapid progression to overwhelming sepsis may occur. The following are important warning signs of infection: respiratory difficulty, poor feeding, vomiting, abdominal distension and tenderness, drowsiness, floppiness, pallor, apnoea, seizures, temperature instability, tender limb. In particular, poor feeding is a frequent early sign of infection.

Investigations

If one or more of the warning signs are present it is important to investigate infection. This includes

- Blood culture: arterial or venous – at least 2–4 mL.
- Urine: suprapubic aspiration (SPA) under ultrasound imaging if possible. If unsuccessful pass a catheter using a size-5 French gauge tube after adequate preparation of the genitalia. A bag collection of urine is rarely helpful.
- Throat and rectal swabs and swabs of any obviously infected lesion.
- Cultures or specific PCR for viral infections.
- Lumbar puncture if meningitis is suspected. This should always be performed in the presence of fever in a newborn.

Management

Any ill neonate should be admitted to hospital for investigation and treatment.

- Start with IV benzylpenicillin and gentamicin.
- Add IV cefotaxime if meningitis is suspected (see Antimicrobial guidelines) and IV metronidazole if abdominal sepsis is suspected.
- If there is any possibility that the baby may have HSV (i.e. the mother has active genital herpes) give acyclovir.
- Antibiotics may be subsequently tailored according to culture results.
- Careful attention to temperature stability, respiratory status, fluid and electrolytes, blood pressure, blood glucose and haematology parameters is essential.

Neonatal seizures
Clinical features
- Subtle: deviation of the eyes, staring, abnormal sucking, lip smacking or cycling movements of the limbs.
- Tonic: stiffening of limbs, frequently associated with apnoea and eye deviation.
- Clonic: movement of one or all limbs that persists despite holding the limb.
- Benign sleep myoclonus: occurs in neurologically normal infants only during sleep. The electroencephalogram (EEG) is normal and no treatment is necessary. It can be exacerbated by benzodiazepines and usually resolves by 2 months of age.

Aetiology
The aetiology can usually be determined for neonatal seizures. Causes include

- Hypoxic ischaemic encephalopathy: seizures occur within 24 hours of the hypoxic episode, often within the first 4–6 hours.
- Stroke.
- Intracranial haemorrhage.
- Infection: bacterial or viral meningitis.
- Metabolic
  - Hypoglycaemia.
  - Hypocalcaemia/hypomagnesaemia.
  - Hyponatraemia or hypernatraemia.
  - Kernicterus
    - Inborn errors of metabolism (characterised by intractable seizures, with progressive loss of consciousness, or metabolic acidosis).
- Drug withdrawal.
- Developmental brain abnormalities.
- Autosomal dominant neonatal seizures.

Investigations
Consider

- Bloods
  - Immediately check blood glucose.
  - Electrolytes including calcium and magnesium.
  - Blood gases.
  - Blood cultures.
- Metabolic screen: blood ammonia, lactate, amino acids, carnitine and urinary organic acids.
- Urine analysis including ketones and reducing substances.
- Lumbar puncture and viral investigations.
- Cranial ultrasound.
- Where there are focal neurological signs on examination a cranial CT scan should be considered to exclude intracranial haemorrhage that may warrant neurosurgical intervention.
- MRI brain scan to determine extent of injury in HIE (usually performed around day 5); to exclude stroke where focal seizures are occurring, or for suspected developmental brain abnormality.
- EEG to detect seizure activity and to aid prognosis. Where conventional EEG is not immediately available, bedside amplitude integrated EEG (aEEG) may be useful in the detection of some seizures.

Management
Admission to a neonatal intensive care unit is mandatory for all neonates with seizures. Attention to temperature and glucose stability, optimal ventilation, blood pressure control, and fluid and electrolyte balance is essential.
Anticonvulsants

- Phenobarbitone: 20 mg/kg IV over 30 minutes (beware this dose may cause apnoea in a non-ventilated baby). A further 10 mg/kg may be given for refractory seizures followed by 5 mg/kg per day.
- Phenytoin: 20 mg/kg IV over 1 hour.
- Midazolam: 200 mcg/kg IV bolus followed by intravenous infusion at 1–5 mcg/kg/min.

- Clonazepam: up to 0.25 mg. This may cause apnoea. Careful monitoring and the availability of mechanical ventilation are essential.
- Pyridoxine: 50–100 mg IV or p.o. should be considered for intractable seizures. Where possible, conventional EEG should be obtained both before and after administration of the first dose of pyridoxine.

Neonatal abstinence syndrome

Neonatal abstinence syndrome occurs in babies born to women who are chemically dependent and who may use multiple substances. These babies exhibit signs of withdrawal and may require treatment. The features of withdrawal are assessed using a standardised scoring system (commonly adapted from the system devised by Finnegan). **Do not use Naloxone at delivery in these babies, it may precipitate acute withdrawal associated with seizures.**

The onset of withdrawal is variable:

- Heroin: 48–72 hours.
- Methadone: may be delayed for up to 1–2 weeks.

Withdrawal may be less evident in premature infants.

Clinical features

Neurological signs

- Hypertonia, tremors, hyperreflexia.
- Myoclonic jerks, seizures (1–2% heroin, 7% methadone).
- Irritability, restlessness, high-pitched cry.
- Sleep disturbance.

Autonomic system dysfunction

- Nasal stuffiness, sneezing, yawning
- Low grade fever, sweating
- Skin mottling
- Gastrointestinal abnormalities:
  ○ Regurgitation, vomiting, diarrhoea
- Poor feeding, dysmature swallowing
- Failure to thrive
- Respiratory symptoms:
  ○ Tachypnoea
  ○ Apnoea
- Excoriations (especially around the anus)

Management of opiate withdrawal may involve the administration of morphine to assist gradual withdrawal.

Note: The Selective Serotonin Reuptake Inhibitors (SSRIs) commonly used to treat depression were once thought to be entirely safe from the perspective of the foetus. However a minority of exposed newborns will develop seizures in the first few days of life as a consequence of withdrawal from SSRIs. These seizures are usually short lived (days) and the long-term neurodevelopmental outcome is thought to be normal.

Postnatal depression

Mild-to-moderate postnatal depression (PND) occurs in about one in six women and also occurs in men. The diagnosis may not always be obvious, so a high level of awareness is required when assessing any baby in the first months of life. Infants may present with feeding problems, failure to thrive or excessive crying. The Edinburgh Postnatal Depression Scale is a useful screening instrument that is easy to administer, score and interpret (http://www.beyondblue.org.au/resources/for-me/pregnancy-and-early-parenthood/edinburgh-postnatal-depression-scale).

If you suspect that the mother or father has PND, refer them to their GP or mental health professional.

Maternal mastitis

Mastitis is common in breastfeeding women.

- The organism is usually *S. aureus.*
- It presents with aches, pains and fever.
- Examination reveals a tender engorged segment in one or both breasts.

Management
- Prompt treatment is important to prevent abscess formation.
- Oral antibiotics – flucloxacillin 500 mg p.o. 6 hourly.
- Paracetamol and increased fluids.
- Breastfeeding should continue.

Problems of the extremely very low birthweight infant
While it is not the intention of this chapter to discuss the problems of managing very low birthweight (VLBW) infants (birthweight <1500 g), it is important to be aware of some of the problems that occur after discharge from the neonatal unit.

Chronic lung disease (bronchopulmonary dysplasia)
This is a common chronic lung disease occurring for a few months in very premature infants after RDS. It is characterised by an abnormal chest x-ray and oxygen dependency after 36 weeks' gestation. The majority of infants with bronchopulmonary dysplasia can be weaned from oxygen treatment within 4 weeks of the expected date of delivery. A small number require oxygen therapy for months and some are managed at home in oxygen. Timely immunisation should be given to these infants, against influenza as these babies are particularly susceptible to respiratory infections in the first 18 months of life. The first dose is given after 6 months chronological age, at the appropriate season, with a booster one month later. Pavilizumab (monoclonal antibody to RSV) is also considered in some infants.

Necrotising enterocolitis
This is due to inflammation of the intestine in the early neonatal period. While many babies recover with conservative management (nil orally, intravenous alimentation and antibiotics), some develop necrosis that necessitates bowel resection. The risks to these babies after discharge from hospital are
- Stricture formation: this can present weeks or months after the initial episode. The presenting features of obstruction include bile-stained vomiting, distension, constipation and failure to thrive.
- Gastroenteritis: this can produce severe dehydration very rapidly in a baby who has had a bowel resection. Admission to hospital for intravenous fluids is mandatory.

Hearing and visual deficits
These are common problems and must be carefully screened and assessed soon after discharge from hospital.

Further common problems
- Inguinal hernias: require prompt surgical referral as they frequently strangulate. See Chapter 2, *Surgical conditions*.
- Immunisation: hepatitis B vaccination is recommended just after birth or at 32 weeks if born prematurely. All other immunisations are given at the appropriate postnatal age as per the immunisation schedule. Refer to Chapter 18, *Infectious diseases and immunisation*, p. 296.
- Apnoea: this is a common problem until about 34 weeks' gestation. However, ex-VLBW infants are at increased risk of apnoea until 3 months past their due date, after general anaesthesia, or with respiratory infections. Close monitoring is advised at these times.
- Haemangiomas (strawberry naevus): these appear after birth as small raised, red, lobulated and compressible lesions that increase in size over a few months. They are more common in premature infants, but also occur in term babies. Most involute during the first 2 years. Failure to involute or difficult locations (e.g. near the eye) require urgent referral to a dermatologist for laser or intralesional steroid therapy (see Chapter 17, *Dermatologic conditions*). Involvement of the laryngeal opening causing stridor requires involvement of ENT.

Apparent life-threatening events
Infants with an apparent life-threatening event (ALTE) often presents with a colour change, a perception of a lack of breathing, floppiness and possibly choking or gagging. No explanation will be found in approximately 50%. This engenders enormous anxiety for affected parents, and whilst there is currently no evidence that home monitoring will prevent SIDS, many will request some form of home monitoring to provide reassurance.

The possible causes for ALTE can be considered in the following groups:
1. Gastrointestinal, for example gastro-oesophageal reflux, aspiration, infection, intussusception
2. Neurological, for example seizures, infection, breath-holding

3. Respiratory, for example airway/pulmonary infection, airway obstruction (Pierre Robin Sequence)
4. Cardiovascular, for example Wolff–Parkinson–White syndrome, long QT syndromes, structural anomalies, myocarditis
5. Metabolic and endocrine, for example medium chain acyl-CoA dehydrogenase deficiency (MCAD)
6. Other – overfeeding, medications, non-accidental injury, Munchausen by proxy syndrome
7. Idiopathic ALTE

A detailed history and examination should occur. Investigations should be targeted but generally include a full septic screen, an ECG and an arterial blood gas, with further metabolic testing if there are derangements in blood sugar or acid–base balance. Infants will usually require admission for at least 24 hours with full cardiorespiratory and oxygen saturation monitoring. Once initial investigations and monitoring are returned negative, parents should be reassured and discharged without home monitoring if possible. Parents should receive some basic first aid training about infant resuscitation and be counselled about measures to reduce SIDS risk. A summary of the recommendations by the American Academy of Pediatrics is

- Put infants on their back to sleep.
- Use a firm sleep surface.
- Keep soft objects and loose bedding out of the crib.
- Do not smoke during pregnancy and avoid exposure of infants to second-hand tobacco smoke.
- A 'separate but proximate' sleep environment is recommended, for example crib in the parents' bedroom.
- Avoid overheating.
- Avoid commercial devices marketed to reduce the risk of SIDS.
- Do not use home monitors as a strategy to reduce the risk of SIDS.
- Avoid the development of positional plagiocephaly, for example by using tummy time when awake and varying the position of the infant's head.

American Academy of Pediatrics. Policy Statement. The changing concept of sudden infant death syndrome: diagnostic coding shifts, controversies regarding the sleeping environment, and new variables to consider in reducing risk. *Pediatrics*. 2005; 116:1245–1255.

USEFUL RESOURCES
- *www.rwh.org.au/nets/handbook* – Victorian Newborn Emergency Transport Services Handbook.

CHAPTER 22
Adolescent health

Susan Sawyer
Michelle Telfer
Sonia Grover

Adolescence is no longer considered the healthiest time of life. Dramatic improvements in infant and child mortality have brought greater visibility – and greater concern – about adolescents as they have experienced far less improvement in their health. Far-reaching social and economic changes appear to have contributed to higher rates of emotional and mental disorders, obesity, substance use and misuse and increased rates of sexually transmitted infections (STIs) in the young.

Definition of adolescence
Earlier onset of puberty (onset of adolescence) and later completion of the social role transitions to adulthood (end of adolescence) such as completion of education, commencement of work, financial independence, marriage and childbearing have resulted in an extended period of adolescent and young adult development in countries like Australia and increasingly across the world.

The WHO uses the term 'adolescent' to refer to 10–19 years olds and 'youth' to refer to 15–24 year olds. The terms 'young people' and 'adolescents and young adults' are increasingly used to refer to 10–24 years olds. Informally, these terms tend to be used fairly interchangeably.

Major biological and neurocognitive maturation occurs during adolescence which underpin the growing interest and relevance for young people around:
- autonomy and independence from family;
- personal identity, self-esteem and body image;
- peer relationships;
- educational and vocational goals;
- financial independence; and
- sexuality.

Adolescence and adolescent health care
The burden of disease in adolescents differs greatly from infants and children. Many causes of ill health in adolescents reflect unhealthy patterns of behaviour that are largely preventable, as well as mental disorders. Young people with chronic disease and disability can be especially disadvantaged.

Marginalised young people who are poorly connected to their families and schools have poorer health outcomes. High-risk vulnerable young people include those with
- significant health risk behaviours (e.g. regular drug use);
- mental health problems (e.g. severe depression, psychosis, eating disorders);
- families who are chaotic; and
- parents who have a mental illness or substance use issue.

High-risk young people commonly experience a range of co-morbidities for which they uncommonly receive appropriate health care. Close consultation and liaison with case managers in the community is a priority and is generally more effective than referral to new services.

Understanding adolescent friendly health care is the key to providing the best care possible for young people. Clinicians should recognise the dynamic changes that occur across adolescence and reflect this in the care they

Paediatric Handbook, Ninth Edition. Edited by Amanda Gwee, Romi Rimer and Michael Marks.
© 2015 John Wiley & Sons, Ltd. Published 2015 by John Wiley & Sons, Ltd.

provide. Key steps to achieving adolescent friendly health care include:

- Actively engaging young people in their health care;
- Assessing psychosocial concerns even if not the presenting problem;
- Promoting self-management and adherence to treatment regimens, including medication;
- Supporting the process of transition to adult health care;
- Liaising with health and community professionals involved in the young person's care;
- Ensuring the physical environment is appropriate and welcoming for young people.

When young people require admission to hospital they prefer to be nursed with other people of their own age. Adolescent inpatient wards provide developmentally appropriate nursing, recreation and peer support. They also facilitate links to educational and mental health support.

Starting the consultation

Building an independent relationship with adolescents while respectfully engaging parents is a key challenge in consulting with young people. Key steps include

- Greet the young person by name. When parents are present, greet the young person first, then introduce yourself to the parents.
- If parents are present spend time with both the parents and child together to understand the presenting complaint, past history and parent concerns.
- Explain the issue of confidentiality at the beginning of the first contact with every adolescent (see Table 22.1 below). It is important for parents to hear this as well.
- Spend some time alone with the young person as they must learn to increasingly function independently of their parents.
- Allow adequate time.
- Listen and acknowledge the young person's viewpoint and opinions.
- Always attempt to confidentially 'go beyond' the presenting complaint to identify wider psychosocial risks – as it is uncommon for these to be the presenting complaint.
- A clinician who listens respectfully and acknowledges a young person's point of view will have made an excellent start in establishing a therapeutic relationship.
- Young people benefit from reminders about confidentiality when sensitive information is discussed (see Table 22.1).

Psychosocial screening and developmental assessment

Every consultation should go beyond the presenting complain to identify broader psychosocial concerns (e.g. bullying at school, academic failure, anxiety, disordered eating, family illness).

One approach to taking a psychosocial history is to use the HEADSS framework (see Table 22.2). Questions can be asked in any order, although the first three domains generally involve less sensitive questions than the last three. Taking a psychosocial history is a powerful way of engaging a young person and establishing rapport. It also provides an opportunity to assess developmental stage (maturity), identify the balance of health risk and protective factors, and identify opportunities for early intervention and health promotion.

Table 22.1 Explaining confidentiality

- Define the term at the start of the interview[a].
- Consider all information from an adolescent as confidential until discussed or clarified.
- In most Australian States, confidentiality is a legal requirement over 16 years of age.
- Negotiation or compromise may be required for adolescents under 16 years.
- Exceptions to confidentiality are when the adolescent is at risk of significant harm, such as risk of suicide or if they are subject to physical or sexual abuse.
- Ensure that information to be kept confidential from parents is appropriately highlighted in the medical record.

[a]For example: 'In addition to spending time with you and your parents together, we also spend time with young people alone without their parents. This part of a consultation is confidential. That means that I cannot talk about anything we discuss today with your parents or anyone else, unless you and I have agreed to do so. However, there are some exceptions. I cannot maintain confidentiality if you are at risk of harm, such as threat of suicide, self-harm, or sexual abuse.'

Table 22.2 Adolescent developmental screening: the 'HEADSS' psychosocial assessment

Domains	Potential topics to discuss	Tips on contextualising and addressing these domains
Home	• Where they live, with whom • Housing security (tenure), recent moves • Physical environment and resources (e.g. electricity, transport, phone) • Social environment, key supports	Physical living arrangements and social and psychological supports available to young people at home are all key to understanding and addressing health conditions, especially chronic conditions (such as mental health). Living arrangements of young people can be quite complex – it is important not to make any assumptions.
Education/employment	• Current education/employment • Educational performance, literacy, and numeracy • Relationships with peers and superiors • Employment, finances, and financial security/supports • Future aspirations and needs	Education and employment are important determinants of health and well-being. Health status is also a significant determinant of young people's capacity to engage in education and employment. In addressing this domain, it is important to appreciate how hard it can be for young people to be honest about bullying at school, or to acknowledge that they are not as academically successful as they or their families expected.
Eating/exercise	• Number and nature of meals • Body image; satisfaction, are others concerned? • Exercise patterns	Capitalize on the opportunity to address nutrition and exercise: both under- and over-nutrition are important determinants of individual and intergenerational health. Avoid using language like 'fat', 'chubby', or 'bony'– young people are sensitive about their weight and body image, irrespective of their body habitus.
Activities	• Activities and interests, including weekends/holidays • Family contact, shared activities, supports • Friend and peer networks, including social media	Personal, peer, and family activities are all important determinants of health. Interests and hobbies may also provide a lever for change (e.g. ability to play sport may be an incentive to take asthma medication). Marginalized youth may have limited supports and friends – it is important to ask questions sensitively.
Drugs	• Peer and family substance use • Individual substance use, recent changes • Effects of substance use and regrets • Injected substances (blood-borne virus risk) • Knowledge gaps	Family, peer, and personal drug use all impact on health outcomes and behaviours. Adolescence is a period of experimentation, and drug use is often modifiable. Before asking these questions, reaffirm confidentiality. Asking first about family and peer substance use helps normalize and contextualize this. Use this opportunity to provide education and advice around harm reduction.
Sexuality	• Sexual activity, orientation, and identity • Concerns around sex (coercion, unplanned pregnancy, STI) • Contraception and safe sex • Females: menstrual periods • Knowledge gaps	Sexual debut is common during adolescence. STIs and unplanned pregnancy disproportionally affect adolescents. Explain why you are asking these questions, and use the opportunity to educate and promote sexual reproductive health and rights. Do not assume that young people are heterosexual. Be sensitive; sexual coercion is common and not all sexual experiences may be desired or pleasurable.

(continued)

Table 22.2 (*Continued*)

Domains	Potential topics to discuss	Tips on contextualising and addressing these domains
Suicide and depression	• Sleep, appetite, energy, emotions (depression symptom screen) • Common mental health problems (anxiety) • Self-harm/suicidal thoughts, attempts, plans	Poor mental health is a significant health issue but an uncommon reason for accessing health care. Additionally, mental health is an important determinant of many other health outcomes. In addressing this domain, be cognizant of the stigma of mental illness; a sensitive approach and reassurance of confidentiality (and its exceptions) are important. There is no evidence that asking about suicide or self-harm increases risk of these behaviours.
Safety	• Safety at home, school, and within the community • Reasons for not feeling safe (e.g. driving with someone affected by alcohol or drugs) • Personal weapons • Use of seatbelts, bicycle helmuts, off road motorbikes etc.	Injury is a leading contributor to the burden of disease experienced by young people globally. Health consultations provide an opportunity to identify key risk behaviours and can help the young person identify ways to improve their safety.
Strengths and spirituality	• Culture and identity • Strengths, both as identified by the individual, and strengths that others identify	Culture and identity can be powerful protective factors. This domain also promotes a strengths-based approach and may help reassure young people of the skills and strengths they have and the active role they can play in improving their health. Importantly, culture and identity of young people can be different to that of their family or community.

Source: Modified from Azzopardi PS, Creati MB, Sawyer SM. Adolescent Health. In: Nelson B, ed. Essential Clinical Global Health Medicine. Wiley Blackwell Publishing. 2015. p. 168. (Nelson 2014. Reproduced with permission of Wiley & Sons Ltd.)

Physical examination

- Conduct a thorough physical examination whenever appropriate.
- Ensure privacy from others and protect modesty as much as possible.
- Reassure and explain the reason for the particular exam.
- Many young people are anxious about many aspects of normal development and benefit from reassurance.
- Provide feedback on examination findings as much as possible.
- Monitor height, weight and pubertal development. Plot growth on a growth chart then explain what this means in the context of normal growth patterns.

Common issues when working with young people with chronic diseases and disabilities

Young people with chronic conditions are typically the most experienced consumers of the paediatric health system. Most young people greatly benefit from the support provided by parents around looking after their health. However, as young people mature, they should be supported to take on increasing responsibility for managing their health. Both clinicians and parents need to have appropriate expectations of what adolescents can (and can't) do – while supporting greater self-management over time.

Specific elements of self-management that young adults need to be able to take responsibility for, independent of their parents, include being able to

- Name and explain their condition.
- Explain why each medication is necessary.

- Remember to take their medication.
- Arrange repeat prescriptions before medication runs out.
- Be able to consult with doctors (see the doctor alone, ask and answer questions, arrange and cancel appointments).
- Develop a desire to be independent with health care.
- Prioritise their health over (some) other desires.

Adolescents with intellectual disability (and their families) should also be supported to develop greater self-management capacities as they have variable potential for independent living as young adults.

Conflict of priorities

At times there may be a conflict of priorities between the therapeutic goals of the clinician (focused on disease control and management) and the developmental goals that are frequently the main concern of young people. For example, a young person with persistent asthma who goes on a school camp may be too embarrassed to take their preventer medication while on camp, preferring instead to put up with the unknown consequences (and the unspoken wishful thinking that their asthma will be fine).

Practical tips include

- Negotiate management approaches in ways that the young person is developmentally comfortable with.
- Provide the young person with a choice of acceptable management options.

Adherence

Promoting adherence with treatment regimens is a challenge for clinicians irrespective of the age of the patient. It can be especially difficult with adolescents with chronic disease, as they are generally less influenced by long-term health goals than adults. There may be conflict between the young person's (developmentally appropriate) pursuit of increasing autonomy and independence, and the clinician and parents' desire to improve their health. Don't assume adolescents are informed, even if their parents are.

Practical tips include

- Provide a clear rationale for all treatments.
- Simplify the treatment regimen (e.g. choose daily dosing rather than b.i.d dosing options when available).
- Use simple language and write down all instructions.
- Don't use threats.
- Help the adolescent develop routines about each treatment. Use technology, for example phones can assist with reminders.
- Discuss the acceptability of treatment in relationship to peers and education.
- Work with both parents and young people. Parents may need to be more involved, or encouraged to 'back off' and be less overprotective.

Working across teams and across sectors

- Multidisciplinary team input can be very valuable, especially for young people with complex health conditions.
- Excellent communication is required – different team members need to repeat the same key messages to the young person and family.
- It can be valuable gaining information from others who know the young person better, both within the health sector (e.g. Mental health counsellor) and beyond (e.g. schools).
- Young people must provide their consent for doctors to contact school-based professionals.

Transition to adult health care

Transition is the purposeful and planned movement of adolescents with chronic diseases and disability from child-centred to adult-oriented health care systems. 'Transition' refers to the process of facilitating developmentally appropriate self-management and generally requires the acquisition of knowledge, attitudes and skills over time. This skill set starts to develop well before transfer to adult health care, the actual timing of the physical move, with the process of transition continuing well after transfer. From the time of diagnosis, anticipation of transfer to an adult setting is one way of ensuring that the physical move is truly part of a broader transition process.

Practical tips for successful transition

- Start seeing young people alone for at least part of the health consultation from about the age of 14 years. This helps remind parents that their children are growing up, can prompt young people 'stepping up' within health consultations and facilitate successful transition to adult health care.
- Use a checklist and resources to support success transition (See http://www.rch.org.au/transition/).
- Planning and coordination of transfer to adult health care is essential. Young people may be transferred from specialist paediatric service to primary care, while others will transfer to adult specialist services in public hospitals or to private specialists, including psychiatrists. In all cases, GPs are a critical resource.
- When adult tertiary care is indicated, identify an adult specialist team that is both interested and capable of providing tertiary care. This is fundamental, but sometimes challenging.
- Documentation to support the transfer is important: a detailed health care summary should be compiled and clearly communicated to adult providers. It is important the adolescent and their GP also receive a summary of this information.

Management of specific health problems in adolescence
Fatigue

Fatigue is a common presenting complaint in adolescent medical consultations. It is often accompanied by other constitutional and neuropsychological symptoms (commonly sleep disturbance, headaches, abdominal pain, nausea, postural and depressive symptoms).
Differential diagnoses include

- Depression
- Inadequate sleep (e.g. obstructive sleep apnoea, excessive nocturnal computer use)
- Hypothyroidism
- Anaemia
- Malabsorption syndromes (e.g. coeliac disease)
- Chronic Illness (e.g. inflammatory bowel disease, connective tissue disease, renal disease)
- Chronic fatigue syndrome (CFS). This is a clinical diagnosis. Many patients have a preceding history of suspected or confirmed viral illness although examination and investigations are usually normal.

The management of CFS involves a multidisciplinary approach with engagement of the GP and school based professionals.

- A multidisciplinary approach. Ongoing consultation with the patient, family, school/education providers and the local doctor.
- A graded return to normal life via a balanced reintroduction of activities including social contact.
- Support a graded return to function via the balanced introduction of activities including learning and social engagement.
- Symptomatic treatment of focal symptoms (e.g. sleep disturbance) is required.
- Pay close attention to the psychosocial aspects of the illness.
- A majority of patients with CFS will recover with normal function but it may take several years.

Substance use and misuse

- Assess other psychosocial risks as adolescents who use substances are more likely to experience other health risks, including mental health concerns.
- Take a non-judgemental, 'harm minimisation' approach to preserve rapport. Over time, important health messages can be conveyed and reasons for using drugs explored.
- Referral to specialist drug services is generally not helpful unless the young person wishes to reduce substance use.

Mental health

Adolescence is characterised by a marked increase in a wide range of emotional and mental health disorders. The presence or extent of these may not be appreciated by adolescents themselves or by their parents, hence the importance of opportunistic assessment.

Eating Disorders

Eating disorders typically arise in the early to mid-teens. Dieting is a common antecedent to a clinical presentation. More severe dieting behaviours are associated with a greater risk of developing an eating disorder, although the majority of those who go on to develop an eating disorder have more moderate levels of dieting. Abnormal eating behaviour and a preoccupation with weight or body shape that interferes with normal adolescent social or emotional functioning requires further assessment, especially when it is associated with significant weight loss (even if the adolescent is not underweight).

Anorexia nervosa

The diagnostic criteria of anorexia nervosa include

- Restriction of energy intake leading to a markedly low body weight.
- Intense fear of gaining weight or becoming fat or persistent behaviour to avoid weight gain, even though at a markedly low weight.
- Body image disturbance or persistent lack of recognition of the seriousness of the current low body weight.
- A typical anorexia nervosa describes those who have lost significant weight (e.g. 5–20 kg in 6–12 months) and have all the diagnostic features of anorexia nervosa except they are not underweight.

Anorexia nervosa can be of either restricting type or binge-eating/purging type (self-induced vomiting or the misuse of laxatives, diuretics or enemas in the last 3 months).

Differential diagnoses include physical disorders (e.g. thyrotoxicosis, malabsorption) and other psychiatric disorders (e.g. major depression, obsessive compulsive disorder).

Physical complications are potentially very severe, especially if the onset of the disorder occurs during the prepubertal or peripubertal stages where growth retardation and osteoporosis are of particular concern. Cardiac arrhythmias, substance abuse, self-harm and suicide contribute to a mortality rate that is greater than that of any other psychological disorder.

Management

- Confirm diagnosis by careful medical and mental health assessment (not electrolytes).
- Provide multidisciplinary outpatient care utilising family-based treatment which aims to empower the parents/carers to refeed the adolescent to a healthy body weight within the home environment.
- Brief hospital admission is required when evidence of physiological compromise (e.g. bradycardia or postural hypotension) signals lack of physical safety.
- Refeeding is the mainstay of acute admissions that aim to achieve physiological stability. The adolescent is supported to eat the meals provided to them; nasogastric feeding is required if the adolescent is unable to eat enough to appropriately gain weight.
- Refeeding syndrome is a common and potentially fatal acute complication that requires careful monitoring of electrolyte and cardiovascular status, especially within the first 72 hours following increased caloric intake.

Bulimia nervosa

Bulimia Nervosa is characterized by repeated episodes of bingeing (excessive or compulsive consumption of food) and purging (getting rid of food), eating beyond the point of fullness, feeling out of control during a binge, inappropriate compensatory behaviors following a binge, frequent dieting, and extreme concern with body weight and shape. Diagnostic criteria are:

- Recurrent episodes of binge eating characterised by lack of control during the episode.
- Recurrent inappropriate compensatory behaviour in order to prevent weight gain (e.g. self-induced vomiting, misuse of laxatives, diuretics, other medications, fasting or excessive exercise).
- The binge eating and inappropriate compensatory behaviours both occur, on average, at least once per week for 3 months, and
- Self-evaluation is unduly influenced by body shape and weight.

Common co-morbidities and complications

- Depression.
- Anxiety.
- Difficulties with impulse control in other areas (e.g. alcohol and substance use, self-harm).

Potential complications

- Dental erosion.

- Oesophagitis.
- Potentially severe electrolyte abnormalities leading to cardiac arrhythmias can occur.

Management
- Usually occurs on an outpatient basis.
- Focal psychotherapies such as cognitive-behavioural therapy are effective both in individual and group treatment settings.
- Antidepressant medication such as selective serotonin reuptake inhibitors (SSRIs) are indicated when severe depressive symptoms are present.

Binge Eating Disorder
Diagnostic criteria for binge eating disorder include
- Recurrent episodes of binge eating characterised by a sense of lack of control during the episode.
- The binge eating episodes are associated with eating more rapidly than normal, eating until uncomfortably full, eating large amounts of food when not feeling hungry, eating alone due to embarrassment and feeling disgusted with oneself, depressed or very guilty after overeating.
- Marked distress regarding binge eating is present.
- The binge eating occurs, on average, at least once per week for 3 months and is not associated with recurrent use of inappropriate compensatory behaviour (e.g. purging).

While overeating is commonly seen within the general population, binge eating disorder is much less common, is far more severe and is associated with significant complications relating to the physical and psychological problems of obesity (see Chapter 14, *Growth and puberty*, p. 205).

Menstrual problems
Menorrhagia (heavy menses)
Menorrhagia is a common and often distressing symptom for adolescent females. It may occur as a result of anovulation particularly in the first few years post menarche, or more rarely from bleeding diatheses, pregnancy-related causes, or endometritis, secondary to chlamydia.

Assessment
Take a menstrual history which includes
- Frequency of periods.
- Date of menarche.
- Heaviness of loss (number of pads, passage of clots); heavy loss usually includes changing pads more frequently than 2 hourly, or overnight changes or overflow; missing school due to heaviness.
- Bleeding history (bruising, epistaxis, gum bleeds, post-operative bleeding and family history of bleeding).
- Assess if sexually active (see HEADSS, Table 22.2).
- Exercise.
- Stress.

Investigations
- FBE
- Iron studies
- Consider further haematological testing for underlying bleeding disorder
- If sexually active consider
  - β-HCG (for pregnancy-related heavy bleeding, ectopic pregnancy or miscarriage)
  - Chlamydia PCR

Management
- Iron supplements if required.
- Non-steroidal anti-inflammatory drugs (reduce menstrual loss by 30%).
- Tranexamic acid (antifibrinolytic agent, reduce menstrual loss by 50%).
- Oral contraceptive pill. This can be used continuously to skip menses, or used cyclically with tranexamic acid.
- Depot medroxyprogesterone acetate.
- Levonorgestrel intrauterine system (reduces menstrual loss by 95% and requires a general anaesthetic for insertion in non-sexually active adolescents).

Amenorrhoea

Primary amenorrhoea

Causes of primary amenorrhoea include

- Obstructive anomalies (see Chapter 10, *The urogenital tract*).
- Uterovaginal agenesis. Clinical features include
  - Postpubertal adolescent with absent menses.
  - No uterus seen on ultrasound.
  - Treatment: surgical dilatation to form a vagina.
- Hormonal causes include (see Chapter 13, *The endocrine system* and Chapter 14, *Growth and puberty*)
  - Central/hypothalamic causes: underweight (anorexia, elite athlete), secondary to a medical condition (Crohn's disease, post irradiation).
  - Pituitary causes: hyperprolactinaemia, thyroid disease, panhypopituitarism.
  - Ovarian failure: gonadal dysgenesis, premature ovarian insufficiency.
  - Adrenal causes: poorly controlled congenital adrenal hyperplasia (CAH), late onset CAH.
  - Absent hormone receptor: androgen insensitivity syndrome.

Management

The management of adolescents with significant reproductive diagnoses (gonadal dysgenesis, ovarian insufficiency, uterovaginal agenesis, androgen insensitivity syndrome) requires a sensitive approach and recognition of the significant impact of the diagnosis on future fertility/infertility. Referral to a specialist familiar with these issues is recommended.

Secondary amenorrhoea

Causes of secondary amenorrhoea include

- Hormonal causes – as listed above.
- Overweight /obesity – see Chapter 14, *Growth and puberty*, p. 205.
- Pregnancy – the identification of a pregnant adolescent should alert the clinician to other risk behaviours associated with sexual activity in young people. A HEADSS screen should be performed and consideration given to screening for chlamydia infection. Appropriate referral for discussion of pregnancy options is required.
- Strenuous exercise.
- Stress (e.g. exams, social/family or travel).
- Polycystic ovary syndrome.

Treat the symptoms for each of these problems as required.

Polycystic ovary syndrome (PCOS) (The international criteria for this condition are for adult women, not adolescents)

- Irregular menses or multiple follicles found on pelvic ultrasound AND
- Signs of excess androgen (severe acne and/or hirsutism);
- Obesity is a common association.

The diagnosis of PCOS (particularly in adolescents) can be difficult as normal variants overlap. Many teenagers who have multiple follicles on pelvic ultrasound are inappropriately told they have PCOS. Multiple follicles (15–20) are completely normal in this age group. Many adolescents in the first 1–3 years after menarche have irregular menses due to immature hypothalamic-pituitary–ovarian axis.

Management

Treat the symptoms as required. There is little benefit from a label of PCOS and there is a risk of unplanned pregnancy when contraception is stopped or not used due to perceived infertility.

- Address obesity (see Chapter 14, *Growth and puberty*, p. 205). This can significantly improve the irregular menses, and hirsutism.
- Amenorrhoea itself does not need treatment, but associated problems may require intervention. Oligomenorrhoea may require treatment on its own merits (heavy, painful, unpredictable).
- Hirsutism responds to the oral contraceptive pill due to improved oestrogen levels. This may be further aided by an oral contraceptive pill containing cyproterone acetate (an antiandrogen). This initiates withdrawal bleeds, which are lighter and more regular.

- Infertility: irregular ovulation may impede fertility. Specialist advice is recommended when planning conception.
- Osteopenia: prolonged amenorrhoea associated with low oestrogen levels potentially leads to a negative effect on bone mineral density. The addition of hormonal treatment may then be indicated.

Menstrual related pain/dysmenorrhea

Period pain is very common in adolescents. There are a number of potential causes of dysmenorrhea such as:

- prostaglandin-related dysmenorrhea;
- retrograde bleeding;
- congenital urogenital anomalies; and
- endometriosis.

Assessment

Obtain a clear history to understand the pattern of the pain and associated symptoms. The pattern of pain may give clues to the underlying cause

- Pain may begin a few days prior to menses, with maximum pain usually just before or on the first few days of menses.
- Pain may radiate to thighs and low back.
- Associated symptoms such as nausea, vomiting, diarrhoea, lethargy, fainting and dizziness occur frequently, and may support a diagnosis of *prostaglandin-related dysmenorrhea*.
- Stress will often precipitate more severe episodes of dysmenorrhoea.
- Pain can also occur due to *retrograde bleeding* which occurs in >90% of menstruating women. Free fluid (blood) in the peritoneal cavity may cause symptoms of peritoneal irritation such as pain with movement, voiding and defaecation.
- Pain due to an *obstructive anomaly* usually increases with each cycle and is worse towards the end of the period.

Prostaglandin induced/primary dysmenorrhea is diagnosed predominantly on clinical history.

Vaginal examination is not done if the young woman is not sexually active, and even then only with careful consent. Occasionally, vaginal examination in young women who are using tampons may be possible, but alternatives such as a transabdominal pelvic ultrasound examination will usually provide all the required information (obstructive anomaly).

Management

Treatment options for dysmenorrhoea include

- Prophylactic non-steroidal anti-inflammatory drugs and/or tranexamic acid. These can reduce menstrual loss if the adolescent has heavy menses or symptoms of peritoneal irritation.
- The oral contraceptive pill will reduce menstrual loss and pain. This can be used continuously to skip menses and avoid painful withdrawal bleeds.
- If an obstructive anomaly is identified, corrective surgical intervention may be required.

Other treatment options include

- Depot medroxyprogesterone acetate to suppress menses.
- Levonorgestrel intrauterine system (Mirena IUS) or etonorgestrel implant (may reduce menstrual loss, although may cause irregular bleeding in 30%).

Endometriosis

Endometriosis is usually caused by retrograde bleeding and is more common in women with heavy menstrual loss. Reducing menstrual loss will reduce the amount of retrograde bleeding.

Management

- Symptom management and menstrual suppression.
- Surgery can usually be avoided as there is no evidence that an early laparoscopy will alter long-term outcome.

Sexual health

Respectful inquiry about a young person's sexual health may identify individuals who are at risk because of unsafe sexual relationships (physical risks; e.g. STIs; unplanned pregnancy; emotional risks; e.g. rape, sexual abuse). It also offers the opportunity for sexual health education.

Adolescents, both male and female, who are sexually active at a young age are also more likely to be involved in other health risk behaviours and careful screening for these is appropriate. An initial screen can be done using HEADSS (see Table 22.2). Remind the young person that the discussion and any tests are confidential. It is important to understand the legal context of sexual intercourse in minors. For example, in Victoria, statutory rape refers to sexual intercourse when a person is under 16 years old and has sexual intercourse (consensual or not) with someone who is 2 years older.

Do not assume knowledge regarding sexual activity, safe sex and contraception.

Be opportunistic and discuss immunisation (e.g. HPV vaccine), contraceptive options, STI prevention and PAP smears.

Chlamydia screening is recommended annually
Contraception: best options for young women

Condoms

Condoms offer the advantage of protection from STIs, as well as fairly good contraception. They may not be a reliable form of contraception if alcohol and drug-taking are issues.

Oral contraceptive pill

Contraindications

- Thromboembolic disease
- Liver disease
- Oestrogen-dependent tumours
- Migraines with neurological signs

Note: Migraines can be oestrogen-induced (onset with commencement of OCP) or secondary to oestrogen withdrawal (onset with menses) in which case menses should be avoided through continuous use of the OCP.

Short-term side effects

- Nausea. this tends to settle, although a lower oestrogen dose pill is an alternative option.
- Breast tenderness.
- Mood-related problems may relate to the type of progestagen. Altering the oral contraceptive pill (or progestagen) may help.
- Breakthrough bleeding (this should resolve with continuing usage or change of pill type).

Types

- Constant dose (e.g. Microgynon 30ED and Nordette): for the patient who suffers erratic, heavy periods, premenstrual moodiness or irregular lifestyle routines (there is a slightly greater leeway in the time of taking such pills).
- Higher oestrogen content: if using anticonvulsants (which increases hepatic metabolism of OCP) or if there is persistent breakthrough bleeding.

Note: A higher oestrogen dose OCP is required for individuals using anticonvulsants.

Other forms of contraception

- Implanon: hormonal implant inserted under the skin in the upper arm. Very effective contraception that lasts 3 years. Often associated with a reduction in menstrual loss, although irregular periods occur in up to 30% of young women. Amenorrhoea occurs in 20%.
- Etonorgestrel implant: subdermal implant to upper arm. Lasts for 3 years. Reliable contraception but 30% may experience irregular bleeding.
- Depo Provera: a 150 mg, 3-monthly injection. This often causes irregular bleeding initially but amenorrhoea after 6–9 months. Very reliable contraception. Long-term usage in teenagers may have some impact on bone density although this appears to be reversible. Depo Provera – 3 monthly injection. Reliable contraception. Irregular bleeding in the first 6 months, then most are amenorrhoeic.

- Mirena IUS: very reliable, lasts 5 years. This is associated with reduced menstrual loss and reduced period pain.
- Progesterone-only pill: Not often used in adolescents as it is less reliable than combined OCP and must be taken at the same time every day to be effective.

Emergency contraception
Prostinor 2 (levonorgestrel 75 mcg, 2 tablets).
- Take both tablets at once, as soon as possible after intercourse.
- Available over the counter.
- Can be used up to 72 hours after unprotected intercourse. Some evidence for its use up to 5–7 days, although with reduced efficacy.

These treatments are >90% effective, but do not provide continuing contraception. It is essential to plan ongoing contraception, STI prevention, PAP smears and follow-up strategies to ensure that the emergency treatment has worked.

Pelvic Inflammatory disease
Common causative organisms of Pelvic Inflammatory disease (PID) include Neisseria gonorrhoea, coliforms, *Gardnerella vaginalis*, *Haemophilus influenzae*, group B *Streptococcus* and *Bacteroides* species.

Assessment
Consider PID in a sexually active young woman with pelvic pain. It is often associated with vaginal discharge, dyspareunia and fever.

Investigations
- Do endocervical and high vaginal swabs for culture and PCR. (Consider blood cultures if febrile).
- If unable to do speculum – urine PCR for chlamydia and gonorrhoea.

Management
- Broad spectrum antibiotic cover required (see local Therapeutic guidelines).
- Admit for IV antibiotics if febrile.

CHAPTER 23

Child development and disability

Daryl Efron
Catherine Marraffa
Sheena Reilly
Dinah Reddihough

Developmental delay and disability

Approximately 3–5% of children have developmental delay of at least mild–moderate severity that may remain undiagnosed unless specific assessment is undertaken. In general, problems affecting motor development and speech present early, and problems affecting receptive language, socialisation and cognition present later. The clinician's role is to ascertain whether a child's development is aberrant for their age and to determine if there are underlying reasons for this. The term "delay" can be misleading for families of children who have a condition which is known to cause long-term functional impairment. Where this is the case, a sensitive explanation of the use of "developmental disability" is often helpful.

Developmental surveillance

Developmental surveillance is a flexible, continuous process of skilled observation as part of providing routine health care. It should occur opportunistically whenever a child comes into contact with a health professional.

If a parent is concerned about a child's development it is likely that evaluation will confirm developmental delay; however, a lack of concern from parents is no guarantee that the child's development is normal.

Screening methods

- Informal clinical judgement – mostly unreliable. Milestone checklists (see Table 23.1) serve as a memory aid but do not take into account the wide range normal development.
- PEDS (Parents' Evaluation of Developmental Status) – used in the primary care setting and consists of 10 questions aimed to elicit parental concern. It is validated from birth to 8 years.
- Formal screening (e.g. Denver II, the Australian Developmental Screening Tests, the Brigance) – allows the objective discrimination of the child who *probably* has a developmental delay from the child who *probably* does not. A fail on such a test requires referral of the child for formal developmental assessment.
- Formal assessment (e.g. Bayley Scales of Infant Development, the Griffiths Mental Development Scales) – test used depends on the child's risk factors (see Table 23.2).

Children with developmental delay or disability, have the same basic needs as all children. They have the potential for further development and the principles of normal development apply.

Specific disabilities in one area may cause secondary disabilities in other areas (e.g. children who have motor disabilities with reduced opportunity for exploration may suffer delayed development of their comprehension abilities).

Developmental delay may be associated with

- Prematurity
- Physical illness
- Prolonged hospitalisation
- Family stress
- Lack of opportunities to learn

Persistent developmental disabilities include

- Language disorders

Paediatric Handbook, Ninth Edition. Edited by Amanda Gwee, Romi Rimer and Michael Marks.
© 2015 John Wiley & Sons, Ltd. Published 2015 by John Wiley & Sons, Ltd.

Table 23.1 Developmental milestones

Age[a]	Gross motor	Fine motor adaptive	Language	Personal–social
1 m	Lifts head momentarily while prone (0–3 w)	Visual following to mid-line (0–5 w)		Watches face (0–4 w)
2 m	Lifts head momentarily to erect position when sitting	Hands predominantly open	Vocalises (0–7 w)	Smiles responsively (0–7 w)
3 m	Lifts head to 90° while prone (0–10 w)	Visual following past mid-line (0–10 w)	Laughs (6–10 w)	
4 m	Head steady when held erect (6–17 w)	Plays with hands together (6–15 w)	Coos and gurgles	Excited by approach of food
5 m	No head lag when pulled to sitting (3–6 m). Rolls over	Grasps rattle (10–18 w) Reaches for object with palmar grasp (3–5½ m)	Squeals (6–18 w)	Smiles spontaneously (6 w–5 m)
6 m	Lifts head forward when pulled to sit (9–19 w)	Passes block hand to hand (4½–7½ m)	Turns to voice (3½–8½ m)	Friendly to all comers
8 m	Maintains sitting position without support		Repetition of syllables (e.g. baba, Dada)	Feeds self-biscuit (5–8 m) Tries to get toy out of reach (5–9 m)
10 m	Stands holding on (5–10 m)	Index finger approach	'Mama', 'Dada' without meaning (6–10 m)	Shy with strangers Plays peek-a-boo
12 m	Walks holding on to furniture (7½–12½ m)	Crude finger–thumb grasp (7–11 m)	Imitates speech sounds (6–11 m)	Gives up a toy
15 m	Walks alone (11½–15 m)	Neat pincer grasp of pellet (9–15 m)	'Mama', 'Dada' with meaning (9–15 m)	Indicates wants (10½–14½ m)
1½ y	Walks well (11½–18 m)	Builds tower of two blocks (12–20 m)	Three words other than 'Mama', 'Dada' (12–20 m)	Drinks from cup (10–17 m)
2 y	Walks up steps without help (14–22 m)	Scribbles (12–24 m)	Points to one named body part (14–23 m)	Feeds self with spoon (12–24 m)
2½ y	Throws ball (15–32 m)	Builds tower of four blocks (15–26 m)	Combines two words (14–27 m)	Helps in house – simple tasks (15–24 m)
3 y	Pedals tricycle (21 m–3 y)	Imitates vertical line (18 m–3 y) Copies circle (2½–3½ y)	Uses three word sentences	Puts on clothes (2–3 y)
4 y	Balances on one foot (2³⁄₄–4½ y)	Copies square	Gives first and last name (2–4 y)	Dresses with supervision (2½–3½ y)
5 y	Hops on one foot (3–5 y)	Draws person in three parts (3–5 y)	Knows some colours (3–5 y) Knows age	Dresses without supervision (2½–5 y)

w, weeks; m, months; y, years.

[a]Age indicates when at least 90% of a normal group of children will achieve the test. Figures in parentheses represent the range from 25th to 90th centiles for achievement.

- Intellectual disability
- Cerebral palsy
- Autism spectrum disorder
- Hearing impairment
- Visual impairment
- Degenerative disorders
- Neuromuscular disorders

Once concern regarding a child's development has been raised, a detailed paediatric consultation is required. This should include full details of the family, obstetric, neonatal, developmental and social histories. Liaison with the GP and a maternal and child health nurse to obtain background information is often helpful. A history of loss of previously attained developmental skills is suggestive of regression rather than delay and requires more comprehensive investigation to exclude neurodegenerative conditions. Observation of how the child looks, listens, moves, explores, plays, communicates and socialises is essential before the formal examination. Understandably, parents will be anxious and a sensitive approach is essential at all times.

Developmental assessment provides the family with an understanding of the child's developmental status and outlines developmental goals and strategies. Further assessment and management may include input from physiotherapists, speech pathologists, occupational therapists, psychologists, specialist teachers and social workers.

Principles of assessment

These include

- Utilisation of play as a fundamental assessment tool.
- Involvement of the parents in the assessment process.
- Promotion of optimal performance of the child.
- Gearing the assessment towards remediation rather than merely producing a profile.
- Close linking of the assessment with services offering support.

Early intervention

The aims of early intervention are to minimise the handicapping effects of the child's disability and to support the family in understanding and providing for their child's individual needs. Services include individual teaching and therapy (speech therapy, physiotherapy and occupational therapy), family support and counselling as well as providing resources and support to childcare, preschools and respite carers. Services are usually regionally based and are provided by government and non-government agencies. Unfortunately, waiting lists for these Early Childhood Intervention Services can be many months and it is important to enlist other locally available services while awaiting these specialist services.

The Australian government has a number of initiatives which help fund services for certain developmental conditions.

Education

There is a range of special educational strategies to optimise learning and development, dependent on the child's abilities and disabilities. Paediatricians should liaise with the school in order to best support the child and his/her family. This may include applying for government funding for aides, management of physical disability, seizure management and behavioural support. GPs may assist in these processes.

Family supports

Parents need to be informed of the services that are available to them. Supports include social security benefits, home help, respite care and community residential units. Consumer organisations can provide parent support, information and advocacy.

Learning difficulties

A specific learning disability is defined as a discrepancy between a child's intellectual ability and their academic achievement. There are many reasons why a child may experience learning difficulties, and often multiple factors are involved. These include specific learning disabilities (commonly language–literacy based), intellectual

Table 23.2 Children at risk of developmental problems

Risk group	Risk factors	Action
High	Developmental regression Abnormal neurology Dysmorphism Chromosomal abnormality Hearing or vision problems	Bypass developmental screening Refer for comprehensive developmental assessment

Moderate	Parents suspect developmental delay
	History of severe prenatal or perinatal
	    insult
	Very low birthweight (<1500 g)
	Family history of developmental delay
	Severe socio-economic or family
	    adversity
		Administer a formal screening test
		Pass – reassure that development is within normal
		    range and continue surveillance through local
		    doctor/maternal and child health nurse
		Questionable – repeat the test 4 weeks later
		Fail – refer for comprehensive paediatric
		    consultation and developmental assessment

Low	No parental or professional concerns
	No other risk factors
		Developmental surveillance by local
		    doctor/maternal and child health nurse is
		    recommended
		Should there be later parental or professional
		    concerns, a formal screening test is
		    recommended
		If there are no further concerns, continue
		    surveillance monitoring

disabilities, attention deficits, sensory impairments (hearing, auditory processing, vision), emotional disturbance, chronic illness, family and social difficulties, and suboptimal teaching or educational environments.

Assessment
- Obtain information from both parents and teachers (including previous reports).
- Neurodevelopmental assessment.
- Formal educational psychology assessment.

Management
- The doctor has an important role in excluding treatable contributing medical factors (e.g. sleep deprivation, iron deficiency, ADHD, depression, epilepsy), as well as advocating for the child.
- Liaise closely with the school to ensure appropriate assessments are undertaken and that an individualised educational plan is devised and reviewed periodically.
- In severe cases an application for disability programme-funded assistance should be made via the school to the education department.
- Some children benefit from remedial tuition either within or outside school hours. It is important for parents not to overburden children, who also need normal recreational time.
- Parents need support in understanding their child's potential and ways in which they can help optimise their child's learning. Identifying and enhancing the child's strengths is important in maintaining self-esteem.

Speech and language impairment
Language impairment can involve receptive skills (ability to understand spoken language), expressive skills (language production), pragmatic skills (the social use of language) or a combination of these (Table 23.3). Articulation/phonological problems may also occur, resulting in reduced speech intelligibility.

Background
- Approximately 20% of 2-year olds have smaller vocabularies than would be expected (i.e. <50 words and few or no word combinations) yet only 30% are still delayed at 4 years.
- The prevalence of language impairment at school entry is between 5% and 16% depending on how impairment is defined.

Table 23.3 Speech and language milestones: indicators of concern

Age (years)	Reason for concern
6 months	No response to sound, not cooing, laughing or vocalising
12 months	Not localising to sound or vocalising. No babbling or babbling contains a low proportion of consonant vowel babble (e.g. baba). Doesn't understand simple words (e.g. 'no' and 'bye'), recognise names of common objects or responds to simple requests (e.g. clap hands) with an action Does not respond reliably to name by turning head
18 months	No meaningful words except 'mum/dad'. Doesn't understand and hand over objects on request
2 years	Expressive vocabulary <50 words and no word combinations. Cannot find 2–3 objects on request
3 years	Speech is not understood within the family. Not using simple grammatical structures (e.g. tense markers). Doesn't understand concepts such as colour and size
4 years	Speech is not understood outside the family. Not using complex sentences (4–6 words). Not able to construct simple stories
5 years	Speech is not intelligible. Does not understand abstract words and ideas. Cannot reconstruct a story from a book

- It is not possible to predict with any certainty which children will go on to have persistent speech and language problems.

Prognosis
- Children with isolated expressive language impairment tend to have positive outcomes.
- Children with mixed or receptive language impairments, and those with social communication difficulties are at higher risk and should be referred to speech pathologists as early as possible.
Preschool children with persistent speech and language impairment tend to have
- Learning and social difficulties when starting formal schooling.
- Increased risk for later literacy and numeracy problems.
- Increased rate of emotional and behavioural disorders.
These problems may persist into adolescence and adulthood and affect employment opportunities.

Factors raising concern about speech and language
- Parental concern regarding speech and language development.
- History of hearing loss.
- Delay in both receptive and expressive language skills.
- Concern about other aspects of development and lack of developmental progress.
- Autistic features.
- Parental report of regression in babbling or language.
- Family history of speech and language problems.

Management
- Assess other areas of the child's development.
- Refer to an audiologist to exclude hearing loss.
- Refer to a speech pathologist as early as possible.
- In cases where regression in language is suspected, refer promptly to a paediatrician.

Stuttering
Stuttering is a disorder that affects the fluency of speech production. It has a strong genetic link, with 50–75% having at least one relative who also stutters. While the exact cause of stuttering is still not known, recent research has found that onset is not associated with anxiety, stress or personality differences.

Stuttering behaviours can include repeated speech movements, such as 'I w-w-w-w-w-w-w-was saying ... ' and fixed postures which include stretching out a sound in a word (prolongations) or not being able to produce any sound (blocks). Other features include are superfluous behaviours, such as visible tension in the head and/or neck.

Approximately 12% of children will stutter at some point by 4 years of age. While the majority of children will recover eventually, it is not possible to predict which children will recover. Current best practice recommends waiting for up to 12 months before commencing treatment. However, if the child is distressed, there is parental concern or the child becomes reluctant to communicate then refer to a speech pathologist to assess the child and make appropriate recommendations.

Management

- Treatment of preschool children who stutter should be undertaken by speech pathologists trained in the Lidcombe Program, which has the best evidence in this age group.
- Parents should be advised to converse with their children normally and not draw attention to stuttering. If the child is visibly frustrated, recommend they acknowledge this in a sensitive manner. For example, your speech seems 'bumpy' today.
- Stuttering is more difficult to treat in older children.

Intellectual disability

Intellectual disability affects up to 2.5% of children. It is defined as a significantly subaverage general intellectual functioning (i.e. two standard deviations below the mean of the intelligence quotient) which

1. Exists concurrently with deficits in adaptive behaviour; and
2. Manifests itself during the developmental period.

Causes of intellectual disability

Prenatal

- Chromosomal: e.g. trisomy 21, fragile X syndrome and velocardiofacial syndrome.
- Genetic: e.g. tuberous sclerosis and metabolic disorders.
- Major structural anomalies of the brain.
- Syndromes: e.g. Williams, Prader–Willi, Rett.
- In-utero infections: e.g. cytomegalovirus.
- Drugs: e.g. alcohol.

Perinatal

- CNS infections
- Brain trauma
- Metabolic abnormalities
- Very low birth weight

Postnatal

- Head injury
- Meningitis or encephalitis
- Poisons

In people with mild intellectual disability, the cause is identifiable in <20% of individuals. Where a cause is identified, the majority are caused by problems during the prenatal period. The three most common identifiable causes of intellectual disability are trisomy 21, fragile X syndrome and velocardiofacial syndrome.

Investigations

It is important to establish aetiology where possible in order to understand prognosis, provide genetic counselling and to ensure that associated problems are detected.

The following investigations should be considered:

- Screening for congenital infections
- Thyroid function testing
- Chromosomal microarray testing
- Fragile X testing

- Creatinine kinase
- Metabolic screen
- MRI Brain

Despite thorough investigation, the cause is often not identified.

Management

- Support and information for parents.
- Referral to and liaison with other practitioners.
- Early intervention, family support and educational services.
- Child advocacy.
- Regular assessment of vision and hearing.
- Investigation for associated anomalies (e.g. cardiac, hearing, thyroid and coeliac status for children with trisomy 21).
- Treatment of associated disorders (e.g. epilepsy, behavioural problems).
- Monitoring of development.

Cerebral palsy

Cerebral palsy (CP) describes a group of permanent disorders of movement and posture causing activity limitation, following an insult to the developing foetal or infant brain. The motor disorders of CP are often accompanied by disturbances of sensation, perception, cognition, communication and behaviour, by epilepsy and by secondary musculoskeletal problems. It has a prevalence of 1.5–2.5 per 1000 live births.

Aetiology

There are many risk factors (e.g. low birthweight and prematurity) but few definite causes. Perinatal asphyxia accounts for <10% of cases and post-neonatal illnesses or injuries for a further 10%.

Classification

CP is classified according to the

- Type of motor disorder (e.g. spasticity, dyskinesia (includes dystonia and athetosis), ataxia, mixed).
- Distribution of the motor disorder (e.g. hemiplegia, diplegia and quadriplegia).
- Severity of the motor disorder on gross motor function and mobility, using the Gross Motor Function Classification System (GMFCS).

Presentation

Children with CP may present with

- delayed motor milestones
- asymmetric movement patterns
- abnormal muscle tone
- associated problems (e.g. severe feeding difficulties and irritability)

Investigation

CP is a clinical diagnosis.

- An MRI brain scan should be undertaken if the cause is unknown. This may provide information about underlying neuropathology and timing of the brain injury.
- Testing for genetic and metabolic conditions is sometimes necessary, particularly in the presence of a normal MRI brain scan.
- Progressive neurodevelopmental conditions may present in a similar manner to CP and must be excluded.

Management

A multidisciplinary team approach with family input is essential. Remember the usual childhood needs for immunisation and good dental health.

Associated impairments

- **Communication difficulties** include receptive and expressive language delays and dysarthria. Some children require an alternative means of communication such as an electronic device. The Communication Function Classification System rates a child's everyday communication performance regardless of the method used.
- **Intellectual disability and specific learning problems** occur in about 50% of children with CP. Children benefit from cognitive assessment particularly at school entry. Perceptual problems may also be identified.
- **Manual limitations** in grasping, releasing or manipulating objects, which impact on a child's ability to perform everyday tasks. For children aged 4–18 years, manual ability levels are classified using the Manual Abilities Classification System.
- **Visual problems** are found in about 45% of children with CP. All children require a visual assessment.
- **Hearing deficits** of at least moderate degree are found in about 7% of children with CP. All children require a hearing assessment.

Health problems

- Provide advice about **constipation** resulting from immobility, low-fibre diet and poor fluid intake.
- Monitor for risk of **aspiration** and subsequent **chronic lung disease**. Coughing or choking during mealtimes or wheeze during or after meals may signal the presence of aspiration. It can also occur without symptoms or signs. Videofluoroscopy may be useful.
- **Growth** should be monitored. Poor weight gain, major feeding problems or aspiration are indications for non-oral feeding by nasogastric or gastrostomy tube. Conversely obesity can occur particularly in children with GMFCS levels I,II and III.
- **Gastro-oesophageal reflux**, oesophagitis with associated pain, bleeding and resulting anaemia are common in CP.
- Undescended testes are more frequent in this group.
- Manage **epilepsy** with optimal medication regimes.
- **Osteopenia** is frequent. Monitor vitamin D levels, especially in children with limited sun exposure and watch for pathological fractures.
- Pay careful attention to **psychological** and **social** difficulties.

Consequences of the motor disorder

- **Poor saliva control** can be improved by speech pathology input, the use of medication and occasionally surgery.
- **Incontinence** may be due to cognitive deficits, lack of opportunity, and detrusor overactivity.
- **Spasticity** and **dystonia** should be managed with the aim of improving function, comfort and care. A team approach is required. Options include
  - ○ Prescription of appropriate aides and equipment to facilitate function.
  - ○ Oral medications, for example diazepam, baclofen and L-Dopa.
  - ○ Botulinum toxin for localized spasticity or focal dystonia. Botulinum toxin may be followed by serial casting to increase joint range.
  - ○ Intrathecal baclofen for a small number of children with severe spasticity or dystonia.
  - ○ Selective dorsal rhizotomy for a selected group of children with severe spastic diplegia.
- **Orthopaedic intervention**: Surgery is mainly undertaken on the lower limb, but is occasionally helpful in the upper limb. Some children also require surgery for scoliosis. Physiotherapy is an essential part of postoperative management with advice from occupational therapists regarding equipment for home use. Gait laboratories are useful in planning the surgical program for ambulant children.
  - ○ **The hips**: non-walkers (GMFCS IV, V) and those ambulant only with mobility devices (GMFCS III) are prone to hip subluxation and eventual dislocation. Early detection is vital. Hip x-rays should be performed according to hip surveillance guidelines at http://www.ausacpdm.org.au/_data/assets/pdf_file/0007/14569/consensus_statement.pdf. Dislocation causes severe pain, is extremely difficult to treat and can usually be prevented by timely orthopaedic surgery.

○ **The knees**: flexion contractures may require hamstring surgery.
○ **The ankles**: equinus deformity is the most common orthopaedic problem in children with CP. It is treated conservatively in young children with orthoses, and botulinum toxin. Older children may require surgery. A range of other problems around the foot and ankle may benefit from orthopaedic assessment.

Referrals
Liaising with the kindergarten, school and family doctor (GP) is important. Referral to and ongoing liaison with allied health professionals is essential to enable children to achieve their optimal potential and independence.

- **Physiotherapists** aim to reduce impairments and optimise function. They also give advice regarding mobility aids, the use of orthoses and special seating.
- **Occupational therapists** provide parents with advice on developing their child's upper limb and self-care skills. They design and make arm and hand splints, can provide advice on specialized equipment (such as car seats and adapted cutlery) and recommend home modifications.
- **Speech pathologists** assist with severe eating and drinking difficulties, as well as communication and augmentative communication systems for children with limited verbal skills.
- **Orthotists** design, fabricate, fit and maintain various orthoses (braces). Orthoses are used to improve function, support, align, prevent or correct musculoskeletal deformities and improve function in different parts of the child's body, most commonly the lower limbs.
- Other professionals who may be helpful include **social workers, nurses, psychologists and special education teachers**.

Irritability in children with profound disability
Irritability in children with disabilities can present the clinician with diagnostic uncertainty, amplified in patients with difficulties in communication or complex medical illness. The following differentials should be considered:

- Hunger
- Seizures
- Sleep deprivation
- Pain
  ○ Consider all the usual sites of infection (e.g. ears, throat, respiratory tract, urine and skin).
  ○ Muscle spasms
  ○ Gastro-oesophageal reflux.
  ○ Dental abscess/caries.
  ○ Corneal abrasion/foreign body in the eye.
  ○ Pancreatitis.
  ○ Renal colic.
  ○ Surgical – appendicitis, intussusception, torted testes.
  ○ Severe constipation.
  ○ Subluxing or dislocated hips.
  ○ Fractures – accidental or inflicted.
  ○ Side effects of medication, for example anticonvulsants.
  ○ Gynaecological.
  ○ Increased intracranial pressure (many children with disabilities have VP shunts which may become obstructed).
  ○ Anxiety and/or depression.

Neural Tube Defects/Myelomeningocele
The Neural Tube Defects (NTDs) comprises a spectrum of disorders of abnormal folding and closure of the embryonic neural tube and are the most common severe congenital malformation of the nervous system. Of these, spina bifida with a myelomeningocoele is the most prevalent and causes multi-system dysfunction. The degree of impairment from the spinal cord pathology varies. Most children have some lower limb motor weakness, sensory loss and a neurogenic bladder and bowel. Eighty per cent have an Arnold Chiari malformation leading to

progressive hydrocephalus and requiring CSF diversion surgery. Many children with NTDs have specific learning problems (even in the absence of hydrocephalus).

Prevention

Folic acid supplementation in the month before conception and in the first 3 months of pregnancy has been shown to reduce the risk of recurrence in any at-risk family (by ~75%). Recommended doses are

- 0.5 mg daily: low-risk women (no family history of NTDs).
- 5 mg daily: if there is a family history of NTD *or* if the woman is taking anticonvulsant medications.

Fewer children are now being born with NTDs, mainly due to antenatal diagnosis and termination of pregnancy. In this context the magnitude of effect of folate supplementation on incidence is not clear.

Note: Multivitamin supplements are not recommended because of the potential risks of vitamin overdose to the developing foetus.

Management

Management requires collaboration between the child and family as well as an interdisciplinary team. Ideally, this includes a GP, maternal and child health nurse, paediatrician, neurosurgeon, urologist, orthopaedic surgeon, neuropsychologist, physiotherapist, orthotist, occupational therapist, social worker, continence and stomal therapists. Most children with NTDs attend regular schools.

Initial management

- Discuss the diagnosis, natural history and prognosis with the family.
- Neurosurgical and paediatric assessment of the newborn infant to determine if early surgery could close the spinal defect. Clinical and ultrasound observation to detect and monitor hydrocephalus is important. Insertion of a ventriculoperitoneal shunt is often necessary.
- Urological consultation and investigations in the neonatal period provide baseline information for subsequent management. A small number of infants require early management of a high-pressure neurogenic bladder.
- Orthopaedic assessment includes clinical examination and hip ultrasound. Infants with spina bifida have a higher than usual prevalence of developmental dysplasia of the hips and talipes.

Specific aspects of management

Regular monitoring of

- Mobility:
  - Independent mobility is the primary goal of the orthopaedic surgeon, physiotherapist and orthotist. Upright experience in the early years, use of gait aides, improves independence in adulthood, even if the person has progressed to using a wheelchair for ambulation.
- Urinary tract
  - Neonates with myelomeningocoele are born with normal, functioning kidneys. The primary goal is the maintenance of satisfactory renal function and the secondary goal is the establishment of urinary continence.
  - Abnormal innervation can cause a range of bladder dysfunction. At the extremes, the neuropathic bladder may be small and non-compliant, or compliant and floppy with poor emptying. The function of the sphincter and degree of reflux also influence the degree of leaking (incontinence) and intravesical pressures, which may render the kidneys at 'high risk' of long-term damage.
  - Renal function is monitored by checking creatinine.
  - Renal tract ultrasound (US) is regularly repeated to monitor for changes, such as hydronephrosis, bladder trabeculation and to assess normal renal structure. Initially every 6–12 weeks, then 6 monthly in toddlers and children.
  - Urinary tract infection (UTI) is common and tested via midstream or catheter specimen urine.
  - Urodynamic studies establish the filling and emptying pressures of the bladder to gauge 'risk' to kidneys and to inform treatment.

- o Clean intermittent catheterisation (CIC) can be started in the neonatal period. Additional support may be necessary in the form of medication (e.g. oxybutynin 8–12 hourly), protective clothing and sometimes condom drainage.
- o Surgical interventions are aimed at protecting renal function and achieving continence (includes 'social dryness' – not wetting between CIC).
  - ▪ Vesicostomy – performed when high pressure bladder is causing hydronephrosis despite CIC, or where UTI is frequent, (usually in infancy).
  - ▪ Bladder augmentation.
  - ▪ The Mitrofanoff procedure (fashioning a conduit from the bladder to the abdominal wall by using the appendix) is also used more frequently to facilitate independence in catheterisation.
  - ▪ Insertion of artificial sphincter.
- o People with spina bifida who have undergone bladder augmentation, those with Mitrofanoff and those who perform daily CIC, have an increased risk of malignant change. Lifelong surveillance by a urologist is recommended.
- Neuropathic Bowel
  - o Difficulties in managing soiling, incontinence and chronic constipation affect the quality of life of patients and their carers.
  - o Constipation is common, and dietary advice, laxatives, enemas and even irrigation may be required.
  - o For children with severe incontinence anal plugs can be used following careful assessment by a stomal therapist.
  - o The Malone procedure is the fashioning of a non-refluxing appendicocaecostomy so that an antegrade continence enema can be performed to regularly evacuate the bowels and prevent soiling.
- Neurological functioning
  - o Children with shunts should have neurosurgical assessment regularly (in infancy every 6–9 months; in childhood and adolescence at least every 1–2 years). See also Chapter 33, *Neurologic conditions*, p. 470.
  - o Tethering of the spinal cord to surrounding structures occurs in most children. In a small number, traction on the cord causes deterioration in neurological functioning. Surgical de-tethering may be required.
  - o Children often have specific cognitive difficulties and a neuropsychological assessment is usually carried out before school entry and repeated before transition to secondary school.
- Co-morbid medical problems
  - o Scoliosis is a common management problem.
  - o Pressure sores occur in all children with spina bifida at some time, most commonly on the feet or the buttocks.
  - o Epilepsy occurs in 15% of people with myelomeningocoele.
  - o Latex allergy is much more common in children with spina bifida and has serious implications. Testing is offered to all children.
  - o Obesity is increasingly prevalent, especially as mobility changes, usually at puberty. Obesity can have significant implications for independence, making it more difficult to do independent transfers, to self-catheterise and care for skin. In ambulant people the increased load on joints affects gait, joint integrity and may cause loss of walking. The increased metabolic complications of obesity are probably contributing to the rising rates of cardiovascular death in adults with myelomeningocoele.
- Adolescent issues
  - o Puberty may be delayed or precocious.
  - o Specific adolescent issues including sexuality, relationship difficulties and contraception should be addressed.
  - o Mental health should be monitored.
  - o Vocational support is important.
  - o Transition and transfer to adult services is a major challenge and needs careful planning and support for the young person.

Autism spectrum disorders

Autism is now seen as part of a spectrum of disorders with multiple causes. In 2013 DSM-5 was launched after 19 years of consultation, research and discussion around the world. It replaces DSM-IV. Of particular note, there will no longer be the subdiagnoses of autistic disorder, Asperger syndrome, pervasive developmental disorder not otherwise specified, childhood disintegrative disorder or Rett syndrome

Prevalence
Estimates vary with definitions used, but autism spectrum disorder is now thought to affect 1% of the population with a sex ratio of 3 or 4 males:1 female.

Aetiology
The aetiology of autism is complex. Factors involved may include

- Genetic: recurrence rate in families is now estimated to be between 2% and 18%.
- Syndromal: there is an association with tuberous sclerosis, fragile X syndrome and congenital rubella.
- Structural: subtle brain abnormalities are described in some children.

Associated disorders
- Intellectual disability (50%).
- Epilepsy (20–30%).
- Other: ADHD, aggression and disruptive behaviours, anxiety disorders and depression, obsessive compulsive disorder, Tourette syndrome.

Clinical features
Parents will often identify that something is different about their child well before the second birthday. Early features include *lack of*

- Pretend play
- Pointing out objects to another person
- Social interest
- Joint attention
- Social play
- Response to name when called

Language development is delayed or disordered, and there may be unusual social use of language. Regression of language may be seen.

Diagnosis
There is no single test for autism spectrum disorders. Diagnosis is best made by a skilled, multidisciplinary team of a paediatrician/child psychiatrist, speech pathologist and psychologist.

Management
Management is multidisciplinary. It includes

- Parent support and education.
- Appropriate screening of vision/hearing, investigation for associated disorders/syndromes if suspected.
- Early intervention programmes, including a well-structured and predictable environment with
  - behavioural modification;
  - speech therapy; and
  - special education.
- A combination of educational, developmental and behavioural treatments has been shown to improve a child's rate of progress.
- Teaching social skills and friendship skills.
- Drug therapy is sometimes used to treat co-morbid psychopathology (e.g. attentional and behavioural problems, anxiety, self-injury). It does not affect the core autistic symptoms.
- Advice regarding educational options.
- Support groups.
- Access to respite care.

Families of children with autism spectrum disorder will often seek alternative health care, sometimes at considerable cost. It is important for parents to be aware and informed of what is available and the evidence supporting/refuting such strategies so that an educated choice can be made.

USEFUL RESOURCES

- *www.pedstest.com* – Parent's evaluation of developmental status.
- *www.disabilitycareaustralia.gov.au*

CHAPTER 24

Sleep problems

Margot Davey

Sleep physiology
Sleep is a major challenge to the respiratory system, because it causes changes in respiratory mechanics and control of breathing leading to

- Decreased ventilation
- Decreased functional respiratory capacity (loss of intercostal muscle tone)
- Increased upper airways resistance (hypotonia of dilating muscles of upper airway)
- Depression of respiratory drive (REM > NREM > awake)
- Decreased response to hypoxia and hypercarbia

Sleep stages
- Two sleep states are rapid eye movements (REMs) and non-rapid eye movement (NREM) sleep. NREM sleep is further divided into three stages – NREM1 (light sleep) through to NREM3 (deep sleep) via EEG changes.
- REM/NREM cycles occur at intervals of 60 minutes in the infant and lengthen to 90 minutes in the preschooler.

Sleep patterns
- Newborn infants sleep around 16 hours per day, reducing to 14.5 hours by 6 months and to 13.5 hours by 12 months.
- Around 3 months of age, the infant's circadian rhythm is emerging, with sleeping patterns becoming more predictable and most sleep occurring at night.
- By 6 months of age, most full-term healthy infants have the capacity to go through the night without a feed.
- Towards the end of the first year of life, the child's sleep architecture becomes similar to that of an adult, with most of the NREM3 occurring in the first third of the night and REM sleep concentrated in the second half of the night.
- Infants who develop the ability to transition from sleep cycle to sleep cycle without parental assistance appear to sleep through the night.
- In toddlers, the total sleep duration is around 12–13 hours and in preschoolers 11–12 hours. The majority of children stop regular naps by 5 years, providing they receive sufficient good quality sleep overnight.
- In school-aged children, total sleep time is between 9–11 hours.

Assessment
One-third of families will complain of difficulties with their child's sleeping patterns. Assessment should include

- Detailed sleep history over 24 hours, including how and where the child goes to sleep, frequency and character of wakings, snoring and daytime functioning.
- Sleep patterns during weekends/holidays and with different caregivers.
- A sleep diary may help clarify the situation (see Fig. 24.1).
- Family and social history to examine the presence of contributing problems, such as parental depression, relationship problems and drug or alcohol abuse.
- Exclude medical conditions contributing to disrupted sleep patterns such as obstructive sleep apnoea (OSA), asthma, eczema, nocturnal seizures, gastro-oesophageal reflux, otitis media with effusion, and nasal obstruction.

Paediatric Handbook, Ninth Edition. Edited by Amanda Gwee, Romi Rimer and Michael Marks.
© 2015 John Wiley & Sons, Ltd. Published 2015 by John Wiley & Sons, Ltd.

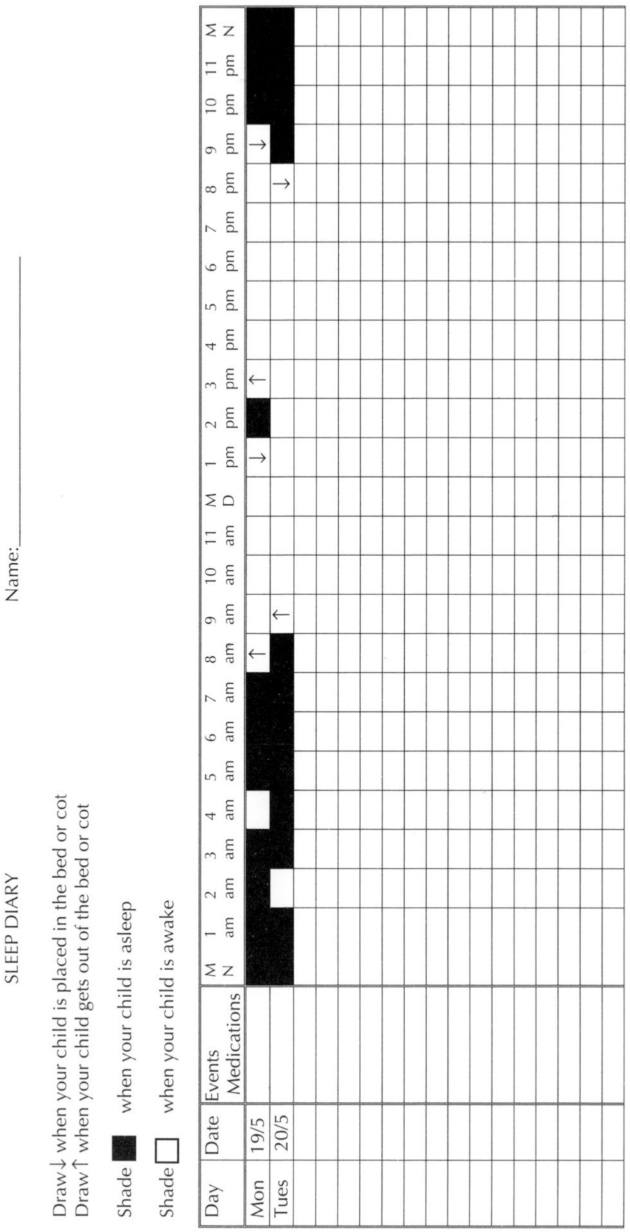

SLEEP DIARY

Name: _____

Draw ↓ when your child is placed in the bed or cot
Draw ↑ when your child gets out of the bed or cot

Shade ■ when your child is asleep

Shade □ when your child is awake

Day	Date	Events Medications	M N	1 am	2 am	3 am	4 am	5 am	6 am	7 am	8 am	9 am	10 am	11 am	M D	1 pm	2 pm	3 pm	4 pm	5 pm	6 pm	7 pm	8 pm	9 pm	10 pm	11 pm	M N
Mon	19/5										→↑	←↑				→↓		←↑									
Tues	20/5																						→↑	→↑			

Fig. 24.1 Sleep diary

Bedtime struggles and night-time waking

For infants <6 months of age, no interventions other than schedule manipulation (ensuring the infant is not overtired and that sleep times are adequately spaced) and anticipatory guidance are used. If parents want their infant to learn to settle by him/herself then they can try to leave the infant settled in their cot – leaving before he/she is asleep. In the first 3 months of life, some infants sleep better swaddled.

For older children, treatment plans must be individualised and adapted for each family.

Aetiology

- Sleep associations occur when a child learns to fall asleep in a particular way, so that every time the child has a normal arousal he/she wakes up fully and is unable to put him/herself back to sleep unless those particular conditions are replicated. Examples include rocking, feeding or falling asleep in the pram or car.
- Frequent feeding can cause wakings both by sleep associations and by the child developing a 'learned hunger' response. Some children can develop patterns that lead to consumption of large quantities of milk which affects not only their sleep patterns but eating during the day. Most healthy full-term babies can go without a night-time feed by 6 months.
- Erratic routines can contribute to sleep disturbance by inappropriate timing of naps and lack of a regular bedtime routine.
- Inconsistent limit setting in toddlers and preschoolers can exacerbate bedtime struggles and night-time wakings.

Management

- Detailed explanation about normal sleep and sleep cycles in a non-critical manner.
- Strategies to deal with inappropriate sleep associations all aim to provide the child with the opportunity to learn to fall asleep without parental assistance. Interventions range from extinction (letting the child cry it out), graduated extinction or controlled crying (checking the child at increasing periods of time until they fall asleep by themselves) to a more gradual approach (including the presence of a caregiver all night and progressively changing settling patterns).
- If frequent night feeding is a problem, discuss reducing the amount of fluid over 7–10 days and allowing the child to develop other ways to settle to sleep. Increasing the interval between breastfeeds, decreasing the volume in bottles and offering water instead of milk or other fluids are all useful strategies.
- A regular day–night routine needs to be established. An age-appropriate, enjoyable bedtime routine should be introduced to help the child learn to anticipate going to bed. Sometimes a gate is useful when the child has graduated to a bed and the newfound freedom creates bedtime struggles.
- There is a trend towards the use of melatonin in behavioural insomnia in childhood, either as an adjunct to behavioural management, or when behavioural interventions have failed. In this scenario, melatonin is being used for its hypnotic properties rather than its circadian rhythm effects. Melatonin has been found to be helpful in children with developmental disorders, ADHD and autism, but evidence is lacking for use in younger, typically-developing children. Best practice supports behavioural interventions as first-line management in all children.
- Sedative medication is not recommended for children <2 years. Promethazine or trimeprazine as single night-time dose – each 0.5 mg/kg (max 10 mg) – may be used in conjunction with behavioural techniques over a short time period or for blocks of parental respite.

Night-time fears and anxiety

Aetiology

Night-time fears may present in the preschool and school-age child with bedtime struggles and refusal to sleep by themselves. There may be a precipitant (frightening movie, bullying at school) or it may be a manifestation of an anxiety disorder.

Management

- Address separation issues for the child, which may include the introduction of a transitional object.
- Camper bed technique: a camper bed and a parent are moved into the child's room. The parent spends the entire night in the child's bedroom for 2 weeks helping them overcome their fears and gaining confidence in their own bed and room. This is often used in conjunction with a reward/sticker chart. Once the child is

Table 24.1 **Characteristics of night terrors, seizures and nightmares**

Characteristic	Night terrors	Nightmares	Epilepsy
Sleep stage	NREM 3	REM	NREM2 but can occur all stages
Time of night	First 1/3	Last 1/2	Any time
Wakefulness	Unrousable	Easily aroused	Usually unrousable
Amnesia	Yes	No	Yes, or may have some recall
Return to sleep	Easy	Difficult	Easy
Family history	Yes	No	Possibly

sleeping through the night in their own bed and room, attention can be directed at encouraging the child to fall asleep by themselves at the beginning of the night. Once a child has gained that skill, the parent can gradually move out of the child's bedroom.

- Self-control techniques including relaxation, guided imagery and positive self-statements may also be used, again often in conjunction with reward/sticker chart.
- Make sure that the child is not in bed too early, allowing them the opportunity to further fuss and worry, which will interfere with sleep onset.

Night-time arousal phenomena and differentials
Aetiology
Sleepwalking and night terrors are disorders of partial arousal from NREM3 and therefore occur in the first third of the night. They share common characteristics such as the child is confused and unresponsive to the environment, they have retrograde amnesia and varying degrees of autonomic activation (dilated pupils, sweating, tachycardia). See Table 24.1.

- **Sleepwalking** occurs at least once in 15–30% of healthy children and is most common between 8 and 12 years. It can range from quiet walking, performance of simple tasks such as rearranging furniture or setting tables, to more frenetic and agitated behaviour. At times children open doors/windows and walk outside the home.
- **Night terrors** are most common between 4 and 8 years of age and have a prevalence of 3–5%. They usually begin with a terrified scream and the child may either thrash around in bed or get up and run around the house. Efforts to calm or contain the child often make the episode worse.

Differentials
- **Nightmares** generally occur during REM sleep and are thus more common in the second half of the night. They are vivid dreams accompanied by feelings of fear which wake the child up from sleep. They are most common in 3–6 year olds.
- **Nocturnal frontal lobe epilepsy (NFLE).** This can present with brief repetitive stereotypical movements ± vocalizations throughout the night which can be associated with awareness by the patient. Alternatively, NFLE can present with bizarre complex stereotypic dystonic movements which typically last <2 minutes.

Management
- Obtain detailed history including the timing and duration of events, and the exact nature of movements (rhythmic or stereotypical) and behaviours.
- Completion of a sleep diary.
- A home video may be useful to aid diagnosis.
- All but NFLE are generally self-limiting. Explain reassure and discuss safety issues.
- Avoid sleep deprivation as this can precipitate events. Ensure regular bedtime routines and sleep patterns. If children are having difficulties settling due to night-time fears and worries, techniques discussed in previous section maybe applicable.

- If events occur at a consistent time then scheduled awakening (waking the child 30 minutes before an event) may be useful.
- Sleep studies are required only if the history is unclear; if the nocturnal events are very frequent, violent or atypical; or if there is impaired sleep quality. The latter may be a clue to unrecognised OSA.
- Medication is rarely needed. In situations where no aetiology has been found and there are very frequent and disruptive events, low-dose clonazepam before bedtime may be useful for 4–6 weeks.
- If NFLE is suspected then a sleep-deprived EEG or prolonged video EEG may be required. Most NFLE responds to carbamazepine.

Snoring and sleep-disordered breathing

- Sleep provides a physiological stress to breathing which can unmask respiratory difficulties that may not be apparent during wakefulness.
- Snoring is the most common symptom of sleep-disordered breathing in children and can be associated with primary snoring (PS) through to OSA.
- PS refers to snoring not associated with sleep or ventilatory disturbances and occurs in up to 20% of children.

Obstructive sleep apnoea

- OSA is defined as repeated episodes of partial or complete upper airway obstruction that disrupt normal ventilation and sleep.
- Incidence is 3% of children with peak incidence at 2–6 years due to adenotonsillar hypertrophy.
- Complications of severe OSA include growth failure and cor pulmonale, with the most common morbidity being impairment of behaviour and neurocognitive functioning.
- Symptoms include snoring, difficult or laboured breathing, apnoeas, mouth breathing, excessive sweating and restless or disturbed sleep. Children less commonly present with tiredness and lethargy. In older children, daytime symptoms may include behavioural and learning difficulties.
- Increased risk of OSA is associated with
  - Adenotonsillar hypertrophy
  - Obesity
  - Syndromes (e.g. Down syndrome, Prader–Willi)
  - Craniofacial abnormalities (e.g. Pierre-Robin, Crouzons)
  - Mucopolysaccharidoses
  - Achondroplasia and skeletal abnormalities
  - Neuromuscular weakness (e.g. Duchenne)
  - Hypotonia, hypertonia (e.g. cerebral palsy)
  - Prematurity
  - Previous palatal surgery (repaired cleft palate)
- Examination involves assessment of predisposing conditions and complications of OSA:
  - Growth: either failure to thrive or obesity
  - Craniofacial structure (retro/micrognathia, midface hypoplasia)
  - Mouth breathing
  - Nasal patency, septum, turbinates, allergic rhinitis
  - Tongue, pharynx, palate, uvula, tonsils
  - Pectus excavatum
  - Right ventricular hypertrophy, pulmonary hypertension
- Investigation by nasal endoscopy or lateral neck radiograph may have a place in assessing adenoidal size.

Investigation

- Overnight oximetry is the most useful screening tool, with positive oximetry being diagnostic of OSA. Positive oximetry is defined as >3 clusters of SpO_2 desaturations, with at least 3 desaturations to <90%. It is important that the averaging time of the oximeter is short (i.e. 2–3 seconds). Negative or normal oximetry does not exclude OSA, although it may provide reassurance that the child is unlikely to have severe OSA while awaiting further assessment.

- Oximetry is limited in that it does not provide any information on the type of events associated with oxygen desaturations, CO_2 retention or sleep disruption. Oximetry should not be used to diagnose OSA in children less than 12 months,
- Overnight polysomnography (sleep study) continues to be the gold standard for diagnosis of OSA and should be performed if uncertainty persists in high-risk children, children <2 years of age, or those with co-morbid conditions where there is a risk of central sleep-disordered breathing in addition to OSA.

Management
- Adenotonsillectomy is the first-line treatment, being curative in majority of children. The role of adenoidectomy alone is unclear.
- Adenotonsillectomy is associated with a 2-week recovery period and there is a 2–3% risk of secondary haemorrhage especially 5–10 days post-operatively.
- Non-invasive ventilation (usually continuous positive airway pressure CPAP) may be used for residual OSA, if there is a delay in surgery, or if surgery is contraindicated.
- Medical treatments of OSA include treatment of allergic rhinitis (intranasal steroids) and management of obesity.

Polysomnography (sleep study)
Polysomnography involves the continuous and simultaneous recording of multiple physiological parameters related to sleep and breathing. Sleep studies are indicated for:
- OSA; primary snoring versus sleep-disordered breathing.
- Central sleep disordered breathing.
- Monitoring non-invasive ventilation requirements.
- Excessive daytime sleepiness (include multiple sleep latency testing if narcolepsy suspected).
- Atypical night-time disruptions including very frequent or violent wakings.
- A full EEG montage is required if seizures are suspected.
- Periodic limb movement disorder.

USEFUL RESOURCES
- *www.raisingchildren.net.au* – evidence-based parenting website with step-by-step instructions for behavioural techniques including graduated extinction, adult fading, phasing out dummies and overnight feeding. Parent handouts for sleepwalking, night terrors, bedtime struggles and separation anxiety.
- *www.sleepforkids.org* – launched by National Sleep Foundation aimed to provide information to children aged 7–12 years.
- *www.rch.org.au/ccch/profdev.cfm* – Practice Resources Online – RCH Community Child Health Centre. Evidence-based settling and sleep problems practice resource.

CHAPTER 25

Behaviour and mental health

Chidambaram Prakash
Lionel Lubitz
Daryl Efron

Toddler behaviour problems

Behavioural difficulties in children can be highly distressing for parents and often lead them to seek medical advice. Doctors can be very helpful by listening supportively to parents' concerns and suggesting management strategies. It is often best to begin either with a problem that is relatively easy to fix so that the parent gains confidence in themselves; or the most distressing problem for them; or alternatively a problem which may be exacerbating other behaviours (e.g. sleep deprivation).

The developmental stage of toddlerhood, characterised by marked egocentricity and the growing need for autonomy, needs to be explained to the parents as the symptoms are often an expression of the child negotiating this stage. It is normal for toddlers to try to control what they eat, to resist bedtime and to become frustrated if they do not get their way or fail in a task. In the process parents can sometimes feel that they are losing control, or are disempowered, or even defeated by a feisty toddler.

The doctor's role is to assist the parents to regain control, so that the toddler can develop a healthy sense of themselves without diminishing the parents' self-efficacy. Additionally, child behavioural problems can often generate or exacerbate conflict between parents. Calm and practical professional advice can help improve strained relationships.

Evaluation

- History: listen carefully to what the parent is telling you. Why is this a problem for them? Why have they come now? What resources and supports do they have to help manage the problem? Are there developmental concerns, such as communication or social-emotional delay? Are there family issues, such as separation, parental mental illness, recent death or other stressors?
- Examination: perform a thorough general examination to rule out significant health problems (uncommon).

There are three main types of problematic behaviour that often concerns parents of small children:

1. Sleep issues
2. Food issues
3. Tantrum behaviours

Sleep issues

This is a common complaint and one that causes a great deal of distress. There may be problems with sleep onset, night wakings or both. Such sleep patterns may result in parental sleep deprivation, which can make everyday life very difficult.

Principles in managing sleep problems in toddlers include

- Establish predictable routines e.g. dinner, bath, story and good night cuddles.
- Ensure the toddler is left awake in the cot/bed to fall asleep on their own, with transitional objects of their choice. Sleep associations are commonly problematic (e.g. the child needing to have a parent or bottle present as they fall asleep). The child will then demand the same conditions to be present to resettle when they wake overnight, causing disturbance.
- If toddlers come out of bed at night and go to the parent they should be put back to bed. If the child lays awake in a cot, the parent should reassure them briefly and then leave them to settle back to sleep. This may

Paediatric Handbook, Ninth Edition. Edited by Amanda Gwee, Romi Rimer and Michael Marks.
© 2015 John Wiley & Sons, Ltd. Published 2015 by John Wiley & Sons, Ltd.

need to be repeated many times over. Some parents find the crying very difficult to tolerate, so supportive strategies may need to be developed which suit this particular parent to get through the first few nights. If parents persist, the problem usually greatly improves or even resolves, over days to weeks.

- Medications are rarely helpful. They may offer temporary relief but do not change behaviour patterns.

Make yourself available for contact once a management plan has commenced. A follow-up phone call can be very helpful.

Food issues

Many parents worry that their toddlers do not eat enough and mealtime battles often ensue. It is most unlikely that an otherwise healthy child will become significantly malnourished from poor eating. If the history does not indicate a structural or functional oromotor problem, a swallowing disorder or developmental disorder, the best approach is to reduce the stress around food:

- Plan a balanced toddler diet.
- Offer three meals and three snacks per day so that there is only about 2 hours between eating opportunities.
- Present the food/drink on a high chair tray or low table.
- Allow sufficient but limited time for finishing the meal (e.g. 20 minutes).
- Give the child a 5-minute warning before the food is taken away so that they can complete their meal.
- Take the unfinished food away until the next 'meal'.
- Offer no food in between the set meal and snack times so that the child develops an appetite.
- Try not to become upset if the child chooses not to eat.

Once again, phone contact during this process can be very reassuring and supportive, as it can be counter-intuitive for a parent to resist 'feeding' their toddler.

Tantrum behaviours

Toddler tantrums are almost universal as an expression of frustration, and sometimes as a more controlled attention-seeking strategy. However, when frequent or intense, these behaviours can be very distressing and embarrassing for parents.

Tantrums can be minimised by applying some simple strategies:

- Try to prevent tantrums by distraction or avoidance of triggers.
- Ignore tantrums until they resolve.
- During a tantrum, avoid eye contact, say nothing and walk away. Try not to convey to the child that you are upset. Never engage a child who is having a tantrum, as it simply 'adds fuel to the fire'. This can be challenging in public places, such as supermarkets, but is important in order to reduce tantrums.
- Time out is a good strategy for more severe antisocial behaviours, such as physical aggression. Removing the child from the social group conveys the message that this behaviour is unacceptable. Place the child in an uninteresting place for a time-limited period, such as 1 minute per year of age. A corner, time out spot or separate room can be used, depending on the parent's preference. It is OK to close the door as long as the toddler can get out. If they come out, return them to the room or corner until they calm down. Once the tantrum is over, there is no need for discussion, simply re-engage with the child in enjoyable play.

Remember, toddlers respond well to positive reinforcement. Parents should be advised to 'catch the child being good' and reward them with praise, physical affection and/or a tangible reward, such as a sticker. This is important to promote more socially acceptable behaviours.

The objective of these behaviour strategies is not just to modify problematic behaviour and make the toddler comply with parental wishes, but also to help foster a loving relationship between the parent and child and reduce conflict. Sometimes, parental expectations of what is 'normal' may need to be addressed so that the toddler can be helped to develop strong self-esteem and reach their potential.

Tics/Tourette's disorder

Tics are sudden, rapid, involuntary, non-rhythmic movements or vocalisations which occur repeatedly. Patients usually have some degree of voluntary control over the tics, such that they can suppress them for minutes to hours, at the cost of a build-up of tension which is relieved when the tics are permitted to be expressed. They may occur many times through the day. Typically there are periods of intense and frequent tic activity, and other periods when they are hardly noticed at all. They tend to be less severe when the child is engaged in a task requiring concentration.

Simple motor tics are the commonest type, where one muscle group twitches repeatedly, for example, eye blinking, limb jerking. Some children experience more complex motor tics, with stereotypic patterns of movement involving multiple muscle groups or limbs, sometimes recruiting the whole body. In some cases these can be difficult to differentiate from stereotypies or seizures, which may co-occur. Vocal tics are also common, including sniffing, throat clearing and various vocalisations. These are often misdiagnosed as medical problems such as allergies or upper respiratory infections. Complex vocal tics are less common. These involve repeating one's own sounds or the last heard word or phrase, or rarely socially unacceptable words or insults.

Tics are common in childhood and affect boys approximately four times more frequently than girls. The incidence of tics in boys is more than 10%. It is substantially more common in children with neurodevelopment disorders such as attention deficit hyperactivity disorder (ADHD) and autism spectrum disorder. Onset is typically in the preschool or early primary school years. Most cases are transient, but some run a chronic course. Tourette's disorder can be diagnosed when both motor and vocal tics have been present for at least 12 months.

The nature of the tics usually shifts over time, with one tic or repertoire of tics being replaced by another. They tend to be more severe with stress, sleep deprivation and over-excitement. The natural history of tics is to wax and wane over some years, before usually disappearing in adolescence. Only a small proportion persists into adulthood.

Most children with tics do not need any specific treatment. Although parents are often upset by them and may tell the child to stop, the child is not usually bothered by the tics. In these cases it is best to try to distract the child and ignore the tics. In severe cases tics can cause embarrassment and social exclusion, emotional disturbance, muscle pain and interference with function. These cases warrant intervention.

The mainstay of treatment is pharmacological. There are a number of medications which have been shown to reduce the frequency of tics; however, effect sizes are generally small over and above the natural fluctuation in severity. The most effective medications are the antipsychotics, particularly haloperidol, risperidone and olanzapine. These are associated with a risk of significant side effects, in particular acute dystonic reactions, sedation and weight gain (Table X). In some children anxiety is a major driving factor, and anti-anxiety medication such as fluoxetine can be helpful. Other medications with some anti-tic activity include clonidine, clonazepam and tetrabenazine. Botulinum toxin injections can be effective for disabling focal motor tics. New therapies under investigation include transcranial magnetic stimulation and deep brain stimulation surgery.

Behavioural approaches such as habit reversal therapy can have benefits in some children. This involves helping the child to identify the premonitory urge sensation and to develop an alternative response,for example, slow stretch of arms rather than a rapid jerk. Another technique is called exposure and response prevention, aimed at actively suppressing the urge.

At this stage there is insufficient evidence to support the theory that group A streptococcal infections can precipitate or exacerbate tics and obsessive compulsive disorder (OCD), a hypothesised condition called Paediatric Autoimmune Neuropsychiatric Disorders Associated with Streptococcal Infection (PANDAS). The use of long-term antibiotics or immune-modifying therapies such as plasma exchange or intravenous immunoglobulin are not currently justified.

Children with tics commonly have associated problems, particularly ADHD and OCD. These conditions are often more functionally impairing than the tics and are more likely to require treatment.

Attention deficit hyperactivity disorder

ADHD is the most common neurodevelopmental disorder in childhood, with a prevalence of approximately 3–5%. It is highly heritable and approximately twice as common in boys than girls. Delays or deficits in executive brain functions lead to the core features of poor impulse control and limited sustained attention to tasks. Younger children with ADHD often exhibit motor hyperactivity. Many children with ADHD also exhibit poor emotional regulation. Common associated problems include oppositional defiant disorder, anxiety disorders, learning disorders, autism spectrum disorder and tics. Risk factors include family history, prematurity, very lowbirth weight, in-utero exposure to neurotoxins such as alcohol, and environmental deprivation in infancy.

The DSM-5 diagnostic criteria for ADHD are provided in Table 25.1. Approximately two-thirds of children with ADHD have the combined presentation, that is, both inattention and hyperactive-impulsive symptoms. The predominantly inattentive subgroup often present later with academic difficulties.

Table 25.1 DSM-5 diagnostic criteria for ADHD

A A persistent pattern of inattention and/or hyperactivity-impulsivity that interferes with functioning or development as characterized by (1) and/or (2)

1. *Inattention*: At least six or more of the following symptoms have persisted for at least 6 months to a degree that is inconsistent with developmental level and that negatively impacts on social and academic/occupational activities.
   Note: The symptoms are not solely a manifestation of oppositional behaviour, defiance, hostility, failure to understand tasks or instructions. For older adolescents and adults (17 years and above) at least five symptoms are required.
   - Often fails to give close attention to details or makes careless mistakes in schoolwork, at work or during other activities (e.g. overlooks or misses details, work is inaccurate)
   - Often has difficulty sustaining attention in tasks or play activities (e.g. has difficulty remaining focused during lectures, conversations or lengthy readings)
   - Often does not seem to listen when spoken to directly (e.g. mind seems elsewhere even in the absence of any obvious distractions)
   - Often does not follow through on instructions and fails to finish schoolwork chores or duties in the workplace (e.g. starts tasks but quickly loses focus and is easily side tracked)
   - Often has difficulty organising tasks and activities (e.g. difficulty managing sequential tasks; difficulty keeping materials and belongings in order; messy disorganized work; has poor time management; fails to meet deadlines)
   - Often avoids or dislikes tasks that require sustained mental effort (e.g. schoolwork or homework; for older adolescents and adults, preparing reports, completing forms, reviewing lengthy papers)
   - Often loses things necessary for tasks or activities (e.g. school materials, pens, pencils, books, tools, wallet, keys, paperwork, eyeglasses, mobile telephones)
   - Is often easily distracted by extraneous stimuli (for older adolescents and adults may include unrelated thoughts)
   - Is often forgetful in daily activities(e.g. doing chores, running errands; for older adolescents and adults, returning calls, paying bills, keeping appointments)

2. *Hyperactivity/impulsivity*: Six of the following symptoms have persisted for at least 6 months to a degree that is inconsistent with developmental level and that negatively impacts directly on social, academic/occupational functioning:*Note*: The symptoms are not solely a manifestation of oppositional behaviour, defiance, hostility, failure to understand tasks or instructions. For older adolescents and adults (17 years and above) at least five symptoms are required.
   - Often fidgets with or taps hands or feet and squirms in seat
   - Often leaves seat situations in which remaining seated is expected (e.g. leaves his or her place in classroom, in the office or other workplace, or in other situations requiring remaining in place)
   - Often runs about or climbs excessively in situations where it is inappropriate (in adolescents or adults may be limited to feelings of restlessness)
   - Often has difficulty playing or engaging in leisure activities quietly
   - Is often 'on the go' and acts as if 'driven by a motor' (e.g. is unable to be or uncomfortable being still for extended time, as in restaurants, meetings, may be experienced by others as being restless or difficult to keep up with)
   - Often talks excessively
   Impulsivity:
   - Often blurts out answers to questions before the questions have been completed(e.g. completes people's sentences, cannot wait for turn in conversations)
   - Often has difficulty awaiting his or her turn (e.g. while waiting in line)
   - Often interrupts or intrudes on others (e.g. butts into conversation, games or activities; may start using other people's things without asking or receiving permission; for adolescents and adults, may intrude into or take over what others are doing)

B Several inattentive or hyperactive-impulsive symptoms were present prior to age 12 years.

C Several inattentive or hyperactive-impulsive symptoms must be present in two or more settings (e.g. at school, at home or at work; with friends or relatives; in other activities).

D There is clear evidence that the symptoms interfere with or reduce the quality of social, academic or occupational functioning.

E The symptoms do not occur exclusively during the course of schizophrenia, or another psychotic disorder, and are not better accounted for by another mental disorder (e.g. mood disorder, anxiety disorder, dissociative disorder, personality disorder, substance intoxication or withdrawal).

(*continued*)

Table 25.1 (*Continued*)

Specify whether:
Combined presentation (criteria A1 and A2 are met for the past 6 months)
Predominantly inattentive presentation (criteria A1 are met but A2 are not met for the past 6 months)
Predominantly hyperactivity-impulsivity (criteria A1 are not met but A2 are met for the past 6 months)
Specify:
In partial remission: When full criteria were previously met, fewer than full criteria have been met for the past 6months and the symptoms still result in impairment in social, academic/occupational functioning
Specify current severity:
Mild: Few if any symptoms in excess of those required for diagnosis are present and symptoms result in no more than minor impairments in social, academic/occupational functioning
Moderate: Symptoms or functional impairments between mild and severe are present
Severe: Many symptoms in excess of those required for diagnosis are present or several symptoms that particularly severe or the symptoms result in marked impairments in social, academic/occupational functioning

Assessment

- History: A detailed history is essential, focusing on early development, academic progress, social skills and the family context. The timing and nature of initial concerns along with secondary effects such as depression, low self-esteem and social ostracism should be noted. It is important to identify the child's strengths as well as their weaknesses, and to gather information from the child's teacher(s) about behaviour and performance in the classroom and playground. School reports may be of some value; however, standardised behaviour rating scales completed by parents and teachers are more useful (e.g. Connors, Achenbach). Exacerbating factors such as sleep deprivation or nutritional deficiencies should be identified and managed. Diagnosis is less reliable before school entry because of variability in the normal development of self-regulation and unpredictable future trajectories.
- Physical examination: A detailed examination should be performed to exclude medical conditions or genetic syndromes. A neurodevelopment assessment, including tests of fine and gross motor coordination, visual-motor integration, auditory and visual sequencing, often identifies so-called soft neurological signs, indicating delayed neuromaturation. Inviting the child to read some text and sampling handwriting may provide valuable information regarding literacy competence.
- Psychoeducational assessment: Children with significant learning difficulties should be referred to an educational psychologist for a formal assessment to identify their learning strengths and weaknesses. This can be arranged through the education department (via the school) or privately.
- Hearing should be tested with formal audiology. Other investigations are not helpful unless there are clinical indicators.

Management

The functional impairments, management priorities and intervention targets tend to change over time. The child and family need sustained support over many years. This requires the doctor to work in collaboration with other health, educational and community professionals. A multimodal strategy is usually required.

Behaviour modification

- The methods described previously under aggression/oppositionaldefiant behaviour (p. 377) are generally helpful.
- Parents and teachers need to apply structured behavioural modification strategies as calmly and consistently as possible. Good communication between home and school is important, with best progress made when parents and teachers work together using similar strategies.

Educational strategies

- An individualised plan should be developed to optimise learning and promote appropriate behaviour.
- Classroom adaptations include seating the child at the front of the classroom near a good role model, minimising distractions, and using written lists and other visual prompts. Some children need individualised instructions and reminders to complete tasks, with increased adult one-to-one supervision such as a teacher's aide or volunteer classroom helper. Jobs such as collecting lunch orders break up the work and are also good for self-esteem.
- Clear rules and predictable routines are important.
- Positive reinforcement should be provided for acceptable behaviour.

Medication

Stimulants

Psychostimulant medication is the single most effective intervention for children with ADHD (see Table 25.2). It provides effective symptom reduction in about 80% of cases, improving impulse control and sustained attention. Secondary benefits including improved academic progress, peer status, family functioning and self-esteem accrue over time. The main side effect of stimulants is appetite suppression. Anxiety and tics may be increased. A small minority of patients exhibit withdrawn behaviour or subdued personality. This resolves when the medication is stopped. Weight, height and blood pressure need to be monitored. Stimulant medications are not addictive in the doses used to treat ADHD.

Other medications

A number of other medications are useful in some children with ADHD. These include:

- Atomoxetine, a selective noradrenaline reuptake inhibitor, which is given once daily.
- Clonidine, which can with sleep onset, explosive behaviour and tics. If clonidine is used in combination with a stimulant, twice-daily dosing is preferable and the total daily dose should not exceed 200 mcg.
- Antidepressants (SSRI, SNRI, tricyclics) are beneficial to treat associated impairing anxiety.

Other strategies

The parents of children with ADHD commonly try a range of unproven complementary therapies, including dietary modifications, behavioural optometry, EEG biofeedback, chiropractic, etc. There is no evidence that these interventions are helpful in real-life settings such as the classroom or playground. Elimination of synthetic food colourings and preservatives is beneficial in some children with irritable mood. There is some evidence that fish oil may be helpful for some children.

Table 25.2 Medications for ADHD

Trade name	Generic name	Formulation	Duration of action	Usual dosing times
Dexamphetamine	Dexamphetamine	5 mg tab	4–5 h	Morning and lunchtime
Ritalin 10	Methylphenidate	10 mg tab	2.5–4 h	Morning, lunchtime ± after school
Ritalin LA	Methylphenidate biphasic release	10, 20, 30, 40 mg caps	6–8 h	Morning
Concerta	Methylphenidate extended release	18, 27, 36, 54 mg tabs	10–12h	Morning
Strattera	Atomoxetine	10, 18, 25, 40, 60, 80, 100 mg caps	Steady state	Morning (occasionally given in evening)

Notes:
1. All items are available in Australia on the PBS by authority prescription. In most states the prescribing of these medications is restricted to paediatricians, child psychiatrists and neurologists.
2. If the main symptom is inattention then medication may be needed only for school.
3. Drug holidays (planned treatment interruptions over school holidays) are not necessary for most children; consider if suboptimal growth.

As indicated above, most children with ADHD have one or more comorbidities. These often need to be managed alongside the ADHD.

Prognosis

Most children with ADHD will continue to have some difficulties through adolescence and into adulthood, although many develop compensating strategies and function well. A significant minority have adverse long-term outcomes including academic underachievement, delinquency, vocational disadvantage, relationship difficulties, substance abuse, mental health disorders and motor vehicle accidents. Children with ADHD treated with stimulant medication appear to be less likely to develop substance abuse in adolescence and adult life than those left untreated.

Mental health

Mental health is defined as a state of emotional and social well-being in which individuals realise their own abilities, cope with the normal stresses of life, work productively and are able to make a contribution to their community.

One in five people will experience mental health problems in their lifetime. The prevalence of mental health problems among children and adolescents in Australia (including subclinical symptoms) is approximately 14%. Most are managed in their community.

Childhood and adolescent mental health problems are predominantly managed by GPs, paediatricians, schools and community services. A relatively smaller number of children and adolescents with mental health problems of significant severity are treated by specialist mental health services/professionals. As medical practitioners are often well placed to identify mental health problems and facilitate management, it is important that they develop skills in mental health assessments.

The recognition and early diagnosis of child and adolescent mental health disorders is a clinical challenge. Presenting features may be different to those in an adult population. Many child and adolescent mental health problems continue into adulthood resulting in long lasting morbidity, hence the need for early diagnosis and referral for treatment.

Child mental health problems may have their origins in biological, attachment, developmental or family issues. Additionally, adolescent mental health problems may arise in the context of interpersonal and social problems. Critical life phases, such as puberty, are significant as these are stages of transition that are marked not only by biological changes but also major psychosocial stress.

Key skills required by medical practitioners:

- Listen and engage children, adolescents and their families to discuss emotional and psychological issues in a comfortable manner.
- Manage common and less complex mental health problems either independently or in consultation with mental health professionals.
- Identify when mental health issues are serious, more complex and/or chronic in order to facilitate appropriate referral.

Approach to mental health problems
History taking, interview and assessment

- Presenting problem: duration, severity, exacerbating and relieving factors
  - What are the parents' ideas about this problem?
  - In adolescents, what are their ideas about the problems?
- School history (including types of school, class sizes, academic performance now and previously, social relationships, attendance and behaviour in school, history of being bullied or bullying at school).
- The child's feeding, sleeping and toileting habits where appropriate.
- In adolescents also explore
  - substance use (type, amount, frequency, who with, motivation for change);
  - sexual history;
  - social relationships (including the type of peer group—related activities, closeness to peers, position in the peer group); and
  - eating habits, patterns of exercise, self and body image in adolescents.

- Also look for self-harm and risk-taking behaviours.
- Friendships, relationships within the family.
- Perinatal history (including experience of the pregnancy, delivery and the child's early months).
- Family history (both medical and psychiatric).
- Possible traumatic events at home and school (directly experienced or witnessed). Consider physical or sexual abuse and ask sensitive questions directly where appropriate.

Each interview of a child or adolescent and family should lead to an assessment and evaluation (including their strengths and difficulties) and the contributions of the family, peers and significant others to these difficulties and capacity to help overcome them. The child/adolescent and family should come to feel the problem is taken seriously and understood by the clinician. The following points are general guidelines and must be applied according to individual situations:

- See preschool and early primary age school child with their parents. See older children (7–11 years) with their parents initially but where possible, also interview and observe them in the room without their parents. Aim to speak with the child directly and engage other family members. This enables a therapeutic relationship to be established with the child.
- See adolescents both with their families and alone. This helps to give them a private space to discuss matters that they deem confidential. It also reinforces their efforts at separation from their parents and the developmental process of individuation. Inform them of your professional responsibility to keep matters discussed with them confidential but also explain the exceptions to this rule where they may be at risk to their own self (suicidal ideas or plans, serious self-harm, sexual abuse) or pose a risk to others.
- Get the family/parents to identify and specify the main issue or two that they feel needs attention. At the conclusion of the assessment, come back to this and see if your assessment of the main issues to be addressed matches the family's view.
- Assess the presenting problem, noting the language and narrative used by the child/adolescent and family.
- Observe the verbal and non-verbal interaction between the child/adolescent and each parent and sibling present.
- Aim to make a formulation of the problems based on the initial assessment, decide on an initial management plan and whether to refer for specialist mental health assessment.
- A clinician needs to be able to answer the following questions:
  - What is the problem now? Is the problem in the child/adolescent or is the child a symptom bearer for family/parental psychological issues?
  - Why is the child/adolescent presenting at this stage?
  - What is this child/adolescent usually like?
  - In an adolescent, ascertain if the symptoms are part of an evolving major mental illness such as major depression, anxiety disorder or psychosis, the effects of psychoactive substances or a reaction to the psychosocial stressors that they are living with.

Consider
- Stresses arising from family problems.
- Inability of children and adolescents to cope with the demands of their developmental stage or phase of life.
- Problems within the parental/carer support system including losses, conflicts, grief (e.g. death or illness in the family).
- Bullying, academic and social difficulties in school.
- In adolescents conflict (e.g. victimisation by peers or arguments with parents) relationship breakdowns, problems with school work and a lack of emotional and interpersonal skills to deal with the developmental tasks of adolescence (e.g. difficulties in initiating social contact, dealing with new sexual feelings and negotiating greater independence within the family) contribute to mental health problems.

Mental state examination in children
See Table 25.3.

Principles of intervention
At the conclusion of the therapeutic assessment, the clinician should form a provisional diagnosis and assess the severity and urgency of the presenting problem.

Table 25.3 Mental state examination

Observe the child's play and behaviour before, during and after the formal consultation. The young child communicates through play. Access to simple toys (e.g. a doll, a ball, or pencil and paper) allows the clinician to assess the child's level of self-organisation as well as their inner world of imagination and thought. Ask the child to draw a person or a house. Interview with the parents.

1. General appearance and behaviour
   - Observe the child's appearance, demeanour, gait, motor activity and relationship with examiner.
   - What is the child's apparent mood?
   - Do they seem sad, happy, fearful, perplexed, angry, agitated?
2. Speech
   - How does the child communicate?
   - Consider rate, volume (amount), tone, articulation and reaction time.
3. Affect
   - Observe the range, reactivity, communicability, and appropriateness to the context and congruence with the reported mood state.
4. Thought
   - Stream: Are there major interruptions to flow of thinking?
   - Content: What is the child thinking about?
   - Do they seem preoccupied by inner thoughts, obsessional ideas, delusions, fears or have suicidal ideation?
5. Perception
   - Are there hallucinations, illusions, imagery in various sensory modalities?
6. Cognition
   - Conscious state and orientation: Does the child know where they are, what time it is, who they are and who is around them?
   - Concentration: Is the child able to concentrate on developmentally appropriate tasks?
   - Memory: How well do they remember things of the recent and more distant past?
   - Do they understand questions posed to them and how well do they problem-solve?
7. Insight
   - Does the child seem aware of their illness?
8. Judgement
   - Personal (as inferred from answers to questions about themselves), social (as inferred from social behaviour) and test situation (answers to specific questions).

Much of this information can be obtained from the child in a non-threatening way by asking them directly in detail about things such as their family, home, school, address, telephone number and their immediate context.

Options for intervention

- Explain and reassure if the problem is transient or minor. Suggest further contact with the GP or community counsellor.
- Further mental health intervention through paediatric or primary care service. Offer a follow-up appointment or telephone contact.
- Telephone consultation with regional mental health service or a colleague.

Available interventions in specialist child and youth mental health services

- Brief therapies – family or individual
- Crisis intervention
- Cognitive behavioural therapy (CBT)
- Interpersonal therapy in adolescents
- Acceptance and commitment therapy
- Dialectical behaviour therapy
- Psychodynamic psychotherapy
- Family and parent therapy
- Supportive intervention for the child and family (clinic, school or home based)
- Psychopharmacology

When and how to make a mental health referral

Referral to mental health services should be discussed with families. The manner in which this is done can influence their engagement with these services, their expectations and understanding and even treatment outcome.

- Avoid coercion (unless the patient is at serious risk to themselves or others).
- Ensure an open and honest discussion about why you believe a mental health referral would be helpful.
- Explain what the child or adolescent and family should expect from an initial mental health consultation in clear and simple language.
- Examine your own responses/feelings about mental health and ensure you do not impose these views on a child/adolescent or family (e.g. being sceptical about the usefulness of mental health services but referring anyway, or presenting the mental health clinician as the potential cure to all current and future difficulties).
- Where appropriate, continue your involvement and interest in a child and family.

Some children/adolescents and families accept mental health referral readily, whereas others are wary or even openly opposed to referral. In the latter, referral may be discussed over a period of weeks or months before being made. Stigma around mental health continues to be a powerful influence. Adolescents and families may interpret the suggestion of a referral as an indication that you think they are 'mad' or 'crazy'. Such beliefs may not necessarily be overt and reassurance is helpful.

Children who are hospitalised or have been subjected to significant medical interventions need to be reassured that the mental health clinician is a talking person (rather than someone who gives needles). In adolescents who are admitted to hospital with a medical illness and need to see a mental health clinician, it is important to reiterate that the role of this clinician is to assist them in coping with their condition and strengthen their resilience. Terms such as 'the talking doctor' can be useful. Similarly, talking to parents about mental health 'colleagues' as you would talk about other medical/surgical referrals can help reduce stigma or concerns.

Common childhood and adolescent mental health problems

Anxiety disorders

Fear is a normal response to a frightful stimulus. Anxiety is a fear response that is abnormal in either context or extent. Common symptoms of anxiety disorders are listed in Table 25.4.

- In infants and toddlers, anxiety often manifests at separation from parents.
- Preschoolers and school-age children may be fearful of the dark or specific situations.
- Older children and adolescents may exhibit performance anxiety associated with exams, social situations, interpersonal relationship situations etc. Anxiety is most commonly experienced at times of transition (e.g. moving house, starting or changing schools).

Anxiety disorders may be characterised by

- Persistent fears and/or developmentally inappropriate fears.
- Irrational worries or avoidance of specific situations that trigger anxiety.
- Impaired ability to perform normal activities (e.g. inability to attend school).
- Anxiety disorders are common (4–9% in children and adolescents). This risk is greatly increased if a parent has/had an anxiety disorder or substance abuse disorder.

General management principles

- A thorough history should include details of anxiety symptoms, length of time anxiety has persisted, the degree to which the child is impaired in their day-to-day activities and their relationships.
- Behavioural analysis: how does the problem manifest in their behaviour?
- Cognitive analysis: what are the thoughts and emotions associated with the problem?
- Family, school and developmental assessment.

Generalised anxiety disorder

Generalised anxiety disorder is persistent and pervasive anxiety that is not contextually based. This includes feeling 'on edge' at most times, with bodily symptoms such as tachycardia, palpitations, dizziness, headache and 'butterflies in the tummy'.

Management

- If symptoms are mild, explore behavioural and/or family support interventions with the child and family, then review.

Table 25.4 Common symptoms of anxiety disorders in children

Symptoms
Distress and agitation when separated from parents and home
School refusal
Pervasive worry and fearfulness
Restlessness and irritability
Timidity, shyness, social withdrawal
Terror of an object (e.g. dog)
Associated headache, stomach pain
Restless sleep and nightmares
Poor concentration, distractibility and learning problems
Reliving stressful event in repetitive play
Family factors
Parental anxiety, overprotection, separation difficulties
Parental (maternal) depression and agoraphobia
Family stress: marital conflict, parental illness, child abuse
Family history of anxiety

Source: Reproduced with permission from Tonge B. Common child and adolescent psychiatric problems and their management in the community. *Medical Journal of Australia* 1998;168:241–248. (Tonge 1998. Reproduced wtih permission of AMPCo.)

- CBT techniques such as the F (Feelings) E (Expectation) A (Attitude/action) R (Reward) for generalised anxiety and systematic desensitisation and modelling for specific phobias are highly recommended.

Anxiety-based school refusal

School refusal is often an indicator of separation difficulties, where the child/adolescent is frightened to leave their parent or home. Children refusing to attend school often present with somatic complaints such as abdominal pain.

Ascertain the basis of the child's/adolescent's anxiety. These may be related to factors at home, including a parent's physical or mental health, difficulties with parental or peer relationships, or school factors (such as bullying or academic performance).

Management

- Conduct a physical examination if the child/adolescent presents with somatic symptoms.
- Assess the source of the anxiety and consider whether further management is required (e.g. family therapy, school counsellor etc.).
- Returning to school is a high priority. If necessary, this can be done by gradually increasing the time at school over a short period of time.
- Evidence supports CBT in group settings and educational support therapy. The latter involves having a nominated teacher or aide support the child through participation in the therapeutic intervention and then assisting them practice the learnt strategies in school.

Obsessive-compulsive disorder

Obsessive-compulsive disorder (OCD) is one of the more severe forms of anxiety disorders. Although it is relatively rare (1–2% of children and adolescents, more commonly in males), OCD can be associated with childhood anxiety, as well as depressive and pervasive developmental disorders.

Symptoms include intrusive thoughts and a variety of compulsive/ritualistic behaviours. Common co-morbid conditions include social anxiety disorder, separation anxiety, agoraphobia and generalised anxiety disorder.

Management
- Provide support and explanation to the patient and family.
- Refer for assessment and management by a mental health specialist.
  - ○ Principles of treatment are symptom control, improvement and maintenance of function.
  - ○ For children and adolescents with mild symptoms, CBT is the treatment of choice.
  - ○ For children and adolescents with more severe symptoms, a combination of CBT and medication (SSRI) in relatively higher doses is indicated.

Post-traumatic stress disorder

Trauma can directly contribute to mental health difficulties and can manifest as post-traumatic stress disorder (PTSD). See Table 25.5 for common symptoms of PTSD in children.

Background
- Children and adolescents show a variable response to trauma.
- PTSD is not an expected outcome of trauma.
- It is not strongly correlated to the perceived severity of the trauma.
- The cluster of symptoms is intrusion, avoidance and arousal.
- The criteria are not particularly sensitive to trauma effects in very young children.
- It is more common in girls than boys.
- Common co-morbid conditions include specific phobia, social phobia and agoraphobia.

Assessment
- PTSD can be diagnosed only when the traumatic event *precedes* the symptoms and symptoms are present for >1 month.
- Co-morbid mental health disorders such as anxiety disorder or depressive disorder can occur. Hence, some presenting symptoms may be indicative of these co-morbid disorders rather than PTSD.
- When symptoms have persisted beyond a period of a few days or weeks, refer to mental health services for further assessment and management.

Table 25.5 Common symptoms of post-traumatic stress disorder in children

Intrusive thoughts and 're-experiencing' of the event(s) – may be demonstrated through play, enactment or drawings
Fear of the dark
Nightmares
Difficulties getting to sleep and/or nocturnal waking
Separation anxiety
Generalised anxiety or fears
Developmental regression, for example continence, language skills
Social withdrawal
Irritability
Aggressive behaviour
Attention and concentration difficulties
Memory problems
Heightened sensitivity to other traumatic events

Source: Reproduced with permission from Tonge B. Common child and adolescent psychiatric problems and their management in the community. *Medical Journal of Australia* 1998;168:241–248. (Tonge 1998. Reproduced wtih permission of AMPCo.)

Management
- Trauma-focused CBT has been shown to be effective. Techniques include graded exposure, cognitive processing, psychoeducation, training in stress reduction, relaxation and positive self-talk.
- Medication is not first-line treatment unless co-morbid conditions such as depression are present. In such circumstances, propranolol, clonidine, risperidone and citalopram (an SSRI) can be used.

Paediatric medical traumatic stress

Children, adolescents and families may experience a traumatic stress response as a result of their experiences associated with pain, injury, serious illness, medical procedures or invasive medical treatment. This cluster of symptoms has been referred to recently as paediatric medical traumatic stress (PMTS). This trauma may be chronic, repetitive, predictable (such as associated with medical procedures), and involve interpersonal interaction. This is referred to as *complex trauma*.

Background
- The child, adolescent and/or family may experience symptoms of arousal, re-experiencing and avoidance in response to a medical event.
- Symptoms may vary in intensity but may impact on general functioning.
- Symptoms may not reach diagnostic criteria of PTSD or acute stress disorder (ASD) but can occur along a continuum of intensity (from normative stress reactions to persistent and distressing symptoms).
- *Subjective* appraisals of threat rather than *objective* disease/medical factors seem more predictive of stress responses.
- There is debate regarding the need to acknowledge complex trauma experienced by some children as a distinct form of trauma stress disorder.

Management
Prevention is the best cure. Health care providers are well placed to modify stress experiences of patients and families in the medical context, subsequently reducing the risk of persistent symptoms. This can be done by
- Explaining procedures in a developmentally appropriate manner
- Checking their understanding of the explanation
- Teaching parents how to comfort and reassure their children
- Looking for opportunities for the child to make decisions in their management (e.g. in young children ask if they would prefer to sit up or lie down or if they would like for a parent to hold their hand during procedures; involving adolescents in the discussions regarding the diagnosis and treatment processes to give them a sense of ownership)
- Implementing good pain management practice (see Chapter 3, *Pain management*)
- Screening for persistent symptoms of distress post injury/illness

Depression

Child and adolescent depression is common. There is a 2% incidence in children with a cumulative incidence of 20% by 18 years of age. Whilst it is twice as common in females during adolescence, there is no gender bias in younger children. Depression is a chronic, highly relapsing, recurrent and debilitating disorder.

Symptoms vary according to the age and developmental stage of the child.

Infants and younger children: irritable mood, failure to gain weight and lack of enjoyment in play and other activities.

Children and younger teenagers: more symptoms of anxiety (e.g. phobias, separation anxiety), somatic complaints, irritability with temper tantrums and behavioural problems. See Table 25.6 for common symptoms of childhood depression.

Older adolescents: more 'adult like' symptoms of depression including insomnia, easy fatiguability, loss of interest in pleasurable activities and then in all activities, loss of appetite and weight, psychomotor slowing, in severe cases delusional thinking, self-harming and suicidal behaviours.

Co-morbidities
- These are common and include anxiety disorder, conduct disorder or attention deficit hyperactivity disorder (ADHD).

Table 25.6 Common symptoms of childhood depression

Symptoms
Persistent depressed mood, unhappiness and irritability
Loss of interest in play and friends
Loss of energy and concentration
Deterioration in school work
Loss of appetite and no weight gain
Disturbed sleep
Thoughts of worthlessness and suicide (suicide attempts are rare before age 10 years, then increase)
Somatic complaints (headaches, abdominal pain)
Co-morbid anxiety, conduct disorder, ADHD, eating disorders or substance abuse
Family factors
Family stress (ill or deceased parent, family conflict, parental separation)
Repeated experience of failure or criticism
Family history of depression

Source: Reproduced with permission from Tonge B. Common child and adolescent psychiatric problems and their management in the community. *Medical Journal of Australia* 1998;168:241–248. (Tonge 1998. Reproduced wtih permission of AMPCo.)

- Incidence of co-morbidities:
  - In patients with anxiety disorder, 10–20% have co-morbid depression.
  - In patients with depressive disorder, >50% have co-morbid anxiety.
  - In patients with disruptive behaviour disorders, 15–30% have co-morbid anxiety.

Assessment
- Recognition is important, as untreated childhood and adolescent depression increases the risk for depression in adulthood.
- Depression in childhood and particularly in adolescence increases the risk of suicide and self-harming behaviours.

Management
There are three phases of treatment:
1. Acute phase lasting 6–12 weeks (stages 1 and 2 of treatment)
2. Continuation phase 6–12 months (stage 3 of treatment)
3. Maintenance phase 1 year or more
Most treatment effectiveness studies in children and teenagers have focused on the acute phase and some on the continuation phase and relatively few if any studies have focused on the maintenance phase.

Acute phase
Stage 1
Form a therapeutic alliance to assist in making a thorough assessment (including biopsychosocial antecedents) and diagnosis. Psychoeducation can be particularly effective in involving the child and parents in this process.

Stage 2
Target areas for intervention such as reduced self-care, social and occupational activity, ineffective coping with stressors, correcting the problem-solving deficits, reducing the social impairment and inadequate self-esteem.

Psychotherapy is the first-line treatment for mild to moderate mood disorder. Effective psychotherapies include CBT and interpersonal therapy for adolescents.

Whilst some studies have shown positive outcomes in the placebo group alone, a combination of CBT and SSRI medication (fluoxetine, ciatlopram escitalopram, sertraline) provides good outcomes. Fluoxetine appears to have the lowest number needed to treat. Fluoxetine is FDA approved in USA for the treatment of childhood depression. Fluoxetine and escitalopram are approved for adolescent depression.

Continuation phase

Stage 3 focuses on relapse prevention. GPs can play an important role in this. Referral to local mental health services may also be required. Carefully monitor for self-harm, suicide, ideas of hopelessness, deterioration in overall functioning.

SSRIs and suicidality

SSRIs are prescribed for a variety of childhood problems including anxiety disorders and major depressive episodes. Prescribing rates are increasing in Australia, USA and Europe.

There has been some concern regarding increased risk of suicidality and deliberate self-harm associated with SSRI use in children, although the evidence to date is relatively weak.

Risk of deliberate self-harm appears to be highest in the first 2–4 weeks of starting an SSRI. The following guidelines should be adhered to

- Start with a low dose and increase slowly. Side effects are dose-dependent, but efficacy is not. Always use the lowest effective dose.
- Only use as an adjunct to psychotherapy.
- Explain to parents (and child if appropriate) about possible adverse effects of antidepressants. Discuss the issues of deliberate self-harm and suicidality and the need for close monitoring, especially in the first 2–4 weeks.
- Explain the discontinuation syndrome, which occurs when an SSRI is withdrawn abruptly. This can result in irritability, mood lability, insomnia, anxiety, vivid dreams, nausea, vomiting, headache, dizziness, tremor, dystonia, fatigue, myalgia, rhinorrhoea and chills.
- Monitor closely for adverse effects in the first 4 weeks; consider using structured rating instruments.

Psychosomatic problems

Somatic responses to stressful situations are common (e.g. sweating during a job interview or diarrhoea before taking an exam). Somatic complaints in children are also believed to be relatively common and appear as physical sensations related to affective distress.

Psychosomatic or somatoform disorders refer to the presence of physical symptoms suggesting an underlying medical condition without such a condition being found, or where a medical problem cannot adequately account for the level of functional impairment.

Common symptoms:

- Headache
- Abdominal pain
- Limb pain
- Fatigue
- Pain/soreness
- Disturbance of vision
- Symptoms suggestive of neurological disorders

Conversion disorder may present with dramatic symptoms such as

- Gait disturbance
- Paraesthesia
- Paralysis
- Pseudoseizures

In this situation, the onset of the symptom is closely associated to a psychological stressor. Conversion disorders are generally relatively short-lived. They are often alleviated by identification and management of the stressor(s) and in some instances, symptomatic treatment of the physical problem.

Somatisation disorders may present in children whose families have a history of illnesses or psychosomatic disorders. Such patterns may be evident at a multigenerational level where physical symptoms appear to be the 'currency' by which affective states are communicated. Possible family relationship difficulties (including sexual abuse) should be considered as part of a thorough assessment.

Management

- Assess symptoms to determine lack of clear 'medical pattern'.
- Validate the symptom(s) as a real issue for the patient.
- Assess how the symptom(s) affect the life of the child and family.
- If medical tests are normal, bring up the possibility of a somatoform problem not in exclusion to medical causes but alongside it.
- Assess the patient's awareness of the psychological nature of the symptoms.
- Give the child (using age appropriate language and content) and parents an explanation.
- Explain that stress results in an 'organic' bodily response. Use examples such as anxiety causing increased heart rate.
- Explain that the treatment is psychotherapy.

Mental health problems associated with chronic illness

Children and adolescents with chronic illnesses may present with exacerbations of their physical symptoms that relate to their affective state. Such responses may be related to a precipitating stressor or may reflect the child's changing responses to their illness.

Children and adolescents may be angry, resentful of the limitations their condition imposes, or be particularly sensitive to being different from their peers. Additionally, responses by their parents (e.g. over- or under-protectiveness) may contribute to adjustment problems. Along with somatisation, other difficulties may emerge, such as non-adherence with treatment and family relationship problems.

Management

Management depends on the nature, severity and duration of the problem. Some general principles are

- It is important to recognise that the physical symptoms as genuine and distressing.
- Thorough clinical examination, investigation and mental health assessment is usually required. Hospital admission may be required to facilitate this.
- Discussion of mind–body interactions can be useful. Discuss early on the possibility that psychological factors are contributing to symptoms or well-being. This may allow the patient and family to begin to discuss possible psychological stressors, reducing resistance to mental health input.
- Symptomatic treatment (e.g. heat packs, relaxation exercises, physiotherapy, mild analgesia) may be appropriate, along with supportive counselling and/or mental health referral.
- Avoid medical over-investigation based on the family's coercion or unwillingness to consider psychological factors.
- It is important that the patient and family do not feel they have 'wasted your time' if there is no evident medical problem. Maintain an interest in the patient and family with a review appointment or follow-up telephone enquiry as appropriate.

Developmental and family psychiatry
Infant mental health

Infant mental health is an area of clinical work aimed at understanding the psychological and emotional development of infants from birth to 3 years and the particular difficulties that they and their families might face.

Babies come into the world with a range of capacities and vulnerabilities and together with their parents, negotiate their way through the next months and years. This process of attachment, growth and development may be challenged by a range of experiences that stress or interrupt this course. Examples include traumatic events, developmental concerns, hospitalisation of the infant or parent, prematurity, illness or disability, an experience of loss, changing family circumstances or postnatal depression.

Consider referral to a mental health clinician for

- Persistent crying, irritability or 'colic'
- Gaze avoidance
- Bonding difficulties
- Slow weight gain
- Persistent feeding or sleeping difficulties
- Persistent behavioural symptoms, for example tantrums, nightmares, aggression
- Family relationship problems

- Infants with chronic ill health
- Premature babies and their families

Family relationship difficulties

A family-sensitive approach is crucial to the assessment and management of childhood mental health issues. Behavioural and/or emotional difficulties in a child can occur in the context of chronic family dysfunction. Conversely, such difficulties can arise in the context of well-functioning families where the child's temperament, personality or precipitating stressors may lead to behavioural or emotional difficulties for the child and/or parent–child relationship difficulties. When a child is presenting with behavioural and/or emotional difficulties, assessment should include an understanding of the family situation including

- Family tree, living arrangements and caregiving roles
- Quality of family relationships
- Early attachments/relationships
- History of significant losses, stressors, precipitating factors
- Social/family support networks
- Identifiable 'risk' factors such as poverty, illnesses, absent social supports

Children can be symptom-bearers for family relationship difficulties. In such instances, treatment of the presenting symptom is unlikely to be successful in the long term without appropriate family and/or couple counselling.

When working with families

- Conduct at least one family interview when dealing with a child with significant behavioural or emotional difficulties.
- Interview all family members (including siblings, who are often insightful commentators on family life) and provide an empathic response to each member's point of view. In the case of young children, observing and commenting upon play themes is useful.
- Do not assume that different family members agree on what is the presenting problem. It is often useful to ask family members to rank their concerns such as
  - What is the problem you are most worried about today?
  - What is the number 1 worry you have at the moment ... number 2 ... number 3?
  - Who in the family is most worried about this problem? Who is the least worried?
- If family members are not present, seek further understanding by questions such as
  - If your husband were here today, what would he say about this problem?
  - Who else in the family has noticed the changes that you have described today?
- Encouraging families to find solutions to their difficulties is more likely to provide long-term change. This may involve helping families identify negative or unhelpful patterns of interaction, helping families identify strengths and resilience and noting small changes/improvements.

Grief and loss

Experiences of grief and loss are inevitable. Where losses are severe or traumatic or where a child has preexisting vulnerabilities, these experiences can contribute to mental health problems or result in complicated grief reactions.

Children may believe that they caused a loved one's death or illness. Adolescents may find it difficult to speak about the loss as it may be intricately linked in with their sense of self. Bereaved children or adolescents may feel different from others, thus feel isolated or have difficulty managing the reactions of their peers.

In most instances, the bereaved child or adolescent can be supported through family, school, community and religion. Where the loss is within the family, family-based counselling/therapy can be helpful to address the young person's grief in the context of other family members' reactions.

Grief and loss experiences for children or adolescents may also occur in situations other than bereavement (e.g. chronic illness, refugee status or having a parent with a mental illness). Parental divorce is a common source of grief and loss in young people. Grief associated with this situation can be complicated and often remains unacknowledged by significant adults. Young people may experience feelings of guilt and self-blame, harbour fantasies of a parental reunion, struggle with divided loyalties and feel anxious about their own future relationships. Feelings of anger, rejection and sadness may lead to behavioural or emotional manifestations of their grief.

Breaks ups with friends or the break up of a romantic relationship can be severely testing for adolescents, sometimes leading to depressed feelings, thoughts and acts of aggression or self-harm. There may be self-blame, an over focus on the importance of this lost relationship to their lives and catastrophising, displacement of the negative feelings towards loved ones at home or authority figures such as parents and teachers. Help the young person see how such changes in relationships are common, that they can and will survive this and that they, as well as their lives, are bigger and more resilient than they may fear or imagine.

Management

- Acknowledge the child's loss in an empathic and appropriate manner. This can be helpful even when a loss is not recent.
- Where a grieving child presents with behavioural or emotional difficulties, gently probe their beliefs about why the loss occurred. This can help the clinician understand the child's predicament. For example:
  - Sometimes, when I see young people who have lost their mum/brother, etc., they feel like it's their fault that they died or got sick. Does it ever feel like that for you?
  - How do you imagine your life would be different if your mum and dad were still together?
  - Why do you think people get cancer, etc.?
- Assist the family in gaining access to appropriate support and counselling.
- Seek further specialist mental health services when a young person continues to exhibit extreme distress or prolonged behavioural or emotional difficulties.

Psychosis

Psychosis is a general term for states in which mental function is grossly impaired. Symptoms consist of two main groups:

1. *Positive symptoms*: reality testing and insight are lacking; delusions; hallucinations; incoherence; thought disorder and disorganised behaviour
2. *Negative symptoms*: inexpressive faces; blank looks; monotone; reduced and monosyllabic speech; few gestures; seeming lack of interest in the world and other people; inability to feel pleasure or act spontaneously

In the case of 'organic' psychosis, there may also be a clouding of consciousness, confusion and disorientation, as well as perceptual disturbances. Short-term memory impairment is common in organic brain syndromes. Organic brain syndromes may follow even minor head injury.

Negative symptoms are much more pervasive and have a much greater effect on a patient's quality of life. About 25% of patients with schizophrenic psychosis have a condition called the deficit syndrome, defined by severe and persistent negative symptoms.

Substances associated with psychotic reactions:

- Anticholinergics
- Anticonvulsants
- Antidepressants
- Antimalarials
- Benzodiazepines
- Illicit drugs (amphetamines, cocaine, marijuana, opiates and hallucinogens)
- Cannabis in particular has been associated with significant mental state changes that could lead to a psychotic disorder

Adolescents may occasionally present in an acutely psychotic state with no prior history of drug ingestion or head injury. In this case, the possibility of a 'functional' psychosis, schizophrenia or bipolar disorder should be considered. The latter often presents with an elated mood, grandiose ideas, increased energy and reduced sleep requirements.

Management

- Admit to hospital for a full psychiatric and medical assessment to rule out an organic cause.
- The use of antipsychotic medications should be discussed with a child and adolescent psychiatrist.

Psychiatric emergencies

The most common underlying problem that leads to psychiatric emergency presentations in children and adolescents is emotional (affective) dysregulation.

Emotional dysregulation is a set of poorly modulated responses to a situation that is not socially acceptable. They are characterised by verbal and/or physical aggression, threats and acts of self-harm, suicidal gestures, substance use, disinhibited sexualised behaviours and dissociation. Self-harm, aggression, substance use and dissociation may be means by which the patient avoids or distracts from internal psychological distress.

Young people of all ages may have emotional dysregulation; however, it is more pronounced in adolescence. Possible associations include neurobiological vulnerability, attachment disorders, trauma, experiences of abuse or victimisation and neglect.

Suicidal gestures and deliberate self-harming

After motor vehicle accidents, suicide is the next most common cause of death in 15–25 year olds in Australia. Children have a well formed idea of death as being final, from around the age of 9–10 years.

Factors most commonly associated with completed suicide are

- history of suicidal gestures and/or deliberate self-harm;
- major depression;
- psychosis with command hallucinations;
- substance abuse;
- homelessness; and
- antisocial behaviour.

In most instances, deliberate self-harm is not true suicidal behaviour with the intent of causing death; however, most self-harm is associated with a degree of psychiatric disturbance.

Adolescent suicide differs from adult suicide in that it is more likely to be

- Motivated by revenge or a feeling of loss of peer supports
- An act of anger or irritation
- Impulsive
- Romantically and idealistically driven
- Related to low self-esteem

Assessment

Assess the patient's intentionality to end their life.

- Assess the risk of current and further suicidal behaviour, the precipitants and context of the suicide attempt, as well as the presence of coexisting psychopathology (e.g. depression, psychosis, bipolar disorder, severe anxiety).
- Enquire about past history of suicidal gestures including their circumstances and their lethality, deliberate self-harm without suicidal intent.
- Ask about their expectations of death from this suicide attempt (e.g. there is life after death or that after punishing others by their suicide they can come back).
- Assess the 'finality' of their attempt (e.g. whether they left notes saying goodbye to loved ones, gave away possessions, completed commitments).
- When seeing the patient after a failed suicide attempt, check the individual's risk of trying other strategies to end their life.
- Assess the capacity of the patient to reflect on what effect their suicide might have on loved ones.

Look for other relevant historical factors such as a history of the patient showing sudden changes in relationships, history of exhibiting violent and disruptive behaviour, withdrawing from friends and social involvements, look for episodic stressful precipitants, troubles with school authorities or police, feared pregnancy, major family dysfunction, recent break up with boyfriend or girlfriend, refusal by significant others to provide anticipated help, support or love.

Immediate interventions

- Estimate immediate to short-term risk.
- Decide whether or not to hospitalise.

- Assess the availability of supports if the patient will not be hospitalised.
- If the patient can be managed at home, negotiate a management plan with the patient and family/caregivers.

Management plan
- Define the level of support to be provided by the family/carers and relevant services (e.g. parents to watch all the time or check in with the patient every few minutes/hours).
- Document a list of precipitating factors and early warning signs of another suicide attempt or escalating distress in the patient.
- Write a crisis plan that lists strategies on managing early warning signs and written information on how to seek further help.
- Provide a 24-hour telephone number and name of a contact person.
- Confirm a date and time for a reassessment.
- Convey this information to the mental health service/provider to whom the patient is referred for further care and treatment.

Medium term interventions
- Work with the young person.
- Develop a caring and empathic relationship.
- Instil hope.
- Provide education to the patient and their family/carers about depression or other associated psychiatric condition.
- Provide advice on sleep, diet, hygiene and exercise where there are problems.
- Exploring the incidents with the person looking at motivation and circumstances.
- Ensure the environment is safe.
- Increase support from family and friends.
- Contact other professionals involved to ensure support is provided and coordinated.
- Ensure basic needs are met (food, shelter).
- Identify individual risk and protective factors.
- Develop contingency and relapse plans.
- Arrange ongoing assessment of capacity of the family to manage the young person's safely.
- Family treatment.

Psychoeducation
- Communication skills
- Conflict resolution
- Affect regulation within the family

Behaviour management
- Orientate the parents toward limit setting in a non-coercive way.
- Help the parents change their ways of interacting with the patient, improve cohesion and increase supportive gestures by the parents towards the adolescent.
- Reinforce non-suicidal, adaptive responses.
- Interventions in specialist mental health services would include
  - CBT
  - Problem-solving therapy
    - Social skills training
    - Effective communication
    - Affect management
    - Recognition and regulation of anger before it escalates to suicidal behaviour
    - Tension recognition (feeling thermometer)
    - Interpersonal therapy
    - Improvement of distress tolerance and mindfulness skills through dialectical behaviour therapy
    - Relapse prevention
    - Treatment of co-morbidities

Non-suicidal self-injury

Non-suicidal self-injury (NSSI) is more common than suicidal gestures in children and adolescents. Self-injury or self-harm may indicate anger, a response to perceived rejection by loved ones and peers, a coping mechanism to deal with states of internal distress or emptiness that may be associated with disturbed self-image. It may also be done as an alternative to suicidal gestures by those who are distressed by having suicidal urges. NSSI may occur acutely at times of significant stress such as family and peer relationship problems, a loss of self-esteem through a break up of a relationship or failure in exams. NSSI may also be a chronic problem in some adolescents with distressing and intrusive trauma-related images and memories or emerging borderline personality disorder.

Interventions include

- Teaching emotional regulation skills
- Identifying emotions and obstacles to changing emotions
- Reducing vulnerability to stress
- Increasing positive emotional events
- Applying distress tolerance techniques
- Problem solving
- Identifying the current problem
- Generating, evaluating and implementing alternative solutions that might have been used or could be used in the future

Adolescents with chronic NSSI may benefit from highly specialised psychological therapies.

Associated disorders such as depression must be treated.

The violent young person and emergency restraint

See also Chapter 1, *Medical emergencies*.

As physical restraint and sedation deprives the patient of autonomy, it should only be contemplated as a last resort for safety and/or treatment. A patient who is 'acting out' and who does not need acute medical or psychiatric care should be discharged from hospital to a safe environment rather than be restrained.

Alternative means of calming a patient

- Crisis prevention.
- Anticipate and identify early irritable behaviour (and past history).
- Involve mental health expertise early for assistance.
- Provide a safe 'containing' environment.
- Give a confident reassuring approach without added stimuli.
- Listen and talk simply and in a calm manner.
- Offer planned 'collaborative' sedation (e.g. ask the patient if they would take some oral medication to regain some control of their behaviour).

When physical restraint is required, a coordinated team approach is essential, with roles clearly defined and swift action taken. Unless contraindicated, sedation should usually accompany physical restraint.

Indications for restraint

- Other methods to control the behaviour (such as de-escalation techniques) have failed
- The patient displays aggressive or combative behaviour which arises from a medical or psychiatric condition (including intoxication)
- The patient requires urgent medical or psychiatric care
- The behaviour involves a proximate risk of harm to the patient or others, or risk of significant destruction of property

Cautions to physical restraint and emergency sedation

- A patient who is 'acting out' and who does not need acute medical or psychiatric care should be discharged to a safe environment (e.g. home, child protection services, police) rather than be restrained.
- Be aware of previous medications and possible substance use.
- Safe containment may possible via alternative means (including voluntary, collaborative oral sedation).

Contraindications to physical restraint and emergency sedation

- Inadequate personnel/unsafe setting/inadequate equipment.
- Situation is judged as too dangerous (e.g. patient has a weapon).

Emergency chemical restraint

See Emergency chemical restraint CPG (http://www.rch.org.au/clinicalguide/guideline_index/Emergency_chemical_restraint_%E2%80%93_Medication_options/).

If at all possible, the patient should be given the option of taking an oral medication. Benzodiazepines are generally the medication of first choice, particularly in cases of known intoxication. If the patient has a known psychiatric disorder, consider using top-up doses of their regular medication.

Give one option, wait for an effect and then consider further medication. If a drug from one group has had a poor therapeutic response after two doses, try a different drug and reconsider your diagnosis (e.g. underlying organic pathology) and indications for using emergency sedation (Table 25.7).

If the patient can tolerate oral medications

- Diazepam (oral): 0.2–0.4 mg/kg (max 10 mg per dose if benzodiazepine naïve); OR
- Lorazepam (oral): 0.5–1 mg (if <40 kg); 1–2.5 mg (if >40 kg); OR
- Olanzapine wafer (sublingual): 2.5–5 mg (if <40 kg); 5–10 mg (if >40 kg).

If the patient cannot tolerate oral medications

- Midazolam IM/IV: 0.1–0.2 mg/kg (max 10 mg per dose); OR
- Olanzapine IM only : 5 mg (if <40 kg); 10 mg (if >40 kg); OR
- Haloperidol IM/IV: 0.1–0.2 mg/kg (max 5 mg per dose); OR
- Midazolam/haloperidol combination (IM): as above combined in one syringe.

The following antidotes should be readily available for reversal of potential side effects:

- **Benztropine** – 0.02 mg/kg (max 2 mg per dose) given IV/IM for reversal of dystonic reactions associated with haloperidol and olanzapine. Repeated doses may be required.

Table 25.7 Drug-specific information

Drug	Time to review clinical effect before second med	Adverse effects
Midazolam	IM: 10–20 minutes IV: almost immediate	Respiratory depression[a] and airway compromise, paradoxical reactions.[d]
Olanzapine	Oral: 20–30 minutes IM: 15–30 minutes	Respiratory depression,[a] hypotension, ↑HR. Do not use if history suggestive of prolonged QTC, extrapyramidal reactions,[b] neuroleptic malignant syndrome,[c] may reduce seizure threshold.
Haloperidol	IM/IV: 15–30 minutes	Respiratory depression,[a] hypotension, ↑HR. Do not use if history suggestive of prolonged QTC, extrapyramidal reactions,[b] neuroleptic malignant syndrome,[c] may reduce seizure threshold.
Diazepam	Oral: 30–60 minutes	Respiratory depression[a] (unlikely to see immediate complications as longer half-lives) and paradoxical reactions.[d]
Lorazepam	Oral: 20–40 minutes	Respiratory depression[a] (unlikely to see immediate complications as longer half-lives) and paradoxical reactions.[d]

[a] **Respiratory depression** – More commonly seen with benzodiazepines but can also occur with olanzapine and haloperidol.
[b] **Extrapyramidal reactions** – More commonly seen with haloperidol but may be seen with olanzapine after only one dose. Reversible with benztropine.
[c] **Neuroleptic malignant syndrome** – A rare complication of typical and atypical antipsychotics. If suspected, get immediate help and check serum CK as it is invariably elevated.
[d] **Paradoxical reactions** – Administration of a benzodiazepine results in increasing agitation and anxiety as opposed to its normal sedating effect. This is more commonly seen in patients with developmental delay and/or a history of aggressive behaviour.

- **Flumazenil** – 10 mcg/kg (max 200 mcg per dose) repeated at 1 minute intervals p.r.n. for up to five doses, to treat reversal of respiratory depression associated with benzodiazepines only. **Do not give unless you are sure the patient is not on long-term benzodiazepines.**

Psychotropic medications

Medication may be prescribed as part of the management plan for some children with development and mental health disorders, alongside behavioural and therapies. Psychotropic medications can treat symptoms, improve function and quality of life for children with a range of development and mental health disorders, including ADHD, anxiety disorders, OCD, psychosis, Tourette's disorder, and moderate to severe depression. The target of medication is often a symptom rather than a diagnosis. For example, there is no medication to treat autism; however, children with autism often benefit from medications to treat symptoms such as anxiety, severe aggression or sleep disturbance (Table 25.8). Some conditions such as mild depression and oppositional defiant disorder do not respond as well to medications but will benefit from behavioural and/or talking therapies.

As with all therapies, the decision regarding prescribing psychotropics involves weighing up the potential benefits against potential harms. In general, medications should only be considered when the child has significant impairment which is not responding to non-pharmacological therapies. The main prescribers of psychotropic medications for children in Australia are paediatricians and child and adolescent psychiatrists. Some medications are restricted to these groups, while others can also be prescribed by general practitioners.

Where possible decisions to prescribe should be discussed with the child or adolescent in developmentally appropriate terms. This includes discussions about the effectiveness and side effects of medication, and decisions to continue or terminate treatment.

Table 25.8 Psychotropic medications for children and adolescents

Drug group	Indications	Common or serious side effects	Monitoring
Stimulants, e.g. methylphenidate	ADHD	Appetite suppression, anxiety, tics	Exclude cardiac disease on personal and family history, examination before prescribing; weight, height, blood pressure
Noradrenergic agents, e.g. atomoxetine, tricyclic anti-depressants	ADHD, anxiety, sleep disturbance	Gastrointestinal upset, sedation, for tricyclics also look for urinary retention, constipation	Tricyclics – ECG at baseline and after some weeks on treatment
SSRI, e.g. fluoxetine, sertraline	Anxiety, OCD, severe adolescent depression	GI upset, sleep disturbance; agitation/increased self-harm or suicidality (soon after starting)	Monitor closely in first weeks; avoid sudden cessation (discontinuation syndrome – flu-like symptoms)
Atypical antipsychotics, e.g. risperidone, olanzapine	Severe aggression, agitated obsessionality especially in children with autism spectrum disorder; Tourette's disorder; adolescent psychosis	Sedation, weight gain, metabolic syndrome, hyperprolactinaemia; QTc prolongation, acute dystonic reaction, chronic extrapyramidal symptoms	Weight/BMI, waist circumference during every clinic visit; fasting lipid profile, oral glucose tolerance test every 3 months, liver function tests if excessive weight gain; prolactin level only if symptoms
Mood stabilisers, e.g. valproate, lamotrigine	Mood dysregulation/irritability	Specific to drug used	Specific to drug used
Alpha-2 agonists, e.g. clonidine	Sleep disturbance, explosive aggression	Sedation	Heart rate, blood pressure

Principles of safe and effective prescribing of psychotropic medications

- Be clear about a priori target, in order to evaluate effectiveness.
- Warn of common and serious side effects, provide clear written information on side effects in plain English/language of the patient.
- Start with a low dose, and increase gradually until benefits are seen or unacceptable side effects restrict use.
- Avoid sedation (where symptom change may be the goal) and over sedation (where some sedation may be the goal).
- Ensure adequate dose and duration of medication trial. This is particularly important for anti-depressants and atomoxetine.
- Be available for contact.
- Monitor regularly.
- Optimise non-medication management.
- Consider a trial off treatment when symptoms are well controlled for a period of time.

USEFUL RESOURCES
- *www.nctsnet.org* – National Child Traumatic Stress Network. Excellent website containing practical resources for families and healthcare professionals.
- *www.aacap.org* – American Academy of Child & Adolescent Psychiatry. Contains useful practice parameters for doctors and information for families.
- *www.nimh.nih.gov* [Health & Outreach > Topics > Children & Adolescents] – National Institute of Mental Health in USA with parent information.
- *www.zerotothree.org* – Excellent resource for infant mental health in this Washington-based organisation.

CHAPTER 26

Prescribing for children

Noel Cranswick
Antun Bogovic

Knowledge of drug administration in children and infants is essential to the practice of paediatrics. Most registered medicines do not have licensed (official medication body) indications or dosing for children, and we rely on specialist paediatric information sources to provide guidance.

Drug choice and dose

There are many issues that influence drug choice and dose in paediatric practice. Pharmacokinetic parameters change with age and dosage regimens need to take into account factors such as growth, organ development and sexual maturation. (Sexual maturation corresponds to pubertal changes, with significant impact on physiology and pharmacokinetics).

Unlicensed and off-label drug use

These are commonplace in paediatric practice as a result of inadequate paediatric data.

- *Unlicensed drug* use is the use of
  - a drug that has not been approved by the Therapeutic Goods Administration (TGA), **or**
  - an untested formulation of an approved drug, **or**
  - a non-pharmacopoeial substance as a medicine.
- *Off-label prescribing* is the use of a drug in a manner other than that recommended in the manufacturer's product information.

Dosing considerations

- Most medicines in children are dosed by weight. Always attempt to obtain accurate weight and height data before calculating the appropriate initial dose.
- Consider using ideal body weight in obese children (BMI >95th% for age and sex).
- A few medications, especially cytotoxic drugs, may only have dosing information by body surface area (see Appendix 4).
- A child's weight (in kg) can be estimated by the formula (age + 4) × 2 for children aged from 1 to 8 years. **Remember to confirm an accurate weight at the first available opportunity**.
- In emergencies, standardised centile charts for weight and height may be utilised for these calculations.
- See general guidelines in Table 26.1.

Adverse drug reactions

- Are common but under-recognised in children.
- All suspected and proven adverse drug reactions (ADRs) should be reported, even if seemingly trivial.
- Suspected allergic reactions should be assessed and followed up (e.g. by a drug allergy clinic).
- When an avoidable ADR is identified, patients should be given a permanent record (e.g. card or medical alert bracelet) as appropriate.
- There may be variation in the ADRs experienced in different age group (e.g. neonates, children, adolescents). Some specific examples include
  - Jaundice (hyperbilirubinaemia) in neonates or very young children taking sulfur-containing drugs, such as cotrimoxazole.

Paediatric Handbook, Ninth Edition. Edited by Amanda Gwee, Romi Rimer and Michael Marks.
© 2015 John Wiley & Sons, Ltd. Published 2015 by John Wiley & Sons, Ltd.

Table 26.1 Guidelines for best prescribing practice

DO check the dose:
- Use a calculator for dosing by weight/BSA
- Ensure it does not exceed the maximum adult dose

DO check for allergies and contraindications

DO write legibly

DO write UNITS (not IU) after insulin doses – and other medications where the dose is expressed as 'units'

DO include generic drug name. Generic names should always be used – avoid trade names if possible. Dose, frequency, route and date of start, finish or review should also be provided.

DO only use recognized abbreviations for prescription instructions

Do refer to accepted RCH and paediatric prescribing and dosing

DO write a leading zero before a decimal point, for example 0.6 mg not .6 mgreferences, including local clinical practice guidelines.

DO NOT write a trailing zero after a whole number, for example 8 mg not 8.0 mg

DO NOT abbreviate drug names, for example AZT could be azathioprine or azithromycin

Source: RCH Medication Management Procedure – http://ww2.rch.org.au/policy_rch/?doc_id=6570. Reproduced with permission of The Royal Children's Hospital Clinical.

- Renal damage from ACE inhibitors and NSAIDs.
- Biliary sludging with neonates/very young children receiving ceftriaxone.
- Grey baby syndrome associated with chloramphenicol – although this drug is now rarely prescribed.
- Reye syndrome in patients receiving moderate to high doses of aspirin.
- **D**rug **R**eaction (or Rash) with **E**osinophilia and **S**ystemic **S**ymptoms (DRESS syndrome) – This usually presents as eosinophilia associated with a rash, fever or organ dysfunction. It is associated with a wide range of medications with anticonvulsants being the most common group.

The important points to document on history are
- The specific illness the medication was prescribed for (intercurrent viral infections may also cause urticaria).
- The name of the medication and preparation.
- Whether this was the first exposure to the medication.
- How many doses were given before a reaction occurred?
- The time of onset of the reaction from the last dose given.
- The symptoms of the reaction and its total duration.
- Any other reactions or allergies the child may have OR a family history of reaction/allergy?

Types of adverse drug reactions
Type A adverse drug reaction
- These are predictable from the known pharmacology of the drug and are dose-dependent.
- Examples include opiate sedation and tachycardia with β_2-agonists.

Type B adverse drug reaction
- These are less common, unpredictable (idiosyncratic) and dose-independent.
- They are often serious and usually require ceasing the drug, for example Stevens–Johnson syndrome (most commonly associated with anticonvulsants).

Suspected allergic skin reactions to antibiotics
One of the most common ADR presentations in children is a non-specific skin rash following the commencement of an antibiotic. These patients should be followed up with confirmatory tests (e.g. intradermal or controlled oral re-challenge in a specialist facility). The majority of children who are tested are found not to be allergic to or intolerant of the antibiotic.

Therapeutic drug monitoring
- Relatively few drugs need therapeutic drug monitoring (TDM).
- It is beneficial in drugs with a narrow therapeutic index, or where serum levels correlate with efficacy or toxicity.

- TDM can be useful for
  - Antibiotics, for example gentamicin, vancomycin.
  - Anticonvulsants, for example phenytoin, phenobarbitone.
  - Immunosuppressants, for example tacrolimus, cyclosporin, methotrexate.
  - Drug overdose, for example paracetamol, iron.
- Routine testing is not beneficial for
  - Carbamazepine
  - Valproate
- Timing of samples for monitoring will vary depending upon the actual drug but accurate recording of the drug dose, administration time and sample time is essential.
- Most benefit will be derived from reference to specific monitoring programs and guidelines (link to vancomycin clinical practice guideline), or through liaison with specialist services. As a general rule, consider increasing the dose amount if the blood level is low or increasing the dose interval (i.e. giving less frequently) if the blood level is high.

Dose adjusting following TDM

Most drugs (the significant exception being phenytoin) involved in TDM have linear kinetics. That is, a doubling in dose will result in a proportionate doubling in serum concentration. For example, if the measured drug concentration is 6 and the target concentration is 12, a doubling in dose would be needed to achieve the required target. Examples requiring this approach include aminoglycosides (gentamicin, tobramycin) and vancomycin.

Drug errors

- Paediatric patients are at high risk of drug errors.
- Certain drugs are commonly associated with medication errors in all patients, and some more frequently in children (e.g. opiates, paracetamol, antibiotics, 50% dextrose, heparin and electrolytes such as K^+ and IV Ca^{2+} and Mg^{2+}). Extra care should be taken when prescribing or administering these medicines.
- Errors in the prescription of IV fluids are more frequently seen in paediatric patients with the outcomes more severe. Administration rate of IV fluids (including parenteral nutrition) has to take into account the concurrent administration of oral and enteral fluids.
- A safety check that is frequently effective in adult – to reassess the dose if more than one ampoule of the drug is required – does not provide as much assurance with paediatrics. A small patient can be severely overdosed on administration of less than a single ampoule.
- When prescribing for children, the following factors should be taken into consideration:
  - Children's doses vary widely and so there is no standard dose (as there is with adults).
  - Clarify if drug doses are given in mg/kg per day in divided doses (or mg/kg per dose given x times per day). When prescribing, always write as **mg/kg per dose given x times per day.**
  - Calculations are required for most childhood dosing and errors may occur during this step.
  - Some paediatric preparations may cause confusion in those unfamiliar with their use, for example IV versus enteral paracetamol, or Painstop Night-Time which contains three active agents.
  - The small doses used in children may cause measuring and administration errors.
  - Misplacing or misreading of decimal points can lead to error.

Drug interactions

- Drug interactions are always possible when using more than one medicine.
- Only a few drug combinations result in clinically significant sequelae.
- Be aware that drug interactions are more common when
  - More drugs are prescribed – where possible, aim for monotherapy.
  - Patients are sick, especially with multiple organ pathologies.
- Drugs with a narrow therapeutic window are more likely to result in more significant interactions.
- Drug interactions do not just occur between drugs that are recognized as traditional pharmaceutical products. They can occur between drugs and feeds, fluids, supplements and other agents, for example IV administration of ceftriaxone to neonatal patients receiving fluids containing calcium can cause widespread precipitation, with severe and possibly fatal consequences.

- Interactions listed in reference books can be difficult to interpret. Likelihood and consequences may best be assessed through discussion with specialist pharmacologists or medicines information pharmacists.

Complementary medicines
Specific history of these should be sought, as
- Complementary medicines and many herbal products are available 'over the counter' or through alternative medicine practitioners.
- Families often do not offer this information – either feel uncomfortable in admitting they use such products or do not consider something 'natural' could cause harm.
- Such products can be involved in ADRs and interactions.

Examples of potential drug interactions
- *St John's wort:* anticoagulants, antidepressants, digoxin, MAO inhibitors, dextromethorphan, decreases effects of cyclosporin and antiviral drugs, and prolongs effect of general anaesthetics.
- *Ginseng:* anticoagulants, stimulants, antihypertensives, antidepressants, phenelzine, digoxin, potentiates effects of corticosteroids and oestrogens.
- *Ginger:* anticoagulants, antihypertensives, cardiac drugs, hypoglycaemic drugs and enhances effects of barbiturates.

USEFUL RESOURCES
- *http://www.drugdoses.net* – For information regarding and purchase of Frank Shann's drug doses book.
- *http://www.australianprescriber.com/* – An independent journal with articles relevant to both paediatric and adult prescribing.
- *https://childrens.amh.net.au/* – Australian Children's Dosing Guide cover commonly used medicines.
- *http://www.tga.gov.au/hp/medicines-pregnancy.htm* — Prescribing medicines in pregnancy.
- *http://www.bnf.org/bnf/org_450055.htm* – BNF for Children with recently updated dosing information.
- *http://www.micromedex.com/* – Micromedex: a US-based comprehensive database of drug monographs (subscription required).

CHAPTER 27

Immigrant health

Georgia Paxton

Definitions

A refugee is someone who 'owing to a well-founded fear of being persecuted for reasons of race, religion, nationality, membership of a particular social group or political opinion, is outside the country of his/her nationality, and is unable to, or owing to such fear, is unwilling to avail himself/herself of the protection of that country'.

An asylum seeker is someone who has applied for refugee status and who is awaiting a decision on this application.

In this chapter, **refugee background** is used to describe both refugees and asylum seekers.

Introduction

There have been significant changes in refugee and asylum seeker policy and settlement in Australia in recent years. They include

- Changes in the composition of the Humanitarian program, which includes places for
  - Refugees arriving from overseas (Offshore – Refugee Program).
  - Refugees arriving from overseas who are sponsored by someone living in Australia (Offshore – Special Humanitarian Program).
  - Asylum seekers who have been granted permanent status (Onshore arrivals).
- Large numbers of asylum seekers arriving by boat over 2012 and 2013.
- Increased numbers of people (including children) held in immigration detention and the reintroduction of offshore processing on Manus Island and Nauru.
- The use of community detention, with preference given to families with children.
- Changes in source countries for refugees and asylum seekers – current arrivals are predominantly from Afghanistan, Burma, Iran, Iraq and Sri Lanka.
- Changes in the health requirements under Migration law – with an expected increase in offshore Humanitarian entrants with disability and HIV.

People of a refugee background

- Are usually resourceful and resilient
- Will have experienced conflict and transitions with migration and resettlement, including disruption to family, schooling and community
- May be separated from immediate family members
- May have witnessed or experienced physical or sexual violence, including torture and severe human rights violations
- May have spent long periods in refugee camps or immigration detention
- Usually come from countries where health facilities and programs are minimal or have been disrupted and are more likely to have been exposed to communicable and vaccine-preventable diseases
- Almost always require catch-up immunisations
- Are at increased risk for mental health problems, especially those who have been held in immigration detention

Paediatric Handbook, Ninth Edition. Edited by Amanda Gwee, Romi Rimer and Michael Marks.
© 2015 John Wiley & Sons, Ltd. Published 2015 by John Wiley & Sons, Ltd.

- Have higher rates of dental disease
- May be less familiar with preventive health care
- May be worried about or feel threatened by medical consultations
- Will nearly always require the assistance of an interpreter in the initial (and often later) stages of settlement

Pre-departure screening

Pre-departure screening and treatment is limited for children and young adolescents. It varies with refugee camp, port of departure, means of arrival and services available. Screening for offshore Humanitarian arrivals includes

- **Visa medical assessment** (completed 3–12 months prior to travel, note this assessment is completed for all permanent entrants to Australia)
  - Medical assessment, height and weight.
  - A full ward test of urine in those aged ≥5 years.
  - A chest radiograph (CXR) in those aged ≥11 years or younger if clinical features suggest tuberculosis (TB) or there is a history of TB contact. A diagnosis of active TB delays the issue of a visa until reassessment after treatment.
  - HIV screening in those aged ≥15 years or younger if there is a history of blood transfusion or other clinical indication.
  - Unaccompanied refugee minors are also screened for hepatitis B.
- **Departure health check** (voluntary, completed 3–5 days prior to travel)
  - Malaria testing in endemic areas (and treatment if positive).
  - Albendazole treatment (varies with country of origin).
  - MMR vaccine in those aged 9 months to 54 years.
  - Yellow fever vaccine (varies with country of origin).
  - A 'Fitness to fly' assessment for febrile illnesses, gastrointestinal illness, and any relevant conditions in area of origin.

Health assessment for asylum seekers varies; adults in immigration detention usually have an equivalent check to the visa health assessment, the assessment of children and early adolescents varies widely, and in practice, many children have not had blood tests or screening for TB exposure. Children in immigration detention do usually receive catch-up immunisation, although records may be difficult to access.

In some states of Australia (including Victoria), there are no routine post-arrival health checks. Access to health services is variable. People arriving as refugees have greater settlement support than those arriving under the Special Humanitarian Program, where the onus is on the sponsor to facilitate access to health care. Support and health care for asylum seekers varies widely.

Health care visits need to be handled sensitively, and an interpreter will be needed with a majority of families. It is never appropriate to use a family member as an interpreter. Establishing trust is essential. Recently arrived communities may be small, and interpreters may be known to the family.

Health issues

Refugee background children and adolescents have typical paediatric health problems and also have health issues specific to their background. Common paediatric issues such as iron-deficiency anaemia or constipation may have a more complicated aetiology in this group. Assessment of newly arrived children and adolescents focuses on

- Parent (or self-identified) concerns
- Excluding acute illness
- Immunisation status and catch-up
- TB screening
- Symptoms of parasitic infections (including malaria in people from endemic areas)
- Nutritional status and growth (including iron deficiency, vitamin D and bone health)
- Oral health
- Concerns about development, vision and hearing
- Mental health issues and trauma exposure
- Previous childhood illness or physical trauma
- Issues arising from resettlement in Australia

Children and adolescents need a thorough physical examination. Particular features to note include

- Growth parameters
- Anaemia
- Rickets
- Oral health
- ENT disease
- Presence of a BCG scar (location varies, e.g. forearm, deltoid)
- Respiratory examination
- Lymphadenopathy, hepatosplenomegaly
- Skin (scars, infections)

There may be particular cultural practices such as scarification.

Suggested initial screening investigations

It is important to explain the concepts of health assessment, screening and disease prevention; families need to understand the implications of health screening and give informed consent. Individual counselling and an explanation of the bounds of confidentiality, including interpreter confidentiality, will be required in adolescents.

The following list includes suggested first line investigations; additional investigations may be needed depending on the clinical scenario.

- Full blood examination and film
- Ferritin
- Vitamin D, calcium, phosphate, ALP, in children with risk factors for low vitamin D
- Vitamin A
- Malaria screen (Malaria antigen immunochromatographic test and thick/thin film) in children from endemic areas
- Hepatitis B screen (HBsAg, HBcAb, HBsAb)
- Hepatitis C antibodies
- HIV testing
- Schistosoma serology in children from endemic areas
- Strongyloides serology
- Faecal specimen (ideally fixed) for ova, cysts and parasites (OCP)
- Mantoux test (Quantiferon testing is an alternative in adolescents, but should not be used as initial screening in younger children)
- Sexually transmitted infection (STI) screen (see Chapter 22, *Adolescent health*), depending on age and history. Syphilis screening should be performed in all children where parents are known to have positive syphilis screening

Recently arrived children who are febrile and unwell may require further investigations. Consult an infectious diseases specialist.

Some groups may need additional screening investigations depending on prevalence data from their country of origin or clinical presentation. See http://www.rch.org.au/immigranthealth/clinical/Initial_assessment/

Immunisation

Immunisation records are not a pre-departure requirement and most refugees do not have written records. Check for a BCG scar and a past history of varicella.

For specific information on catch-up vaccination information *The Australian Immunisation Handbook*, 10th edition, http://www.health.gov.au/internet/immunise/publishing.nsf/Content/Handbook10-home.

Principles of catch-up immunisations in refugee background children include

- People of a refugee background should be vaccinated so they are up to date according to the Australian Immunisation Schedule, equivalent to an Australian-born person of the same age.
- Catch-up vaccination is required unless written documentation of immunisation is provided.
- Serology for immunity to VPD is not routinely recommended.

- Vaccination information for children aged ≤7 years should be entered into the Australian Childhood Immunisation Register (ACIR), which can then be cross-checked. Information for asylum seeker children is also entered in ACIR, although this may be difficult to check in children without Medicare cards.
- Provide a written record and a clear plan for ongoing immunisations.

Detailed catch-up guidelines are available: http://www.rch.org.au/immigranthealth/clinical/Catchup_immunisation_in_refugees/

Translated health information sheets are available: http://www.health.vic.gov.au/immunisation/factsheets/anguage.htm

Nutritional issues

Nutritional issues are common; fussy eating and concerns about weight gain (too little or too much) may be a family priority. These are common paediatric concerns and are not specific to refugee background families. Specific issues include vitamin D deficiency, vitamin A deficiency, vitamin B12/folate deficiency, iron deficiency and anaemia.

Monitor growth parameters and clarify the correct birth date/age first. Linear growth is similar in children aged <5 years worldwide. Growth must be considered in the context of parental height and pubertal status; children may have different growth parameters from their Australian-born peers and still have normal growth. An early severe/prolonged nutritional insult or chronic disease during infancy will affect long-term growth and may affect final height ('stunting'). This history is usually easily elicited. In children/adolescents with poor growth also consider gastrointestinal and other infections (including TB), vitamin D deficiency, rickets and thyroid dysfunction. Once an initial screen has been completed and treatment initiated as necessary, a period of monitoring growth is often appropriate.

Fussy eating is often due to high caloric intake in the form of excessive milk/juice consumption at the expense of solids/mealtimes; a good dietary history will elicit this. Consider organic disease early in children of a refugee background, including gastrointestinal infection (*Giardia*, other parasites, *Helicobacter pylori*) and other infections. The principles of healthy eating are universal and should be discussed with families (refer to Chapter 9, *Fluids and nutrition*).

Anaemia

Anaemia is usually multifactorial in the paediatric refugee population. Contributors may include low maternal iron stores, poor food access, iron deficiency, low B12/folate, malaria infection and other parasite infections. Iron deficiency is usually nutritional but there may be a component of gastrointestinal loss. Other causes of anaemia to consider include haemoglobinopathies (more common in African and Asian populations) and lead toxicity (reported in paediatric refugees). See Anaemia, p. 159 in Chapter 22.

Vitamin D

See also Hypocalcaemia, Endocrine conditions, Chapter 13, pp. 199–200.

Vitamin D is essential for bone and muscle health, and there is emerging evidence that it is important in other aspects of health. 'Vitamin D' refers to both D_3 (cholecalciferol; the form produced in the skin and found in fish) and D_2 (ergocalciferol; the form in small amounts in some plant-based foods). Currently available supplements are all D_3. 25-hydroxy vitamin D levels (25(OH)D) are used to measure vitamin D status; the recommended 25(OH)D is ≥50 nmol/L at all ages.

Definitions of vitamin D deficiency

Severe deficiency	<12.5 nmol/L
Moderate deficiency	12.5–29 nmol/L
Mild deficiency	30–49 nmol/L

Most vitamin D is made in the skin through the action of ultraviolet B (UVB) light in sunlight. Adults with dark skin require a longer duration of sunlight exposure (compared to people with light skin) to make adequate vitamin D. The amount of sunlight required in children is unclear. Vitamin D is not naturally available in any great

quantity in diet, and most people only receive 10–25% of their estimated average daily requirements from diet. In the absence of sun exposure, recommended dietary allowances of vitamin D are
- Age <12 months: adequate intake 400 IU daily
- 1–18 years: estimated average requirements 400 IU daily (reflects estimated individual median requirements) and recommended daily allowance 600 IU daily (meets/exceeds the needs of 97.5% of the population)

Note: 1 mcg of vitamin D = 40 International Units (IU).

Risk factors for low vitamin D include
- Lack of skin exposure to UVB in sunlight (time inside, chronic illness/hospitalization, complex disability, covering clothing, southerly latitude)
- Dark skin
- Medical conditions (obesity, liver failure, renal failure, malabsorption) or medications (isoniazid, rifampicin, anticonvulsants) affecting vitamin D metabolism
- In infants: maternal vitamin D deficiency and exclusive breastfeeding combined with at least one other risk factor

The prevalence of low vitamin D in Australian refugee cohorts is 33–100%. Rickets has re-emerged in children born to migrant parents in the southern parts in Australia.

Assess for
- Bone and muscle pain, especially with exercise.
- Irritability, delayed motor milestones (young children).
- Dairy intake, symptoms of low calcium (muscle cramps, stridor, seizures) – hypocalcaemic seizures are rare beyond 6 months of age.
- Sunscreen use, time outside.
- Previous vitamin D levels, previous/current treatment (especially with newer forms of supplementation available).
- Family understanding of vitamin D as a health issue.
- Rickets – deformity in growing bones due to failure of mineralisation of osteoid. The peak incidence is during infancy, although deformity reflects age/growth (and can be in any direction). Consider other causes if asymmetrical. Look for long bone deformity, splaying (wrists, ankles), bossing, delayed fontanelle closure, and rachitic rosary.
- Oral health – delayed dentition (no incisors by 10 months, no molars by 18 months), enamel hypoplasia.

Screening
- Screen children with one or more risk factors for low vitamin D.
- Measure 25(OH)D, calcium, phosphate and ALP. Also measure parathyroid hormone in children with low calcium intake, symptoms/signs of low vitamin D or multiple risk factors.
- In exclusively breastfed infants with at least one other risk factor, it is usually more practical to start supplements without screening (see below).
- Children with rickets require additional investigations to exclude renal pathology and rarer causes of rickets.
- In recent arrivals: if the initial vitamin D level is normal, repeat the level at the end of the first winter in Australia. Levels at the start and end of winter can be useful to make a clinical judgment on frequency of dosing.

Management
- Children with symptomatic rickets or hypocalcaemia require hospital assessment; do *not* give high dose vitamin D in the outpatient setting to this group.
- Children with low vitamin D should be treated to restore their levels to the normal range with either daily dosing or high (stoss) dose therapy. There is inadequate evidence to support the use of high dose therapy in children aged <3 months.
- Ensure adequate calcium intake. Consider calcium supplements if dietary intake is poor (<2 serves of dairy per day)
- Health education and advice about sun protection/sun exposure; encouraging outside activity. Those with dark skin can tolerate intermittent sun exposure without sunscreen.
- Follow-up bloods to check response to treatment at 3 months (earlier in infants with moderate to severe deficiency).

- Children with ongoing risk factors for low vitamin D need to understand this is a lifelong health issue; they require ongoing monitoring, with annual testing and a plan to maintain vitamin D and calcium status through behavioural change where possible, and supplementation where this is inadequate.
- Breastfed babies with at least one other risk factor for low vitamin D should be given 400 IU daily for at least the first 12 months of life. Babies on full formula feeds should receive adequate vitamin D from this source. Consider checking levels or adding daily supplements in babies with risk factors for low vitamin D with mixed feeds or who have appropriately reduced their formula intake after starting solids.
- Clinical photography is useful to monitor bony deformity (nutritional rickets usually corrects after treatment of low vitamin D provided the child has adequate calcium and phosphate intake).

Vitamin A

Vitamin A is required for vision, immune function, growth and maintenance of epithelial cells. Infants rely on breast milk or formula for their vitamin A intake. Vitamin A is contained in yellow/orange fruits and vegetables as well as butter, eggs, cheese and liver. Vitamin A deficiency is not uncommon in recently arrived children and should be treated where present. Specific treatment guidelines are available: http://www.rch.org.au/immigranthealth/clinical/Vitamin_A/. Risk factors for vitamin A deficiency should resolve with good health care and access to fresh food in Australia.

Tuberculosis

See Chapter 18, *Infectious diseases and immunisation*, p. 292.

Hepatitis B infection

See Chapter 18, *Infectious diseases and immunisation*, p. 284.

Intestinal and other parasites

In refugee cohorts, children tend to have a higher prevalence of parasite infections than adults, and they are at increased risk for faecal/oral and horizontal transmission. Parasite infections may last for years and have sequelae for nutrition, growth and wellbeing.

Symptoms may be non-specific, ask about

- Abdominal pain, constipation, diarrhoea, bloody diarrhoea and growth.
- Bladder symptoms and haematuria (seen in *Schistosoma haematobium* infection).
- Macroscopically visible worms are likely to be tapeworms or ascarids.
- *Strongyloides* infection (positive serology) should be regarded as persisting lifelong if not treated. Patients with untreated *Strongyloides* infections can develop a hyperinfection syndrome if given immunosuppressant therapy (including short courses of steroids). Hyperinfection syndrome has a high mortality, even with treatment. Consider, screen (and treat) *Strongyloides* in any child from an endemic area who is commencing immunosuppressive therapy

Management

- Parasite screening should be part of the initial assessment (*see p. 406*).
- In general, treatment is usually short course (often single dose) and well tolerated. See http://www.rch.org.au/immigranthealth/clinical/Intestinal_Parasites/.

Human immunodeficiency virus

See Chapter 18, *Infectious diseases and immunisation*, p. 293.

Many refugee children come from regions with high prevalence of human immunodeficiency virus (HIV) infection (e.g. sub-Saharan Africa, south-east Asia). HIV testing is part of routine post-arrival screening, and should be considered in all children with

- Symptoms of possible HIV infection (e.g. failure to thrive, chronic respiratory infections, persistent thrush, generalised lymphadenopathy)
- Parents who are known or suspected to be HIV positive, regardless of pre-departure screening results
- TB disease
- Viral hepatitis

Informed consent is required for HIV testing, and pre-test counselling for HIV is imperative; an explanation of confidentiality, including interpreter confidentiality is also essential. Phone interpreting (where there is no disclosure of names) may be a useful option.

Oral health

Oral health assessment is important in refugee children, as they may have had poor diet, dental injuries and limited access to dental care/oral health promotion. Oral health is often not an immediate concern, although high rates of caries are reported in refugee cohorts.

Female circumcision/cutting (FGM)

Girls and women from refugee background communities may have been subject to female genital mutilation (FGM). This is rarely disclosed on the initial assessment, even with direct questioning. Assessing for FGM requires sensitive discussion, often over more than one visit. Specialised clinics are available to assess girls/women who have had FGM. It is illegal to practice or to obtain FGM in Australia, or to take a child from Australia for this purpose. Any impending threat of FGM should be reported to a child protection service immediately (mandatory reporting applies). Questions about FGM should be considered in pre-travel assessment, as there may be pressure from family overseas for this procedure.

Development and mental health considerations

Development may be affected by any combination of biological, environmental, social and emotional factors. Additional considerations in children of a refugee background include

- **Biological:** malnutrition, severe infections, malaria (associated with ADHD and learning problems), injury/accidents, chronic disease, hearing impairment, visual impairment.
- **Environmental:** living conditions, access to food, safety, access to health care or schooling, exposure to communicable diseases, trauma exposure, language and migration transitions (and their timing in relation to development milestones).
- **Social:** parenting roles, family disruption, changing roles and responsibilities with settlement.
- **Emotional:** stress, trauma experiences, displacement, uncertainty around future, mental health issues (and parent mental health issues).

See Chapter 25, *Behaviour and mental health*. It is worth considering how children learn English as an additional language (EAL). Immigrants generally achieve conversational proficiency in their new language after 2–3 years; however, the level of language proficiency required for success in school is far higher than the level required for everyday social interaction. It takes at least 5–7 years to achieve academic language proficiency, and contrary to popular belief; younger children do *not* learn languages more quickly than older children. The amount of first language schooling is the most important predictor of success in the new language, and late primary/early secondary age students achieve academic language proficiency the fastest. It is important to encourage the first language (mother tongue) in order to achieve success in the new language, and in school in general, even (and maybe especially) in children with developmental issues.

Available data suggest many refugee children have experienced significant trauma. Family separation, exposure to conflict and witnessing extreme violence are common. Unaccompanied minors are identified as a particular risk group for mental health problems, and for having experienced sexual violence. The migration pathway itself may be a source of trauma, especially for asylum seekers, where perilous boat journeys and immigration detention further affect mental health. Concern for remaining family overseas may be overwhelming, with significant effects on settlement and wellbeing.

Responses to trauma include depression, anxiety, post-traumatic stress, low self-esteem and guilt. These may manifest in a variety of ways including behavioural problems, problems with sleeping and eating, poor school performance, difficulty making friends and psychosomatic symptoms. While it is important to understand the influence of trauma on the refugee journey, it is often inappropriate to ask about trauma directly, children/families may disclose their trauma history once trust is established and other health issues are dealt with.

Consider mental health in the broad family and settlement context. Poverty, housing stress and reduced employment opportunity are common in recently arrived families, and are associated with mental health problems. Parents with mental health issues and stress related to settlement will have reduced coping and parenting skills.

A thorough history and examination will establish risk factors and contributors to the child's current development and mental health status. In reality, developmental and mental health surveillance will usually occur after the initial (health) assessment. If developmental or learning concerns are elicited, organise early vision and hearing assessment, screening for thyroid dysfunction and treatment of iron deficiency. Consider mental health issues as a contributing factor or co-morbidity. In children with a clear history of developmental delay/disability, it is usually appropriate to seek formal IQ assessments early (e.g. at childcare/school) even though there are significant issues with standardised testing. Repeat testing will be needed over time.

Health screening is only one part of promoting health and wellbeing in new immigrants to Australia. Facilitating resettlement in terms of learning English, educational placement and gaining employment are also priorities and will promote physical and psychological health in families. Parents are likely to have their own health needs and will also need appropriate health assessment.

USEFUL RESOURCES
- *www.rch.org.au/immigranthealth* – RCH immigrant health clinic website.
- *www.foundationhouse.org.au* – Victorian Foundation for Survivors of Torture.
- *http://refugeehealthnetwork.org.au/* – Refugee health network.

CHAPTER 28

The death of a child

Jenny Hynson

Parental grief is intense, prolonged and prone to complication. For both the sick child and their family's future well-being, it is crucial that the health care team provide skilled and sensitive care so that the child's suffering is minimised. Potential suffering may be the result of
- the disease itself;
- the interventions being used; and
- insufficient intervention (e.g. inadequate treatment of pain).

What is palliative care?
Palliative care includes, but is not restricted to, terminal care. In fact, it is much more about life than death and can be provided alongside ongoing attempts to modify or even cure disease. Most paediatric patients are involved with the palliative care team for months and sometimes years.

Specialists in palliative care are available in all states in Australia and can help children and families with difficult symptoms, complex decisions and the practical supports they need to get through their illness. They can also help children achieve goals such as returning to school, if that is their wish.

Place of care
Often the death of a child can be anticipated. Most (but not all) children and families wish to spend as much time as possible at home and with appropriate planning and support, most symptoms can be controlled effectively in this environment. Domiciliary care can be provided by community-based palliative care services and the GP in consultation with hospital staff. Most palliative care services also provide after-hours support.

Although home care offers many advantages, it may result in physical, emotional and financial stress. Readmission to hospital or hospice should be easily and readily available. A letter detailing the child's condition, plans in case of sudden deterioration and people to contact will facilitate appropriate care in an emergency.

Decision-making for children with life-limiting conditions
Talking with families about their child's prognosis and making decisions about care can be extremely difficult. Staff need to be aware of how their own feelings of anxiety, sadness and impotence may influence this process. Most families appreciate honest information given in an empathic way and tempered with a sense of hope. Realistic hope may be offered in terms of ongoing support, attention to symptoms and help to maximise the child's quality of life.

Decision-making is a process not an event. The team should talk beforehand to minimise the risk of confusion or delivery of mixed messages. Try to find a quiet place and allow sufficient time to speak with the family. Ensure those who need to be present are, but be mindful of having too many people in the room.

Wherever possible, it is useful to discuss goals of care and key decisions before a crisis occurs. This conversation is often best started by talking in very general terms and asking some fundamental questions. These might include
- Tell me about your child: what does she enjoy? What things frighten her? What is it like for her to be in hospital?
- What do you understand about her condition right now?
- What is most important to you?
- What are the most frightening things for you?

Paediatric Handbook, Ninth Edition. Edited by Amanda Gwee, Romi Rimer and Michael Marks.
© 2015 John Wiley & Sons, Ltd. Published 2015 by John Wiley & Sons, Ltd.

- What are you hoping for now? What else are you hoping for?
- Is there anything you would like us to know that will help us take better care of you and your child?

Medical leadership is very important. Parents should not feel that they are solely responsible for decisions. Clinicians should provide guidance and direction about what they believe to be the best way forward. Where there is disagreement, resolution is usually achieved with time and good communication. Try to avoid 'convincing' parents of the reality of their child's situation. They usually know but strong emotions are at play. Helping them acknowledge, express and explore these emotions can be a helpful intervention. Where disagreement cannot be resolved, a second opinion, consultation with a clinical ethics service and/or legal advice may be helpful. It is always important to tell parents that you can see how much they love their child and that they are trying to do the best they can.

Do not be afraid of sadness or silence – important things are often said after a long pause in the conversation.

Adequate relief of pain and distress for the child

Step 1: Recognition of distress

Children can deny pain for many reasons. It is important to actively observe the child and ask about symptoms.

Step 2: Assessment

What is the most likely cause or mechanism? Are any of these reversible or treatable in their own right (e.g. agitation may be caused by urinary retention; fatigue may be caused by anaemia)?

Step 3: Intervention

Considerations

- Type of medication
  - will depend on cause or mechanism of pain
- Route of administration of medication
  - oral versus IV versus subcutaneous
  - NB: subcutaneous infusions can often be given at home

In general, it is best to prescribe a background level of medication such as morphine and midazolam and ensure provision for breakthrough doses. The breakthrough dose for these medications is calculated as one-sixth to one-tenth the total 24-hour dose. The following is an example.

Serena is 5 years old and weighs 20 kg. She has AML and widespread bone pain, not controlled by paracetamol. Morphine is initially commenced at a dose of 0.2 mg/kg (4 mg) 4 hourly p.r.n. It is effective but she is needing this regularly. She is therefore prescribed 4 mg 4 hourly and can have an additional breakthrough dose of 2.5 mg hourly p.r.n. On review two days later, she has needed only one additional dose so she is changed to a long-acting form of morphine. To do this, the total 24-hour dose (24 mg) is divided by two and this (12 mg) is given b.i.d. The breakthrough dose remains unchanged.

Step 4: Education

There may be concern about the use of opioids and benzodiazepines for fear of hastening the death of the child. There is no evidence that the appropriate use of medications such as morphine alters the timing of death.

Step 5: Planning ahead

Understanding the disease and its natural history is essential in order to plan for potential hurdles down the road.

Step 6: Review and titration

The child's symptoms should be reviewed regularly to ensure comfort. The following is an example of how to titrate morphine.

Serena is now on 10 mg of morphine over 24 hours as a subcutaneous infusion. The breakthrough dose is 1 mg hourly p.r.n. She has needed four breakthrough doses of morphine in the last 24 hours. The background dose therefore needs to be increased to 14 mg over 24 hours and the breakthrough dose needs adjusting so that it is one-sixth to one-tenth the total 24-hour dose (i.e. 1.5 mg). Continue titrating in this way.

Communicating with children about death and dying

Parents may feel compelled to protect their children from 'bad news'. Children often know a great deal about their disease and prognosis even when they have not been 'told'. They may not reveal what they know, for fear of upsetting their parents. Attempts to protect the child from accurate information may leave them feeling anxious and isolated as they sense distress in those around them and generate incorrect explanations for this such as '*I have been bad*' or '*Mummy and Daddy are angry with me*'. In general, it is best to encourage parents to be honest with children, but information needs to be provided in a manner appropriate to their cognitive ability and developmental level. It may be helpful to anticipate questions and work with the family in planning responses.

It is important to listen to what the child is asking. The child who asks '*Am I going to die?*' may actually not be concerned about dying as such but more about who will look after their parents, what their friends will think, or whether they will be in pain. A response such as '*What makes you ask me that?*' will provide further information upon which to base an answer. Children may not wish to express themselves verbally or directly. Stories, artwork, music and play allow expression, build trust and facilitate communication.

Concepts of death

The child's concept of death becomes more complete with development and life experience. Preschoolers typically view death as a reversible phenomenon (e.g. Snow White) and do not yet appreciate that people die as a consequence of age, illness or trauma. Magical thinking may lead them to believe they have caused death through bad behaviour or thoughts. By 7 years of age most children understand the concepts of irreversibility, causality, universality and cessation of bodily functions. Most 8-year olds also understand that dead people cannot feel pain or fear.

Siblings

Siblings of children with life-threatening conditions suffer not only the distress of having a brother or sister who is sick and dying, but the isolation of having parents who are frequently either physically or psychologically unavailable to them. They may feel guilty that they do not have the condition, or may fear for their own health. They may resent the attention being given to the sick child. They may feel they have somehow caused the illness. Siblings often do not want to burden their parents with their concerns and may express distress through developmental regression, school failure and physical symptoms.

Siblings benefit from inclusion in visits to the hospital and where possible, the care of the child. Staff can help by dedicating special time to children in which they may be given information and allowed to ask questions. Specific reassurance that the illness is not their fault may be needed, especially for siblings who have donated organs.

Preparations for death
Time and space

What constitutes a 'good death' varies according to the individual values of children and their families. It is crucial that staff do not impose their ideas of what a good death is on the families they care for. Every family is unique so the best way to ensure respectful care is to ask how you can be most helpful.

Spiritual needs and memory-making

Arrangements may need to be made for baptism, religious support, photographs, videos and other memories of the child.

Information

In most cases, it is possible to be very reassuring that dying is generally peaceful and it is often helpful to talk with parents about what to expect (e.g. reduced consciousness, reduced desire for food and fluids, reduced urine output, changes in breathing). Some parents are also curious about funeral arrangements but feel it is bad to think about such things while their child is alive. Reassurance that many parents share these thoughts and even plan the funeral in advance can be helpful.

The child

Preparation for death is largely dependent on the age and life experience of the child. Just as adults do, children may wish to 'put their affairs in order'. They may want to do and say certain things to those they love and may even wish to give possessions away.

The moment of death

Although usually anticipated, the moment of death is an important event and needs medical confirmation. See http://www.rch.org.au/clinicalguide/guideline_index/Death_of_a_child/.

Taking the deceased child's body home

Some families wish to take their child home after death. Families should be advised to consult with a funeral director before taking the child home as some preparation of the body is likely to be necessary. In most cases parents can transport their child's body from hospital to home, but it is important for the medical team to provide them with a brief document explaining the situation.

Brain death

Brain death is defined as the irreversible cessation of all brain function including that of the brain stem. There are strict clinical criteria for the determination of brain death. Occasionally it becomes clear that a child who is dependent on mechanical ventilation is brain dead. In such a situation

- The senior doctor needs to explain the meaning of brain death. The unambiguous message that death has occurred, together with the distinction between brain death and coma, needs to be clarified.
- It can be helpful to say that, although the child's body is still alive, the brain is dead and therefore the person is dead.
- It frequently helps parents to understand that their child has died by encouraging them to witness some or all of the brain death tests.
- The request for organ donation generally requires a separate interview, made in a positive manner, without coercion and with the clear acknowledgement of the family's vulnerability.

After death

Viewing the body

- A private and comfortable area should be provided where the family can spend uninterrupted time with their child.
- Families should feel able to spend as long as they need with their child.
- Families should be offered the opportunity to wash and dress their child as a last act of love and care.

Autopsy

- The purpose of the autopsy is to seek full information regarding the cause of the child's death, the nature of the illness and the risk of recurrence of the illness in other family members or future children.
- The autopsy may be limited to a system or area or be designated as a full autopsy. Informed consent is essential if removed organs are to be disposed of or retained for teaching purposes.
- The autopsy will be performed on the next working day after the child's death and may interfere with the funeral arrangements. The results are usually not available until approximately 6 weeks later.
- An autopsy will not be performed without parental consent unless required by the coroner.

Coroner's cases

A doctor must report a death to the Coroner as soon as possible if

- The cause of death is unable to be determined.
- The death appears to have been unexpected, unnatural or violent.
- The death appears to have resulted, directly or indirectly, from accident or injury.
- The death occurred during an anaesthetic and is not due to natural cause.
- The deceased person was held in care immediately before death.
- The deceased person's identity is unknown.

The second or subsequent death of a child with the same parent(s) must also be reported to the Coroner's Court.

The Coroner then decides if an autopsy is needed. Parents can request for an autopsy not to be performed. In many cases, where the cause of death is not in doubt (e.g. severe head injury), the Coroner will respect the wish of the family.

Funeral options

The family should be assisted in making arrangements in their own time with a funeral director and religious personnel as appropriate. Encouragement is given to involve siblings in this important ritual.

Breastfeeding

In the case of neonatal death or the death of an infant, advice needs to be given to the breastfeeding mother regarding suppression of lactation. Consultation with a specialist is recommended.

Surviving siblings

Children react in their own way to a sibling's death. They may blame themselves and may fear their own death or that of others close to them. This fear is often unspoken. At times children may not appear to be grieving the death of their sibling as they often grieve in short bursts. Distress may be expressed by regression to an earlier stage, difficulties at school, acting out or in other ways. Parents often need help and support to understand the responses of their surviving children who may need repeated reassurance. Opportunities to talk as a family about the death, their feelings and their day-to-day challenges and achievements are important. A return to family routines can help them to feel more secure.

Availability of the health care team

The health care team should be available to the family after death and follow-up arranged. It is usually important to both families and team members that farewells are made.

Notification of other professionals

Notify the health professionals who have been and who will continue to be involved with the family following the child's death, including the referring doctor or institution, the family's GP and the maternal and child health nurse. This must be done as soon as possible.

Other families

The death of a child often affects the parents of other children in the hospital ward or local community. The acknowledgement of a child's death with these families is very important.

Follow-up
Medical interview

It is essential that an appointment be made for the parents to see the child's treating doctor. Some parents are reluctant to attend, but most see the interview as a 'final farewell'. The discussion should include the autopsy results (if one was performed), the child's period of illness, future childbearing and issues related to bereavement. It is important the family be given information regarding potential sources of support and ongoing counselling if required.

If a family is reluctant to attend this important interview, alternative interviews with other health care providers should be arranged.

Condolences

The value of communication such as a letter or card from the medical practitioner/team involved with the care of the child cannot be overstated.

Ongoing support

The course of parental grief following the death of a child may vary greatly. Many families manage their grief with the support of family and friends and may not utilise more formal supports. The grieving process changes over time, often intensifying after the initial period of shock, around important dates and sometimes unexpected triggers. Over time (usually years, not months) parents develop ways of living with their loss and are able to regain some sense of purpose and happiness in their lives. Factors to consider when assessing the risk of a more complicated grieving process include the preparedness of the family for their child's death, their view of the pre-death care, their perception of available supports, their own physical and mental health, substance use or addiction issues and life stressors. If someone is struggling more than expected, formal referral should be considered.

CHAPTER 29

Forensic medicine

Anne Smith

Background

Health professionals should always consider the possibility of child abuse when they evaluate and treat an injured child and during interactions with children who are vulnerable to harm from abuse and neglect. Whenever a child's living circumstances suggest the possibility of risk of harm, a comprehensive psychosocial assessment should be carried out. Doctors are encouraged to promptly consult with local medical professionals who have expertise in this area.

The body of knowledge related to child abuse and the demand for expert court testimony are increasing. Furthermore, there are expectations that doctors understand their legal obligations and demonstrate skill when providing evidence that will withstand the rigors of cross examination in court.

Mandatory reporting

In most Australian states medical practitioners are legally required to notify the relevant statutory authorities of children who have experienced, or are likely to experience abuse. Medical practitioners should be familiar with the relevant legislation in their own state or territory.

Referral centres

Most major metropolitan paediatric hospitals have established reference centres for the medical assessment and treatment of child abuse. Paediatricians and other medical professionals working in these centres provide expert advice in relation to the assessment and management of suspected child abuse. Seek advice early.

Definitions: types of child abuse and neglect
Child abuse

Child abuse is also termed child maltreatment. It is the words or actions that cause actual, threatened or potential harm (physically, emotionally or sexually), ill treatment, neglect, or deprivation (acts of omission) of any child.

Physical abuse

Child physical abuse is physical trauma inflicted on a child. Objective evidence of this violence may include bruising, burns and scalds, head injuries, fractures, intra-abdominal and intra-thoracic trauma, suffocation and drowning. Injury can be caused by impact, penetration, heat, a caustic substance, a chemical or a drug, but the definition also includes physical harm sustained as a result of fabricated or induced illness by carer.

Child sexual abuse

Child sexual abuse is the involvement of dependent, developmentally immature children and adolescents in sexual activities that they may not fully comprehend and to which they are unable to give consent. Sexual exploitation is included.

Child neglect

Child neglect is the failure of caregivers to adequately provide for and safeguard the health, safety and well-being of the child. It applies to any situation in which the basic needs of a child are not met with respect to nutrition, hygiene, clothing or shelter. It also comprises failure to provide access to adequate medical care, mental health care, dental care, stimulation to promote development, or attendance to a child's moral and spiritual care and education.

Paediatric Handbook, Ninth Edition. Edited by Amanda Gwee, Romi Rimer and Michael Marks.
© 2015 John Wiley & Sons, Ltd. Published 2015 by John Wiley & Sons, Ltd.

Psychological maltreatment

Psychological maltreatment consists of acts that are judged on the basis of a combination of community standards and professional expertise to be psychologically damaging. Such acts are committed by individuals who by their characteristics (e.g. age, status, knowledge and organisational form), are in a position of differential power that renders a child vulnerable. Such acts damage, immediately or ultimately, the behavioural, cognitive, affective or physical functioning of the child. Examples of psychological maltreatment include acts of spurning (hostility, rejecting or degrading), terrorising, isolating, exploiting or corrupting and denying emotional responsiveness. Exposure to interpersonal violence in the home is included in this definition.

Cumulative harm

Subtypes of child abuse and neglect often co-exist in children who are experiencing a range of adverse circumstances and events. The serious and pervasive harm that results from a number of episodes of maltreatment and/or a range of chronically harmful situations is recognized in Victorian legislation by the term 'cumulative harm'. This term reflects the fact that many children are harmed by more than a single episode of physical assault, poor supervision or chronic neglect.

Consent for forensic medical procedures

Valid consent must be obtained:
- For the right procedure.
- From the right person
  - Who understands the nature and purpose of the procedure.
  - Who has considered the consequences of going ahead or not going ahead with the procedure. This includes consideration of rare but important negative outcomes.
  - Who has the capacity to make a choice.
- Consent must be freely given.
- Consent may be withdrawn at any time during the procedure.

Consent for a forensic medical procedure is best obtained in writing (refer http://www.rch.org.au/uploadedFiles/Main/Content/vfpms/child-abuse-proforma.pdf) and should be specific for each aspect of the evaluation process. Consent should be obtained by the medical practitioner who performs the procedure.

Capacity to consent

When a mature minor is assessed in relation to determining his/her capacity to consent to a forensic medical procedure, the assessing doctor should take into consideration:
- Age
- Maturity
- Intelligence
- Capacity to make autonomous decisions (e.g. self-supporting, self-determining in daily life, financial independence, living independently)
- Factors that might impair capacity for decision making, both short-term and long-term
- The possibility of a guardian providing consent in the legal sense with the minor providing written verification of his/her assent

Factors specific to the situation such as pain, fear, emotional upset, intoxication, being drug affected (or affected by drug withdrawal), tiredness, possible intimidation or coercion by others (including professionals) and an acute stress reaction that might resolve within hours. It is wise to defer forensic examination whenever doubt exists about the capacity of a mature minor to consent to a forensic procedure.

Suspects

Determination of fitness for interview, fitness to plead, and collection of 'intimate samples' for forensic analysis from suspects/persons-of-interest should only be undertaken by medical professionals who are working for a forensic medical organisation and who have been trained to do so. Police may collect non-intimate samples from suspects, for example buccal swabs for DNA analysis.

Forensic evaluation of physical injury

When assessing and treating an injured child, there is a duty to accurately diagnose or exclude the diagnosis of child abuse. Table 29.1 lists situations that should generate suspicion regarding non-accidental injury.

Table 29.1 Features on history that generate suspicion about non-accidental injury

- No story is offered to account for injuries
  - No witnessed account
  - Hypothesis based on minimal information or speculation
- The story offered by one individual changes over time
- The story offered by two individuals differs without apparent explanation
- The story is not in keeping with the child's developmental skills
- The postulated injury mechanism involves a young sibling or other child who is alleged to have caused the injury
- The story seems implausible
- An unexplained delay occurred between the alleged time of injury and the time when medical care was sought

Aims of forensic assessment

- Assess and manage the child's medical needs and plan ongoing care.
- Differentiate inflicted trauma from accidents and medical conditions confused with assault. Consider possible causative forces and mechanisms.
- Estimate time of injury.
- Determine the most likely cause of the child's injuries.
- Take action to protect the child or another child in the family from additional harm. This usually involves working in partnership with police, protective workers and support agencies.

Discuss *all* situations of possible child abuse with a paediatrician or colleague with expertise in child abuse.

Interview techniques

- Ensure privacy. Allow adequate time
- Use a non-judgemental, sensitive approach
- Listen
- Ask open, non-directive questions
- Record information sources and information provided. Use verbatim quotes whenever possible
- Do not speculate or suggest possible mechanisms of injury

History of injury

Gather information about the possible mechanism, timing and circumstances of injury:

- Determine when, where and how the injury occurred
- Record
  - Who told the story
  - Where the information came from
  - Who (if anyone) witnessed the event(s) that caused the injury
  - The child's previous injuries, illnesses and emergency department presentations
- Assess the child's developmental capabilities

It is important to obtain details of the child's past medical, social and family history. Explore possible medical causes of easy bruising/excessive bleeding and fragile bones.

Examination

A thorough physical examination must be performed.

- Describe injuries accurately, use body diagrams and photograph all visible injuries.
- Include details of the site, size, colour and shape of ALL injuries and skin lesions.

Look for

- Skin injuries (bruises, petechiae, lacerations, abrasions, puncture wounds). Note injuries that might have been inflicted by a human hand (slap, firm grip or fingertip pressure) or patterned bruising from impact with an implement
- Intra-oral, intranasal and tympanic membrane injuries
- Eye injuries (examine from the lids to the retina)
- Internal injuries (organs in the thorax and abdomen)
- Genital injuries

There are few examination findings that serve as definitive evidence of assault, but there are many examination findings that should generate suspicion about a non-accidental cause. These include

- Bruising or fracture in non-mobile children.
- Bruising over soft parts of the body that are well protected from accidental trauma.
- Patterned bruising suggestive of human bite marks or forceful contact with an object.
- Unexplained encephalopathy in a child aged less than 2 years (consider abusive head trauma).
- Unexplained intracranial bleeding in infants (particularly thin subdural haemorrhages over convexities).
- Metaphyseal fractures at the ends of long bones.
- Immersion-patterned scalds.

Medical investigation of suspicious injury (Fig. 29.1)
Investigation of suspicious bruising
- Basic investigation of bruising
  - FBE, PT (INR), APPT

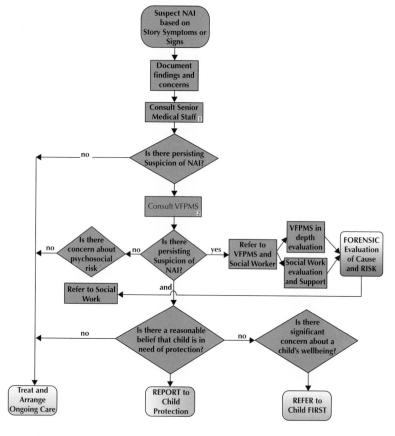

1 REPORT to Child Protection if belief formed that child is in need of PROTECTION

2 REPORT to Child Protection if belief formed that child is in need of PROTECTION

Fig. 29.1 Algorithm to guide decision making regarding suspected non-accidental injury

- Consider
  - U&E, Cr, LFT (proteins), calcium
  - Fibrinogen
- An extended clotting profile might be performed when the child has clinical signs that suggest an inherited/congenital problem or a medical condition that might be associated with bruising. Also consider an extended clotting profile when results to first-line tests are abnormal.
  - Factor VIII, IX, XI, XIII
  - von Willebrand screen (and blood group)
  - Platelet function tests (PFA 100)
  - Lupus anticoagulant (with additional tests for lupus)
  - Inflammatory markers (if vasculitis suspected)

Investigation of intra-abdominal injury
1. Amylase and lipase
2. Ultrasound abdomen
3. CT abdomen if raised amylase or if considering intra-abdominal haemorrhage or traumatic ileus
4. X-ray (erect and supine) if considering perforated hollow viscus

Investigation of suspicious fracture
1. Radiology
   - X-ray sites of clinically suspected fracture(s).
   - Bone scan **and** skeletal survey (together) are recommended in children <3 years of age to search for occult fractures.
   - In children >3 years, bone scans are used only if occult or healing fractures are suspected. A bone scan is unlikely to detect an occult fracture that occurred more than 12 months previously.

Note: A bone scan is not a sensitive tool for the detection of skull fractures; if suspected, obtain a skull x-ray or CT scan. The dose of irradiation must be weighed against the need to determine whether a skull fracture exists.

2. Blood tests
   - First-line tests
     - FBE, U&E, Cr, LFT (including ALP)
     - Calcium, phosphate, vitamin D
   - Second-line tests
     - Magnesium, copper
     - Parathyroid hormone
     - Syphilis serology
     - Urine metabolic screen
     - Inflammatory markers
     - Consider genetic tests for osteogenesis imperfecta (COL1A1 and COL1A2)

Investigation of suspected shaking
In an infant or young child with a history of shaking, an unexplained encephalopathy or unexplained retinal haemorrhages.
- Consider MRI and/or CT brain
- Consider MRI cervical spine, or whole spine
- Investigate as for fracture
- Ophthalmologic examination
- When intracranial bleeding exists
  - Investigate as for bruising
  - Urine metabolic screen

Admission to ICU should be considered whenever an infant presents with altered conscious state and shaking is suspected because of the high risk of further neurological deterioration caused by progressive brain swelling.

Investigation of suspicious burns and scalds
If suspicion exists about intentional thermal injury such as scalds or contact burns in children aged <3 years, then skeletal survey, bone scan and additional investigations for other forms of child abuse should be considered.

Toxicology

- Toxicology tests might be considered when ingestion or poisoning is possible as a result of caregiver neglect or intentional exposure/ingestion. Send samples for forensic drug analysis to forensic toxicology laboratories, not hospital biochemistry laboratories, and preserve the chain of evidence. Samples must be securely sealed and the names recorded of every person who takes possession of the samples between the time of collection and the time of analysis. Consult with forensic experts if uncertain about collecting samples. Collect blood and urine if ingestion or poisoning was within prior 24 hours.
- Collect urine if ingestion or poisoning was more than 24 hours previously.
- Collect hair samples only after discussion with forensic expert.

Photographs

Photography is an important means of documenting injuries and should be obtained in all situations of suspected assault. A colour wheel and a tape measure/ruler should be included when possible, but the absence of these tools should not prevent the photographing of injuries. Photography augments a detailed written description of injuries and body diagrams, but should never replace this.

Child sexual abuse

Aim for a single assessment by a suitably trained medical practitioner (Fig. 29.2). This doctor should have expertise in assessment of sexual assault including genital injury, collection of forensic samples, preparation of medical reports and presentation of evidence in court. In Victoria, the Victorian Forensic Paediatric Medical Service (VFPMS) is responsible for sexual assault examinations of under 18-year olds.

Doctors must ensure that all aspects of the examination and photo-documentation are in accordance with local policies, procedural guidelines and legislation.

History

This should include

- The identity of the alleged perpetrator(s).
- The nature of the sexual contact (digital, penile, vaginal, rectal, oral or a foreign object).
- The time and circumstances of the alleged abuse.
- Whether ejaculation occurred and whether a condom was used.
- Genital symptoms (pain, discharge, bleeding or possible injury).
- Activities such as bathing and toileting that occurred in the interval between the alleged assault and examination. These activities might reduce the likelihood of obtaining DNA or other forensically important material.

Examination

Examination should occur following consultation with VFPMS. The VFPMS proforma is available to use as a tool to guide assessment and medical management. A kit (forensic medical examination kit, FMEK) may be utilized for sample collection.

- Speculum examination is not usually required in girls who are not sexually active.
- Collect the child's clothing (especially underwear) for forensic evaluation.
- Swabs and slides for microbiological tests should be performed as clinically indicated.

Investigations

- At time of examination (optional):
  - Gonorrhoea and Chlamydia PCR (first pass urine)
- Two weeks post assault:
  - Urine gonorrhoea and chlamydia PCR
  - Hep B, Hep C, HIV, syphilis serology
- Three months post assault:
  - Hep C, HIV serology
- Six months post assault:
  - HIV serology

Medical management

- STI prophylaxis: azithromycin 1 g stat
- Pregnancy prophylaxis: Postinor (post coital contraception) within 72 hours of sexual contact. Arrange for a follow-up pregnancy test (see Chapter 22, *Adolescent health*)
- HIV prophylaxis: discuss with ID physician

All abused children and their parents should have access to appropriate counselling.

Samples for forensic analysis must be collected in a room which can be cleaned to a standard that removes a significant amount of DNA on surfaces. When fit-for-purpose facilities are not available and urgent collection of forensic samples is required, consideration should be given to transferring the patient to a suitable facility.

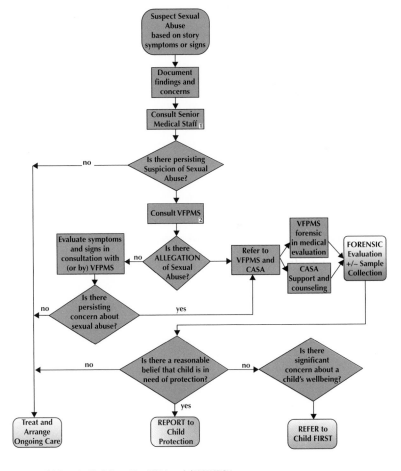

1 REPORT to Child Protection if belief formed that child is in need of PROTECTION
2 REPORT to Child Protection if belief formed that child is in need of PROTECTION

Fig. 29.2 Algorithm to guide decision-making regarding suspected sexual assault

Child neglect

History

This should include

- Child's health, growth, nutrition
- Safety, physical and emotional well-being
- Behaviour and relationships
- Family engagement with family-based intervention and support services
- Events/situations that placed child at risk of harm

Examination

This should include

- Nature and appropriateness of a child's clothing.
- Cleanliness.
- Growth percentiles and nutritional status.
- Developmental skills.
- Evidence of infections and other medical conditions. Take particular notice of undertreated or untreated chronic medical conditions.

Information sharing

Medical staff are expected to attend case conferences with police and protective workers in order to share information and plan intervention.

- SCAN meetings (suspected child abuse and neglect) held within 24 hours of admission to hospital provide useful early opportunities to share information, plan intervention and additional investigations.
- Discharge planning meetings also enable health professionals to jointly plan with child protection for children's safe care, and monitoring of that care, after leaving hospital.

Report writing

Senior medical staff should write (or supervise the preparation of) medical reports. Avoid complex terms and medical jargon. A well-presented, accurate and logically argued opinion within a medical report reflects well the author's credibility. The converse also applies.

Format of medicolegal reports

The recommended format of medicolegal reports varies between jurisdictions. A suggested format is found at http://www.rch.org.au/vfpms/.

All reports should be headed 'Confidential'.

Do not use any identifying patient details apart from name and date of birth.

- Information about author
  Document your credentials clearly. This includes academic qualifications and year of graduation/conferring of degrees, relevant past experience and current position.
- Information about circumstances
  State why, when and where examination took place and who else was present in the room, part or all of the time.
- Consent
  Record the name of the person giving consent for the medical evaluation, and for what (including preparation and release of the report, photo-documentation and treatment).
- Presenting history
- Physical examination
- Investigations
- Conclusions and opinion
  Aim to offer an opinion about the likelihood that the cause of the child's condition is abuse or neglect. If possible, comment on force, mechanism and timing.
- Recommendations
  Professional recommendations about intervention aimed to improve the child's health, safety, growth, development, relationships, behaviour and well-being.

Court testimony

Seek advice from experienced colleagues and/or experts working in your local tertiary level child protection service. Legislation varies significantly between jurisdictions and doctors are encouraged to familiarise themselves with local court procedures and requirements.

Doctors are usually required to take original notes (work-notes or hospital record) of the consultation to court and can be cross-examined about the details of this record. Ensure appropriate permission has been obtained from the health service before records or copies are removed from work premises. Patient records might need to be subpoenaed from the health service.

USEFUL RESOURCES
- *www.rch.org.au/clinicalguide [Child Abuse]* – RCH Clinical Practice Guidelines. Contains useful guidelines for assessment and management of child abuse.
- *http://www.rch.org.au/vfpms/* – Victorian Forensic Paediatric Medical Service. Contains useful relevant literature, educational resources and guidelines.

Growth charts

Paediatric Handbook, Ninth Edition. Edited by Amanda Gwee, Romi Rimer and Michael Marks.
© 2015 John Wiley & Sons, Ltd. Published 2015 by John Wiley & Sons, Ltd.

Girls in utero 24–42 weeks and postnatal 0–3 years

Intrauterine Growth Curves (Composite Male/Female)

Measuring Technique: As for ages 0–36 months (see over page).

Additional Notes: Gestational ages are recorded in completed weeks from the first day of the mother's last menstrual period.
Foetal growth is influenced by many factors including age, body weight, height, parity, ethnic origin of the mother and sex of the foetus.
Corrections for some of these factors are found in the quoted reference.

Data Source: Kitchen, W. H. *et al.* 1983, 'Revised intrauterine growth curves for an Australian hospital population', *Aust. Paediatr. J.* 19: 157–161.

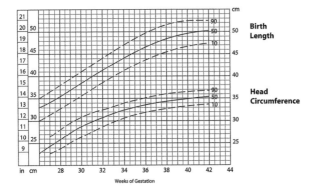

Birth Length

Head Circumference

Weeks of Gestation

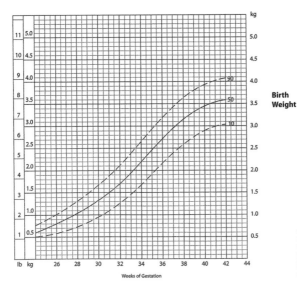

Birth Weight

Weeks of Gestation

The opinions, views and recommendations expressed in this publication do not necessarily reflect those of the sponsor or publisher. Pfizer Australia accepts no responsibility for treatment decisions based upon these charts.

Girls in utero 24–42 weeks and postnatal 0–3 years

Pfizer

AUSTRALIA
Reproduced with
permission of
Pfizer Australia

Surname	Identification No.
Given Names	Date of Birth

Weight Percentile for Girls 0–3 years

Weight should be taken in the nude, or as near thereto as possible. If a surgical gown or minimum underclothing (vest and pants) is worn, then its estimated weight (about 0.1 kg) must be subtracted before weight is recorded. Weights are conventionally recorded to the last completed 0.1 kg above the age of 6 months. The bladder should be empty.

Endorsed By

Australasian **P**aediatric **E**ndocrine **G**roup

DATE	AGE	LENGTH	WEIGHT	HEAD CIRCUM.

Simplified Calculation of Body Surface Area (BSA)

$$BSA\ (m^2) = \sqrt{\frac{Ht\ (cm) \times Wt\ (kg)}{3600}}$$

Reference: Mosteller, R. D. 1987,
'Simplified calculation of body surface area',
N. Engl. J. Med. 317: 1098.

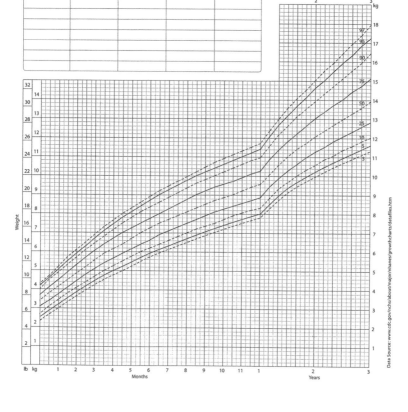

Data Source: www.cdc.gov/nchs/about/major/nhanes/growthcharts/datafiles.htm

Length Percentile for Girls 0–3 years

Mother's Height

Father's Height

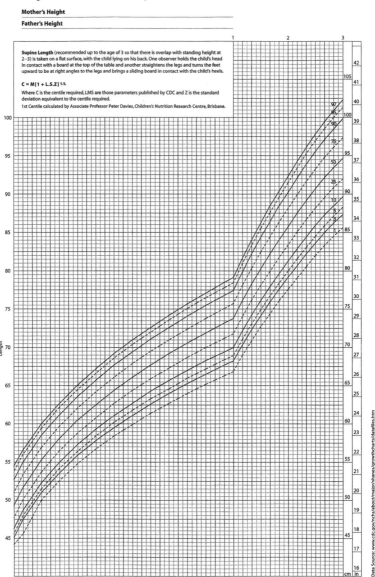

Supine Length (recommended up to the age of 3 so that there is overlap with standing height at 2–3) is taken on a flat surface, with the child lying on his back. One observer holds the child's head in contact with a board at the top of the table and another straightens the legs and turns the feet upward to be at right angles to the legs and brings a sliding board in contact with the child's heels.

$C = M[1 + L.S.Z]^{1/L}$

Where C is the centile required, LMS are those parameters published by CDC and Z is the standard deviation equivalent to the centile required.

1st Centile calculated by Associate Professor Peter Davies, Children's Nutrition Research Centre, Brisbane.

Data Source: www.cdc.gov/nchs/about/major/nhanes/growthcharts/datafiles.htm

Head Circumference

Measuring Technique: The tape should be placed over the eyebrows, above the ears and over the most prominent part of the occiput taking a direct route. A paper tape is preferable to plastic, which stretches unacceptably under tension. The maximum measurement should be recorded to the nearest 0.1 cm.

In utero 28–40 weeks, 0–12 months

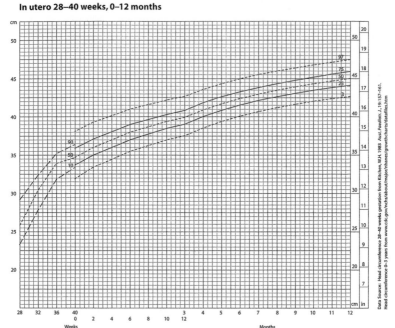

Data Source: Head circumference 28–40 weeks gestation from Kitchen, W.H. 1983. *Aust. Paediatr. J.* 19:157–161. Head circumference 0–3 years from www.cdc.gov/nchs/about/major/nhanes/growthcharts/datafiles.htm

1–3 years

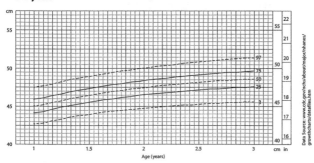

Data Source: www.cdc.gov/nchs/about/major/nhanes/growthcharts/datafiles.htm

Boys in utero 24–42 weeks and postnatal 0–3 years

Intrauterine Growth Curves (Composite Male/Female)

Measuring Technique: As for ages 0–36 months (see over page).

Additional Notes: Gestational ages are recorded in completed weeks from the first day of the mother's last menstrual period.
Foetal growth is influenced by many factors including age, body weight, height, parity, ethnic origin of the mother and sex of the foetus.
Corrections for some of these factors are found in the quoted reference.

Data Source: Kitchen, W. H. *et al.* 1983, 'Revised intrauterine growth curves for an Australian hospital population', *Aust. Paediatr. J.* 19: 157–161.

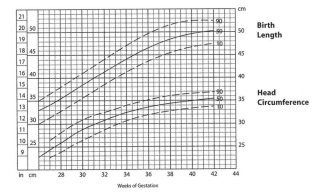

Birth
Length

Head
Circumference

Weeks of Gestation

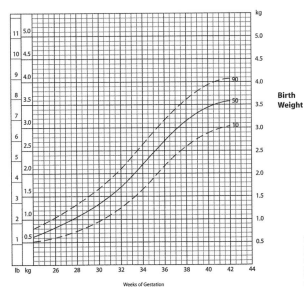

Birth
Weight

Weeks of Gestation

The opinions, views and
recommendations expressed in
this publication do not necessarily
reflect those of the sponsor or
publisher. Pfizer Australia accepts
no responsibility for treatment
decisions based upon these charts.

Boys in utero 24–42 weeks and postnatal 0–3 years

AUSTRALIA
Reproduced with
permission of
Pfizer Australia

Surname _____   Identification No. _____

Given Names _____   Date of Birth _____

Weight Percentile for Boys 0–3 years

Weight should be taken in the nude, or as near thereto as possible. If a surgical gown or minimum underclothing (vest and pants) is worn, then its estimated weight (about 0.1 kg) must be subtracted before weight is recorded. Weights are conventionally recorded to the last completed 0.1 kg above the age of 6 months. The bladder should be empty. .

Endorsed By

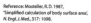

DATE	AGE	LENGTH	WEIGHT	HEAD CIRCUM.

Simplified Calculation of Body Surface Area (BSA)

$$BSA\ (m^2) = \sqrt{\frac{Ht\ (cm) \times Wt\ (kg)}{3600}}$$

Reference: Mosteller, R. D. 1987,
'Simplified calculation of body surface area',
N. Engl. J. Med., 317: 1098.

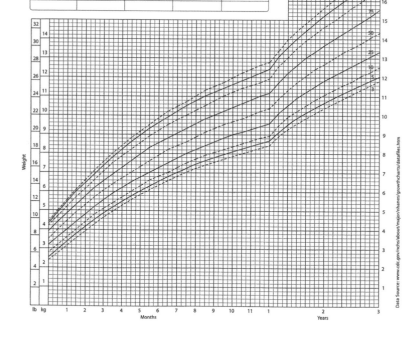

Data Source: www.cdc.gov/nchs/about/major/nhanes/growthcharts/datafiles.htm

Length Percentile for Boys 0–3 years

Mother's Height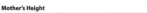

Father's Height

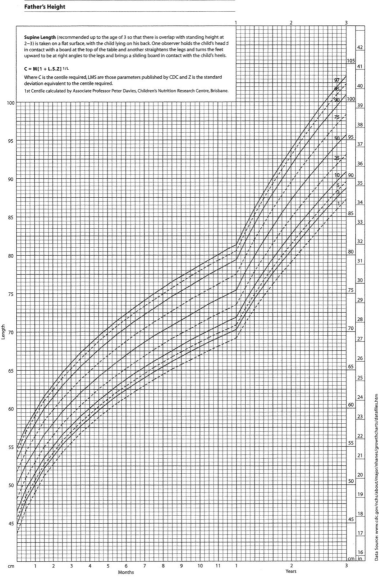

Supine Length (recommended up to the age of 3 so that there is overlap with standing height at 2–3) is taken on a flat surface, with the child lying on his back. One observer holds the child's head d in contact with a board at the top of the table and another straightens the legs and turns the feet upward to be at right angles to the legs and brings a sliding board in contact with the child's heels.

$$C = M[1 + L.S.Z]^{1/L}$$

Where C is the centile required, LMS are those parameters published by CDC and Z is the standard deviation equivalent to the centile required.

1st Centile calculated by Associate Professor Peter Davies, Children's Nutrition Research Centre, Brisbane.

Length

Months

Years

Head Circumference

Measuring Technique: The tape should be placed over the eyebrows, above the ears and over the most prominent part of the occiput taking a direct route. A paper tape is preferable to plastic, which stretches unacceptably under tension. The maximum measurement should be recorded to the nearest 0.1 cm.

In utero 28–40 weeks, 0–12 months

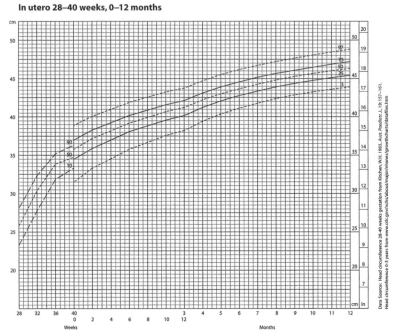

Data Source: Head circumference 28–40 weeks gestation from Kitchen, W.H. 1983. *Aust. Paediatr. J.,* 19: 157–161.
Head circumference 0–3 years from www.cdc.gov/nchs/about/major/nhanes/growthcharts/datafiles.htm

1–3 years

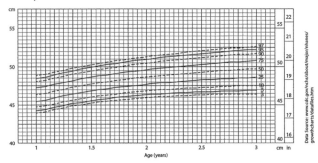

Data Source: www.cdc.gov/nchs/about/major/nhanes/
growthcharts/datafiles.htm

Girls 2 –18 years
Stages of Puberty

Ages of attainment of successive stages of pubertal sexual development are given in the Height Percentile chart.
The stage Pubic Hair 2+ represents the state of a child who shows the pubic hair appearance stage 2 but not stage 3 (see below).

The centiles for age at which this state is normally seen are given, the 97th centile being considered as the early limit, the 3rd centile as the late limit. The child's puberty stages may be plotted at successive ages (Tanner, 1962, *Growth at Adolescence*, 2nd edn).

Pubic Hair Development

Stage 1. Pre-adolescent. The vellus over the pubes is not further developed than that over the abdominal wall that is no pubic hair.

Stage 2. Sparse growth of long, slightly pigmented downy hair, straight or slightly curled, chiefly along labia.

Stage 3. Considerably darker, coarser and more curled. The hair spreads sparsely over the junction of the pubes.

Stage 4. Hair now adult in type, but area covered is still considerably smaller than in the adult. No spread to the medial surface of thighs.

Stage 5. Adult in quantity and type with distribution of the horizontal (or classically 'feminine') pattern. Spread to medial surface of thighs but not up linea alba or elsewhere above the base of the inverse triangle (spread up linea alba occurs late and is rated stage 6).

Breast Development Stages

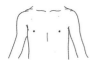

Stage 1. Prepubertal

Stage 2. Elevation of breasts and papilla

Stage 3. Further elevation and areola but no separation of contours

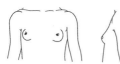

Stage 4. Areola and papilla form a secondary mound above level of the breast

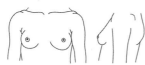

Stage 5. Areola recesses to the general contour of the breast

Pubic Hair Stages

Stage 2

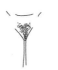

Stage 3

Stage 4

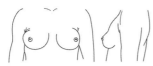

Stage 5

The opinions, views and recommendations expressed in this publication do not necessarily reflect those of the sponsor or publisher. Pfizer Australia accepts no responsibility for treatment decisions based upon these charts.

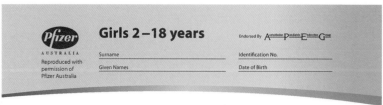

Girls 2–18 years

Endorsed By Australian Paediatric Endocrine Group

Surname _____

Given Names _____

Identification No. _____

Date of Birth _____

Weight Percentile

Weight should be taken in the nude, or as near thereto as possible. If a surgical gown or minimum underclothing (vest and pants) is worn, then its estimated weight (about 0.1 kg) must be subtracted before weight is recorded. Weights are conventionally recorded to the last completed 0.1 kg above the age of 6 months. The bladder should be empty.

Body-Mass Index

DATE	AGE	HEIGHT	WEIGHT	HEAD CIRCUM.	PUBERTAL STAGES		
					BREAST	PUBIC HAIR	MENARCHE

Height Percentile

Mother's Height

Father's Height

Simplified Calculation of Body Surface Area (BSA)

$$BSA\ (m^2) = \sqrt{\frac{Ht\ (cm) \times Wt\ (kg)}{3600}}$$

Reference: Mosteller, R. D. 1987, 'Simplified calculation of body surface area', *N. Engl. J. Med.* 317: 1098.

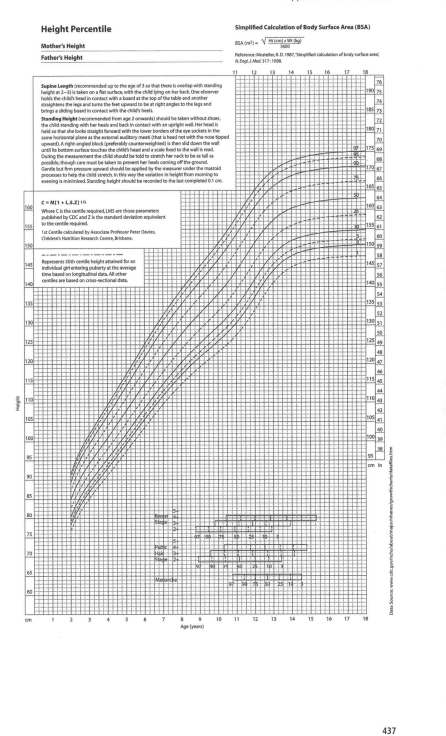

Supine Length (recommended up to the age of 3 so that there is overlap with standing height at 2–3) is taken on a flat surface, with the child lying on her back. One observer holds the child's head in contact with a board at the top of the table and another straightens the legs and turns the feet upward to be at right angles to the legs and brings a sliding board in contact with the child's heels.

Standing Height (recommended from age 2 onwards) should be taken without shoes, the child standing with her heels and back in contact with an upright wall. Her head is held so that she looks straight forward with the lower borders of the eye sockets in the same horizontal plane as the external auditory meati (that is head not with the nose tipped upward). A right-angled block (preferably counterweighted) is then slid down the wall until its bottom surface touches the child's head and a scale fixed to the wall is read. During the measurement the child should be told to stretch her neck to be as tall as possible, though care must be taken to prevent her heels coming off the ground. Gentle but firm pressure upward should be applied by the measurer under the mastoid processes to help the child stretch. In this way the variation in height from morning to evening is minimised. Standing height should be recorded to the last completed 0.1 cm.

C = M[1 + L.S.Z] $^{1/L}$

Where C is the centile required, LMS are those parameters published by CDC and Z is the standard deviation equivalent to the centile required.

1st Centile calculated by Associate Professor Peter Davies, Children's Nutrition Research Centre, Brisbane.

Represents 50th centile height attained for an individual girl entering puberty at the average time based on longitudinal data. All other centiles are based on cross-sectional data.

Data Source: www.cdc.gov/nchs/about/major/nhanes/growthcharts/datafiles.htm

Head Circumference

Measuring Technique: The tape should be placed over the eyebrows, above the ears and over the most prominent part of the occiput taking a direct route. A paper tape is preferable to plastic, which stretches unacceptably under tension. The maximum measurement should be recorded to the nearest 0.1 cm.

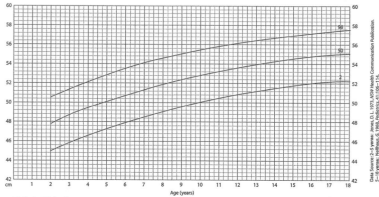

Data Source: 2–5 yeras: Jones, D.L. 1973, *NSW Health Communication Publication*. 5–18 yeras: Nelfhaus, G. 1968, *Pediatrics*, 41:106–114.

Height Velocity

The standards are appropriate for velocity calculated over a whole-year period, not less, since a smaller period requires wider limits (the 3rd and 97th centiles for whole year being roughly appropriate for the 10th and 90th centiles over 6 months). The yearly velocity should be plotted at the mid-point of a year. The centiles given in black are appropriate to children of average maturational tempo, who have their peak velocity at the average age for this event. The red line is the 50th centile line for the child who is **2 years early** in maturity and age at peak height velocity, and the blue line refers to a child who is 50th centile in velocity but **2 years late**. The arrows mark the 3rd and 97th centiles at peak velocity for early and late maturers.

Centiles for girls maturing at average time ———— 97 ———— 50 ———— 3

97 and 3 centiles at peak height velocity for Early (+ 2SD) maturers — · — · — Late (−2SD) maturers ·· — ·· — ··

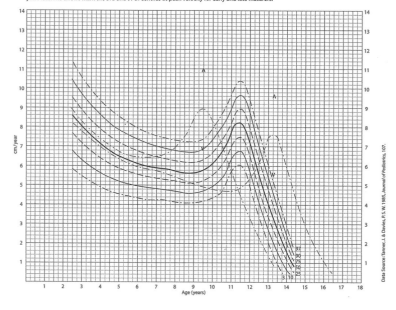

Data Source: Tanner, J. & Davies, P. S. W. 1985, *Journal of Pediatrics*, 107.

Boys 2–18 years
Stages of Puberty

Ages of attainment of successive stages of pubertal sexual development are given in the Height Percentile chart.
The stage Pubic Hair 2+ represents the state of a child who shows the pubic hair appearance stage 2 but not stage 3 (see below).
The centiles for age at which this state is normally seen are given, the 97th centile being considered as the early limit, the 3rd centile as the late limit. The child's puberty stages may be plotted at successive ages (Tanner. 1962, *Growth at Adolescence*, 2nd edn). Testis sizes are judged by comparison with the Prader orchidometer (Zachmann, Prader, Kind, Haflinger & Budliger. 1974, *Helv. Paed. Acta*. 29, 61-72).

Genital (Penis) Development

Stage 1. Pre-adolescent. Testes, scrotum and penis are of about the same size and proportion as in early childhood.

Stage 2. Enlargement of scrotum and testes. Skin of scrotum reddens and changes in texture. Little or no enlargement of penis at this stage.

Stage 3. Enlargement of the penis which occurs at first mainly in length. Further growth of the testes and scrotum.

Stage 4. Increased size of penis with growth in breadth and development of glans. Testes and scrotum larger; scrotal skin darkened.

Stage 5. Genitalia adult in size and shape.

Pubic Hair Development

Stage 1. Pre-adolescent. The vellus over the pubes is not further developed than that over the abdominal wall, that is no pubic hair.

Stage 2. Sparse growth of long, slightly pigmented downy hair, straight or slightly curled at the base of the penis.

Stage 3. Considerably darker, coarser and more curled. The hair spreads sparsely over the junction of the pubes.

Stage 4. Hair now adult in type, but area covered is still considerably smaller than in the adult. No spread to the medial surface of thighs.

Stage 5. Adult in quantity and type with distribution of the horizontal (or classically 'feminine') pattern. Spread to medial surface of thighs but not up linea alba or elsewhere above the base of the inverse triangle (spread up linea alba occurs late and is rated stage 6).

Genital and Pubic Hair Development Stages

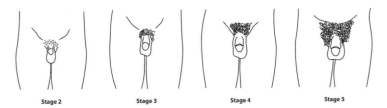

| Stage 2 | Stage 3 | Stage 4 | Stage 5 |

Stretched Penile Length

Measured from the pubo-penile skin junction to the tip of the glans (Shonfeld & Beebe. 1942, *Journal of Urology*, 48, 759–777).

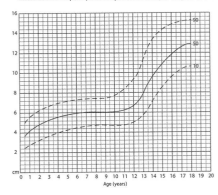

Pfizer

AUSTRALIA

Reproduced with permission of Pfizer Australia

Boys 2–18 years

Endorsed By Australasian Paediatric Endocrine Group

Surname _____

Given Names _____

Identification No. _____

Date of Birth _____

Weight Percentile

Weight should be taken in the nude, or as near thereto as possible. If a surgical gown or minimum underclothing (vest and pants) is worn, then its estimated weight (about 0.1 kg) must be subtracted before weight is recorded. Weights are conventionally recorded to the last completed 0.1 kg above the age of 6 months. The bladder should be empty.

Body-Mass Index

DATE	AGE	HEIGHT	WEIGHT	HEAD CIRCUM.	PUBERTAL STAGES		TESTES	
					GENITAL	PUBIC HAIR	L	R

Height Percentile

Mother's Height _____

Father's Height _____

Simplified Calculation of Body Surface Area (BSA)

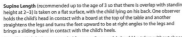

$$BSA\ (m^2) = \sqrt{\frac{Ht\ (cm)\ x\ Wt\ (kg)}{3600}}$$

Reference: Mosteller, R. D. 1987, 'Simplified calculation of body surface area', *N. Engl. J. Med.* 317 : 1098.

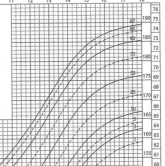

Supine Length (recommended up to the age of 3 so that there is overlap with standing height at 2–3) is taken on a flat surface, with the child lying on his back. One observer holds the child's head in contact with a board at the top of the table and another straightens the legs and turns the feet upward to be at right angles to the legs and brings a sliding board in contact with the child's heels.

Standing Height (recommended from age 2 onwards) should be taken without shoes, the child standing with his heels and back in contact with an upright wall. His head is held so that he looks straight forward with the lower borders of the eye sockets in the same horizontal plane as the external auditory meati (i.e., head not with the nose tipped upward). A right-angled block (preferably counterweighted) is then slid down the wall until its bottom surface touches the child's head and a scale fixed to the wall is read. During the measurement the child should be told to stretch his neck to be as tall as possible, though care must be taken to prevent his heels coming off the ground. Gentle but firm pressure upward should be applied by the measurer under the mastoid processes to help the child stretch. In this way the variation in height from morning to evening is minimised. Standing height should be recorded to the last completed 0.1 cm.

$C = M[1 + L.S.Z]^{1/L}$

Where C is the centile required, LMS are those parameters published by CDC and Z is the standard deviation equivalent to the centile required.

1st Centile calculated by Associate Professor Peter Davies, Children's Nutrition Research Centre, Brisbane.

Represents 50th centile height attained for an individual boy entering puberty at the average time based on longitudinal data. All other centiles are based on cross-sectional data.

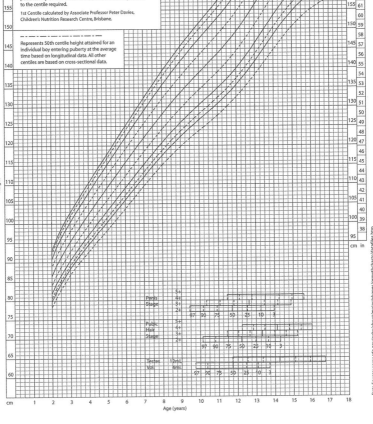

Head Circumference

Measuring Technique: The tape should be placed over the eyebrows, above the ears and over the most prominent part of the occiput taking a direct route. A paper tape is preferable to plastic, which stretches unacceptably under tension. The maximum measurement should be recorded to the nearest 0.1 cm.

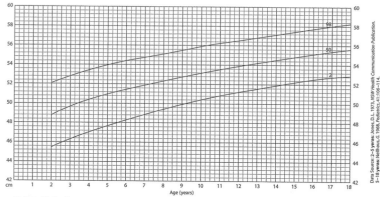

Data Source: 2–5 years: Jones, D.L. 1973, NSW Health Communication Publication. 5–18 years: Nellhaus, G. 1988, Pediatrics, 41:106–114.

Height Velocity

The standards are appropriate for velocity calculated over a whole year period, not less, since a smaller period requires wider limits (the 3rd and 97th centiles for a whole year being roughly appropriate for the 10th and 90th centiles over six months). The yearly velocity should be plotted at the mid-point of a year. The centiles given in black are appropriate to children of average maturational tempo, who have their peak velocity at the average age for this event. The red line is the 50th centile line for the child who is two years early in maturity and age at peak height velocity, and the green line refers to a child who is 50th centile in velocity but two years late. The arrows mark the 3rd and 97th centiles at peak velocity for early and late maturers.

Centiles of a whole year velocity for maturers at average time — 97 / 50 / 3

97 and 3 centile at peak height velocity for Early (+ 2SD) maturers ∧
Late (- 2SD) maturers ∨

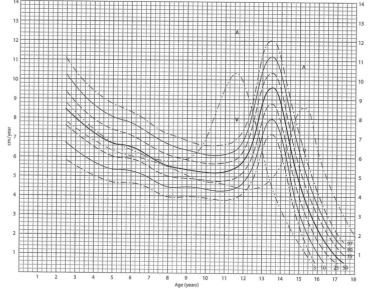

Data Source: Tanner, J. & Davies, P. S. W. 1985, Journal of Pediatrics, 107.

Pharmacopoeia

Drugs are listed by generic name

Acetaminophen   See paracetamol.

Acetazolamide   5–10 mg/kg (adult 100–250 mg) 6–8 H (daily for epilepsy) oral. TB hydrocephalus: 25–50 mg/kg 6–8 H plus frusemide 0.25 mg/kg 6 H; may cause severe alkalosis.

Acetic acid   1% 3 drops/ear 8 H. Box jellyfish: apply vinegar.

Acetylcholine chloride   Adult (NOT/kg): 1% instil 0.5–2 mL into anterior chamber of the eye.

Acetylcysteine   Liver failure, paracetamol poisoning (regardless of delay): 150 mg/kg in 5%D IV over 1 hr; then 10 mg/kg/hr for 20 hr (delay <10 hr), 32 hr (delay 10–16 hr), 72 hr (delay >16 hr) and longer if still encephalopathic; oral 140 mg/kg stat, then 70 mg/kg 4 H for 72 hr. Monitor serum K^+. Give if paracetamol >1000 μmol/L (150 mg/L) at 4 hr, >500 μmol/L 8 hr, >250 μmol/L 12 hr. Lung disease: 20% soltn 0.1 mL/kg (adult 5 mL) 6–12 H nebulised or intratracheal. Meconium ileus equivalent: 5 mL (NOT/kg) of 20% soltn 8 H oral; 60–100 mL of 50 mg/mL for 45 min PR. CF: 4–8 mg/kg 8 H oral. Eye drop 5% + hypromellose 0.35%: 1 drop/eye 6–8 H.

Acetylsalicylic acid   See aspirin.

Aciclovir   EBV, herpes encephalitis, immunodeficiency, varicella: 500 mg/m² IV over 1 hr every 18 H (<30 wk), 12 H (30–32 wk), 8 H (birth to 12 yr); >12 yr 10 mg/kg 8 H IV over 1 hr. Cutaneous herpes 250 mg/m² (birth to 12 yr) 5 mg/kg (>12 yr) 8 H IV over 1 hr. Genital herpes (>12 yr NOT/kg): 200 mg oral x5/day for 10 days, then 200 mg x2–3/day for 6 mo if reqd. Zoster (>12 yr NOT/kg): 400 mg (<2 yr) or 800 mg (≥2 yr) oral x5/day for 7 days. Cold sores: 5% cream x5/day. Eye: 3% oint x5/day.

Actinomycin D   See dactinomycin.

Activated charcoal   See charcoal, activated.

Acyclovir   See aciclovir.

Adalimumab   Adult (NOT/kg): 160 mg SC, 80 mg after 2 wk, then 40 mg every 2 wk.

Adenosine   Arrhythmia: 0.1 mg/kg (adult 3 mg) stat by rapid IV push, incr by 0.1 mg/kg (adult 3 mg) every 2 min to max 0.5 mg/kg (adult 18 mg). Pulmonary hypertension: 50 mcg/kg/min (3 mg/mL at 1 mL/kg/hr) into central vein.

Adrenaline   Asthma, bronchiolitis, croup by inhaltn (<2 yr use 10 L/min gas flow): 1% 0.05 mL/kg diluted to 6 mL, or 1/1000 0.5 mL/kg (max 6 mL) diluted to 6 mL. Cardiac arrest (repeat if reqd): 0.1 mL/kg of 1/10,000 IV or intracardiac; via ETT 0.1 mL/kg of 1/1000. Anaphylaxis: IV 0.05–0.1 mL/kg of 1/10,000, repeat if reqd; IM into thigh: 0.01 mg/kg (0.01 mL/kg of 1/1000) up to 0.1 mg/kg, x3 doses 20 min apart if reqd. IV infsn 0.15 mg/kg in 50 mL at 1–10 mL/hr (0.05–0.5 mcg/kg/min).

Adrenaline 0.1% + fluorouracil 3.33%   Gel: inject into each wart x1/wk for up to 6 wk.

Adrenocorticotrophic hormone (ACTH)   See corticotrophin.

Agar + paraffin 65%   NOT/kg: 6 mo to 2 yr 5 mL, 3–5 yr 5–10 mL, >5 yr 10 mL 8–24 H oral.

Agar + paraffin + phenolphthalein (Agarol)   NOT/kg: 6 mo to 2 yr 2.5 mL, 3–5 yr 2.5–5 mL, >5 yr 5 mL 8–24 H oral.

Agomelatine   Adult (NOT/kg): 25 mg (max 50 mg) daily oral.

Albendazole   Pinworm, threadworm, roundworm, hookworm, whipworm: 20 mg/kg (adult 400 mg) oral once (may repeat after 2 wk). Strongyloides, cutaneous larva migrans, Taenia, H.nana, O.viverrini, C.sinesis: 20 mg/kg (adult 400 mg) daily for 3 days, repeated in 3 wk. 7.5 mg/kg (adult 400 mg) 12 H for 8–30 days (neurocysticercosis); 12 H for three 28-day courses 14 days apart (hydatid).

Albumin   20%: 2–5 mL/kg IV. 4%: 10–20 mL/kg. If no loss from plasma: dose (mL/kg) = 5 × (increase g/L)/(% albumin).

Paediatric Handbook, Ninth Edition. Edited by Amanda Gwee, Romi Rimer and Michael Marks.
© 2015 John Wiley & Sons, Ltd. Published 2015 by John Wiley & Sons, Ltd.

Alclometasone   0.05% cream or ointment: apply 8–12 H.

Alcohol   See ethanol.

Alendronate   0.5 mg/kg (adult 40 mg) daily oral. Post-menopausal osteoporosis (adult, NOT/kg): 10 mg daily, or 70 mg slow release wkly.

Alendronate 70 mg + vitamin D$_3$ 2800 U   1 tab each wk oral.

Alginic acid (Gaviscon single strength)   <1 yr: liquid 2 mL with feed 4 H. 1–12 yr: liquid 5–10 mL, or 1 tab after meals. >12 yr: liquid 10–20 mL, or 1–2 tab after meals.

Aliskiren   Adult (NOT/kg): 150 mg (max 300 mg) daily oral.

Aliskiren + amlodipine 150 mg/5 mg, 150/10, 300/5, 300/10   Adult, NOT/kg: 150 mg/5 daily oral, incr over 2–4 wk to max 300 mg/10 mg daily.

Aliskiren + hydrochlorothiazide 150 mg/12.5 mg, 150/25, 300/12.5, 300/25   Adult NOT/kg: 1 tab daily oral.

Aliskiren + valsarten 150/160 mg, 300/320 mg tabs   Adult (NOT/kg): 1 tab daily oral.

Alitretinoin   0.1% gel: apply 6–12 H.

Allopurinol   10 mg/kg (adult 300 mg) 12–24 H oral. Chemotherapy: 50–100 mg/m^2 6 H IV, oral.

Almotriptan   Adult (NOT/kg): 6.25–12.5 mg oral, repeat in 2 hr if reqd (max 2 doses in 24 hr).

Alogliptin   Adult (NOT/kg): 12.5–25 mg daily oral.

Alogliptin + metformin (12.5 mg/500 mg)   1 tab 12 H oral.

Alogliptin + ploglitazone (25 mg/30 mg)   1 tab daily oral.

Alpha$_1$ proteinase inhibitor   See alpha$_1$ antitrypsin.

Alpha$_1$ antitrypsin   60 mg/kg once wkly IV over 30 min.

Alpha tocopheryl acetate   One alpha-tocopheryl (at) equivalent = 1 mg d-at = 1.1 mg d-at acetate = 1.5 mg dl-at acetate = 1.5 U vit E. Abetalipoproteinaemia: 100 mg/kg (max 4 g) daily oral. Cystic fibrosis: 45–200 mg (NOT/kg) daily oral. Newborn (high dose, toxicity reported): 10–25 mg/kg daily IM or IV, 10–100 mg/kg daily oral.

Alprazolam   0.005–0.02 mg/kg (adult 0.25–1 mg) 8 H oral. Slow release: 0.5–1 mg daily, incr to 3–6 mg (max 10 mg) daily oral.

Alprenolol   1–4 mg/kg (max 200 mg) 6–12 H oral.

Alprostadil (prostaglandin E1, PGE1)   Maintain PDA: 60 mcg/kg in 50 mL 0.9% saline 0.5–3 mL/hr (10–60 ng/kg/min). Erectile dysfunction (adult NOT/kg): 2.5 mcg intracavernous injection, incr by 2.5 mcg if reqd to max 60 mcg (max 3 doses/wk).

Alteplase (tissue plasminogen activator)   0.1–0.6 mg/kg/hr IV for 6–12 hr (longer if no response); keep fibrinogen >100 mg/dL (give cryoprecipitate 1 bag per 5 kg), give heparin 10 U/kg/hr IV, give fresh frozen plasma (FFP) 10 mL/kg IV daily in infants. Local IA infsn: 0.05 mg/kg/hr, give FFP 10 mL/kg IV daily. Blocked central line: 0.5 mg/2 mL (<10 kg) 2 mg/2 mL (>10 kg) per lumen left for 2–4 hr, withdraw drug, flush with saline; repeat once in 24 hr if reqd. Empyema: 4 mg in 40 mL saline intrapleural 1 hr dwell, repeat daily for total 3 doses.

Aluminium acetate   13% soltn (Burrow's lotion): for wet compresses, or daily to molluscum contagiosum.

Aluminium chloride hexahydrate   20% lotion: x1–2/wk.

Aluminium hydroxide   25 mg/kg (adult 0.5–1 g) 4–6 H oral. Gel (64 mg/mL) 0.1 mL/kg 6 H oral.

Aluminium hydroxide 40 mg/mL, Mg hydroxide 40 mg/mL, simethicone 4 mg/mL (Mylanta, Gelusil)   0.5–1 mL/kg (adult 10–20 mL) 6–8 H oral. ICU: 0.5 mL/kg 3 H oral if gastric pH <5.

Aluminium sulphate   20% soltn: apply promptly to sting.

Amantadine hydrochloride   2 mg/kg (adult 100 mg) 12–24 H oral. Flu A prophylaxis (NOT/kg): 100 mg daily (5–9 yr), 100 mg 12 H (>9 yr).

Ambrisentan   Adult (NOT/kg): 5 mg (max 10 mg) daily oral.

Amethocaine   Gel 4% in methylcellulose (RCH AnGel): 0.5 g to skin, apply occlusive dressing, wait 30–60 min, remove gel. 0.5%, 1%: 1 drop/eye.

Amikacin   Single daily dose IV or IM. Neonate: 15 mg/kg stat, then 7.5 mg/kg (<30 wk) 10 mg/kg (30–35 wk) 15 mg/kg (term <1 wk) daily. 1 wk to 10 yr: 25 mg/kg day 1, then 18 mg/kg daily. >10 yr: 20 mg/kg day 1, then 15 mg/kg (max 1.5 g) daily. Trough level <5.0 mg/L.

Amiloride   0.2 mg/kg (adult 5 mg) 12–24 H oral.

Aminobenzoic acid   60 mg/kg (max 3 g) 6 H oral.

Aminocaproic acid   3 g/m^2 (adult 5 g) over 1 hr IV, then 1 g/m^2/hr (adult 1–1.25 g/hr). Prophylaxis: 70 mg/kg 6 H IV, oral.

Aminophylline (100 mg = 80 mg theophylline)   Load: 10 mg/kg (max 500 mg) IV over 1 hr. Maintenance: 1st wk life 2.5 mg/kg IV over 1 hr 12 H; 2nd wk life 3 mg/kg 12 H; 3 wk to 12 mo ((0.12 × age in wk) + 3) mg/kg 8 H; >12 mo and <35 kg, 25 mg/kg at 0.044 mL/kg/hr (1.1 mg/kg/hr) or 6 mg/kg IV over 1 hr 6 H; >35 kg and <17 yr, or >17 yr and smoker, 25 mg/mL at 0.028 mL/kg/hr (0.7 mg/kg/hr) or 4 mg/kg IV over 1 hr 6 H; >17 yr non-smoker 25 mg/mL at 0.02 mL/kg/hr (0.5 mg/kg/hr) or 3 mg/kg IV over 1 hr 6 H; elderly 25 mg/mL at 0.014 mL/kg/hr (0.35 mg/kg/hr) or 2 mg/kg IV over 1 hr 6 H. Level 60–80 µmol/L (neonate), 60–110 (asthma) (x0.18 = mcg/mL).

Aminosalicylic acid (4-aminosalicylic acid, ASA, 4-ASA, para-ASA, PAS)   50–100 mg/kg (adult 4 g) 8 H oral.

5-Aminosalicylic acid   See mesalazine.

Amiodarone   IV: 15 mg/kg in 50 mL 5%D at 5 mL/hr (25 mcg/kg/min) for 4 hr, then 1–3 mL/hr (5–15 mcg/kg/min, max 1.2 g/24 hr). Oral: 4 mg/kg (adult 200 mg) 8 H 1 wk, 12 H 1 wk, then 12–24 H. After starting tablets, taper IV infsn over 5 days. Reduce dose of digoxin and warfarin. Pulseless VF or VT: 5 mg/kg IV over 3–5 min.

Amisulpride   1–6 mg/kg (adult 50–300 mg) daily oral; acute psychosis 5–15 mg/kg (adult 300–800 mg) 12 H.

Amitriptyline   Usually 0.5–1 mg/kg (adult 25–50 mg) 8 H oral. Enuresis: 1–1.5 mg/kg nocte.

Amlodipine   0.05–0.2 mg/kg (adult 2.5–10 mg) daily oral.

Amlodipine + olmesartan (5 mg/20 mg, 5/40, 10/20, 10/40)   Adult (NOT/kg): 1 tablet daily oral.

Amoldipine + telmisartan (5 mg/40 mg, 5/80, 10/40, 10/80)   Adult (NOT/kg): 1 tab daily oral.

Amlodipine + valsartan (5 mg/160 mg, 5/320, 10/160, 10/320)   Adult (NOT/kg): 1 tablet daily oral.

Amodiaquine   Treatment: 10 mg/kg daily for 3 days oral. Prophylaxis: 5 mg/kg once a wk.

Amoxicillin   See amoxycillin.

Amoxycillin   15–25 mg/kg (adult 0.25–1 g) 8 H IV, IM, oral; or 25–40 mg/kg 12 H. Slow release: ≥12 yr 775 mg tab daily oral. Severe inftn: 50 mg/kg (adult 2 g) IV 12 H (1st wk life), 6 H (2–3 wk), 4–6 H or constant infsn (≥4 wk). *H. pylori*: omeprazole.

Amoxycillin + clavulanic acid   Dose as amoxicillin, oral. 4:1 (non-Duo products) 15–25 mg/kg (adult 500/125 mg) 8 H; 7:1 (Duo) 20–30 mg/kg (adult 875/125 mg) 12 H; or 16:1 (XR) 30–50 mg/kg (adult 2000/125 mg) 12 H.

Amphetamine   See dexamphetamine.

Amphotericin B (Fungizone)   Usually 1.5 mg/kg/day (up to 2 mg/kg/day) by continuous infsn IV. Central line: 1.5 mg/kg in 50 mL 5%D at 2 mL/hr (up to 46 kg); 1.5 mg/kg in 1.2 mL/kg 5%D (1.25 mg/mL) at 0.05 mL/kg/hr (over 46 kg). Peripheral IV: usually 1.5 mg/kg in 12 mL/kg 5%D at 0.5 mL/kg/hr (higher concentrations may cause thrombophlebitis). Oral (NOT/kg): 100 mg 6 H, 50 mg 6 H prophylaxis. Bladder washout: 25 mcg/mL. Cream, oint 3%: apply 6–12 H.

Amphotericin, colloidal dispersion (Amphocil, Amphotec)   Usually 3–4 mg/kg (up to 6 mg/kg for aspergillus) daily IV at 2.5 mg/kg/hr.

Amphotericin, lipid complex (Abelcet)   2.5–5 mg/kg daily over 2 hr IV, typically for 2–4 wk.

Amphotericin, liposomal (AmBisome)   3–6 mg/kg (up to 15 mg/kg if severe inftn) daily over 1–2 hr IV, typically for 2–4 wk.

Ampicillin   15–25 mg/kg (adult 0.25–1 g) 6 H IV, IM or oral. Severe inftn: 50 mg/kg (max 2 g) IV 12 H (1st wk life), 6 H (2–4 wk), 3–6 H or constant infsn (4+ wk).

Ampicillin + flucloxacillin   NOT/kg. 125 mg/125 mg or 250/250 (child), 250/250 or 500/500 (adult) 6 H oral, IM or IV.

Ampicillin 1 g + sulbactam 0.5 g   25–50 mg/kg (adult 1–2 g) of ampicillin 6 H IM or IV over 30 min.

Amrinone   <4 wk old: 4 mg/kg IV over 1 hr, then 3–5 mcg/kg/min. >4 wk: 1–3 mg/kg IV over 1 hr, then 5–15 mcg/kg/min.

Amylase   See pancreatic enzymes.

Amylobarbitone   0.3–1 mg/kg (adult 15–50 mg) 8–12 H, or 2–4 mg/kg (adult 200–400 mg) at night, oral.

Anakinra   Adult (NOT/kg): 100 mg daily SC.

Anistreplase   Adult (NOT/kg): 30 U IV over 5 min.

Antihaemophilic factor   See factor 8.

Anti-inhibitor coagulant complex   See factor 8 inhibitor bypassing fraction.

Antilymphocyte globulin   See immunoglobulin, antilym'te.

Antithrombin, antithrombin alfa, antithrombin III, recombinant human antithrombin (rhAT)   Adult: units = (100% − actual %) × Wt/2.2 load, then 23% of this hrly; double dose in pregnancy. Child: **either** 1000 U in 20 mL water diluted to 50 mL with saline: 2.5 mL/kg/hr (50 U/kg/hr) for 3 hr, then 0.3 mL/kg/hr (6 U/kg/hr) **or** 1750 U in 10 mL water diluted to 50 mL with saline: 1.4 mL/kg/hr (49 U/kg/hr) for 3 hr, then 0.17 mL/kg/hr (6 U/kg/hr). Monitor antithrombin activity after 6 hr, then 8–12 H: if <80%, incr dose 30%; if >120%, reduce dose 30%.

Antivenom to Australian box jellyfish, snakes (black, brown, death adder, sea, taipan, tiger), spiders (funnel-web) and ticks   Dose depends on amount of venom injected, not size of patient. Higher doses needed for multiple bites, severe symptoms or delayed administration. Give adrenaline 0.005 mg/kg (0.005 mL/kg of 1 in 1000) SC. Initial dose usually 1 amp diluted 1/10 in Hartmann's soltn IV over 30 min. Do NOT give extra doses for coagulopathy.

Antivenom to black widow spider (USA), red back spider (Australia)   NOT/kg: 1 amp IM, may repeat in 2 hr. Severe: 2 amp diluted 1/10 in Hartmann soltn IV over 30 min. No clear benefit from redback spider anitvenom (Australian Prescriber 35:152).

Antivenom to coral snake (USA)   NOT/kg: 3–6 vials IV over 1–2 hr, repeat if signs progress. Premed with diphenhydramine 5 mg/kg (adult 300 mg) IV, have adrenaline available.

Antivenom to Crotalidae (pit vipers, rattlesnakes – USA)   NOT/kg: 4–6 vials, with higher dose for more severe envenomation, diluted 1/10 in saline IV over 1 hr, repeated 1 hr later if reqd; then 2 vials 6 H for 3 doses.

Antivenom, bark scorpion   NOT/kg: 3 vials IV over 10 min; further 1–2 vials at 30–60 min intervals if reqd.

Antivenom, stonefish   1000 U (2 mL) per puncture IM. Severe: 1000 U/puncture dilutd 1/10 in Hartmann soltn IV over 30 min.

Apomorphine   Adult (NOT/kg): usually 2.4–3.6 mg/dose (max 6 mg) p.r.n. to max 50 mg/day SC. Infsn: 0.02–0.08 mg/kg/hr (max 200 mg/day) SC.

Aprostadil   See alprostadil.

Argatroban   2 mcg/kg/min IV; adjust to maintain APTT x1.5–3.

Arginine hydrochloride   Dose (mg) = BE × Wt (kg) × 70; give half this IV over 1 hr, then repeat if reqd.

Arginine vasopressin, argipressin   See vasopressin.

Aripiprazole   0.1 mg/kg (adult 5 mg) incr if reqd by 0.1 mg/kg (adult 5 mg) each wk to max 0.6 mg/kg (adult 30 mg) daily. Extended release: 6–8 mg/kg (adult 300–400 mg) IM monthly.

Artemether, oily soltn   3.2 mg/kg IM stat, then 1.6 mg/kg daily unitl oral therapy possible.

Artemether 20 mg + lumefantrine 120 mg   NOT/kg: 1 tab (10–14 kg), 2 tab (15–24 kg), 3 tab (25–34 kg), 4 tab (>34 kg) with fatty food (e.g., milk) at 0, 8, 24, 36, 48 and 60 hr. Repeat dose if vomit within 1 hr of ingestion.

Artemisinin   25 mg/kg oral day 1; then 12.5 mg/kg daily for 2 days (with mefloquine 15–25 mg/kg on day 2), or for 4–6 days if mefloquine resistance.

Artesunate + mefloquine   Oral: 2.5 mg/kg at 0, 12, 24 and 48 hr (with mefloquine 15–25 mg/kg on day 2), and daily for another 2–4 days if mefloquine resistance. IM, or IV over 1–2 min: 2 mg/kg stat, then 1 mg/kg in 6 hr if hyperparasitic, then 2 mg/kg daily until oral therapy possible.

Artesunate + pyrimethamine + sulphadoxine   Artesunate 4 mg/kg daily x3 days oral + pyrimethamine 1.25 mg/kg (max 75 mg) and sulphadoxine 25 mg/kg (max 1.5 g) on 1st day.

Articane 40 mg/mL + adrenaline 1:100,000   Adult (NOT/kg) average dose 1.7 mL (max 7 mg/kg = 0.175 mL/kg) by injection.

Ascorbic acid   Burn (NOT/kg): 200–500 mg daily IV, IM, SC, oral. Metabolic dis (NOT/kg): 250 mg (<7 yr) 500 mg (>7 yr) daily oral. Scurvy (NOT/kg): 100 mg 8 H oral for 10 days. Urine acidification: 10–30 mg/kg 6 H.

Asparaginase   See colaspase.

Aspirin 10–15 mg/kg (adult 300–600 mg) 4–6 H oral. Antiplatelet (enteric-coated unreliable absorption): 5 mg/kg (max 100 mg) daily. Kawasaki: 10 mg/kg 6 H (low dose) or 25 mg/kg 6 H (high dose) for 2 wk, then 3–5 mg/kg daily. Arthritis: 25 mg/kg (max 2 g) 6 H for 3 days, then 15–20 mg/kg 6 H. Salicylate level (arthritis) midway between doses 0.7–2.0 mmol/L (x13.81 = mg/100 mL).

Aspirin 25 mg + dipyridamole 200 mg Adult (NOT/kg) 1 sustained release cap 12 H oral.

Atenolol Oral: 1–2 mg/kg (adult 50–100 mg) 12–24 H. IV: 0.05 mg/kg (adult 2.5 mg) every 5 min if reqd (max 4 doses), then 0.1–0.2 mg/kg (adult 5–10 mg) over 10 min 12–24 H.

Atomoxetine 0.5 mg/kg (>70 kg 40 mg) daily oral, incr after at least 3 days to max 1.2 mg/kg (>70 kg 100 mg) as single daily dose or divided 12 H.

Atorvastatin 0.2 mg/kg (adult 10 mg) daily, incr if reqd every 4 wk to max 1.6 mg/kg (adult 80 mg) daily.

Atorvastatin + ezetimibe (10 mg/10 mg, 20/10, 40/10, 80/10) Adult (NOT/kg): 1 tab daily oral.

Atovaquone, micronised Pneumocystis: 3–24 mo 45 mg/kg, >24 mo 30 mg/kg (max 1500 mg) daily oral.

Atovaquone 250 mg + proguanil 100 mg (Malarone) Malaria treat: 20 mg/kg of atovaquone (adult 1 g) daily for 3 days oral; prophylaxis: 5 mg/kg of atovaquone (adult 250 mg) daily.

Atovaquone 62.5 mg + proguanil 25 mg (Malarone paediatric) Malaria prophylaxis: 5 mg/kg (adult 250 mg) daily oral.

Atracurium besylate 0.3–0.6 mg/kg stat, then 0.1–0.2 mg/kg when reqd or 5–10 mcg/kg/min IV.

Atropine 0.02 mg/kg (max 0.6 mg) IV or IM, then 0.01 mg/kg 4–6 H. Organophosphate poisoning: 0.05–1 mg/kg (adult 2 mg) IV, then 0.02–0.05 mg/kg (adult 2 mg) every 15–60 min until atropinised, then 0.02–0.08 mg/kg/hr for several days. Auto-injector (adult, NOT/kg): 2 mg + obidoxime 110 mg IM.

Atropine 25 mcg + diphenoxylate 2.5 mg tab (Lomotil) Adult (NOT/kg): 1–2 tab 6–8 H oral.

Azathioprine 25–75 mg/m² (approx 1–3 mg/kg) daily oral, IV.

Azilsartan 1–2 mg/kg (adult 40–80 mg) daily oral.

Azilsartan + chlorthalidone (40/12.5, 40 mg/25 mg) Adult (NOT/kg): 40/12.5 tab daily, incr to 40/25 daily if reqd.

Azithromycin Oral (only 40% bioavailable): 15 mg/kg (adult 500 mg) on day 1 then 7.5 mg/kg (adult 250 mg) days 2–5, or 15 mg/kg (adult 500 mg) daily for 3 days; trachoma 20 mg/kg (adult 1 g) wkly x3; MAC prophylaxis (adult) 1.2 g wkly; Gp A strep 20 mg/kg daily x3. IV: 15 mg/kg (adult 500 mg) day 1, then 5 mg/kg (adult 200 mg) daily. 1% eye drops: 1 drop 12 H for 2 days, then daily for 5 days.

Aztreonam 30 mg/kg (adult 1 g) 8 H IV. Severe inftn: 50 mg/kg (adult 2 g) 12 H (1st wk life), 8 H (2–4 wk), 6 H or infsn (4+ wk). Nebulised (adult, NOT/kg): 75 mg 8 H.

Bacillus Calmette-Guerin (BCG) vaccine (CSL) Live. Intradermal (1 mg/mL): 0.075 mL (<3 mo) or 0.1 mL (>3 mo) once. Percutaneous (60 mg/mL suspension): 1 drop on skin, inoculated with Heaf apparatus, once.

Bacitracin 500 U/g + polymyxin B 10,000 U/g Eye ointment: apply x2–5/day.

Bacitracin 400 U/g + polymyxin B 5000 U/g + neomycin 5 mg/g (Neosporin) Ointment or eye ointment: apply x2–5/day. Powder: apply 6–12 H (skin inftn), every few days (burns). Eye drops: see gramicidin.

Baclofen 0.2 mg/kg (adult 5 mg) 8 H oral, incr every 3 days to 1 mg/kg (adult 25 mg, max 50 mg) 8 H. Intrathecal infsn: 2–20 mcg/kg (max 1000 mcg) per 24 hr.

Balsalazide Adult (NOT/kg): 2.25 g 8 H oral (= 2.34 g mesalazine daily).

Bambuterol 0.2–0.4 mg/kg (adult 10–20 mg) nocte oral.

Bazedoxifene 20 mg + conjugated oestrogens 0.45 mg Adult (NOT/kg): 1 tab daily.

BCG vaccine See Bacillus Calmette-Guerin vaccine.

Beclomethasone dipropionate Rotacap or aerosol (NOT/kg): 100–200 mcg (<8 yr), 150–400 mcg (>8 yr) x2/day (rarely x4/day). Nasal (NOT/kg): aerosol or pump (50 mcg/spray): 1 spray 12 H (<12 yr), 2 spray 12 H (>12 yr).

Belimumab 10 mg/kg IV over 1 hr every 2 wk x3, then 4 wkly.

Bemiparin Surgery (adult, NOT/kg): 2500 U (orthopaedics 3500 U) SC 2 hr preop or 6 hr postop, then daily for 7–10 days. DVT: 115 U/kg daily 5–9 days (or until oral anticoag).

Benazepril 0.2–0.4 mg/kg (adult 10–20 mg) 12–24 H oral.

Bendroflumethiazide See bendrofluazide.

Bendrofluazide 0.1–0.2 mg/kg (adult 5–10 mg) daily oral.

Benflumetol (lumefantrine)   See artemether.

Benperidol   5–15 mcg/kg (adult 0.25–1.5 mg) 12–24 H oral.

Benserazide   See levodopa + benserazide.

Benzathine penicillin   See penicillin, benzathine.

Benzatropine   See benztropine.

Benzocaine   1–20% topical: usually applied 4–6 H.

Benzoyl peroxide   Liquid, gel 2.5–10%: apply x1–3/day. See also adapalene + benzoyl peroxide.

Benzthiazide 25 mg + triamterene 50 mg   Adult (NOT/kg): 1–2 tab on alternate days, oral.

Benztropine   >3 yr: 0.02 mg/kg (adult 1 mg) stat IM or IV, may repeat in 15 min. 0.02–0.06 mg/kg (adult 1–3 mg) 12–24 H oral.

Benzydamine   3% cream: apply 8 H.

Benzyl benzoate   25% lotion. Scabies: apply neck down after hot bath, wash off after 24 hr; repeat in 5 days. Lice: apply to infected region, wash off after 24 hr; repeat in 7 days.

Benzylpenicillin   See penicillin G.

Beractant (bovine surfactant, Survanta)   25 mg/mL soltn. 4 mL/kg intratracheal 2–4 doses in 48 hr, each dose in 4 parts: body inclined down with head to right, body down head left, body up head right, body up head left.

Besifloxacin   0.6% eye ointment: apply 8 H.

Beta carotene   Porphyria: 1–5 mg/kg (adult 30–300 mg) daily.

Betahistine   0.15–0.3 mg/kg (adult 8–16 mg) 8 H oral.

Betamethasone   0.01–0.2 mg/kg daily oral. Betamethasone has no mineralocorticoid action, 1 mg = 25 mg hydrocortisone in glucocorticoid action. Gel 0.05%; cream, lotion or ointment, 0.02%, 0.05%, 0.1%: apply sparingly 8–24 H. Eye 0.1%: initially 1 drop/eye 1–2 H, then 6 H; or 0.6 cm oint 8–12 H.

Betamethasone acetate 3 mg/mL + betamethasone sodium phosphate 3.9 mg/mL (Celestone Chronodose)   Adult: 0.25–2 mL (NOT/kg) intramuscular, intra-articular, or intralesional injection.

Betamethasone dipropionate 0.064% + calcipotriol 0.005% (Dovonex)   Ointment: apply daily to no more than 30% of body for up to 4 wk (max 100 g/wk in adult).

Betamethasone 0.1% + neomycin 0.5%   1 drop/eye 4–8 H.

Bethanecol   Oral: 0.2–1 mg/kg (adult 10–50 mg) 6–8 H. SC: 0.05–0.1 mg/kg (adult 2.5–5 mg) 6–8 H.

Bicarbonate   Slow IV: dose (mmol) = BE × Wt/4 (<5 kg), BE × Wt/6 (child), BE × Wt/10 (adult). These doses correct half the base deficit. Alkalinise urine: 0.25 mmol/kg 6–12 H oral.

Bisacodyl   NOT/kg: <12 mo 2.5 mg PR, 1–5 yr 5 mg PR or 5–10 mg oral, >5 yr 10 mg PR or 10–20 mg oral. Enema: half daily (6 mo to 3 yr), 1 enema daily (>3 yr).

Bisacodyl 10 mg + docusate sodium 100 mg   <2 yr half suppos, 1–11 yr half to 1 suppos, >11 yr 1 suppos daily.

Bismuth subsalicylte   5 mg/kg (adult 240 mg) 12 H oral 30 min before meal. *H. pylori*, see omeprazole.

Bisoprolol   0.2–0.4 mg/kg (adult 10–20 mg) daily oral.

Bosentan   1 mg/kg (adult 62.5 mg) 12 H oral for 1–4 wk, then 2 mg/kg (adult 125 mg) 12 H. IV: half oral dose.

Botulinum toxin type A   NOT/kg: 50 U IM per site, every 12 wk if reqd. Blepharospasm: 1.25–2.5 U into 3 sites/eye (max 5 U/site) IM, max total 200 U/30 days. Oesoph achalasia: 100 U per session divided between 4–6 sites. Hyperhidrosis: 50 U/2 mL intradermal per axilla (given in 10–15 sites).

Botulinum toxin type B   NOT/kg: usual total dose 2500–10,000 U, repeated every 12 wk if reqd.

Bowel washout   See colonic lavage soltn.

Bretylium tosylate   5 mg/kg IV in 1 hr, then 5–30 mcg/kg/min.

Bromocriptine   0.025 mg/kg (adult 1.25 mg) 8–12 H, incr wkly to 0.05–0.2 mg/kg (adult 2.5–10 mg) 6–12 H oral. Diabetes (adult, NOT/kg): 0.8 mg tab daily oral, incr wkly to max 1.6–4.8 mg daily. Inhibit lactation, NOT/kg: 2.5 mg 12 H for 2 wk.

Brompheniramine   0.1–0.2 mg/kg (adult 5–10 mg) 6–8 H oral, SC, IM or slow IV.

Budesonide   Metered dose inhaler (NOT/kg): <12 yr 50–200 mcg 6–12 H, reducing to 100–200 mcg 12 H; >12 yr 100–600 mcg 6–12 H, reducing to 100–400 mcg 12 H. Nebuliser (NOT/kg): <12 yr 0.5–1 mg 12 H, reducing to 0.25–0.5 mg 12 H; >12 yr 1–2 mg 12 H, reducing to 0.5–1 mg 12 H. Croup: 2 mg (NOT/kg) nebulised. Nasal spray, aerosol (NOT/kg): 64–128 mcg/nostril 12–24 H. Crohn disease, adult (NOT/kg): 9 mg slow-release tab daily for 8 wk, then reduce over 4 wk.

Budesonide + formoterol   NOT/kg: 80 mcg/4.5 mcg or 160 mcg/4.5 mcg, two inhalations 12 H.

Bupivacaine   Max dose: 2–3 mg/kg (0.4–0.6 mL/kg of 0.5%). Intrathecal: 1 mg/kg (0.2 mL/kg of 0.5%). Epidural: 2 mg/kg (0.4 mL/kg of 0.5%) stat intraop, then 0.25 mg/kg/hr (0.2 mL/kg/hr of 0.125%) postop. Intrapleural: 0.5% 0.5 mL/kg (max 20 mL) 8–12 H, or 0.5 mL/kg (max 10 mL) stat then 0.1–0.25 mL/kg/hr (max 10 mL/hr). Epidural in ICU: 25 mL 0.5% + 1 mg (20 mL) fentanyl + saline to 100 mL at 2–8 mL/hr in adult.

Bupropion   2–3 mg/kg (adult 75–150 mg) 8–12 H oral. NOT/kg: sus-tained 100–200 mg 12 H; extended: 150–300 mg daily.

Burrow's solution   See aluminium acetate soltn.

Buspirone   0.1 mg/kg (adult 5 mg) 8–12 H oral, incr to max 0.3 mg/kg (adult 15 mg) 8–12 H.

C1 esterase inhibitor   1 U = activity 1 mL plasma. Prophylaxis (Cinryze): 10–50 U/kg (adult 1000 U) IV over 1 hr every 3–4 days. Treatment: 20 U/kg IV (Berinert).

Cabergoline   10 mcg/kg/wk (adult 0.5 mg) in 1–2 doses, incr if reqd monthly by 10 mcg/kg/wk to usually 20 mcg/kg/wk (adult 1 mg) in 1–4 doses, max 90 mcg/kg/wk (adult 4.5 mg). Inhibit lactation: 1 mg oral stat.

Caffeine citrate   2 mg citrate = 1 mg base. 1–5 mg/kg (adult 50–250 mg) of citrate 4–8 H oral, PR. Neonate: 20 mg/kg stat of citrate, then 5 mg/kg daily oral or IV over 30 min; weekly level 5–30 mg/L midway between doses.

Caffeine 100 mg + ergotamine tartrate 1 mg tabs   Adult (NOT/kg): 2 stat, then $1\frac{1}{2}$ hrly if reqd (max 6/attack, 10/wk).

Calcifediol (25-OH D3)   Deficiency: 1–2 mcg/kg daily oral.

Calciferol (Vitamin D2)   See ergocalciferol.

Calcipotriene   See calcipotriol.

Calcipotriol   50 mcg/g (0.005%) ointment: apply 12–24 H. See also betamethasone + calcipotriol ointment.

Calcitonin   Hypercalcaemia: 4 U/kg 12–24 H IM or SC, may incr up to 8 U/kg 6–12 H. Paget's: 1.5–3 U/kg (max 160 U) x3/wk IM or SC. Nasal spray: 200 U daily.

Calcitriol (1,25-OH vitamin D3)   Renal failure, vitamin D resistant rickets: 0.02 mcg/kg daily oral, incr by 0.02 mcg/kg every 4–8 wk according to serum Ca (adult usually 0.25 mcg 12 H).

Calcium (as carbonate, lactate or phosphate)   NOT/kg. Neonate: 50 mg x4–6/day; 1 mo to 3 yr: 100 mg x2–5/day oral; 4–12 yr: 300 mg x2–3/day; >12 yr: 1000 mg x1–2/day.

Calcium carbimide   1–2 mg/kg (adult 50–100 mg) 12 H oral.

Calcium carbonate   Adult NOT/kg: 1250–1500 mg (500–600 mg calcium) 8 H oral with meals for hyper-phosphataemia.

Calcium chloride   10% soltn (0.7 mmol/mL Ca): 0.2 mL/kg (max 10 mL) slow IV stat. Requirement <16 yr 2 mL/kg/day IV. Inotrope: 0.03–0.12 mL/kg/hr (0.5–2 mmol/kg/day) via CVC.

Calcium edetate (EDTA)   See sodium calciumedetate.

Calcium gluconate   10% soltn (0.22 mmol/mL Ca): 0.5 mL/kg (max 20 mL) slow IV stat. Requirement <16 yr 5 mL/kg/day IV. Inotrope: 0.5–2 mmol/kg/day (0.1–0.4 mL/kg/hr) via CVC.

Calcium heparin   See heparin.

Calcium polystyrene sulfonate (Calcium Resonium)   0.3–0.6 g/kg (adult 15–30 g) 6 H NG (+ lactulose), PR.

Calfactant   35 mg/mL phosphlipids, 0.65 mg/mL proteins: 1.5 mL/kg intratracheal gradually over 20–30 breaths during inspiration with infant lying on one side, then another 1.5 mL/kg with infant lying on other side.

Candesartan   0.1–0.3 mg/kg (adult 4–16 mg) daily oral.

Capreomycin sulphate   20 mg/kg (adult 1 g) IM daily, decr after 2–4 mo to 2–3 times per wk.

Captopril   Beware hypotension. 0.1 mg/kg (adult 2.5–5 mg) 8 H oral, incr if reqd to max 2 mg/kg (adult 50 mg) 8 H. Less hypotension if mixed with NG feeds given continuously (or 1–2 H).

Carbamazepine   2 mg/kg (adult 100 mg) 8 H oral, may incr over 2–4 wk to 5–10 mg/kg (adult 250–500 mg) 8 H. Bipolar disorder (adult, NOT/kg): 200 mg as slow-release cap 12 H oral, incr if reqd to max 800 mg 12 H. Level 20–40 μmol/L (x0.24 = mg/l).

Carbimazole   0.4 mg/kg (adult 20 mg) 8–12 H oral for 2 wk, then 0.1 mg/kg (adult 5–10 mg) 8–24 H.

Carisoprodol   7 mg/kg (adult 350 mg) 6 H oral.

Carnitine, L form   IV: 5–15 mg/kg (max 1 g) 6 H. Oral: 25 mg/kg 6–12 H (max 400 mg/kg/day).

Carvedilol   0.1 mg/kg (adult 3.125 mg) 12 H oral; if tolerated incr by 0.1 mg/kg (adult 3.125 mg) every 1–2 wk to max 0.5–0.8 mg/kg (adult 25 mg) 12 H.

Caspofungin   70 mg/m^2 (max 70 mg) day 1, then neonate 25 mg/m^2, child 50 mg/m^2, adult 50 mg (>80 kg 70 mg) daily IV over 1 hr.

Cefaclor   10–15 mg/kg (adult 250–500 mg) 8 H oral; 12 H used in some mild infectns. Slow-release tab 375 mg (adult, NOT/kg): 1–2 tab 12 H oral.

Cefadroxil   15–25 mg/kg (adult 0.5–1 g) 12 H oral.

Cefalexin   See cephalexin.

Cefamandole   See cephamandole.

Cefazolin   See cephazolin.

Cefdinir   14 mg/kg (adult 600 mg) daily (or 2 divided doses) oral.

Cefditoren   4–8 mg/kg (adult 200–400 mg) 12 H oral.

Cefepime hydrochloride   25 mg/kg (adult 1 g) 12 H IM or IV. Severe inftn: 50 mg/kg (adult 2 g) IV 8–12 H or constant infsn.

Cefixime   5 mg/kg (adult 200 mg) 12–24 H oral.

Cefodizime   25 mg/kg (max 1 g) 12 H IV or IM.

Cefonicid   15–50 mg/kg (adult 0.5–2 g) IV or IM daily.

Cefoperazone   25–60 mg/kg (max 1–3 g) 6–12 H IV in 1 hr or IM.

Cefotaxime   25 mg/kg (adult 1 g) 12 H (<4 wk), 8 H (4+ wk) IV. Severe inftn: 50 mg/kg (adult 2–3 g) IV 12 H (preterm), 8 H (1st wk life), 6 H (2–4 wk), 4–6 H or constant infsn (4+ wk).

Cefotetan   25 mg/kg (adult 1 g) 12 H IM, IV. Severe inftn: 50 mg/kg (max 2–3 g) 12 H or constant infsn.

Cefoxitin   25–60 mg/kg (adult 1–3 g) 12 H (1st wk life), 8 H (1–4 wk), 6–8 H (>4 wk) IV.

Cefpirome   25–50 mg/kg (adult 1–2 g) 12 H IV.

Cefpodoxime   5 mg/kg (adult 100–200 mg) 12 H oral.

Cefradine   See cephradine.

Cefprozil   15 mg/kg (adult 500 mg) 12–24 H oral.

Ceftaroline   15 mg/kg (adult 600 mg) 12 H IV over 1 hr.

Ceftazidime   15–25 mg/kg (adult 0.5–1 g) 8 H IV or IM. Severe inftn, cystic fibrosis: 50 mg/kg (max 2 g) 12 H (1st wk life), 8 H (2–4 wk), 6 H or constant infsn (4+ wk).

Ceftibuten   10 mg/kg (adult 400 mg) daily oral.

Ceftizoxime   25–60 mg/kg (adult 1–3 g) 6–8 H IV.

Ceftriaxone sodium   25 mg/kg (adult 1 g) 12–24 H IV, or IM (in 1% lignocaine). Severe inftn: 50 mg/kg (max 2 g) daily (1st wk life), 12 H (2+ wk). Epiglottitis: 100 mg/kg (max 2 g) stat, then 50 mg/kg (max 2 g) after 24 hr. Meningococ prophylaxis (NOT/kg): child 125 mg, >12 yr 250 mg IM in 1% lignocaine once.

Cefuroxime   Oral (as cefuroxime axetil): 10–15 mg/kg (adult 250–500 mg) 12 H. IV: 25 mg/kg (adult 1 g) 8 H. Severe inftn: 50 mg/kg (max 2 g) IV 12 H (1st wk life), 8 H (2nd wk), 6 H or constant infsn (>2 wk).

Celecoxib   Usually 2 mg/kg (adult 100 mg) 12 H, or 4 mg/kg (adult 200 mg) daily oral. Familial adenomatous polyposis (adult, NOT/kg): 400 mg 12 H oral.

Celiprolol   5–10 mg/kg (adult 200–400 mg) daily oral.

Cephalexin   Skin or UTI: 12.5 mg/kg (adult 250 mg) 6 H, or 25 mg/kg (adult 500 mg) 12 H oral. Otitis: 25 mg/kg 6 H.

Cephalothin   15–25 mg/kg (adult 0.5–1 g) 6 H IV or IM. Severe inftn: 50 mg/kg (max 2 g) IV 4 H or constant infsn. Irrigation fluid: 2 g/L (2 mg/mL).

Cephamandole   15–25 mg/kg (adult 0.5–1 g) 6–8 H IV over 10 min or IM. Severe inftn: 40 mg/kg (adult 2 g) IV over 20 min 4–6 H or constant infsn.

Cephazolin   10–15 mg/kg (adult 0.5 g) 6 H IV or IM. Severe inftn: 50 mg/kg (adult 2 g) IV 4–6 H or constant infsn. Surgical prophylaxis: 50 mg/kg IV at induction.

Cephradine   Oral: 10–25 mg/kg (adult 0.25–1 g) 6 H. IM or IV: 25–50 mg/kg (adult 1–2 g) 6 H.

Certolizumab   Adult (NOT/kg): 400 mg SC every 2 wk for 3 doses, then every 4 wk if response.

Certoparin   Prophylaxis: 60 U/kg (adult 3000 U) 1–2 hr preop, then daily SC.

Cerumol   See arachis oil + chlorbutol + dichlorobenzene otic.

Cetirizine   NOT/kg: 2.5 mg (6 mo-2 yr), 2.5–5 mg (2–5 yr), 5–10 mg (>5 yr) daily oral.

Cetrimide   See chlorhexidine.

Cetrorelix (GnRH antagonist)   Adult (NOT/kg): 0.25 mg SC on stimulation day 5, then daily until hCG given.

Cevimeline   0.6 mg/kg (adult 30 mg) 8 H oral.

Charcoal, activated   Check bowel sounds present. 1–2 g/kg (adult 50–100 g) NG; then 0.25 g/kg hrly if reqd. Laxative: sorbitol 1 g/kg (1.4 mL/kg of 70%) once NG, may repeat x1.

Chenodeoxycholic acid   5–10 mg/kg 12 H oral.

Chickenpox vaccine   See varicella vaccine.

Chlomethiazole   See clomethiazole.

Chloral betaine   1.7 mg = 1 mg chloral hydrate.

Chloral hydrate   Hypnotic: 50 mg/kg (max 2 g) stat (ICU up to 100 mg/kg, max 5 g). Sedative: 10 mg/kg 6–8 H oral or PR.

Chloramphenicol   Severe inftn: 40 mg/kg (max 2 g) stat IV, IM or oral; then 25 mg/kg (max 1 g) daily (1st wk life) 12 H (2–4 wk) 8 H (>4 wk) x5 days, then 6 H. Eye drop, oint: apply 2–6 H. Ear: 4 drops 6 H. Serum level 20–30 mg/L 2 hr, <15 mg/L trough.

Chlordiazepoxide   0.1 mg/kg (adult 5 mg) 12 H oral, may incr to max 0.5 mg/kg (adult 30 mg) 6–8 H.

Chlorhexidine   0.1%: catheterisation prep, impetigo. 0.2%: mouthwash. 1%: skin disinfection. 2–4%: hand wash.

Chlorhexidine 0.5% + alcohol 70%   Skin disinfection.

Chlorhexidine 1.5% + cetrimide 15%   1/30 in water: cleaning tissues, wounds or equipment. 140 mL in 1 L water: disinfecting skin, equipment (soak 2 min, rinse in sterile water).

Chlorhexidine + cetrimide   0.05%/0.5%, 0.1%/1%, 0.15%/0.15% soltn: wound cleaning.

Chlorhexidine 1% + hexamidine 0.15%   Powder: wounds.

Chlormethiazole   See clomethiazole.

Chlormezanone   5 mg/kg (adult 200 mg) 6–8 H, or 10 mg/kg (adult 400 mg) at night oral.

Chloroprocaine   Max 11 mg/kg (max 800 mg). With adrenaline (1/200,000) max 14 mg/kg (max 1000 mg).

Chloroquine, base   Oral: 10 mg/kg (max 600 mg) daily × 3 days. IM: 4 mg/kg (max 300 mg) 12 H for 3 days. Prophylaxis: 5 mg/kg (adult 300 mg) oral x1/wk. Lupus, rheumatoid arthritis: 12 mg/kg (max 600 mg) daily, reduce to 4–8 mg/kg (max 400 mg) daily.

Chloroquine + pyrimethamine + sulphadoxine   Chloroquine base 10 mg/kg (max 600 mg) daily for 3 days oral, plus pyrimethamine 1.25 mg/kg (max 75 mg) and sulphadoxine 25 mg/kg (max 1.5 g) on first day.

Chlorothiazide   5–20 mg/kg (adult 0.25–1 g) 12–24 H oral, IV.

Chlorphenamine   See chlorpheniramine.

Chlorphenesin   1% ointment: apply 12 H.

Chlorpheniramine   0.1 mg/kg (adult 4 mg) 6–8 H oral.

Chlorpheniramine + hydrocodone   NOT/kg: 4/5 mg 6 H oral.

Chlorpheniramine 1.25 mg + phenylephrine 2.5 mg in 5 mL   Syrup (NOT/kg): 1.25–2.5 mL (0–1 yr), 2.5–5 mL (2–5 yr), 5–10 mL (6–12 yr), 10–15 mL (>12 yr) 6–8 H oral.

Chlorpromazine   Oral or PR: 0.5–2 mg/kg (max 100 mg) 6–8 H; up to 20 mg/kg 8 H for psychosis. IM (painful) or slow IV (beware hypotension): 0.25–1 mg/kg (usual max 50 mg) 6–8 H.

Chlorpropamide   Adult (NOT/kg): initially 125–250 mg oral, max 500 mg daily.

Chlorquinaldol   5% paste: apply 12 H.

Chlortalidone   See chlorthalidone.

Chlortetracycline   3% cream or ointment: apply 8–24 H.

Chlortetracycline 115.4 mg + demeclocycline 69.2 mg + tetracycline 115.4 mg   NOT/kg. >12 yr: 1 tab 12 H oral.

Chlorthalidone   2 mg/kg (max 100 mg) 3 times a wk oral.

Chlorzoxazone   5–15 mg/kg (adult 250–750 mg) 6–8 H oral.

Cholecalciferol (Vitamin D3)   1 mcg = 40 U = 1 mcg ergocalciferol (qv). Osteodystrophy: 0.2 mcg/kg (hepatic) 15–40 mcg/kg (renal) daily oral.

Cholera, whole cell plus toxin b subunit recombinant vaccine (Dukoral) Inanimate. Dissolve granules in 150 mL water. 2–6 yr: give 75 mL x3 doses 1 wk apart oral, boost after 6 mo. >6 yr: give 150 mL x2 doses 1 wk apart, boost after 2 yr.

Cholestyramine NOT/kg. 1 g (<6 yr) 2–4 g (6–12 yr) 4 g (>12 yr) daily oral, incr over 4 wk to max 1–2 × initial dose 8 H.

Choline magnesium trisalicylate See aspirin.

Choline salicylate, mouth gel (Bonjela) Apply 3 H p.r.n.

Choline theophyllinate (200 mg = theophylline 127 mg) See theophylline.

Choriogonadotropin alfa Adult (NOT/kg): 250 mcg SC.

Chorionic gonadotrophin NOT/kg. Cryptorchidism all ages: 500–1000 U x1–2/wk for 5 wk. After FSH: 10,000 i.u. IM once. Men: 7000 i.u. IM x2/wk, with 75 i.u. FSH and 75 i.u. LH IM x3/wk.

Chymopapain Adult (NOT/kg): 2000–4000 picokatal units per disc, max 10,000 picokatal units per patient.

Ciclesonide Inhaltn (>12 yr): 80–320 mcg 12–24 H. Nasal: 100 mcg/nostril once daily.

Ciclopirox 1% cream or lotion: apply 12 H.

Cidofovir 5 mg/kg over 1 hr IV on day 0, day 7, then every 14 days (given with probenecid). Papilloma: inject 6.25 mg/mL soltn (max total 0.6 mg/kg) at interval of > = 2 wk.

Ciclosporin See cyclosporin.

Cilazapril Usually 0.02–0.1 mg/kg (adult 1–5 mg) daily oral. Renal hypertension: 0.005–0.01 mg/kg daily oral.

Cimetidine Oral: 5–10 mg/kg (adult 300–400 mg) 6 H, or 20 mg/kg (adult 800 mg) nocte. IV: 10–15 mg/kg (adult 200 mg) 12 H (newborn), 6 H (>4 wk).

Cinacalcet Adult (NOT/kg) 30 mg daily oral, incr every 2–4 wk (to max 180 mg) to control parathyroid hormone level. Parathyroid carcinoma: 30 mg 12 H, incr every 2–4 wk if reqd to control serum Ca to max 90 mg 6 H oral.

Cinchocaine Max dose 2 mg/kg (0.4 mL/kg of 0.5%) by injection. Oint 0.5% with hydrocortisone 0.5%: apply 8–24 H.

Cinnarizine 0.3–0.6 mg/kg (adult 15–30 mg) 8 H oral. Periph vasc dis: 1.5 mg/kg (adult 75 mg) 8 H oral.

Ciprofibrate 2–4 mg/kg (adult 100–200 mg) daily oral.

Ciprofloxacin 5–10 mg/kg (adult 250–500 mg) 12 H oral, 4–7 mg/kg (adult 200–300 mg) 12 H IV. Severe inftn, or cystic fibrosis: 20 mg/kg (max 750 mg) 12 H oral, 10 mg/kg (max 400 mg) 8 H IV; higher doses used occasionally. Meningococcus proph: 15 mg/kg (max 500 mg) once oral.

Ciprofloxacin, eye drops 0.3%. Corneal ulcer: 1 drop/15 min for 6 hr then 1 drop/30 min for 18 hr (day 1), 1 drop 1 H (day 2), 1 drop 4 H (day 3–14). Conjunctivitis: 1 drop 4 H; if severe 1 drop 2 H when awake for 2 days, then 6 H.

Ciprofloxacin, eye ointment 0.3%. Apply 1.25 cm 8 H for 3 days, then 12 H for 3 or more days.

Cisatracurium 0.1 mg/kg (child) or 0.15 mg/kg (adult) IV stat, then 0.03 mg/kg if reqd or 1–3 mcg/min. ICU: 0.15 mg/kg stat, then (1–10 mcg/kg/min) IV.

Cisplatin 60–100 mg/m^2 IV over 6 hr every 3–4 wk × 6 cycles.

Citalopram 0.4 mg/kg (adult 20 mg) daily, incr if reqd over 4 wk to max 0.4 mg/kg (adult 60 mg) daily oral.

Citric acid 0.25 g + potassium citrate 1.5 g Urine alkalinisation >6 yr (NOT/kg): 2 tab 8–12 H oral.

Clarithromycin 7.5–15 mg/kg (adult 250–500 mg) 12 H oral. Slow-release tab, adult (NOT/kg): 0.5 g or 1 g daily. *H. pylori*, see omeprazole.

Clavulanic acid See amoxycillin, ticarcillin.

Clemastine 0.02–0.06 mg/kg (adult 1–3 mg) 12 H oral.

Clenbuterol Adult (NOT/kg): 20 mcg (up to 40 mcg) 12 H oral.

Clevidipine Adult (NOT/kg): 1 mg/hr incr every 5 min to 4–6 mg/hr (max 16 mg/hr) IV.

Clidinium 0.05–0.1 mg/kg (adult 2.5–5 mg) 6–8 H oral.

Clindamycin 6 mg/kg (adult 150–450 mg) 6 H oral. IV over 30 min, or IM: 5 mg/kg 12 H (preterm <1 wk old), 5 mg/kg 8 H (preterm >1 wk, term <1 wk), 7.5 mg/kg 8 H (term >1 wk), >28 days 10 mg/kg (adult 600 mg) 8 H. Severe inftn (>28 days): 15–20 mg/kg (adult 900 mg) 8 H IV over 1 hr. Acne soltn 1%: 12 H.

Clindamycin 1.2% + tretinoin 0.025% Acne gel: apply daily.

Clioquinol 10 mg/g cream, 100% powder: apply 6–12 H.

Clioquinol 1% + flumetasone 0.02% 2–3 drops/ear 8–12 H.

Clobazam   0.1 mg/kg (adult 10 mg) daily oral, incr if reqd to max 0.4 mg/kg (adult 20 mg) 8–12 H oral. Lennox-Gastaut, incr wkly if reqd: <30 kg 5 mg daily, then 5 mg 12 H, then 10 mg 12 H; >30 kg 5 mg 12 H, then 10 mg 12 H, then 20 mg 12 H oral.

Clobetasol   0.05% spray, cream, ointment, gel, solution, foam, lotion, shampoo: apply 12 H.

Clobetasone   0.1% soltn: 1 drop/eye 1–6 H.

Clocortolone   Cream 0.1%: apply 8 H.

Clodronate   10–30 mg/kg (adult 0.6–1.8 g) IV over 2 hr every 2 mo; or 6 mg/kg (adult 300 mg) IV over 2 hr daily x7 days, then 15–30/mg/kg (adult 0.8–1.6 g) 12 H oral.

Clofarabine   52 mg/m^2 IV over 2 hr for 5 days every 2–6 wk.

Clofazimine   2 mg/kg (adult 100 mg) daily oral. Lepra reaction: up to 6 mg/kg (max 300 mg) daily for max 3 mo.

Clofibrate   10 mg/kg 8–12 H oral.

Clomethiazole   Cap (192 mg base) equivalent action to 5 mL syrup (250 mg edisilate). Adult (NOT/kg): 1–2 cap, or 5–10 mL syrup, at bedtime oral. Alcohol withdrawal: IV (edisylate 0.8%): 1–2 mL/kg (8–16 mg/kg) over 15 min, then 0.5–1 mL/kg/hr (4–8 mg/kg/hr); capsule 192 mg base, adult (NOT/kg): 2–4 cap stat (may repeat in 1–2 hr), then 1–2 cap 8 H, oral.

Clomiphene   Adult (NOT/kg): 50 mg daily for 5 days oral, incr to 100 mg daily for 5 days if no ovulation.

Clomipramine   0.5–1 mg/kg (adult 25–50 mg) 12 H oral, incr if reqd to max 2 mg/kg (adult 100 mg) 8 H.

Clonazepam   1 drop = 0.1 mg. 0.01 mg/kg (max 0.5 mg) 12 H oral, slowly incr to 0.05 mg/kg (max 2 mg) 6–12 H oral. Status (may be repeated if ventilated), NOT/kg: neonate 0.25 mg, child 0.5 mg, adult 1 mg IV.

Clonidine   Hypertension: 1–5 mcg/kg slow IV, 1–6 mcg/kg (adult 50–300 mcg) 8–12 H oral. Migraine: start with 0.5 mcg/kg (adult 50–75 mcg) 12 H oral. ADHD (NOT/kg): 0.1 mg daily ER-tab oral, incr to max 0.2 mg 12 H. Analgesia: 2.5 mcg/kg premed oral, 0.3 mcg/kg/hr IV, 1–2 mcg/kg local block; ventld 0.5–2 mcg/kg/hr put 50 mcg/kg in 50 mL saline at 0.5–2 mL/hr (<12 kg), 25 mcg/kg in 50 mL saline at 1–4 mL/hr (>12 kg).

Clopamide 5 mg + pindolol 10 mg   Adult: 1–2 tab (max 3 tab) daily oral.

Clopidogrel   Child 0.2 mg/kg daily, adult 75 mg daily oral (note higher dose in adults). Poor converters to active form (15–30% CYP2C19 variant) need higher doses, or pasugrel.

Clorazepate   0.3–2 mg/kg (adult 15–90 mg) daily at night oral, or 0.1–0.5 mg/kg (adult 5–30 mg) 8 H.

Clostridia antitoxin   See gas gangrene antitoxin.

Clotrimazole   Topical: 1% cream or solution 8–12 H. Vaginal (NOT/kg): 1% cream or 100 mg tab daily for 6 days, or 2% cream or 500 mg tab daily for 3 days. Oral candida (NOT/kg): 10 mg lozenge dissolved in mouth x5/day for 14 days.

Cloxacillin   15 mg/kg (adult 500 mg) 6 H oral, IM or IV. Severe inftn: 25–50 mg/kg (adult 1–2 g) IV 12 H (1st wk life), 8 H (2–4 wk), 4–6 H (>4 wk) or constant infsn (>4 wk).

Clozapine   0.5 mg/kg (adult 25 mg) 12 H oral, incr over 7–14 days to 2–5 mg/kg (adult 100–300 mg) 8–12 H; later reducing to 2 mg/kg (adult 100 mg) 8–12 H.

Coal tar, topical   0.5% incr to max 10%, applied 6–8 H.

Cocaine   Topical: 1–3 mg/kg.

Codeine phosphate   Inactive in ≈10% of adults, poor activity in children <5 yr. Analgesic: 0.5–1 mg/kg (adult 15–60 mg) 4 H oral, IM, SC. Cough: 0.25–0.5 mg/kg (adult 15–30 mg) 6 H.

Codeine + guaiacol   7 mg/75 mg per 5 mL. Adult (NOT/kg): 10 mL 8 H oral.

Co-danthramer, co-danthrusate   See dantron.

Co-dergocrine mesylate   Adult (NOT/kg): 3–4.5 mg daily before meal oral or subling; 300 mcg daily IM, SC or IV infsn.

Coenzyme Q10   See ubidecarenone.

Colchicine   Acute gout: 0.02 mg/kg (adult 1 mg) 2 H oral (max 3 doses/day). Chronic use (gout, FMF): 0.01–0.04 mg/kg (adult 0.5–2 mg) daily oral.

Colestyramine   See cholestyramine.

Colfosceril palmitate (Exosurf Neonatal)   Soltn 13.5 mg/mL. Prophylaxis: 5 mL/kg intratracheal over 5 min straight after birth, and at 12 and 24 hr if still ventilated. Rescue: 5 mL/kg intratracheal over 5 min, repeat in 12 hr if still ventilated.

Colistimethate   See colistin sulfomethate sodium.

Colonic lavage, macrogol-3350 and macrogol-4000 (polyethylene glyol) 105 g/L Poisoning, severe constipation: if bowel sounds present, 25 mL/kg/hr (adult 1.5 L/hr) oral or NG for 2–4 hr (until rectal effluent clear). Before colonoscopy: clear fluids only to noon, 1 whole 5 mg bisacodyl tab per 10 kg (adult 4 tab) at noon, wait for bowel motion (max 6 hr), then macrogol 4 g/kg (adult 200 g) in 40 mL/kg fluid (adult 2 L) over 2 hr oral or NG.

Colony stimulating factors See ancestrim, epoetin, filgrastim, lenograstim, molgramostim, sargramostim.

Coloxyl See docusate sodium.

Conivaptan Adult (NOT/kg): 20 mg over 30 min IV, then 20 mg (max 40 mg) over 24 hr by IV infusion.

Conjugated oestrogens (CO) + medroxyprogesterone (MP) NOT/kg. CO (NOT/kg): 0.625 mg (0.3–1.25 mg) daily continuously, with MP 10 mg (up to 20 mg) daily oral for last 10–14 days of 28-day cycle.

Co-cyprindiol See cyproterone acetate + ethinyloestradiol.

Corifollitropin alfa Adult (NOT/kg): 100 mcg (≤60 kg) 150 mcg (>60 kg) SC, GnRH day 5–6, FSH for 6–18 days from day 8.

Corticorelin 1–2 mcg/kg (max 100 mcg) IV.

Corticotrophin releasing factor, hormone See corticorelin.

Cortisone acetate 1–2.5 mg/kg 6–8 H oral. Physiological: 7.5 mg/m^2 8 H. Cortisone acetate 1 mg = hydrocortisone 1.25 mg in mineralo- and gluco-corticoid action.

Cosyntropin (ACTH subunit) NOT/kg: <2 yr 0.125 mg, >2 yr 0.25–0.75 mg IM, IV, or infused over 4–8 hr.

Cotrimoxazole (trimethoprim 1 mg + sulphamethoxazole 5 mg) TMP 4 mg/kg (adult 80–160 mg) 12 H IV over 1 hr or oral. Renal prophylaxis: TMP 2 mg/kg (max 80 mg) daily oral. Pneumocystis: prophylaxis TMP 5 mg/kg daily on 3 days/wk; treatment TMP 250 mg/m^2 stat, then 150 mg/m^2 8 H (<11 yr) or 12 H (>10 yr) IV in 5%D over 1 hr; in renal failure dose interval (hr) = serum creatinine (mmol/L) × 135 (max 48 hr); 1 hr post-infsn serum TMP 5–10 mcg/mL, SMX 100–200 mcg/mL. IV infsn: TMP max 1.6 mg/mL in 5%D.

Coumarin Oral: 1–8 mg/kg (adult 50–400 mg) daily. Cream 100 mg/g: apply 8–12 H.

Coxiella burnetti vaccine Inanimate. 0.5 mL SC once.

Crisantaspase See colaspase.

Crizotinib Adult (NOT/kg) 250 mg 12 H oral.

Crofelemer Adult (NOT/kg): 125 mg slow-release tab 12 H oral.

Cromoglycate See sodium cromoglycate.

Cromolyn, sodium See sodium cromoglycate.

Crotamiton 10% cream or lotion: apply x2–3/day.

Cryoprecipitate Low factor 8: 1 U/kg incr activity 2% (half-life 12 hr); usual dose 5 mL/kg or 1 bag/4 kg 12 H IV for 1–2 infns (muscle, joint), 3–6 infns (hip, forearm, retroperitoneal, oropharynx), 7–14 infns (intracranial). Low fibrinogen: usually 5 mL/kg or 1 bag/4 kg IV. Bag usually 20–30 mL: factor 8 about 5 U/mL (100 U/bag), fibrinogen about 10 mg/mL (200 mg/bag).

Cyanocobalamin (Vit B12) 20 mcg/kg (adult 1000 mcg) IM daily for 7 days then wkly (treatment), monthly (prophylaxis). IV dangerous in megaloblastic anaemia. Maintenance treatment (adult NOT/kg): 2 mg daily oral; 50 mcg (incr if reqd to 100 mcg) daily, or 500 mcg wkly nasal.

Cyclizine 1 mg/kg (adult 50 mg) 8 H oral, IM or IV.

Cyclizine 30 mg + dipipanone 10 mg Adult (NOT/kg): 1 tab 6 H oral, incr dose by half tab if reqd to max 3 tab 6 H.

Cyclobenzaprine 0.2–0.4 mg/kg (adult 5–15 mg) 8 H oral. Extended-release (adult, NOT/kg): 15 mg or 30 mg daily oral.

Cyclopenthiazide 5–10 mcg/kg (adult 250–500 mcg) 12–24 H.

Cyclophosphamide A typical regimen is 600 mg/m^2 IV over 30 min daily for 3 days, then 600 mg/m^2 IV wkly or 10 mg/kg twice wkly (if leucocytes >3000/mm^3).

Cycloserine 5–10 mg/kg (adult 250–500 mg) 12 H oral. Keep plasma conc <30 mcg/mL.

Cyclosporin 1–3 mcg/kg/min IV for 24–48 hr, then 5–8 mg/kg 12 H reducing by 1 mg/kg/dose each mo to 3–4 mg/kg/dose 12 H oral. Eczema, juvenile arthritis, nephrotic, syndrome, psoriasis: 1.5–2.5 mg/kg 12 H. Usual target trough levels by Abbott TDx monoclonal specific assay (x 2.5 = non-specific assay level) on whole blood: 100–250 ng/mL (marrow), 300–400 ng/mL first 3 mo then 100–300 ng/mL (kidney), 200–250 first 3 mo then 100–125 (liver), 100–400 ng/mL (heart, lung).

Cyclosporin ophthalmic   0.05% 1 drop in each eye 12 H.

Cyclosporine   See cyclosporin.

Cyproheptadine   0.1 mg/kg (adult 4 mg) 6–8 H oral. Migraine 0.1 mg/kg (adult 4 mg), repeated in 30 min if reqd.

Cyproterone acetate   1 mg/kg (adult 50 mg) 8–12 H oral. Prec puberty: 25–50 mg/m^2 8–12 H oral. Hyperandrogenism: 50–100 mg daily days 5–14, with oestradiol valerate 1 mg daily days 5–25. Prostate carcinoma (NOT/kg): 100 mg 8–12 H oral. See also oestradiol + cyproterone.

Cyproterone acetate + ethinyloestradiol (2 mg/35 mcg) × 21 tab, + 7 inert tab   In females for acne, contraception, or hirsutism: 1 tab daily, starting 1st day of mensturation.

Cysteamine bitartrate   0.05 mg/m^2 6 H oral, incr over 6 wk to 0.33 mg/m^2/dose (<50 kg) or 0.5 mg/kg/dose (>50 kg) 6 H.

Cytarabine   Usually 100 mg/m^2 daily for 10 days by IV injn or constant infsn. Intrathecal: 30 mg/m^2 every 4 days until CSF normal (dissolve in saline not diluent).

Cytomegalovirus immunoglobn   See immunoglobn, CMV.

Dabigatran   Adult (NOT/kg): 150 mg 12 H or 220 mg daily oral.

Dabrafenib   Adult (NOT/kg) 150 mg 12 H oral with trametinib.

Dacarbazine   250 mg/m^2 IV daily for 5 days every 3 wk.

Daclizumab   1 mg/kg IV over 15 min every 2 wk for 5 doses.

Dactinomycin   Usually 400–600 mcg/m^2 IV daily for 5 days, repeat after 3–4 wk.

Dalfampridine   Slow release (adult, NOT/kg): 10 mg 12 H oral.

Dalfopristin 350 mg + quinupristin 150 mg (Synercid IV 500 mg vial)   7.5 mg/kg (combined) 8 H IV over 1 hr.

Dalteparin sodium   Prophylaxis (adult): 2500–5000 U SC 1–2 hr preop, then daily. Venous thrombosis: 100 U/kg 12 H SC, or infuse 200 U/kg/day IV (anti-Xa 0.5–1 U/mL 4 h post dose). Haemodialysis: 5–10 U/kg stat, then 4–5 U/kg/hr IV (acute renal failure, anti-Xa 0.2–0.4 U/mL); 30–40 U/kg stat, then 10–15 U/kg/hr (chronic renal failure, anti-Xa 0.5–1 U/mL).

Danaparoid   Prevention: 15 U/kg (adult 750 U) 12 H SC. Heparin induced thrombocytopenia: 30 U/kg stat IV, then 1.2–2 U/kg/hr to maintain anti-Xa 0.4–0.8 U/mL.

Danazol   2–4 mg/kg (adult 100–200 mg) 6–12 H oral.

Dantrolene   Hyperpyrexia: 1 mg/kg/min until improves (max 10 mg/kg), then 1–2 mg/kg 6 H for 1–3 day IV or oral. Spasticity: 0.5 mg/kg (adult 25 mg) 6 H, incr over 2 wk if reqd to 3 mg/kg (adult 50–100 mg) 6 H oral.

Dantron + docusate (co-danthrusate)   NOT/kg. 50/60 mg cap: 7–12 yr 1 cap, adult 1–3 cap at night. 50/60 mg in 5 mL: 1–6 yr 2.5 mL, 7–12 yr 5 mL, adult 5–15 mL at night.

Dantron + poloxamer 188 (co-danthramer)   NOT/kg. 25/200 mg cap: 7–12 yr 1 cap, adult 1–3 cap at night. 25/200 mg in 5 mL: 1–6 yr 2.5 mL, 7–12 yr 5 mL, adult 5–15 mL at night.

Dapagliflozin   Adult (NOT/kg): 5–10 mg daily oral.

Dapoxetine   NOT/kg: 30 mg 1–3 hr before sex, max x1/day.

Dapsone   1–2 mg/kg (adult 50–100 mg) daily oral. Derm herpet: 1–6 mg/kg (adult 50–300 mg) daily oral.

Dapsone 100 mg + pyrimethamine 12.5 mg (Maloprim)   1–4 yr quarter tab wkly, 5–10 yr half tab, >10 yr 1 tab.

Daptomycin   4 mg/kg IV over 30 min daily. Severe inftn: 8–10 mg/kg IV daily.

Darbepoetin alfa   Incr or reduce dose if reqd by 25% every 4 wk. Renal failure: 0.45 mcg/kg wkly or 0.75 mcg/kg 2 wkly (0.75 mcg/kg wkly if not on dialysis) SC or IV. Cancer: 6.75 mcg/kg every 3 wk, or 2.25 mcg/kg every wk, SC or IV.

Darifenacin   Adult (NOT/kg): 7.5–15 mg daily oral.

Darunavir (DRV)   Adult (NOT/kg): 600 mg 12 H with food oral.

Darunavir + ritonavir   20–29 kg: 375/50 mg 12 H with food; 30–39 kg: 450/60 mg 12 H; ≥40 kg: 600/100 mg 12 H. ≥18 yr: 800/100 mg (naïve) 600/100 mg (past Rx) daily with food.

Dasatinib   Adult (NOT/kg): 70 mg (up to 100 mg) 12 H oral.

Daunorubicin   30 mg/m^2 wkly slow IV, or 60–90 mg/m^2 every 3 wk. Max total dose 500 mg/m^2.

DDAVP   See desmopressin.

Decitabine   15 mg/m^2 IV over 3 hr 8 H for 3 days, repeated every 6 wk (minimum of 4 cycles).

Deferasirox   20 mg/kg (15–30 mg/kg) daily oral.

Deferiprone   25 mg/kg 8 H (max 100 mg/kg/day) oral.

Deferoxamine   See desferrioxamine.

Deflazacort   Usually 0.1–1.5 mg/kg (adult 5–90 mg) 24–48 H oral. 1.2 mg = 1 mg prednisolone in glucocorticoid activity.

Degarelix   Adult (NOT/kg): 240 mg in two SC injections, then 80 mg SC every 4 wk.

Delavirdine   Adult (NOT/kg): 400 mg 8 H, or 600 mg 12 H oral.

Delta-9-tetrahydrocannabinol   See cannabidiol.

Demecarium bromide   0.125%, 0.25% ophthalmic soltn. Glaucoma: 1 drop x2/day to x2/wk. Strabismus: 1 drop daily for 2 wk, then 1 drop alternate days for 2–3 wk.

Demeclocycline   >8 yr: 3 mg/kg (adult 150 mg) 6 H, or 6 mg/kg (adult 300 mg) 12 H oral. See also chlortetracycline.

Denileukin diftitox   9–18 mcg/kg daily IV over 15 min for 5 consecutive days every 21 days.

Denosumab   Adult (NOT/kg). Ostoporosis: 60 mg every 6 mo SC, with calcium 1000 mg daily and at least 400 i.u. vitamin D daily. Prostate cancer: 120 mg SC every 4 wk.

Dequalinium   NOT/kg: one 0.25 mg pastile 4 H oral.

Deserpidine   0.005–0.02 mg/kg (adult 0.25–1 mg) daily oral.

Desflurane   Usually child 5–10%, adult 3–8% by inhalation.

Desferrioxamine   Antidote: 10–15 mg/kg/hr IV for 12–24 hr (max 6 g/24 hr) if Fe >60–90 μmol/l at 4 hr or 8 hr; some also give 5–10 g (NOT/kg) once oral. Thalassaemia (NOT/kg): 500 mg per unit blood; and 5–6 nights/wk 1–3 g in 5 mL water SC over 1 hr, 0.5–1.5 g in 10 mL water SC over 5 min.

Desipramine   2–4 mg/kg (adult 100–200), occasionally incr up to 6 mg/kg (adult 300 mg), daily oral.

Desirudin   0.3 mg/kg (adult 15 mg) 12 H SC.

Desloratadine   0.1 mg/kg (adult 5 mg) daily oral.

Desmopressin (DDAVP)   1 U = 1 mcg. Nasal (NOT/kg): 5–10 mcg (0.05–0.1 mL) per dose 12–24 H; enuresis 10–40 mcg nocte. IV: 0.5–2 mcg in 1 L fluid, and replace urine output + 10% hrly (but much better to use vasopressin). Haemophilia, von Wille: 0.3 mcg/kg (adult 20 mcg) IV over 1 hr 12–24 H. More potent and longer acting than vasopressin.

Desogestrel   Contraception: 75 mcg daily oral, starting 1st day of menstruation.

Desogestrel + ethinyloestradiol (150 mcg/30 mcg, 150/20) x21 tab, + 7 inert tab   Contraception: 1 tab daily, starting 1st day of menstruation.

Desonide   0.05% cream, ointment, lotion: apply 8–12 H.

Desoximetasone   See desoxymethasone.

Desoxymethasone   0.05% or 0.25% cream, oint, gel: apply 12 H.

Desoxyribonuclease   See fibrinolysin.

Desvenlafaxine   Adult (NOT/kg): 50–100 mg daily oral.

Dexamethasone   Biological half-life 2–3 days. 0.1–1 mg/kg daily oral, IM or IV. Antiemetic: 0.5 mg/kg (adult 16 mg) daily IM, IV, oral. BPD: 0.4 mg/kg daily for 3 days, then 0.3 mg/kg 3 days, 0.2 mg/kg 3 days, 0.1 mg/kg 3 days, 0.05 mg/kg 7 days. Cerebral oedema: 0.25–1 mg/kg (adult 10–50 mg) stat, then 0.6–1 mg/kg (adult 4–8 mg) daily IV reducing over 3–5 days to 0.1 mg/kg (adult 2 mg) daily. Congen adr hypopl: 0.27 mg/m^2 daily oral. Severe croup, extubation stridor, bronchiolitis: 0.6 mg/kg (max 20 mg) IV or IM stat, then prednisolone 1 mg/kg 8–12 H oral. Eye drops 0.1%: 1 drop/eye 3–8 H. Dexamethasone has no mineralocorticoid action; 1 mg = 25 mg hydrocortisone in glucocorticoid action.

Dexamphetamine   0.2 mg/kg (max 10 mg) daily oral, incr if reqd to max 0.6 mg/kg (max 40 mg) 12 H.

Dexchlorpheniramine maleate   0.05 mg/kg (adult 2 mg) 6–8 H oral. Repetab (adult NOT/kg): 6 mg 12 H oral.

Dextrose   Infant sedation (NOT/kg): 1 mL 50%D oral. Hypo-glycaemia: 0.5 mL/kg 50%D or 2.5 mL/kg 10%D slow IV, then incr maintenance mg/kg/min. Hyperkalaemia: 0.1 U/kg insulin + 2 mL/kg 50%D IV. Neonates: 6 g/kg/day (about 4 mg/kg/min) day 1, incr to 12 g/kg/day (up to 18 g/kg/day with hypoglycaemia). Infsn rate (mL/hr) = (4.17 × Wt × g/kg/day)/%D = (6 × Wt × mg/kg/min)/%D. Dose (g/kg/day) = (mL/hr x%D)/(4.17 × Wt). Dose (mg/kg/min) = (mL/hr x%D)/(6 × Wt). mg/kg/min = g/kg/day/1.44. 0.5 mL/kg/hr of 50% = 6 g/kg/day.

Diazepam   0.1–0.4 mg/kg (adult 10–20 mg) IV or PR. 0.04–0.2 mg/kg (adult 2–10 mg) 8–12 H oral. Do not give by IV infsn (binds to PVC); emulsion can be infused. Premed: 0.2–0.4 mg/kg oral, PR. 2–3 mg = 1 mg midazolam.

Diazoxide   Hypertension: 1–3 mg/kg (max 150 mg) stat by rapid IV injection (severe hypotension may occur) repeat once if reqd, then 2–5 mg/kg IV 6 H. Hyperinsulinism: <12 mo 5 mg/kg 8–12 H oral; >12 mo 30–100 mg/m^2 per dose 8 H oral.

Diclofenac   1 mg/kg (adult 50 mg) 8–12 H oral, PR. Submicron (adult, NOT/kg): 18 mg or 35 mg 8 H oral. Eye drops 0.1%: preop 1–5 drops over 3 hr, postop 1 drop stat, then 1 drop 4–8 H. Topical gel 1% (arthritis) 3% (keratoses): apply 2–4 g 6–8 H. Patch 1.3% (180 mg) 10 × 14 cm: apply 12 H.

Digitoxin   4 mcg/kg (max 0.2 mg) 12 H oral for 4 days, then 1–6 mcg/kg (adult usually 0.15 mg, max 0.3 mg) daily.

Digoxin   15 mcg/kg stat and 5 mcg/kg after 6 H, then 3–5 mcg/kg (usual max 200 mcg IV, 250 mcg oral) 12 H slow IV or oral. Level 6 hr or more after dose: 1.0–2.5 nmol/L (x0.78 = ng/mL).

Digoxin immmune FAB (antibodies)   IV over 30 min. Dose (to nearest 40 mg) = serum digoxin (nmol/L) × Wt (kg) × 0.3, or mg ingested × 55. Give if >0.3 mg/kg ingested, or level >6.4 nmol/L or 5.0 ng/mL.

Dihydrocodeine   0.5–1 mg/kg 4–6 H oral.

Dihydroergotamine mesylate   Adult (NOT/kg): 1 mg IM, SC or IV, repeat hrly x2 if needed. Max 6 mg/wk.

Diltiazem   1 mg/kg (adult 60 mg) 8 H, incr if reqd to max 3 mg/kg (adult 180 mg) 8 H oral. Slow release (adult, NOT/kg): 120–240 mg daily, or 90–180 mg 8–12 H oral.

Diphenhydramine hydrochloride   1–2 mg/kg (adult 50–100 mg) 6–8 H oral.

Diphenoxylate   See atropine + diphenoxylate (Lomotil).

Diphtheria vaccine, adult (CSL)   Inanimate. 0.5 mL IM stat, 6 wk later, and 6 mo later (3 doses). Boost every 10 yr.

Diphtheria vaccine, child <8 yr (CSL)   Inanimate. 0.5 mL IM stat, in 6 wk, then 6 mo (3 doses). Boost with adult vaccine.

Diphtheria + hepatitis B + pertussis (acellular) + polio + tetanus [DaPT-HepB-IPV] (Pediarix)   Inanimate. 0.5 mL IM at 2 mo, 4 mo, 6 mo (3 doses), and (DaPT) 18 mo.

Diphtheria + hepatitis B + pertussis (acellular) + tetanus vaccine [DaPT-hepB] (Infanrix Hep B)   Inanimate. 0.5 mL IM at 2 mo, 4 mo, 6 mo (3 doses), and (without hep B) 18 mo.

Diphtheria + hepatitis B + Hib + pertussis (acellular) + tetanus vaccine [DaPT-hepB-Hib] (Infanrix Hexa)   Inanimate. 0.5 mL IM at 2 mo, 4 mo, 6 mo (3 doses).

Diphtheria + Hib + pertussis (acellular) + polio + tetanus [DaPT-Hib-IPV] (Infanrix Penta, Pediacel)   Inanimate. 0.5 mL IM at 2 mo, 4 mo, 6 mo (3 doses), and (DaPT) 18 mo.

Diphtheria + pertussis (whole cell) + tetanus vaccine [DPT] (Triple Antigen)   Inanimate. 0.5 mL IM at 2 mo, 4 mo, 6 mo, 18 mo and 4–5 yr of age (5 doses).

Diphtheria + pertussis (acellular) + tetanus vaccine [DaPT] (Tripacel)   Inanimate. 0.5 mL IM at 2 mo, 4 mo, 6 mo, 18 mo and 4–5 yr of age (5 doses).

Diphtheria + pertussis (acellular) + tetanus vaccine, adult [daPt] (Adacel, Boostrix)   Inanimate. ≥10 yr: 0.5 mL IM.

Diphtheria + pertussis (acellular) + polio + tetanus vaccine [DaPT-IPV] (Quadracel)   Inanimate. 0.5 mL IM at 2, 4 and 6 mo (3 doses).

Diphtheria + pertussis (acellular) + polio + tetanus vaccine [DaPT-IPV] (Infanrix-IPV)   Inanimate. 16 mo to 13 yr: 0.5 mL IM once as booster.

Diphtheria + pertussis (acellular) + polio + tetanus vaccine [daPT-IPV] (Repevax)   Inanimate. >3 yr: 0.5 mL IM once as booster.

Diphtheria + pertussis (acellular) + polio + tetanus vaccine, adult [daPt-IPV] (Adacel Polio, Boostrix-IPV)   Inanimate. ≥10 yr: 0.5 mL IM once as booster.

Diphtheria + polio + tetanus vaccine [dT-IPV] (Revaxis)   Inanimate. >6 yr: 0.5 mL IM once as booster.

Diphtheria + tetanus vaccine, adult [dt] (ADT Booster)   Inanimate. 0.5 mL IM for revaccination after primary course.

Diphtheria + tetanus vaccine, child <8 yr [DT] (CDT)   Inanimate. 0.5 mL IM, in 6 wk, 6 mo later (3 dose). Boost with ADT.

Dipyridamole   1–2 mg/kg (adult 50–100 mg) 6–8 H oral. See also aspirin + dipyridamole.

Disulfiram   Adult (NOT/kg): 500 mg oral daily for 1–2 wk, then 125–500 mg daily.

Dobutamine   <30 kg: 15 mg/kg in 50 mL saline at 1–3 mL/hr (5–15 mcg/kg/min) via CVC or periph IV; >30 kg: 6 mg/kg made up to 100 mL with saline at 5–15 mL/hr (5–15 mcg/kg/min).

Docusate sodium   NOT/kg: 100 mg (3–10 yr), 120–240 mg (>10 yr) daily oral. Enema (5 mL 18% + 155 mL water): 30 mL (newborn), 60 mL (1–12 mo), 60–120 mL (>12 mo) PR.

Docusate sodium 50 mg + sennoside 8 mg, tab   >12 yr: 1–4 tab at night oral. See also bisacodyl; casanthranol; dantron.

Domperidone   Oral: 0.2–0.4 mg/kg (adult 10–20 mg) 4–8 H. Rectal suppos: adult (NOT/kg) 30–60 mg 4–8 H.

Dopamine   <30 kg: 15 mg/kg in 50 mL at 1–3 mL/hr (5–15 mcg/kg/min) via CVC; >30 kg: 6 mg/kg made up to 100 mL at 5–15 mL/hr (5–15 mcg/kg/min).

Dopexamine   IV infsn 0.5–6 mcg/kg/min.

Dornase alpha (deoxyribonuclease I)   NOT/kg: usually 2.5 mg (max 10 mg) inhaled daily (5–21 yr), 12–24 H (>21 yr).

Dosulepin hydrochloride   See dothiepin.

Dothiepin   0.5–1 mg/kg (adult 25–50 mg) 8–12 H oral.

Doxapram   5 mg/kg IV over 1 hr, then 0.5–1 mg/kg/hr for 1 hr (max total dose 400 mg).

Doxercalciferol (1,25-OH D2 analogue)   Initially 0.2 mcg/kg (adult 10 mcg) oral, or 0.08 mcg/kg (adult 4 mcg) IV, x3/wk at end of dialysis. Aim for blood iPTH 150–300 pg/mL.

Doxycycline   Over 8 yr: 2 mg/kg (adult 100 mg) 12 H for 2 doses, then daily oral. Severe: 2 mg/kg 12 H. Malaria prophylaxis: 2 mg/kg (adult 100 mg) daily oral.

Doxycycline 30 mg + 10 mg slow release (Oracea)   Rosacea in adults (NOT/kg): 1 tab daily oral.

D-penicillamine   See penicillamine.

Droperidol   Antiemetic: postop 0.02–0.05 mg/kg (adult 1.25 mg) 4–6 H IM or slow IV, chemotherapy 0.02–0.1 (adult 1–5 mg) 1–6 H. Psychiatry, neuroleptanalgesia, IM or slow IV: 0.1 mg/kg (adult 2.5 mg) stat, incr to max 0.3 mg/kg (adult 15 mg) 4–6 H. Psychiatry, oral: 0.1–0.4 mg/kg (adult 5–20 mg) 4–8 H.

Econazole nitrate   Topical: 1% cream, powder or lotion 8–12 H. Vaginal: 75 mg cream or 150 mg ovule twice daily.

Eformoterol   Caps 12 mg (NOT/kg): 1 cap (5–12 yr) or 1–2 caps (adult) inhaled 12 H.

Eformoterol + fluticasone (5/50 mcg, 5/125, 10/250)   NOT/kg. ≥12 yr: 2 inhalations 12 H.

Enalapril   0.1 mg/kg (adult 2.5 mg) daily oral, incr over 2 wk if reqd to max 0.5 mg/kg (adult 5–20 mg) 12 H.

Enoxaparin (1 mg = 100 U)   1.5 mg/kg (<2 mo), 1 mg/kg (2 mo to 18 yr), 40 mg (adult) 12 H SC (anti-Xa 0.5–1 U/mL 4 hr post dose). Prophylaxis: 0.75 mg/kg 12 H (<2 mo), 0.5 mg/kg 12 H (2 mo to 18 yr), 20–40 mg 2–12 hr preop, then daily (adult) SC. Haemodialysis: 1 mg/kg into arterial line at start 4 hr session.

Enoximone   IV: 5–20 mcg/kg/min. Oral: 1–3 mg/kg (adult 50–150 mg) 8 H.

Ephedrine   0.25–1 mg/kg (adult 12.5–60 mg) 4–8 H oral, IM, SC, IV. Nasal (0.25%-1%): 1 drop each nostril 6–8 H, max 4 days.

Epoetin alfa, beta, delta, theta, zeta   20–50 U/kg x3/wk, incr to 75–300 U/kg/wk divided into 1–3 doses/wk SC, IV. If Hb >10 g%: 20–100 U/kg x2–3/wk.

Epoprostenol (prostacyclin, PGI2)   Dilute to 2–10 mcg/mL, new syringe every 8 hr. <8 kg: 12 mcg/kg in 10 mL diluent at 0.25–0.75 mL/hr (5–15 ng/kg/min); >8 kg: 500 mcg in 50 mL diluent at 0.03–0.09 mL/kg/hr (5–15 ng/kg/min). ECMO: 5 ng/kg/min IV.Chronic pul ht: 2 ng/kg/min IV, incr to 20–40 ng/kg/min.

Ergocalciferol (Vitamin D2)   40 U = 1 mcg = 1 mcg cholecalciferol (D3). Cystic fib, cholestasis: 10–20 mcg daily oral. Cirrhosis: adult 40–120 mcg daily oral. Deficiency: 50–100 mcg daily for 2 wk oral, then 10–625 mcg daily (more if severe malabs); or 2.5–5 mg (100,000–200,000 U) every 6–8 wk. Monitor serum calcium; measure alk phos and parathyroid hormone after 6–8 wk. See also doxercalciferol.

Ergometrine maleate   Adult (NOT/kg): 250–500 mcg IM or IV; 500 mcg 8 H oral, sublingual or PR.

Ergometrine maleate 0.5 mg + oxytocin 5 U in 1 mL   1 mL IM; may repeat after 2 hr, max 3 doses in 24 hr.

Ergonovine maleate   See ergometrine maleate.

Ergotamine tartrate >10 yr (NOT/kg): 2 mg sublingual stat, then 1 mg/hr (max 6 mg/episode, 10 mg/wk). Suppos (1–2 mg): 1 stat, may repeat once after 1 hr. See also caffeine + ergot.

Erythromycin Oral or slow IV (max 5 mg/kg/hr): usually 10 mg/kg (adult 250–500 mg) 6 H; severe inftn 15–25 mg/kg (adult 0.75–1 g) 6 H. Gut prokinetic: 2 mg/kg 8 H. 2% gel: apply 12 H.

Esmolol 0.5 mg/kg (500 mcg/kg) IV over 1 min, repeat if reqd. Infsn (undiluted 10 mg/mL soltn; or 2.5 g diluted to 250 mL): 0.15–1.8 mL/hr (25–300 mcg/kg/min); rarely given for >48 hr.

Esomeprazole 0.4–0.8 mg/kg (adult 20–40 mg) daily oral. *H. pylori*, see omeprazole.

Esomeprazole + naproxen (375/20, 500 mg/20 mg) Adult (NOT/kg): 1 tab 12 H before meal oral.

Etanercept Adult (NOT/kg): 50 mg wkly SC.

Ethacrynic acid IV: 0.5–1 mg/kg (adult 25–50 mg) 12–24 H. Oral: 1–4 mg/kg (adult 50–200 mg) 12–24 H.

Ethambutol hydrochloride 25 mg/kg once daily for 8 wk, then 15 mg/kg daily oral. Intermittent: 35 mg/kg x3/wk. IV: 80% oral dose.

Ethamsylate 12.5 mg/kg (max 500 mg) 6 H oral, IM, IV.

Ethanol, dehydrated (100%) Vessel sclerosis: inject max of 1 mL/kg.

Ethanolamine oleate 5% soltn, adult (NOT/kg): 1.5–5 mL per varix (max 20 mL per treatment).

Ethionamide TB: 15–20 mg/kg (max 1 g) at night oral. Leprosy: 5–8 mg/kg (max 375 mg) daily.

Ethosuximide 10 mg/kg (adult 500 mg) daily oral, incr by 50% each wk to max 40 mg/kg (adult 2 g) daily. Trough level 0.3–0.7 mmol/L.

Etidocaine 0.5–1.5% soltn: max 6 mg/kg (0.6 mL/kg of 1%) parenteral, or 8 mg/kg (0.8 mL/kg of 1%) with adrenaline.

Etidronate 5–20 mg/kg daily oral (no food for 2 hr before and after dose) for max 6 mo. IV: 7.5 mg/kg daily for 3–7 days.

Etomidate 0.3 mg/kg slow IV.

Factor 8 concentrate (vial 200–250 U), recombinant antihaemophilic factor (rAHF) Joint 20 U/kg, psoas 30 U/kg, cerebral 50 U/kg. 2 × dose (u/kg) = % normal activity, for example 35 U/kg gives peak level of 70% normal. See also Von Willebrand factor/Factor VII concentrate.

Factor 8 inhibitor bypassing fraction IV max 2 U/kg/min: joint 50 U/kg 12 H, mucous membrane 50 U/kg 6 H, soft tissue 100 U/kg 12 H, cerebral 100 U/kg 6–12 H.

Famciclovir Severe infection: 320 mg/m^2 (adult 500 mg) 8 H oral. Zoster, varicella: 160 mg/m^2 (adult 250 mg) 8 H oral for 7 days; immunocompromised 320 mg/m^2 (adult 500 mg) 8 H for 10 days. Genital herpes (adult, NOT/kg): 125 mg 12 H oral for 5 days (treat), 250 mg (suppress) 12 H; immunocompromised 500 mg 12 H for 7 days (treat), 500 mg daily (suppress).

Famotidine 0.5–1 mg/kg (adult 20–40 mg) 12–24 H oral. 0.5 mg/kg (max 20 mg) 12 H slow IV.

Fat emulsion 20% See lipid emulsion.

Felodipine 0.1 mg/kg (adult 2.5 mg) daily, incr if reqd to 0.5 mg/kg (adult 10 mg) daily oral.

Fenoterol Oral: 0.1 mg/kg 6 H. Resp soltn 1 mg/mL: 0.5 mL diluted to 2 mL 3–6 H (mild), 1 mL diluted to 2 mL 1–2 H (moderate), undiluted continuous (severe, in ICU). Aerosol (200 mcg/puff): 1–2 puffs 4–8 H.

Fentanyl Not ventltd: 1–2 mcg/kg (adult 50–100 mcg) IM or IV; infsn 2–4 mcg/kg/hr (<10 kg 100 mcg/kg in 50 mL at 1–2 mL/hr; >10 kg amp 50 mcg/mL at 0.04–0.08 mL/kg/hr). Ventilated: 5–10 mcg/kg stat or 50 mcg/kg IV over 1 hr; infuse amp 50 mcg/mL at 0.1–0.2 mL/kg/hr (5–10 mcg/kg/hr). Patch (lasts 72 hr) in adult (NOT/kg): 25 mcg/hr, incr if reqd by 25 mcg/hr every 3 days. Transmucosal tabs (adult, NOT/kg): 100 mcg between cheek and upper gum until dissolved (15–30 min) 4–8 H, incr if reqd to max 800 mg 4 H. Buccal film: 200 mcg incr to max 1200 mcg x4/day. Nasal spray (adult, NOT/kg): 50, 100 or 200 mcg doses titrated to response. Epidural: 0.5 mcg/kg stat, or 0.4 mcg/kg/hr.

Ferrous salts Prophylaxis 2 mg/kg/day elemental iron oral, treatment 6 mg/kg/day elemental iron oral. Fumarate 1 mg = 0.33 mg iron. Gluconate 1 mg = 0.12 mg iron; so Fergon (60 mg/mL gluconate) prophylaxis 0.3 mL/kg daily, treatment 1 mL/kg daily oral. Sulphate (dry) 1 mg = 0.3 mg iron; so Ferro-Gradumet (350 mg dry sulphate) prophylaxis 7 mg/kg (adult 350 mg) daily, treatment 20 mg/kg (adult 1050 mg) daily oral.

Filgrastim (granulocyte CSF) Idiopathic or cyclic neutropaenia: 5 mcg/kg daily SC or IV over 30 min. Cong neutropaenia: 12 mcg/kg daily SC or IV over 1 hr. Marrow trans: 20–30 mcg/kg daily IV over 4–24 hr, reduce if neutrophil >1×10^9/L.

Flecainide   2–3 mg/kg (max 100 mg) 12 H oral, may incr over 2 wk to 7 mg/kg (max 200 mg) 8–12 H. IV in 5%D over 30 min.

Flucloxacillin   Oral: 12.5–25 mg/kg (adult 250–500 mg) 6 H. IM or IV: 25 mg/kg (adult 1 g) 6 H. Severe inftn: 50 mg/kg (adult 2 g) IV 12 H (1st wk life), 8 H (2–4 wk), 6 H or constant infsn (>4 wk). See also ampicillin + flucloxacillin.

Fluconazole   12 mg/kg (adult 200–400 mg) daily IV, higher doses if very severe infection; if haemofiltered 12 mg/kg (adult 600 mg) 12 H; neonate 12 mg/kg 72 H (<14 days) 48 H (15–28 days). Superficial inftn: 6 mg/kg (adult 200 mg) stat, then 3 mg/kg (adult 100 mg) daily oral or IV.

Flucytosine (5-fluorocytosine)   400–1200 mg/m^2 (max 2 g) 6 H IV over 30 min, or oral. Peak level 50–100 mcg/mL, trough 25–50 mcg/mL (x7.75 = µmol/L).

Fludrocortisone acetate   150 mcg/m^2 daily oral. Fludrocortisone 1 mg = hydrocortisone 125 mg in mineralocorticoid activity, 10 mg in glucocorticoid.

Flumazenil   5 mcg/kg every 60 sec to max total 40 mcg/kg (adult 2 mg), then 2–10 mcg/kg/hr IV.

Flunitrazepam   Adult (NOT/kg): 0.5–2 mg at night, oral.

Fluoxetine   0.5 mg/kg (max 20 mg) daily, incr to max 1 mg/kg (max 40 mg) 12 H oral. Weekly 90 mg cap: 1 per wk.

Fluoxetine + olanzapine (25 mg/6 mg, 25 mg/12 mg, 50 mg/6 mg, 50 mg/12 mg)   Adult (NOT/kg): 1 cap daily oral.

Fluticasone   Inhaled (NOT/kg): 50–100 mcg (child), 100–500 mcg (adult) 12 H. 0.05% soltn: 1–4 sprays/nostril daily. 0.05% cream: apply daily. See also azelastine, eformoterol.

Fluticasone + salmeterol   NOT/kg. Accuhaler: 100 mcg/50 mcg (child), 250/50 or 500/50 (adult) x1–2 inhltn 12 H. MDI: 50/25 (child), 125/25 or 250/25 x1–2 inhltn 12 H.

Fluvastatin   0.4 mg/kg (adult 20 mg) nocte oral, incr to 0.8 mg/kg (adult 40 mg) 12 H if reqd. Slow release: 80 mg nocte.

Fluvoxamine   2 mg/kg (adult 100 mg) 8–24 H oral. Slow release (adult, NOT/kg): 100–300 mg at night oral.

Folic acid   NOT/kg. Deficiency: 50 mcg (neonate), 0.1–0.25 mg (<4 yr), 0.5–1 mg (>4 yr) daily IV, IM, SC or oral. Metabolic dis: 5 mg/day oral. Pregnancy: 0.5 mg (high risk 4 mg) daily oral.

Follicle stimufating hormone (FSH)   Adult (NOT/kg), monitor urinary oestrogen. Anovulation: usually 50–150 i.u. SC daily for 9–12 days. Superovulation (2 wk after starting GnRH agonist): 100–225 iu/kg daily starting day 3 of cycle.

Formoterol   >4 yr (NOT/kg). Powder: 12 mcg inhalation 12 H. Solutn: 20 mcg in 2 mL nebulised 12 H. See also budesonide.

Formoterol + mometasone (5 mcg/100 mcg, 5 mcg/200 mcg)   MDI 2 puffs 12 H.

Foscarnet   20 mg/kg IV over 30 min, then 200 mg/kg/day by constant IV infsn (less if creatinine >0.11 mmol/l) or 60 mg/kg 8 H IV over 2 hr. Chronic use: 90–120 mg/kg IV over 2 hr daily.

Framycetin sulfate (Soframycin)   Subconjunctival: 500 mg in 1 mL water daily x3 days. Bladder: 500 mg in 50 mL saline 8 H × 10 days. 0.5%: eye 1 drop 8 H, ear 3 drops 8 H, ointment 8 H.

Framycetin sulfate 15 mg/g + gramicidin 0.05 mg/g   Cream or ointment (Soframycin topical): apply 8–12 H. See also dexamethasone + framycetin + gramicidin.

Fresh frozen plasma   Contains all clotting factors. 10–20 mL/kg IV. 1 bag is about 230 mL.

Frusemide   Usually 0.5–1 mg/kg (adult 20–40 mg) 6–24 H (daily if preterm) oral, IM, or IV over 20 min (max 0.05 mg/kg/min IV). IV infsn: 0.1–1 mg/kg/hr (<20 kg 25 mg/kg in 50 mL 0.9% saline with heparin 1 U/mL at 0.2–2 mL/hr; >20 kg amp 10 mg/mL at 0.01–0.1 mL/kg/hr); protect from light.

Fusidic acid   Fusidic acid (susp) absorption only 70% that of sodium fusidate (tabs). Suspension: 15–20 mg/kg (adult 750 mg) 8 H oral. Eye%: 1 drop/eye 12 H. For tablets and IV, see sodium fusidate.

Gabapentin   Anticonvulsant: 10 mg/kg (adult 300 mg) once day 1 oral, 12 H day 2, 8 H day 3 then adjusted to 10–20 mg/kg (adult 300–1200 mg) 8 H. Premed: 25 mg/kg (adult 1200 mg) 1 hr preop. Analgesia: 2 mg/kg (adult 100 mg) 8 H, incr if reqd to 15 mg/kg (adult 800 mg) or higher if tolerated. Adult (NOT/kg) with evening meal oral: restless legs 600 mg dialy, postherpetic neuralgia 300 mg incr over 4 wk to 1800 mg daily.

Ganciclovir   5 mg/kg 12 H IV over 1 hr for 2–3 wk; then 5 mg/kg IV daily, or 6 mg/kg IV on 6 days/wk, or 20 mg/kg (adult 1 g) 8 H oral. Congenital CMV: 7.5 mg/kg 12 H IV over 2 hr.

Gentamicin   IV or IM. 1 wk to 10 yr: 8 mg/kg day 1, then 6 mg/kg daily. >10 yr: 7 mg/kg day 1, then 5 mg/kg (max 240–360 mg) daily. Neonate, 5 mg/kg dose: <1200 g 48 H (0–7 days of life), 36 H (8–30 days), 24 H (>30 days); 1200–2500 g 36 H (0–7 days of life), 24 H (>7 days); term 24 H (0–7 days of life), then as for 1 wk to 10 yr. Trough level <1.0 mg/L.

Gentamicin, eye drops   0.3% 1 drop/eye every 15 min if severe, reducing to 1 drop 4–6 H.

Glibenclamide   Adult (NOT/kg): initially 2.5 mg daily oral, max 20 mg daily.

Glibenclamide + metformin   Adult (NOT/kg): 1.25 mg/250 mg 12–24 H oral, incr if reqd to 2.5 mg/500 mg or 5 mg/500 mg (max 10 mg/1000 mg) 12 H.

Glucagon   1 U = 1 mg. 0.04 mg/kg (adult 1–2 mg) IV or IM stat, then 10–50 mcg/kg/hr (0.5 mg/kg in 50 mL at 1–5 mL/hr) IV. Beta-blocker overdose: 0.1 mg/kg IV stat, then 0.3–2 mcg/kg/min.

Glucarpidase   50 U/kg IV over 5 min.

Glucosamine   Adult (NOT/kg): 1500 mg daily oral.

Glucose   See dextrose.

Glucose electrolyte solution   Not dehydrated: 1 heaped teaspoon sucrose in large cup of water (4% sucrose = 2% glucose); do NOT add salt. Dehydrated: 1 sachet of Gastrolyte in 200 mL water; give frequent sips, or infuse by NG tube.

Glutamic acid   10–20 mg/kg (adult 0.5–1 g) oral with meals.

Glyceryl trinitrate   Adult (NOT/kg): sublingual tab 0.3–0.9 mg/dose (lasts 30–60 min); sublingual aerosol 0.4–1.2 mg/dose; slow-release buccal tab 1–10 mg 8–12 H; transdermal 0.5–5 cm of 2% ointment, or 5–15 mg patch 8–12 H; anal fissure 2.5 cm 0.4% ointment 12 H. IV infsn 0.5–5 mcg/kg/min (<30 kg 3 mg/kg in 50 mL at 0.5–5 mL/hr; >30 kg 3 mg/kg made up to 100 mL at 1–10 mL/hr); use special non-PVC tubing.

Glycopyrrolate   To reduce secretions or treat bradycardia: 5–10 mcg/kg (adult 0.2–0.4 mg) 6–8 H IV or IM. With 0.05 mg/kg neostigmine: 10–15 mcg/kg IV. Anticholinergic: 0.02–0.04 mg/kg (max 2 mg) 8 H oral.

Glycopyrronium   Dose as for glycopyrrolate. Inhaled (adult, NOT/kg): 50 mcg daily.

Gramicidin 25 mcg/mL + neomycin 2.5 mg/mL + polymyxin B 5000 U/mL (Neosporin)   Eye drops: 1 drop/eye every 15–30 min, reducing to 6–12 H. See also dexamethasone.

Griseofulvin (Grisovin, Fulcin)   10–20 mg/kg (adult 0.5–1 g) daily oral.

Haemophilus influenzae type b, vaccines   Inanimate. <12 mo: give diphtheria protein conjugate (HibTITER, ProHIBiT), or tetanus conjugate (Act-HIB, Hiberix) 0.5 mL IM at 2 mo, 4 mo, 6 mo and 15 mo; or meningococcal conjugate (Pedvax HIB) 0.5 mL IM at 2 mo, 4 mo and 15 mo. If 1st dose >18 mo: give 1 dose of HibTITER or Pedvax HIB.

Haemophilus influenzae type b + hepatitis B vaccine (Comvax)   Inanimate. 0.5 mL IM 2 mo, 4 mo, 12–15 mo (3 doses).

Haemophilus influenzae type b + meningococcus type c vaccine (Menitorix)   Inanimate. 0.5 mL IM 2 mo, 3 mo, 4 mo (3 doses); boost from 12 mo.

Haloperidol   0.01 mg/kg (max 0.5 mg) daily, incr up to 0.1 mg/kg 12 H IV or oral; up to 2 mg/kg (max 100 mg) 12 H used rarely. Acutely disturbed: 0.1–0.2 mg/kg (adult 5–10 mg) IM. Long-acting decanoate ester: 1–6 mg/kg IM every 4 wk.

Heparin   1 mg = 100 U. Low dose: 75 U/kg IV stat, then 500 U/kg in 50 mL 0.9% saline at 1–1.5 mL/hr (10–15 U/kg/hr) IV. Full dose: 75 U/kg (adult 5000 U) IV stat, then 500 U/kg in 50 mL saline at 2–4 mL/hr (20–40 U/kg/hr)<12 mo, 2–3 mL/hr (20–30 U/kg/hr) child, 1.5–2 mL/hr (15–20 U/kg/hr) adult; adjust to give APTT 60–85 sec, or anti-Xa 0.3–0.7 U/mL. Hep lock: 100 U/mL.

Heparin calcium   Low dose: 75 U/kg SC 12 H.

Heparin, low molecular weight   See certoparin, dalteparin, danaparoid, enoxaparin, nadroparin.

Hepatitis A vaccine (Havrix)   Inanimate. 0.5 mL (child) or 1 mL (adult) IM stat, and in 6–12 mo (2 doses). Boost every 5 yr.

Hepatitis A vaccine (VAQTA)   Inanimate. 0.5 mL (child) or 1 mL (>17 yr) IM stat, and after 6–18 mo (2 doses).

Hepatitis A + hepatitis B vaccine (Twinrix)   Inanimate. 1–15 yr 0.5 mL, >15 yr 1 mL IM stat, after 1 mo, and after 6 mo (3 doses). Boost every 5 yr.

Hepatitis B immune globulin   See immunoglobulin, hep B.

Hepatitis B vaccine (Engerix-B, HB Vax II) Inanimate. Engerix-B 10 mcg/dose (<10 yr), 20 mcg (>9 yr); HB Vax II 2.5 mcg/dose (<10 yr), 5 mcg (10–19 yr), 10 mcg (>19 yr), 40 mcg (dialysis) IM stat, after 1 mo, and after 6 mo (3 doses). Boost every 5 yr. See diphtheria and haemophilus vaccines.

Herpes zoster vaccine (Zostavax) Live. Age 50 yr or more: 0.65 mL SC once. See also Immunoglobulin, zoster.

Homatropine 2%, 5% soltn: 1 drop/eye 4 H.

Hydralazine 0.1–0.2 mg/kg (adult 5–10 mg) stat IV or IM, then 4–6 mcg/kg/min (adult 200–300 mcg/min) IV. Oral: 0.4 mg/kg (adult 20 mg) 12 H, slow incr to 1.5 mg/kg (max 50 mg) 6–8 H.

Hydrochloric acid Use soltn of 100 mmol/L (0.1 M = 0.1 N = 100 mEq/L); give IV by central line only. Alkalosis: dose(mL) = BE × Wt × 3 (give half this); maximum rate 2 mL/kg/hr. Blocked central line: 1.5 mL/lumen over 2–4 hr.

Hydrochlorothiazide 1–1.5 mg/kg (adult 25–50 mg) 12–24 H.

Hydrochlorothiazide + quinapril 10/12.5, 20/12.5 Adult (NOT/kg): 10/12.5 tab daily oral, incr if reqd to 20/12.5 tab, max two 10/12.5 tab daily.

Hydrocortisone Usually 0.5–2 mg/kg (adult 25–50 mg) 6–8 H oral, reducing as tolerated. 0.5%, 1% cream, ointment: apply 6–12 H. 1% cream + clioquinol: apply 8–24 H. 10% rectal foam: 125 mg/dose. 2.5% eye ointment: apply 6 H.

Hydrocortisone sodium succinate 2–4 mg/kg 3–6 H IM, IV reducing as tolerated. Physiological: 5 mg/m^2 6–8 H oral; 0.2 mg/kg 8 H IM, IV. Physiological, stress: 1 mg/kg 6 H IM, IV.

Hydrogen peroxide 10 volume (3%). Mouthwash 1:2 parts water. Skin or ear disinfectant 1:1 part water.

Hydromorphone Oral: 0.05–0.1 mg/kg (adult 2–4 mg) 4 H. IM, SC: 0.02–0.05 mg/kg (adult 1–2 mg) 4–6 H. Slow IV: 0.01–0.02 mg/kg (adult 0.5–1 mg) 4–6 H. Palliative care: incr to 40–50 mg/day (up to 500 mg/day) oral in divided doses. 1 mg = 4 mg oxycodone.

Hydroxocobalamin (Vit B12) 20 mcg/kg (adult 1000 mcg) IM daily for 7 days then wkly (treatment), then every 2–3 mo (prophylaxis); IV dangerous in megaloblastic anaemia. Homocystinuria, methylmalonic acidur: 1 mg daily IM; after response, some patients maintained on 1–10 mg daily oral.

Hydroxychloroquine sulphate Doses as sulphate. Malaria: 10 mg/kg (max 600 mg) daily for 3 days; prophylaxis 5 mg/kg (max 300 mg) once a wk oral. Arthritis, SLE: 3–6.5 mg/kg (adult 200–600 mg) daily oral.

Hydroxyzine 0.5–2 mg/kg (adult 25–100 mg) 6–8 H oral. 0.5–1 mg/kg (adult 25–100 mg) 4–6 H if reqd IM.

Hyoscine hydrobromide (scopalamine hydrobromide) 6–8 mcg/kg (adult 400–600 mcg) 6–8 H IV, IM, SC. Motion sickness 300 mcg tab (NOT/kg): 0.25 tab (2–7 yr), 0.5 tab (7–12 yr), 1–2 tab (>12 yr) 6–24 H oral 30 min before, may repeat in 4 hr. Transdermal (1.5 mg patch): >10 yr 1 every 72 hr.

Hyoscine hydrobromide (0.4 mg/mL) + papaveretum (20 mg/mL) 0.008 mg/kg (H) + 0.4 mg/kg (P) = 0.02 mL/kg/dose IM.

Hyoscine methobromide (methscopalamine) 0.2 mg/kg (adult 2.5–5 mg) 6 H oral.

Hyoscyamine (L-atropine) 2–5 mcg/kg (adult 100–300 mcg) 4–6 H oral, sublingual, IM or IV.

Ibuprofen 5–10 mg/kg (adult 200–400 mg) 4–8 H oral, IV. Arthritis: 10 mg/kg (adult 400–800 mg) 6–8 H. Cystic fibrosis: 20–30 mg/kg 12 H. PDA: 10 mg/kg stat, then 5 mg/kg after 24 and 48 hr IV over 15 min. See also famotidine + ibuprofen.

Imipenem (+ cilastatin) 15 mg/kg (adult 500 mg) 6 H IV over 30 min. Severe inftn: 25 mg/kg IV over 1 hr (adult 1 g) 12 H (1st wk life), 8 H (2–4 wk), 6–8 H or constant infsn (4+ wk).

Imipramine 0.5–1.5 mg/kg (adult 25–75 mg) 8 H oral. Enuresis: 5–6 yr 25 mg, 7–10 yr 50 mg, >10 yr 50–75 mg nocte.

Immunoglobulin See also antivenoms.

Immunoglobulin, CMV 100–200 mg/kg IV over 2 hr. Transplant: daily for first 3 days, wkly x6, monthly x6.

Immunoglobulin, diphtheria 250 U IM once.

Immunoglobulin, hepatitis B 400 U IM within 5 days of needle stick, repeat in 30 days; 100 U IM within 24 hr birth to baby of Hep B carrier.

Immunoglobulin, antilymphocyte (thymocyte) Horse (Atgam): 10–15 mg/kg daily for 3–5 days IV over 4 hr; occasionally up to 30 mg/kg daily. Rabbit (ATG-Fresenius): 2.5–5 mg/kg daily over 4–6 hr IV.

Immunoglobulin, normal, human Hypogammaglobulinaemia: 10–15 mL/kg of 6% soltn (600–900 mg/kg) IV over 5–8 hr, then 5–7.5 mL/kg (300–450 mg/kg) over 3–4 hr monthly; or 0.6 mL/kg of 16% soltn (100 mg/kg) every 2–4 wk IM. Sepsis: 0.5 g/kg IV over 4 hr. Kawasaki, Guillain-Barre, ITP, myasth gravis, Still's dis: 35 mL/kg of 6% soltn (2 g/kg) IV over 16 hr stat, then if required 15 mL/kg (900 mg/kg) IV over 8 hr each month. Prevention hep A: 0.1 mL/kg (16 mg/kg) IM. Prevention measles: 0.2 mL/kg (32 mg/kg) IM (repeat next day if immunocompromised).

Immunoglobulin, rabies (Hyperab, Imogam) 20 i.u. (0.133 mL)/kg IM once (half SC around wound), with rabies vaccine.

Immunoglobulin, Rh (anti-D) 1 mL (625 iu, 125 mcg) IM within 72 hr of exposure. Large transfusion: 0.16 mL (100 iu, 20 mcg) per mL RH positive red cells (maternal serum should be anti-D positive 24–48 hr after injection).

Immunoglobulin, respiratory syncytial virus 750 mg/kg every month IV (50 mg/mL: 1.5 mL/kg/hr for 15 min, 3 mL/kg/hr for 15 min, then 6 mL/kg/hr).

Immunoglobulin, subcutanoeus (SCIG) Multiply previous IV immunoglobulin dose by 1.37, and divide this into weekly doses. Usually 100–200 mg/kg by SC infusion weekly.

Immunoglobulin, tetanus (TIG) IM preparation, prophylaxis: 250–500 i.u. (1–2 amp). IV preparation, treatment: 4000 i.u. (100 mL) at 0.04 mL/kg/min for 30 min, then 0.075 mL/kg/min IV; intrathecal usually 250 iu.

Immunoglobulin, zoster 1 i.u. ≈ 1.5 mg. Within 96 hr of exposure: 0–10 kg 300 mg, 11–30 kg 600 mg, >30 kg 900 mg IM.

Indomethacin 0.5–1 mg/kg (adult 25–50 mg) 8 H (max 6 H) oral or PR. PDA: 0.1 mg/kg (<1 kg) or 0.2 mg/kg (> = 1 kg) day 1, then 0.1 mg/kg daily days 2–7 oral or IV over 1 hr.

Infliximab 3 mg/kg (arthritis, with methotrexate) 5 mg/kg (Crohn's) IV over 2 hr, then (if response) after 2 wk, 6 wk, and then 5–10 mg/kg every 8 wk.

Influenza A and B vaccine (Fluvax, Vaxigrip) Inanimate. 0.125 mL (3 mo-2 yr), 0.25 mL (2–6 yr), 0.5 mL (>6 yr) SC stat and 4 wk later (2 doses). Boost annually (1 dose).

Influenza A and B live nasal vaccine (Flumist) >5 yr: 0.25 mL/nostril; repeat after 6 wk if aged 5–8 yr and previously unimmunised. Boost annually (1 dose).

Insulin Regular insulin IV: 0.025–0.1 U/kg p.r.n., or 0.025–0.1 U/kg/hr (2.5 U/kg in 50 mL 4% albumin at 0.5–2 mL/hr); later 1 U/10 g dextrose. For hyperkalaemia: 0.1 U/kg insulin and 2 mL/kg 50% dextrose IV. In TPN: 5–25 U/250 g dextrose. SC insulin (onset/peak/duration): glulisine, lispro 10–15 min/1 hr/2–5 hr; aspart 15–20 min/1 hr/3–5 hr; inhaled 10–15 min/1 hr/6 hr; regular $\frac{1}{2}$–1 hr/2 hr/6–8 hr; detemir 1–2 hr/flat/24 hr; glargine 1–2 hr/flat/24 hr; isophane (NPH) 2–4 hr/4–12 hr/18–20 hr; zinc (lente) 2–3 hr/7–15 hr/24 hr; crystalline zinc (ultralente) 4–6 hr/10–30 hr/24–36 hr; protamine zinc 4–8 hr/15–20 hr/24–36 hr.

Insulin (Exubera) Initially 30–39 kg 1 mg, 40–59 kg 2 mg, 60–79 kg 3 mg, 80–99 kg 4 mg, inhaled 10 min before meal.

Interferon alfa-2a, recombinant Haemangioma: 1 million u/m^2 daily SC or IM incr over 4 wk to 2–3 million u/m^2 daily for 16–24 wk, then x3/wk. Hep B, C: 3–6 million u/m^2 x3/wk SC or IM for 4–6 mo; higher doses may be reqd in hep B.

Interferon alfa-2b, recombinant Condylomata: 1 million unit into each lesion (max 5) x3/wk for 5 wk. Haemangioma: as for interferon alfa-2a. Hep B: monotherapy as for interferon alfa-2a. Hep C (adult, NOT/kg) 3 million unit x3/wk SC, plus ribavirin 1000 mg (1200 mg if >75 kg) daily oral, for 24–48 wk.

Interferon alfa-2a/alfa-2b, pegylated See peginterferon.

Interferon alfa-n3 Warts (NOT/kg): 250,000 U injected into base of wart (max 10 doses/session) x2/wk for max 8 wk.

Interferon alfacon-1 Hepatitis C (adult, NOT/kg): usually 9 mcg (7.5 mcg if not tolerated) x3/wk SC for 24 wk; if relapse 15 mcg x3/wk SC for 6 mo.

Interferon beta-1a Mult scler (adult, NOT/kg): Avonex 30 mcg (6 million IU) once a wk IM, Rebif 44 mcg x3/wk SC.

Interferon beta-1b Mult scler (adult, NOT/kg): 250 mcg (8 million IU) SC alternate days.

Interferon gamma-1b Chronic gran dis: 1.5 mcg/kg (body area < = 0.5 m^2) or 50 mcg/m^2 (area >0.5 m^2) x3/wk SC.

Ipecacuanha syrup (total alkaloids 1.4 mg/mL)   1–2 mL/kg (adult 30 mL) stat oral, NG. May repeat once in 30 min.

Ipratropium bromide   Resp soltn (250 mcg/mL): 0.25–1 mL diluted to 4 mL 4–8 H; severe attack every 20 min for 3 doses, then 4–6 H. Aerosol 20 mcg/puff: 2–4 puffs 6–8 H. Nasal: 84 mcg/nostril 6–12 H.

Iron   See ferric salts, ferrous salts.

Iron dextran, iron polymaltose, iron sucrose   Fe 50 mg/mL: dose (mL) = 0.05 × Wt in kg × (15 − Hb in g%) IM (often in divided doses). IV infsn possible (but dangerous).

Isoconazole   1% cream 12 H. Vaginal: 600 mg (2 tab) once.

Isoetharine   Inhaltn soltn (1%): 0.5 mL diltd to 4 mL 3–6 H (mild), 1 mL diltd to 4 mL 1–2 H (moderate), undiltd constant (severe, in ICU). Aerosol 340 mcg/puff: 1–2 puffs 4–6 H.

Isoniazid (INAH)   10 mg/kg (max 300 mg) daily oral, IM or IV. Intermittent: 15 mg/kg 3 times a week. TB meningitis: 15–20 mg/kg (max 500 mg) daily.

Isoprenaline   IV infsn: <33 kg 0.3 mg/kg in 50 mL at 0.5–10 mL/hr (0.05–1 mcg/kg/min); >33 kg give 1/5000 (0.2 mg/mL) soltn at 0.015–0.15 mL/hr (0.05–0.5 mcg/kg/min).

Isosorbide dinitrate   Sublingual: 0.1–0.2 mg/kg (max 10 mg) 2 H or as needed. Oral: 0.5–1 mg/kg (max 40 mg) 6 H or as needed. Slow-release tab, adult (NOT/kg): 20–80 mg 12 H. IV infsn 0.6–2 mcg/kg/min.

Isotretinoin   Adult: 0.5–1 mg/kg daily oral for 2–4 wk, reducing if possible to 0.1–0.2 mg/kg daily for 15–20 wk. 0.05% gel: apply sparingly at night.

Isradipine   0.05 mg/kg 12 H oral, may incr after 2–4 wk gradually to 0.1–0.2 mg/kg (max 10 mg) 12 H.

Itraconazole   2–5 mg/kg (adult 100–200 mg) 12–24 H oral after food. Trough level >0.5 mcg/mL at 10–14 days.

Ivermectin   0.2–0.4 mg/kg (adult 12–24 mg) oral; for head lice, repeat after 7–10 days. Head lice: 0.5% lotion to hair for 10 min then rinse; repeat after 7–10 days.

Japanese encephalitis vaccine, inanimate   Ixiaro: adult 0.5 mL IM stat and 28 days later. JE-Vax: 0.5 mL (1–3 yr), 1 mL (>3 yr) SC stat, 7–14 days later, and (optionally) 1 mo later. Boost after 1 yr.

Japanese encephalitis vaccine, live   Imojev: ≥12 mo 0.5 mL SC, boost after 1–2 yr (age 1–17 yr) or 5 yr (adult).

Kanamycin   Single daily dose IV or IM. Neonate: 15 mg/kg stat, then 7.5 mg/kg (<30 wk) 10 mg/kg (30–35 wk) 15 mg/kg (term <1 wk) daily. 1 wk to 10 yr: 25 mg/kg day 1, then 18 mg/kg daily. >10 yr: 20 mg/kg day 1, then 15 mg/kg (max 1.5 g) daily. Trough level <5.0 mg/L.

Keppra   See levetiracetam.

Ketamine   Sedation, analgesia: 2–4 mg/kg IM; infsn 2–6 mcg/kg/min IV (6 mg/kg in 50 mL at 1–3 mL/hr). Anaesthesia: 5–10 mg/kg IM, 1–2 mg/kg IV, infsn 15 mg/kg in 50 mL at 2–8 mL/hr (10–40 mcg/kg/min). Premed: 5 mg/kg oral. Incompatible with aminophylline, magnesium and salbutamol.

Ketoconazole   Oral: 5 mg/kg (adult 200 mg) 12–24 H. 2% cream: apply 12–24 H. 2% shampoo: wash hair, apply liquid for 5 min, wash off.

Ketoprofen   1–2 mg/kg (adult 50–100 mg) 6–12 H (max 4 mg/kg or 200 mg in 24 hr) oral, IM, PR. Slow release, adults (NOT/kg): 200 mg daily.

Ketorolac   Oral: 0.2 mg/kg (adult 10 mg) 4–6 H (max 0.8 mg/kg/day or 40 mg/day). IV or IM: usually 0.2 mg/kg (adult 10 mg) 6 H; but may use 0.6 mg/kg (max 30 mg) stat, then 0.2–0.4 mg/kg (max 20 mg) 4–6 H for 5 days, then 0.2 mg/kg (max 10 mg) 6 H. Nasal 15.75 mg/spray: adult 1 each nostril (≥65 yr 1 nostril). Eye drop 0.5%: 1 drop 8 H.

Ketotifen   Child >2 yr (NOT/kg): 1 mg 12 H oral with food. Adult (NOT/kg): 1–2 mg 12 H oral with food.

Labetalol   Oral: 1–2 mg/kg (adult 50–100 mg) 12 H, may incr wkly to max 10 mg/kg (max 600 mg) 6 H. IV: 0.25–0.5 mg/kg (adult 20 mg) over 2 min repeated every 10 min if reqd, then 0.25–3 mg/kg/hr.

Lactulose   3.3 g/5 mL soltn. Laxative: 0.5 mL/kg 12–24 H oral. Hepatic coma: 1 mL/kg hrly until diarrhoea, then 6–8 H.

Lamotrigine   0.2 mg/kg (adult 25 mg) oral daily, double dose every 2 wk if reqd to max 1–4 mg/kg (adult 50–200 mg) 12 H. Double dose if taking carbamazepine, phenobarbitone, phenytoin or primidone; halve dose if taking valproate.

Latanoprost   50 mcg/mL: 1 drop/eye daily.

Levodopa + benserazide (4:1)   Adult (NOT/kg): initially levodopa 100 mg 8 H oral; if not controlled, incr wkly by 100 mg/day to max 250 mg 6 H.

Levodopa + carbidopa   250 mg/25 mg and 100 mg/10 mg tabs. Adult (NOT/kg): initially one 100/10 tab 8 H oral; if not controlled, substitute one 250/25 tab for one 100/25 tab every 2nd day; if not controlled on 250/25 8 H, incr by one 250/25 tab every 2nd day to max 6–8 tab/day.

Levonorgestrel   Contraception: 30 mcg daily oral, starting 1st day menstruation. Intrauterine T-system 52 mg or 13.5 mg: insert within 7 days of start of menstruation, replace after 3 yr. Post-coital: 1.5 mg oral within 72 hr; or 0.75 mg within 72 hr, repeat after 12 hr; or 0.5 mg + ethinyloestradiol 100 mcg oral within 72 hr, repeat in 12 hr. See also ethinyloestradiol + levonorgestrel, oestradiol + levonorgestrel.

Levonorgestrel + oestradiol (7 mcg/50 mcg, 15 mcg/45 mcg per day) patch   Post-menopausal (NOT/kg): 1 patch/wk.

Lignocaine   IV: 1% soltn 0.1 mL/kg (1 mg/kg) over 2 min, then 0.09–0.3 mL/kg/hr (15–50 mcg/kg/min); or 30 mg/kg in 50 mL at 50 mL/hr for 2 min, then 1.5–15 mL/hr (15–50 mcg/kg/min). Nerve block: without adrenaline max 4 mg/kg (0.4 mL/kg of 1%), with adrenaline 7 mg/kg (0.7 mL/kg of 1%). Topical spray: max 3–4 mg/kg (Xylocaine 10% spray pack: about 10 mg/puff). Topical 2% gel, 2.5% compound mouth paint/gel (SM-33), 2% and 4% soltn, 5% ointment, 10% dental ointment: apply 3 H p.r.n.

Lignocaine 2.5% + prilocaine 2.5%   Cream (EMLA): 1.5 g/10 cm^2 under occlusive dressing for 1–3 hr.

Lincomycin   10 mg/kg (adult 600 mg) 8 H oral, IM or IV over 1 hr. Severe inftn: 15–20 mg/kg (adult 1.2 g) IV over 2 hr 6 H.

Lindane   1% cream, lotion. Scabies: apply from neck down, wash off after 8–12 hr. Lice: rub into hair for 4 min, then wash off; repeat after 24 hr (max x2/wk).

Liothyronine sodium (T3)   Oral: 0.2 mcg/kg (adult 10 mcg) 8 H, may incr to 0.4 mcg/kg (adult 20 mcg) 8 H. IV: 0.1–0.4 mcg/kg (adult 5–20 mcg) 8–12 H. Septic shock: 0.1–0.2 mcg/kg/hr (adult 100–200 mcg/day) IV infsn.

Lipid   20%: 1–3 g/kg/day IV (mL/hr = g/kg/day × Wt × 0.21).

Lisinopril   0.1 mg/kg (adult 5 mg) daily oral, may incr over 4–6 wk to 0.2–1 mg/kg (adult 10–20 mg) daily.

Lithium (salts)   5–20 mg/kg 8–24 H oral. Slow-release tab 450 mg (adult, NOT/kg): 1–2 tab 12 H. Maintain trough level 0.8–1.6 mmol/L (>2 mmol/L toxic).

Loperamide   0.05–0.1 mg/kg (adult 2–4 mg) 8–12 H oral, incr if reqd to max 0.4 mg/kg (max 4 mg) 8 H.

Lorazepam   0.02–0.06 mg/kg (adult 1–3 mg) 8–24 H oral. IV: 0.05–0.2 mg/kg IV over 2 min, then 0.01–0.1 mg/kg/hr.

Lypressin (lysine-8-vasopressin)   1 spray (2.5 iu) into 1 nostril 4–8 H, may incr to 1 spray both nostrils 4–8 H.

Macrogol 3350, 105 g/L   2–11 yr 6.563 g in 60 mL water, >11 yr 13.125 g in 125 mL water: 1 sachet daily oral, incr to 2–3/day if reqd. Faecal impactn >2 yr: one 13.125 g sachet in 125 mL water per 5 kg body wt (adult 8 sachet) consumed in <6 hr (max 3 days therapy). See also colonic lavage.

Macrogol 3350 powder 255 g in 2 L Gatorade   Adult 1 L oral over 1 hr night before, 1 L next morning 5 hr pre-colonoscopy.

Macrogol 400 (polyethylene glycol) 1% + tetrahydrozoline 0.05%   1 drop/eye 8–12 H.

Macrogol 4000   ≥8 yr (NOT/kg): 10–20 g daily oral.

Magnesium chloride 10%   0.48 g/5 mL = Mg 1 mmol/mL. Low Mg: 0.4 mL/kg slow IV, then 0.3 mL/m^2/hr. My infarct (NOT/kg): 5 mL/hr IV for 6 hr, then 1 mL/hr for 24–48 hr. VF: 0.06 mL/kg IV.

Magnesium hydroxide   58 mg = Mg 1 mmol. Low Mg: 7.5 mmol/m^2/day oral (1.4 mL/m^2 6 H of 78 mg/mL soltn). Antacid: 10–40 mg/kg (max 2 g) 6 H oral. Laxative: 50–100 mg/kg (max 5 g). See also Al hydroxide + Mg hydroxide + simethicone.

Magnesium sulphate 50% (2 mmol/mL)   Low Mg: 0.2 mL/kg IM or slow IV, then 0.16 mL/m^2/hr. Asthma, digoxin tachycardia, eclampsia, prem labour, pul ht: 0.1 mL/kg (50 mg/kg) IV over 20 min, then 0.06 mL/kg/hr (30 mg/kg/hr); keep serum Mg 1.5–2.5 mmol/l (pul ht 3–4 mmol/L). Myocardial infarction (NOT/kg): 2.5 mL/hr (5 mmol/hr) IV for 6 hr, then 0.5 mL/hr (1 mmol/hr) for 24–48 hr. VF: 0.05–0.1 mL/kg (0.1–0.2 mmol/kg) IV. Incompatible with aminophylline, ketamine, salbutamol. Laxative: 1 mL/kg = 0.5 g/kg (max 15 g) as 10% soltn 8 H for 2 days oral.

Maldison   0.5% liquid: 20 mL to hair, wash off after 12 hr.

Mannitol   0.25–0.5 g/kg IV (2–4 mL/kg of 12.5%, 1.25–2.5 mL/kg of 20%, 1–2 mL/kg of 25%) 2 H p.r.n., provided serum osmolality <320–330 mmol/L.

Measles vaccine (Attenuvax)   Live. >12 mo: 0.5 mL SC once.

Measles + mumps vaccine (Rimparix)   Live. >12 mo: 0.5 mL SC once.

Measles + mumps + rubella vaccine (MMRII, Priorix)   Live. >12 mo: 0.5 mL SC.

Mebendazole   NOT/kg: 100 mg 12 H × 3 days. Enterobiasis (NOT/kg): 100 mg once, may repeat after 2–4 wks.

Mebeverine   135 mg tab: adult (NOT/kg) 1–3 tab daily oral.

Mefenamic acid   10 mg/kg (adult 500 mg) 8 H oral.

Mefloquine   15 mg/kg (adult 750 mg) stat, then 10 mg/kg (adult 500 mg) after 6–8 hr. Prophylaxis: 5 mg/kg (adult 250 mg) wkly.

Meningococcus gp A, C, W135, Y vaccine (Mencevax ACWY)   Inanimate. >2 yr: 0.5 mL SC. Boost 1–3 yrly.

Meningococcus gp A, C, W135, Y conjugate vaccines   Inanimate. Menactra 2–55 yr 0.5 mL IM. Menveo 11–55 yr 0.5 mL IM. Menomune ≥2 yr 0.5 mL SC.

Meningococcus gp B, conjugate vaccine (Bexsero)   Inanimate. 0.5 mL IM: 2 mo, 3 mo, 4 mo, boost 12–23 mo; 6–11 mo 2 doses ≥2 mo apart, boost 12–23 mo; 1–10 yr 2 doses ≥2 mo apart; 11–50 yr 2 doses ≥1 mo apart.

Meningococcus gp C, conjugate vaccine (Meningitec, Menjugate, NeisVac-C)   Inanimate. 0.5 mL IM: 3 doses 1–2 mo apart (6 wk to 6 mo), 2 doses (6–12 mo), 1 dose (>12 mo).

Mercaptamine   See cysteamine.

Meropenem   10–20 mg/kg (adult 0.5–1 g) 8 H IV over 5–30 min. Severe inftn: 20–40 mg/kg (adult 1–2 g) 12 H (1st wk life) 8 H (>1 wk) or constant infsn.

Metaraminol   IV: 0.01 mg/kg stat (repeat p.r.n.), then 0.15 mg/kg in 50 mL 5% dextrose (no heparin) at 1–10 mL/hr (0.05–0.5 mcg/kg/min) and titrate dose against BP. SC: 0.1 mg/kg.

Metformin   Adult (NOT/kg): initially 500 mg 8–24 H oral, max 1 g per dose 8 H. See also glibenclamide, alogliptin.

Metformin + rosiglitazone (500/2, 1000/2, 1000 mg/4 mg)   Adult: 1000/2 (1000/4 after 8 wk if reqd) 1 tab 12 H oral.

Metformin + saxagliptin (500/5, 1000/5, 1000 mg/2.5 mg) extended-release   Adult (NOT/kg): 1 tab daily oral.

Metformin + sitagliptin (500/50, 1000, 1000 mg/50 mg)   1–2 cap 12 H (max 2000 mg/100 mg per day) oral.

Metformin + vildagliptin   50 mg/850 mg or (if tolerated) 50 mg/1000 mg 12 H oral.

Methadone   0.1–0.2 mg/kg (adult 5–10 mg) 6–12 H oral, SC, IM.

Methionine   50 mg/kg (max 2.5 g) oral 4 H for 4 doses. Prophylaxis: 1 mg to paracetamol 5 mg.

Methylcellulose   Constipation: 30–60 mg/kg (adult 1.5–3 g) with at least 10 mL/kg (adult 300 mL) fluid 12 H oral. Obesity: 30 mg/kg (adult 1.5 g) with 5 mL/kg water $\frac{1}{2}$ hr before a meal.

Methylene blue   1–2 mg/kg (G6PD deficiency 0.4 mg/kg) IV p.r.n. Septic shock: 2 mg/kg stat IV, then 0.25–2 mg/kg/hr.

Methylphenidate   0.1 mg/kg oral 8 a.m., noon and (occasionally) 4 p.m.; incr if reqd to max 0.5 mg/kg/dose (adult 20 mg). Long acting (NOT/kg): child 10–60 mg (adult 10–80 mg) in morning. Transdermal patch: apply for up to 9 hr; start with 12.5 cm^2, and incr to 18.75 cm^2, 25 cm^2, and 37.5 cm^2 if rqd.

Methylprednisolone   Asthma: 0.5–1 mg/kg 6 H oral, IV or IM day 1, 12 H day 2, then 1 mg/kg daily, reducing to minimum effective dose. Severe croup: 4 mg/kg IV stat, then 1 mg/kg 8 H. Severe sepsis before antibiotics (or within 4 hr of 1st dose): 30 mg/kg IV once. Spinal cord injury (within 8 hr): 30 mg/kg stat, then 5 mg/kg/hr 2 days. Lotion 0.25%: apply sparingly 12–24 H. Methylpred 1 mg = hydrocortisone 5 mg in glucocorticoid activity, 0.5 mg in mineralocorticoid.

Methylprednisolone aceponate   0.1% cream, ointment: apply 12–24 H.

Methyltestosterone   NOT/kg: 2.5–12.5 mg/day buccal.

Methysergide   0.02 mg/kg (adult 1 mg) 12 H oral, incr if reqd to max 0.04 mg/kg (adult 2 mg) 8 H for 3–6 mo.

Metoclopramide   0.15–0.3 mg/kg (adult 10–15 mg) 6 H IV, IM, oral; 0.2–0.4 mg/kg (adult 10–20 mg) 8 H PR. Periop: 0.5 mg/kg (adult 15–20 mg) IV stat, then 0.2 mg/kg (adult 10 mg) 4–6 H if reqd. With chemotherapy: up to 1–2 mg/kg 4 H IV.

Metolazone   0.1–0.2 mg/kg (adult 5–10 mg) daily oral. Up to 0.5 mg/kg (adult 30 mg) daily short term.

Metoprolol   IV: 0.1 mg/kg (adult 5 mg) over 5 min, repeat every 5 min to max 3 doses, then 1–5 mcg/kg/min. Oral: 1–2 mg/kg (adult 50–100 mg) 6–12 H.

Metronidazole   15 mg/kg (max 1 g) stat, then 7.5 mg/kg (max 1 g) 12 H in neonate (1st maintenance dose 48 hr after load if <2 kg, 24 hr in term baby), 8 H (4+ wk) IV, PR or oral. Giardiasis: 30 mg/kg (adult 2 g) daily x3 oral. Amoebiasis: 15 mg/kg (adult 750–800 mg) 8 H oral for 10 days, usually followed by diloxanide furoate 10 mg/kg (adult 500 mg) 8 H oral for 10 days. C.difficile: 10 mg/kg (adult 500 mg) 8 H oral. Topical gel 0.5%: apply daily. Level 60–300 μmol/mL (x0.17 mcg/mL).

Mianserin   0.2–0.5 mg/kg (adult 10–40 mg) 8 H oral.

Micafungin   Infant 10 mg/kg, child 8 mg/kg, adult 50–150 mg daily IV over 1 hr. Prophylaxis: 1 mg/kg (adult 50 mg) daily IV over 1 hr.

Miconazole   7.5–15 mg/kg (adult 0.6–1.2 g) 8 H IV over 1 hr. Topical: 2% cream, powder, lotion, tincture or gel 12–24 H. Vaginal: 2% cream or 100 mg ovule daily x7. Oral candida (NOT/kg): buccal tab 50 mg apply to gum above upper incisor on alternate sides daily x14.

Microlax enema   <12 mo 1.25 mL, 1–2 yr 2.5 mL, >2 yr 5 mL.

Midazolam   Sedation: usually 0.1–0.2 mg/kg (adult 5 mg) IV or IM, up to 0.5 mg/kg used in children; 0.2 mg/kg (repeated in 10 min if reqd) nasal; 0.5 mg/kg (max 20 mg) oral. Infusion (ventltd): 3 mg/kg in 50 mL at 1–4 mL/hr (1–4 mcg/kg/min); fitting usually 2–4 mL/hr (range 1–24 mL/hr). 1 mg = 2–3 mg diazepam.

Milrinone   <30 kg: 1.5 mg/kg in 50 mL, 2.5 mL over 1 hr (75 mcg/kg), then 1–1.5 mL/hr (0.5–0.75 mcg/kg/min). >30 kg: 1.5 mg/kg made up to 100 mL, 5 mL over 1 hr (75 mcg/kg), then 2–3 mL/hr (0.5–0.75 mcg/kg/min).

Minocycline   Over 8 yr: 4 mg/kg (max 200 mg) stat, then 2 mg/kg (max 100 mg) 12 H oral or IV over 1 hr. Sustained release tabs (NOT/kg): 45 mg (45–59 kg), 90 mg (60–89 kg), 135 mg (90 kg or more) daily oral.

Mometasone   0.1% cream or oint: apply daily. 50 mcg spray: adult 2 sprays/nostril daily.

Montelukast   NOT/kg: 4 mg (2–5 yr) 5 mg (6–14 yr) 10 mg (>14 yr) daily at bedtime, oral.

Morphine   Half life 2–4 hr. IM: neonate 0.1 mg/kg, child 0.1–0.2 mg/kg, adult 10–20 mg; half this IV over 10 min. IV (ventltd): 0.1–0.2 mg/kg/dose (adult 5–10 mg). Infsn of 1 mg/kg in 50 mL: ventltd neonate 0.5–1.5 mL/hr (10–30 mcg/kg/hr), child or adult 1–4 mL/hr (20–80 mcg/kg/hr). Patient controlled: 20 mcg/kg boluses (1 mL of 1 mg/kg in 50 mL) with 5 min lockout time + (in child) 5 mcg/kg/hr. Oral double IM dose; slow release: start with 0.6 mg/kg 12 H and incr every 48 hr if reqd.

Morphine + naltrexone (20 mg/0.8 mg, 30/1.2, 50/2, 60/2.4, 80/3.2, 100/4)   1 capsule 12–24 H oral.

Mumps vaccine (Mumpsvax)   Live. >12 mo: 0.5 mL SC once. See also measles + mumps + rubella vaccine.

Mupirocin   2% ointment: apply 8–12 H.

Nalidixic acid   15 mg/kg (adult 1 g) 6 H oral, reducing to 7.5 mg/kg (adult 500 mg) 6 H after 2 wk.

Nalmefene   Opiate intoxication: 0.007 mg/kg IV, and 0.0014 mg/kg after 2–5 min (15 min if IM, SC) if reqd. Postop sedtn: 0.25 mcg/kg every 2–5 min (max 4 doses). Half-life 10 hr.

Naloxone   Postop sedtn: 0.002 mg/kg/dose (0.4 mg diluted to 20 mL, give 0.1 mL/kg/dose) repeat every 2 min x4 if reqd, then 0.3 mg/kg in 30 mL at 1 mL/hr (0.01 mg/kg/hr) IV. Opiate overdose (including newborn): 0.01 mg/kg (max 0.4 mg) (0.4 mg diluted to 10 mL, give 0.25 mL/kg/dose), repeated every 2 min (15 min if IM or SC) x4 if reqd, then 0.3 mg/kg in 30 mL at 1 mL/hr (0.01 mg/kg/hr) IV; intranasal (adult, NOT/kg) 1 mg mist per nostril, repeated if reqd after 3–5 min.

Naltrexone   0.5 mg/kg (adult 25 mg) stat, then 1 mg/kg (adult 50 mg) daily oral. Adult (NOT/kg): 380 mg every 4 wk IM.

Naproxen   1 mg = 1.1 mg naproxen sodium. >2 yr: 5–10 mg/kg (adult 250–500 mg) 8–12 H oral. Adult: 500 mg 12 H PR.

Naproxen + esomeprazole   See esomeprazole + naproxen.

Nedocromil   Inhltn: 4 mg (2 puffs) 6 H, reducing to 12 H when imporoved. 2% eye drops: 1 drop/eye 6–24 H.

Neomycin   1 g/m^2 4–6 H oral (max 12 g/day). Bladder washout: 40–2000 mg/L. See also colistin; dexamethasone; gramicidin.

Neomycin 0.5% + prednisolone sodium phosphate 0.5%   1 drop/eye 4–6 H.

Neostigmine   Reverse relaxants: 0.05–0.07 mg/kg (adult 0.5–2.5 mg) IV; suggested dilution: neostigmine (2.5 mg/mL) 0.5 mL + atropine (0.6 mg/mL) 0.5 mL + saline 0.5 mL, give 0.1 mL/kg IV. Myasth gravis (NOT/kg): neonate 0.05–0.25 mg, child 0.2–0.5 mg, adult 1–2.5 mg 2–4 H IM, SC.

Netilmicin   IV or IM. 1 wk-10 yr: 8 mg/kg day 1, then 6 mg/kg daily. >10 yr: 7 mg/kg day 1, then 5 mg/kg (max 240–360 mg) daily. Neonate, 5 mg/kg dose: <1200 g 48 H (0–7 days of life), 36 H (8–30 days), 24 H (>30 days); 1200–2500 g 36 H (0–7 days of life), 24 H (>7 days); term 24 H (0–7 days of life), then as for 1 wk to 10 yr. Trough level <1.0 mg/L.

Nicardipine   0.4–0.8 mg/kg (adult 20–40 mg) 8 H oral. 1–3 mcg/kg/min (max 20 mg/hr) IV.

Niclosamide   50 mg/kg (adult 2 g) oral.

Nicotinamide   4% gel: apply sparingly 12–24 H

Nicorandil   0.1–0.6 mg/kg (adult 5–30 mg) 12 H oral.

Nicotinic acid   Hypercholesterolaemia and hypertriglyceridaemia: 5 mg/kg (adult 200 mg) 8 H, gradually incr to 20–30 mg/kg (adult 1–2 g) 8 H oral. See also laropiprant.

Nicoumalone   0.2 mg/kg (adult 10 mg) day 1, 0.12 m/kg (adult 6 mg) day 2, then 0.02–0.25 mg/kg (adult 1–12 mg) daily oral. INR 2–2.5 for prophylaxis, 2–3 for treatment.

Nifedipine   Caps 0.25–0.5 mg/kg (adult 10–20 mg) 6–8 H, tabs 0.5–1 mg/kg (adult 20–40 mg) 12 H oral or sublingual.

Nimodipine   10–15 mcg/kg/hr (adult 1 mg/hr) IV for 2 hr, then 10–45 mcg/kg/hr (adult 2 mg/hr). Adult: 60 mg 4 H oral.

Nisoldipine   Slow release: 0.2 mg/kg (adult 10 mg) daily oral, incr to 0.4–0.8 mg/kg (adult 20–40 mg) daily.

Nitazoxanide   100 mg (12–47 mo) 200 mg (4–11 yr) 500 mg (>11 yr) 12 H for 3 days oral.

Nitisinone   0.5–0.75 mg/kg 12 H oral.

Nitrazepam   Child epilepsy: 0.125–0.5 mg/kg 12 H oral. Hypnotic (NOT/kg): 2.5–5 mg (child) 5–10 mg (adult) nocte.

Nitric oxide   1–40 ppm (up to 80 ppm used occasionally). 0.1 L/min of 1000 ppm added to 10 L/min gas gives 10 ppm. [NO] = Cylinder [NO] × (1 − (Patient FiO_2/Supply FiO_2)). [NO] = Cylinder [NO] × NO flow/Total flow.

Nitrofurantoin   1.5 mg/kg (adult 50–100 mg) 6 H oral. Prophylaxis: 1–2 mg/kg (adult 50–100 mg) at night.

Nitrofurazone   0.2% cream, soltn: apply every 1–3 days.

Nitroglycerine   See glyceryl trinitrate.

Nitroprusside   See sodium nitroprusside.

Nizatidine   3–5 mg/kg (adult 150 mg) 12 H oral for max 8 wk, then daily. *H. pylori* (adult): 300 mg 12–24 H.

Noradrenaline   0.15 mg/kg in 50 mL 5%D at 1–10 mL/hr (0.05–0.5 mcg/kg/min); flow <2 mL/hr may cause swings in blood pressure. Low dose: 0.06 mg/kg in 50 mL at 1–10 mL/hr (0.02–0.2 mcg/kg/min).

Norepinephrine   See noradrenaline.

Norethindrone   See norethisterone.

Norethisterone   Contraception: 350 mcg daily, starting 1st day of menstruation; or 200 mg oily soltn IM in 1st 5 days of cycle, repeated once after 8 wk. Menorrhagia: 10 mg 3 H until hge stops, then 5 mg 6 H for 1 wk, then 5 mg 8 H for 2 wk; or 5 mg 8–12 H on days 19–26 of cycle. See also ethinyloestradiol, mestranol, and oestradiol with norethisterone.

Norethisterone + oestradiol (0.1 mg/0.5 mg, 0.5/1, 0.7/2, 1/2)   Post-menopause (NOT/kg): 1 tab daily.

Norethisterone + oestradiol patches   Post-menopause (NOT/kg): none/4 mg (50 mcg/24 hr) patch x2/wk for 2 wk, then 30 mg/10 mg (170/50, 250/50 mcg in 24 hr) patch x2/wk for 2 wk; 0.14 mg/0.05 mg patch: 1 patch x2 per wk.

Norfloxacin   10 mg/kg (adult 400 mg) 12 H oral.

Norgestimate   See ethinyloestradiol + norgestimate.

Norgestrel   See levonorgestrel.

Normacol granules   6 mo to 5 yr half teaspoon 12 H, 6–10 yr 1 teaspoon 12 H, >10 yr 1 teaspoon 8 H.

Nortriptyline   0.5–1.5 mg/kg (adult 25–75 mg) 8 H oral.

Nystatin   100,000 U <12 mo, 500,000 U (1 tab) >12 mo 6 H NG or oral. Prophylaxis 50,000 U <12 mo, 250,000 U >12 mo 8 H. Topical: 100,000 U/g gel, cream or ointment 12 H. Vaginal: 100,000 U 12–24 H. See also gramicidin + neomycin + nystatin + triamcinolone cream and ointment.

Octreotide   Diarrhoea: 1 mcg/kg (adult 50 mcg) 12–24 H SC, may incr to 10 mcg/kg (adult 250 mcg) 8 H. IV: 1 mcg/kg stat, then 1–5 mcg/kg/hr. Chyle: 5 mcg/kg/hr IV. Acromegaly (NOT/kg): 0.05–0.1 mg 8–12 H SC incr if reqd to max 0.5 mg 8 H for 4 wk, then slow release 20 mg (10–30 mg) every 4 wk deep IM.

Oestradiol   NOT/kg. Post-menopausal (add a progestogen for 14 days/mo if uterus intact): tab 1–2 mg/day oral; patch 0.1% (release 25, 37.5, 40, 50, 75, 80, 100 mcg/day) to thigh x1–2/wk; metered-dose pump (0.52 mg/dose of 0.06%; 1.53 mg/dose of 1.7%) 1–3 doses/day to arm; vaginal tab 25 mcg: 1 tab daily for 2 wk, then 1 tab x2/wk. Oestoporosis: every wk apply a patch releasing 12.5 mcg/day. Induction puberty: 0.5 mg alternate days oral, incr over 2–3 yr to 2 mg/day (add progestogen for 14 days/mo when dose 1.5 mg/day or when bleeding occurs). Tall stature: 12 mg/day oral until bone age >16 yr (add progestogen for 14 days/cycle). Gonadal failure: 2 mg/day oral (add progestogen for 14 days/cycle). See also bazedoxifene, dienogest, dydrogesterone, levonorgestrel, medroxyprogesterone, and norethisterone with oestradiol.

Oestriol   Inductn puberty: 0.25 mg/day incr to 2 mg/day (+ progestogen 12 days/cycle) oral. Epiphyseal maturation: 10 mg/day (+ progestogen 12 days/cycle). Vaginal: 0.5 mg daily, reducing to x2/wk. Patch (Menorest) 37.5 (3.28 mg), 50 (4.33 mg), 75 (6.57 mg), 100 (8.66 mg): apply 1 patch x2/wk (adjust dose monthly), with medroxyprogesterone acetate (if uterus intact) 10 mg × 10 days/mo.

Oestrogen   See ethinyloestradiol.

Oestrone   Adult (NOT/kg). Menopause: oral 0.625–5 mg daily; vaginal 0.1–1 mg daily, decr to 1 mg x2–3/wk. Hypogonadism: 1.25–7.5 mg daily oral.

Ofloxacin   5 mg/kg (adult 200 mg) 8–12 H, or 10 mg/kg (adult 400 mg) 12 H oral or IV over 1 hr. 0.3%: 1 drop/eye hrly for 2 days (4 H overnight), reducing to 3–6 H.

Olanzapine   0.1–0.2 mg/kg (adult 5–10 mg) daily oral; slow incr to 0.4 mg/kg (adult 20 mg) daily if reqd. See also fluoxetine.

Olmesartan   0.4–0.8 mg/kg (adult 20–40 mg) daily oral. See also amlodipine + olmesartan.

Olpadronate   0.5 mg/kg daily oral.

Olsalazine   NOT/kg: 250 mg 12 H, incr to max 500 mg 6 H oral. Maintenance: 500 mg 12 H.

Omeprazole   Usually 0.4–0.8 mg/kg (adult 20–40 mg) 12–24 H oral. ZE synd: 1 mg/kg (adult 60 mg) 12–24 H oral, incr up to 3 mg/kg (adult 120 mg) 8 H if reqd. IV: 2 mg/kg (adult 80 mg) stat, then 1 mg/kg (adult 40 mg) 8–12 H. *H. pylori* quadruple therapy (adult NOT/kg): 20 mg 12 H + bismuth subcitrate potassium 420 mg 6 H + metronidazole 375 mg 6 H + tetracycline hydrochloride 375 mg 6 H oral for 10–14 days. *H. pylori* triple therapy (adult, NOT/kg): 20 mg + amoxycillin 500 mg + clarithromycin 500 mg 12 H oral for 7 days. See also ketoprofen + omeprazole.

Ondansetron   IV: prophylaxis 0.15 mg/kg (adult 4 mg); treatment 0.2 mg/kg (adult 8 mg) over 5 min, or 0.2–0.5 mcg/kg/min. Chemotherapy: 0.15 mg/kg (max 16 mg) 4 H x3 doses IV. Oral: 0.1–0.2 mg/kg (usual max 8 mg) 6–12 H.

Oral rehydratn soltn (ORS)   See glucose electrolyte soltn.

Orciprenaline   Oral: 0.25–0.5 mg/kg (adult 20 mg) 6 H. Resp soltn (2%): 0.5 mL diltd to 4 mL 3–6 H (mild), 1 mL diltd to 4 mL (moderate), undiluted continuously (severe, in ICU). Aerosol 750 mcg per dose: 2 puffs 4–6 H.

Orlistat   1.5–3 mg/kg (adult 60–120 mg) with each main meal con-taining fat (max 3 doses/day).

Ornipressin (POR 8)   IV: 0.1 U/kg/hr (max 6 U/hr) for max 4 hr, then 0.03 U/kg/hr (max 1.5 U/hr). SC: 5 U in 30 mL saline, max total dose 0.1 U/kg.

Orphenadrine   1–2 mg/kg (adult 50–100 mg) 8 H oral.

Oseltamivir   2 mg/kg (adult 75 mg) 12 H for 5 days oral. Prophylaxis: 2 mg/kg (adult 75 mg) daily.

Oxacillin   15–30 mg/kg 6 H oral, IV, IM. Severe inftn: 40 mg/kg (max 2 g) 12 H (1st wk life), 8 H (2nd wk), 6 H or infsn (>2 wk).

Oxandrolone   0.1–0.2 mg/kg (adult 2.5–20 mg) daily oral. Turner's synd: 0.05–0.1 mg/kg daily.

Oxaprozin   Usually 20 mg/kg (max 1200 mg), range 10–26 mg/kg (max 1800 mg), daily oral.

Oxazepam   0.2–0.5 mg/kg (adult 10–30 mg) 6–8 H oral.

Oxcarbazepine   4–5 mg/kg (adult 300 mg) 12 H oral; incr wkly by max 5 mg/kg/dose (adult 300 mg) to usually 15 mg/kg/dose (adult 750 mg), max 25 mg/kg/dose (adult 1200 mg).

Oxitropium   Inhaltn: 200 mcg (NOT/kg) 8–12 H.

Oxprenolol   0.5–2 mg/kg (adult 30–120 mg) 8–12 H oral.

Oxybuprocaine   4 mg/mL (0.4%): 1 drop/eye 8–12 H. Deep anaes: 1 drop/eye every 90 sec × 3 doses. See also fluorescein + oxybuprocaine.

Oxybutynin   <5 yr: 0.2 mg/kg 8–12 H oral. >5 yr (NOT/ kg): 2.5–5 mg 8–12 H oral. Slow release: adult 5–30 mg daily oral. Adult (NOT/kg): apply 39 cm² patch (3.9 mg/day) x2/wk; apply 100 mg gel sachet daily.

Oxycodone   0.1–0.2 mg/kg (adult 5–10 mg) 4–6 H oral, SC or IV (beware hypoventilation); incr if reqd. IV infsn: 0.05 mg/kg/hr (adult 2 mg/hr) adjusted. Slow release: 0.6–0.9 mg/kg (adult 10 mg) 12 H oral, incr if reqd. Suppos: adult 30 mg 6–8 H PR.

Oxymetazoline   0.25 mg/mL = 0.025% (<6 yr), 0.5 mg/mL = 0.05% (>6 yr): 2–3 drops or sprays in each nostril 8–12 H.

Oxymetholone   1–2 mg/kg (up to 5 mg/kg) daily oral.

Oxymorphone   Usually 0.02–0.03 mg/kg (adult 1–1.5 mg) 4–6 H IM or SC. Slow IV: 0.01 mg/kg (adult 0.5 mg) 4–6 H. Oral: 0.1–0.4 mg/kg (adult 5–20 mg) 4–6 H; slow-release adult 5 mg 12 H. PR: 0.1 mg/kg (adult 5 mg) 4–6 H.

Oxytetracycline   >8 yr (NOT/kg): 250–500 mg 6 H oral, or 250–500 mg 6–12 H slow IV.

Oxytocin   Labour (NOT/kg): 1–4 mU/min IV, may incr to 20 mU/min max. Lactation: 1 spray (4 iu) into each nostril 5 min before infant feeds.

Paclitaxel   175 mg/m² IV every 3 wk, x3–6 doses. Albumin-bound: 260 mg/m² IV every 3 wk.

Palivizumab   15 mg/kg IM once a month.

Paliperidone (3 mg, 6 mg, 9 mg slow release)   Adult (NOT/kg): usually 6 mg daily oral; may incr by 3 mg every 5–7 days; Injection 234 mg IM, 156 mg after 1 wk, then 117 mg monthly.

Palonosetron   Adult: 0.25 mg IV 30 min before chemo.

Pamidronate   Osteoporosis, OI: 3–7 mg/kg daily oral, 1 mg/kg (adult 15–90 mg) IV over 4 hr daily x3 every 4 mo, or once every 3–4 wk. Hypercalcaemia 20–50 mg/m² (depending on Ca level) IV over 4 hr every 4 wk.

Pancreatic enzymes   Cotazyme, Creon, Nutrizym, Pancrease, Pancrex, Ultrase, Viokase. NOT/kg: usually 1–5 caps with meals. Max lipase 10,000 U/kg/day.

Pancuronium   ICU: 0.1–0.15 mg/kg IV p.r.n. Theatre: 0.1 mg/kg IV, then 0.02 mg/kg p.r.n. Infsn: 0.25–0.75 mcg/kg/min.

Pantoprazole   1.0 mg/kg (adult 40 mg) 12–24 H oral, IV. GI hge, adult: 80 mg stat, then 8 mg/hr. ZE: 80 mg 8–12 H adjusted to achieve acid <10 mmol/L.

Para-aminobenzoic acid   See aminobenzoate.

Para-aminohippuric acid   See aminohippuric acid.

Paracetamol   Oral, IV: 20 mg/kg stat, then 15 mg/kg 4–6 H (max 4 g/day); child usual daily max 60 mg/kg (up to 90 mg/kg for 48 hr). Neonate: 7.5 mg/kg (<10 days) 15 mg/kg (>10 day) 6 H. Rectal: 40 mg/kg stat, then 30 mg/kg 6 H (max 5 g/day).

Paraffin   Liquid: 1 mL/kg (adult 30–45 mL) daily oral. Liquid 50% + white soft 50%, ointmnt: apply 6–12 H. See also agar.

Paraldehyde   IM: 0.2 mL/kg (adult 10 mL) stat, then 0.1 mL/kg 4–6 H. IV: 0.2 mL/kg (adult 10 mL) over 15 min, then 0.02 mL/kg/hr (max 1.5 mL/hr). Rectal, NG: 0.3 mL/kg (adult 10 mL) dilute 1:10.

Parathyroid hormone   Adult (NOT/kg): 100 mcg daily SC. See also teriparatide.

Parecoxib   Adult (NOT/kg): 40 mg stat IM or IV, then 20–40 mg 6–12 H; max 80 mg/day.

Paromomycin   Amoebiasis: 10 mg/kg 8 H oral for 5–10 days. Hepatic coma: 20 mg/kg (adult 1 g) 6 H oral.

Paroxetine   0.4 mg/kg (adult 10 mg) daily oral, incr if rqd over 4 wk to 1 mg/kg (adult 20–60 mg) daily. Hot flushes (NOT/kg) 7.5 mg at night oral.

Pegfilgrastim   >44 kg: 6 mg SC 24 hr after chemo.

Pemoline   >6 yr (NOT/kg): 20–120 mg daily oral.

Penicillamine (d-penicillamine)   Arthritis: 1.5 mg/kg (adult 125 mg) 12 H oral, incr over 3 mo to max 3 mg/kg (adult 375 mg) 6–8 H. Wilson's dis, lead poisoning: 5–7.5 mg/kg (adult 250–500 mg) 6 H oral. Cystinuria: 7.5 mg/kg (adult 250–1000 mg) 6 H oral, titrated to urine cystine <100–200 mg/day.

Penicillin, benzathine   1 mg = 1250 U. Usually 25 mg/kg (max 900 mg) IM once. Venereal disease: 40 mg/kg (max 1.8 g) IM once. Strep prophylaxis: 25 mg/kg (max 900 mg) IM 3–4 wkly, or 10 mg/kg IM 2 wkly.

Penicillin, benzathine + procaine   900 mg/300 mg in 2 mL: 0–2 yr half vial, 3 yr or more 1 vial IM once.

Penicillin, benzyl (penicillin G, crystalline)   1 mg = 1667 U. 30 mg/kg 6 H. Severe inftn: 50 mg/kg (max 2 g) IV 12 H (1st wk life), 6 H (2–4 wk), 4 H or constnt infsn (>4 wk).

Penicillin, procaine   1 mg = 1000 U. 25–50 mg/kg (max 1.2–2.4 g) 12–24 H IM. Single dose: 100 mg/kg (max 4.8 g).

Penicillin V   See phenoxymethylpenicillin.

Pentaerythritol tetranitrate   0.2–1 mg/kg (adult 10–60 mg) 6–8 H oral.

Pentagastrin   6 mcg/kg SC, or 0.6 mcg/kg/hr IV.

Pentamidine isethionate   3–4 mg/kg (1.7–2.3 mg/kg base) IV over 2 hr or IM daily for 10–14 days (1 mg base = 1.5 mg mesylate = 1.74 mg isethionate). Neb: 600 mg/6 mL daily for 3 wk (treatment), 300 mg/3 mL every 4 wk (prophylaxis).

Pentazocine   Oral: 0.5–2.0 mg/kg (adult 25–100 mg) 3–4 H. SC, IM or slow IV: 0.5–1 mg/kg (adult 30–60 mg) 3–4 H. PR: 1 mg/kg (adult 50 mg) 6–12 H.

Pentobarbital   See pentobarbitone.

Pentobarbitone   0.5–1 mg/kg (adult 30–60 mg) 6–8 H oral, IM, slow IV. Hypnotic: 2–4 mg/kg (adult 100–200 mg).

Pericyazine   0.5 mg/yr of age (1–10 yr) 10 mg (>10 yr) daily oral, incr if reqd to max 1 mg/yr (1–10 yr) 25 mg (>10 yr) 8 H.

Perindopril   0.05–0.15 mg/kg (adult 2–8 mg) daily oral. See also indanapamide + perindopril.

Permethrin   1% creme rinse (head lice): wash hair, apply creme for 10 min, wash off; may repeat in 2 wk. 5% cream (scabies): wash body, apply to whole body except face, wash off after 12–24 hr.

Perphenazine   0.1–0.3 mg/kg (adult 5–20 mg) 8–12 H oral.

Pethidine   0.5–1 mg/kg (adult 25–50 mg) IV, 0.5–2 mg/kg (adult 25–100 mg) IM (half life 2–4 hr). Infsn: 5 mg/kg in 50 mL at 1–4 mL/hr (0.1–0.4 mg/kg/hr). PCA 5 mg/kg in 50 mL: usually bolus 2 mL with lockout 5 min, optional background 0.5 mL/hr.

Phenindamine   0.5–1 mg/kg (adult 25–50 mg) 8–12 H oral.

Pheniramine   0.5–1 mg/kg (adult 25–50 mg) 6–8 H oral. Slow-release tab 75 mg at night.

Phenobarbital   See phenobarbitone.

Phenobarbitone   Loading dose in emergency: 20–30 mg/kg IM or IV over 30 min stat. Ventilated: repeat doses of 10–15 mg/kg up to 100 mg/kg per day (beware hypotension). Usual maintenance: 5 mg/kg (adult 300 mg) daily IV, IM or oral. Level 60–172 μmol/L (x0.23 = mcg/mL).

Phenolphthalein   0.5–5 mg/kg (adult 30–270 mg) at night oral. See also agar + paraffin + phenolphthalein.

Phenoperidine   0.03–0.05 mg/kg (adult 1 mg) every 40–60 min. Ventilated: 0.1–0.15 mg/kg (adult 2–5 mg) every 40–60 min.

Phenothrin   Apply; shampoo after 30 min (0.5% mousse) 2 hr (0.2% lotion), 12 hr (0.5% emulsion); comb hair when wet.

Phenoxybenzamine   0.2–0.5 mg/kg (adult 10–40 mg) 8–12 H oral. Cardiac surgery: 1 mg/kg IV over 1–4 hr stat, then 0.5 mg/kg 8–12 H IV over 1 hr or oral.

Phenoxymethylpenicillin (penicillin V)   7.5–15 mg/kg (adult 250–500 mg) 6 H oral. Prophylaxis: 12.5 mg/kg (adult 250 mg) 12 H.

Phentolamine   15 mg/kg in 50 mL saline at 1–10 mL/hr (5–50 mcg/kg/min) IV. May accumulate (half-life 19 min, longer if renal impairment).

Phenylbutazone   Initially 2 mg/kg (adult 100 mg) 4 H, reducing to 1–2 mg/kg (adult 50–100 mg) 6–8 H oral.

Phenylephrine   IV: 2–10 mcg/kg stat (adult 500 mcg), then 1–5 mcg/kg/min. SC or IM: 0.1–0.2 mg/kg (max 10 mg). Oral: 0.2 mg/kg (max 10 mg) 6–8 H. 0.15%, 10% eye drops: 1 drop/eye 6–8 H. 0.25%, 0.5% nose drops: 1–3 drops/sprays per nostril 6–8 H. See also chlorpheniramine.

Phenylephrine 0.12% + prednisolone acetate 1%   1 drop per eye 6–12 H.

Phenyltoloxamine   1 mg/kg (adult 50 mg) 8 H oral.

Phenytoin   Loading dose in emergency: 15–20 mg/kg (max 1.5 g) in saline IV over 1 hr. Initial maintenance, oral or IV: 2 mg/kg 12 H (preterm); 3 mg/kg 12 H (1st wk life), 8 H (2 wk-4 yr), 12 H (5–12 yr); 2 mg/kg (usual max 100 mg) 8 H >12 yr. Level 40–80 μmol/L (x0.25 = mcg/mL).

Phosphate, potassium (1 mmol/mL)   Usually 0.06 mmol/kg/hr for 6 hr IV (max 70 mmol/day).

Phosphate, sodium   Laxative, diluted, NOT/kg: 250 mg (2–4 yr) 250–500 mg (>4 yr) 6 H oral.

Phosphate, sodium (Fleet enema)   Na 1.61 mEq/l + PO$_4$ 4.15 mEq/l + P 1.38 mEq/l: 33 mL (2–5 yr), 66 mL (5–11 yr), 133 mL (adult) rectal.

Phosphatidylcholine   Usually 60 mg/kg (max 3 g) daily oral.

Physostigmine   0.02 mg/kg (max 1 mg) IV every 5 min until response (max 0.1 mg/kg), then 0.5–2.0 mcg/kg/min.

Phytomenadione (vitamin K1)   Deficiency with hge: FFP 10 mL/kg, then 0.3 mg/kg (max 10 mg), IM or IV over 1 hr. Prophylaxis in neonates (NOT/kg): 1 mg (0.1 mL) IM at birth. Warfarin reversal: 0.1 mg/kg (max 5 mg) SC or oral (repeat if reqd); if severe hge 0.3 mg/kg (max 10 mg) with FFP 10 mL/kg. Mitochondrial disease (NOT/kg): 10 mg 6 H oral.

Phytonadione   See phytomenadione.

Pilocarpine   0.1 mg/kg (adult 5 mg) 4–8 H oral. 0.5%, 1%, 2%, 3%, 4% eye drops: 1 drop/eye 6–12 H.

Pimecrolimus   1% cream: apply 12 H.

Pimozide   0.04 mg/kg (adult 20 mg) daily oral, incr if reqd to max 0.4 mg/kg (adult 20 mg) daily.

Pindolol   0.3 mg/kg (adult 15 mg) 8–24 H oral.

Pine tar   Gel, solution: 5 mL to baby bath, 15–30 mL to adult bath; soak for 10 min.

Pioglitazone   Adult (NOT/kg): 15–45 mg daily oral. See also glimepiride, alogliptin.

Pipecuronium   20–85 mcg/kg IV stat, then 5–25 mcg/kg p.r.n.

Piperacillin   50 mg/kg (adult 2–3 g) 6–8 H IV. Severe inftn: 100 mg/kg (adult 4 g) 8 H (1st wk life) 6 H (2–4 wk) 4–6 H (>4 wk) or constant infsn.

Piperacillin 4 g + tazobactam 0.5 g   As for piperacillin.

Piperaquine   See dihydroartemisinin + piperaquine.

Piperazine   75 mg/kg (max 4 g) oral daily for 2 days (ascaris), 7 days (pinworm).

Piperazine oestrone sulphate   See estropipate.

Piperonyl butoxide bioallethrin   Apply enough to wet scalp or body, leave 30 min, wash off.

Pipotiazine   Oily injtn: initially 0.5 mg/kg (adult 25 mg), then gradual incr to 1–4 mg/kg (adult 50–200 mg) every 4 wk IM.

Piracetam   15 mg/kg (max 800 mg) 8 H oral, IM or IV.

Piroxicam   0.2–0.4 mg/kg (adult 10–20 mg) daily oral. Gel 5 mg/g: apply 1 g (3 cm) 6–8 H for up to 2 wk.

Pizotifen   NOT/kg: 0.5 mg daily oral, incr if reqd to max 0.5 mg morning and 1 mg at night.

Podofilox   See podophyllotoxin.

Podophyllotoxin   0.5% paint: apply 12 H for 3 days, then none for 4 days; 4 wk course.

Podophyllum   15–25% soltn, oint: apply to wart x2/day.

Poloxamer   10% soltn: <6 mo 10 drops, 6–18 mo 15 drops, 18 mo to 3 yr 25 drops 8 H oral.

Polyethylene glycol   See colonic lavage, macrogol.

Polymyxin B   See bacitracin; dexamethasone.

Polythiazide   0.02–0.1 mg/kg (adult 1–4 mg) daily oral.

Poractant alfa (porcine surfactant, Curosurf)   Intratracheal: 200 mg/kg stat, then up to 4 doses of 100 mg/kg 12 H if reqd.

Potassium   Deficiency: usually 0.3 mmol/kg/h (max 0.4 mmol/kg/hr) for 4–6 hr IV, then 4 mmol/kg/day. Max oral dose 1 mmol/kg (<5 yr), 0.5 mmol/kg (>5 yr). Maintenance 2–4 mmol/kg/day. If peripheral IV, max 0.05 mmol/mL. 1 g KCl = 13.3 mmol K, 7.5% KCl = 1 mmol/mL.

Potassium citrate   See citric acid + potassium citrate.

Potassium guaiacolsulfonate   1–3 mg/kg (adult 50–160 mg) 4–6 H oral.

Potassium iodide   Nuclear accident (NOT/kg): 16.25 mg (<1 mo), 32.5 mg (1 mo to 3 yr), 65 mg (4–18 yr and <70 kg), 130 mg (adult) daily oral.

Povidone-iodine   Cream, oint, paint, soltn: apply 6–12 H.

Pramlintide   Reduce insulin dose by 50% initially. Adult, NOT/kg. Type 1 diabetes: 15 mcg SC before meals (x4/day), incr if tolerated to 30–60 mcg/dose. Type 2: 60 mcg SC before meals (x4/day), incr if tolerated to 90–120 mcg/dose.

Pravastatin   Adult (NOT/kg): 20–80 mg at bedtime oral.

Praziquantel   20 mg/kg oral once (tapeworm), 4 H x3 doses (schistosomiasis), 8 H x6 doses (other flukes), 8 H 14 days (cysticercosis).

Prazosin   5 mcg/kg (max 0.25 mg) test dose, then 0.025–0.1 mg/kg (adult 1–5 mg) 6–12 H oral.

Prednisolone   Oral. Alopecia, autoimm liver, Crohn's, epilepsy, SLE, ulcerative col: 2 mg/kg daily, gradually reducing. Asthma: 0.5–1 mg/kg 6 H for 24 hr, 12 H x2, then 1 mg/kg daily. Croup: 1 mg/kg stat and in 12 hr; severe 4 mg/kg stat, then 1 mg/kg 8 H. ITP: 4 mg/kg dai-ly. Nephrotic: 60 mg/m^2 (max 80 mg) daily, reducing over several months. Physiological: 4–5 mg/m^2 daily. Eye 0.5%: initially 1 drop/eye 2 H, then 6–12 H. 1 mg = hydrocortisone 4 mg in glucocorticoid activity, 0.8 mg in mineralocorticoid. See also methylprednisolone, neomycin + prednisolone, phenyl-ephrine + prednisolone.

Prednisolone sodium phosphate   0.5%: ear 2–3 drops/ear, eye 1 drop/eye 2–6 H.

Prednisone   Action equivalent to prednisolone.

Pregabalin   Adult (NOT/kg): 50 mg 8 H oral, incr gradually if reqd to max 200 mg 8 H.

Pridopidine   Adult (NOT/kg): 45 mg 12 H oral.

Prilocaine   Max dose 6 mg/kg (0.6 mL/kg of 1%). With adrenaline max dose 9 mg/kg (0.9 mL/kg of 1%).

Primaquine   Usually 0.3 mg/kg (adult 15 mg) daily for 14–21 days oral. Gameteocyte: 0.7 mg/kg (adult 45 mg) once.

Primidone   Initially 2.5 mg/kg (adult 125 mg) at night, incr if reqd to max 15 mg/kg (adult 750 mg) 12 H oral. Trough level (phenobarbitone) 60–120 µmol/L.

Probenicid   25 mg/kg (adult 1 g) stat, then 10 mg/kg (adult 500 mg) 6 H oral.

Procainamide   IV: 0.4 mg/kg/min (adult 20 mg/min) for max 25 min, then 20–80 mcg/kg/min (max 2 g/day). Oral: 5–8 mg/kg 4 H. Level 3–10 mcg/mL.

Procaine   Max dose 20 mg/kg (1 mL/kg of 2%).

Procarbazine   1 mg/kg (adult 50 mg) daily oral, incr over 4–6 days to 4–6 mg/kg (adult 200–300 mg) daily until remission, then 1–2 mg/kg (adult 50–100 mg) daily. Suspend if leucocytes <3000/mm^3 or platelets <80,000/mm^3.

Prochlorperazine   1 mg base = approx 1.5 mg edisylate, maleate or mesylate. Only use if >10 kg. Oral (salt): 0.2 mg/kg (adult 5–10 mg) 6–8 H, slow incr if reqd to max 0.6 mg/kg (max 35 mg) 6 H in psychosis. IM, slow IV (salt): 0.2 mg/kg (adult 12.5 mg) 8–12 H. Buccal (salt): 0.05–0.1 mg/kg (max 6 mg) 12–24 H. PR (base): 0.2 mg/kg (adult 25 mg) 8–12 H.

Progesterone   Adult (NOT/kg). Post-menopausal: 100 mg daily on days 1–25 of cycle, or 200 mg daily on days 15–26. Premenstrual syndome: 200–400 mg PV or PR 12–24 H (last half of cycle). Dysf ut hge: 5–10 mg/day IM for 5–10 days before menses. Prevent abrtn: 25–100 mg IM every 2–4 days.

Proguanil   3.5 mg/kg (adult 200 mg) daily oral after food. See also atovaquone + proguanil.

Promazine   Oral: 2–4 mg/kg (adult 100–200 mg) 6 H. IM 0.7 mg/kg (max 50 mg) 6–8 H.

Promethazine   Antihist, antiemetic: 0.2–0.5 mg/kg (adult 10–25 mg) 6–8 H IV, IM or oral. Sedative, hypnotic: 0.5–1.5 mg/kg (adult 25–100 mg).

Propacetamol   IV preparation: 1 g = 0.5 g paracetamol.

Propafenone   Oral: 70 mg/m^2 (adult 150 mg) 8 H, incr if reqd to max 165 mg/m^2 (adult 300 mg) 8 H. IV: 2 mg/kg over 2 hr, then 4 mcg/kg/min incr if reqd to max 8 mcg/kg/min.

Propamidine   0.1%: 1 drop/eye 6 H for up to 2 days.

Propantheline   0.3–0.6 mg/kg (adult 15–30 mg) 6 H oral.

Propiverine   0.3 mg/kg (adult 15 mg) 6–12 H oral.

Propofol   Sedation in ICU: 1–3 mg/kg/hr (max 4 mg/kg/hr) IV, for no longer than 48 hr. Short-term anaes-thesia: child 2.5–3.5 mg/kg stat, then 7.5–15 mg/kg/hr IV; adult 1–2.5 mg/kg stat, then 3–12 mg/kg/hr IV.

Propoxyphene   See dextropropoxyphene.

Propranolol   0.2–0.5 mg/kg (adult 10–25 mg) 6–12 H oral, incr to max 1.5 mg/kg (max 80 mg) 6–12 H if reqd. IV: 0.02 mg/kg (adult 1 mg) test dose then 0.1 mg/kg (adult 5 mg) over 10 min (repeat x1–3 p.r.n.), then 0.1–0.3 mg/kg (adult 5–15 mg) 3 H.

Propylthiouracil   50 mg/m^2 8 H oral, reduce with response.

Proscillaridin   10–15 mcg/kg (adult 500–750 mcg) 8–12 H oral.

Prostacyclin   See epoprostenol.

Prostaglandin   See alprostadil (PGE1), carboprost (15-Me-PGF2-alpha), dinoprost (PGF2-alpha), dinopros-tone (PGE2), epoprostenol (PGI2, prostacyclin), gemeprost (PGE1 analogue), and misoprostol (PGE1 ana-logue).

Protamine   IV 1 mg/100 U heparin (0.5 mg/100 U if >1 hr since heparin dose) slow IV stat; subsequent doses of protamine 1 mg/kg (max 50 mg). 1 mg per 25 mL pump blood. Heparin 1 mg = 100 U (half-life 1–2 hr).

Protein C, activated   See drotrecogin alfa.

Protein C and S   See factor 9 complex (Beriplex, Octaplex).

Prothionamide   TB: 15–20 mg/kg (adult 0.75–1 g) at night oral. Leprosy: 5–8 mg/kg (adult 250–375 mg) daily.

Prothrombin complex   See factor 9 complex.

Protionamide   See prothionamide.

Protirelin   NOT/kg: 200 mcg IV stat.

Protriptyline   0.1–0.4 mg/kg (adult 5–20 mg) 6–8 H oral.

Proxymetacaine   0.5% soltn: 1 drop/eye stat, then 1 drop every 10 min for 5–7 doses.

Pseudoephedrine   1 mg/kg (adult 60 mg) 6–8 H oral. Slow-release: adult (NOT/kg) 120 mg 12 H.

Pseudoephedrine 60 mg + triprolidine 2.5 mg (Actifed)   10 mL elixir = 1 tab. NOT/kg: 2.5 mL (<2 yr), 2.5–5 mL (2–5 yr), 0.5 tab (6–12 yr), 1 tab (>12 yr) 6–8 H oral.

Psyllium   Usually 0.1–0.2 g/kg (adult 5–10 g) 8–24 H oral.

Pumactant (ALEC)   Preterm babies (NOT/kg): disconnect ETT, rapidly inject 100 mg in 1 mL saline via catheter at lower end ETT, flush with 2 mL air; repeat after 1 hr and 24 hr. Prophylaxis if unintubated: 100 mg into pharynx.

Pyrantel   Threadworm: 10 mg/kg (adult 750 mg) once oral, may repeat 2 wkly x3 doses. Roundworm, hookworm: 20 mg/kg (adult 1 g) once, may repeat in 7 days. Necator: 20 mg/kg (adult 1 g) daily x 2–3 doses.

Pyrazinamide   30–40 mg/kg (max 1.5 g) daily oral, or 75 mg/kg (max 3 g) x2/wk.

Pyrethrins + piperonyl butoxide   Lice: apply enough shampoo to wet hair, wash off in 15 min; repeat in 10 days.

Pyridostigmine   Myas gravis: 1 mg/kg (adult 60 mg) 4–6 H oral, incr to max 2–3 mg/kg (adult 120–180 mg) 4–6 H if reqd. 180 mg slow-release tab (Timespan), adult (NOT/kg): 1–3 tab 12–24 H oral. 1 mg IV, IM or SC = 30 mg oral.

Pyridoxine   With isoniazid or penicillamine (NOT/kg): 5–10 mg daily IV, oral. Fits: 10–15 mg/kg daily IV or oral. Siderobl an: 2–8 mg/kg (max 400 mg) daily IV or oral. See also doxylamine.

Pyrimethamine   Adult (NOT/kg): 25 mg tab weekly oral.

Pyrimethamine 25 mg + sulphadoxine 500 mg (Fansi-dar)   <4 yr $\frac{1}{2}$ tab once, 4–8 yr 1 tab, 9–14 yr 2 tab, >14 yr 3 tab. Prophylaxis: <4 yr $\frac{1}{4}$ tab wkly, 4–8 yr $\frac{1}{2}$ tab, 9–14 yr $\frac{3}{4}$ tab, >14 yr 1 tab. See also artesunate, chloroquine, dapsone.

Quetiapine   Adult (NOT/kg) 12 H oral per dose: 25 mg day 1, 50 mg day 2, 100 mg day 3, 150 mg day 4, then 150–250 mg (range 75–400 mg) 12 H. Beware long QTc interval.

Quinalbarbitone   Sedative 5 mg/kg. Premed 10 mg/kg.

Quinapril   0.2–0.8 mg/kg (adult 10–40 mg) daily oral. See also hydrochlorothiazide.

Quinidine, base   10 mg/kg stat, then 5 mg/kg (max 333 mg) 4–6 H oral. IV: 6.3 mg/kg (10 mg/kg of gluconate) over 2 hr, then 0.0125 mg/kg/min. IM: 15 mg/kg stat, then 7.5 mg/kg (max 400 mg) 8 H. NOTE: 1 mg base = 1.2 mg sulphate = 1.3 mg bisulphate = 1.6 mg gluconate.

Quinine, base   Oral: 8.3 mg/kg (max 500 mg) 8 H for 7–10 days. Parenteral: 16.7 mg/kg (20 mg/kg of dihydrochloride) IV over 4 hr or IM, then 8.3 mg/kg 8 H IV over 2 hr or IM for 2–3 days, then 8.3 mg/kg 8 H oral for 5 days. NOTE: 1 mg base = 1.7 mg bisulphate = 1.2 mg dihydrochloride = 1.2 mg ethyl carbonate = 1.3 mg hydrobromide = 1.2 mg hydrochloride = 1.2 mg sulphate.

Quinupristin   See dalfopristin + quinupristin.

Rabeprazole   Adult (NOT/kg): 20 mg daily oral 4–8 wk (DU), 6–12 wk (GU), 4 wk then 10–20 mg daily (reflux). ZE: 60 mg daily, incr if reqd to 12 H. *H. pylori*, see omeprazole.

Raltegravir   8 mg/kg (adult 400 mg, max 600 mg) 12 H oral.

Ramipril   0.05 mg/kg (adult 2.5 mg) oral daily, may incr over 4–6 wk to 0.1–0.2 mg/kg (adult 5–10 mg) daily.

Ranitidine   IV: 1 mg/kg (adult 50 mg) slowly 6–8 H, or 2 mcg/kg/min. Oral: 2–4 mg/kg (adult 150 mg) 8–12 H, or 300 mg (adult) at night.

Ranitidine bismuth citrate   8 mg/kg (adult 400 mg) 12 H oral. *H. pylori*, see omeprazole.

Rapacuronium   Initially 2 mg/kg (child), 1.5 mg/kg (adult), 2.5 mg/kg Caesar); maintenance 33–50% initial.

Rasagiline   Adult (NOT/kg): 0.5–1 mg daily oral.

Rasburicase   0.15–0.2 mg/kg IV daily for 5–7 days.

Reboxetine   Adult (NOT/kg): 2–4 mg 12 H oral, incr gradually if reqd to max 10 mg 12 H.

Recombinant antihaemophilic factor   See factor 8.

Recombinant human antithrombin   See antithrombin.

Remifentanil   0.05–0.2 mcg/kg/min. Ventilated: usually 0.5–1 mcg/kg/min; occasionally up to 8 mcg/kg/min if reqd.

Repaglinide   Adult (NOT/kg) before main meals, oral: initially 0.5 mg, incr every 1–2 wk to 4 mg (max 16 mg/day).

Reserpine   0.005–0.01 mg/kg (adult 0.25–0.5 mg) 12–24 H oral.

Residonrate   Adult (NOT/kg): 5 mg daily oral; slow release 35 mg once a week.

Resonium   See sodium polystyrene sulphonate.

Reteplase   Adult (NOT/kg) for myocardial infarction: give heparin 5000 U IV + aspirin 250–350 mg oral; then reteplase 10 U IV over 2 min + 2nd dose 30 min later; then heparin 1000 U/hr for 24–72 hr and aspirin 75–150 mg/day until discharge.

Retinol A   See vitamin A.

Ribavirin   Inhltn (Viratek nebulizer): 20 mg/mL at 25 mL/hr (190 mcg/L of gas) for 12–18 hr/day for 3–7 days. Oral: 5–15 mg/kg 8–12 H. Hepatitis C: see interferon alfa-2b.

Riboflavine   NOT/kg: 5–10 mg daily oral. Organic acidosis (NOT/kg): 50–200 mg daily oral, IM or IV.

Rifabutin   Pulmonary TB: 3–5 mg/kg (adult 150–300 mg) daily oral. Resistant pul TB: 5–7.5 mg/kg (adult 300–450 mg) daily. Mycobact avium complex: 7.5–12 mg/kg (adult 450–600 mg) daily; prophylaxis 5 mg/kg (adult 300 mg) daily.

Rifampicin   10–20 mg/kg (max 600 mg) daily oral fasting, or IV over 3 hr (monitor AST). Prophylaxis: N.meningitidis 10 mg/kg daily (neonate), 10 mg/kg (max 600 mg) 12 H for 2 days; H.influenzae 10 mg/kg daily (neonate), 20 mg/kg (max 600 mg) daily for 4 days.

Rifampin   See rifampicin.

Risedronate   Osteoporosis: 0.1 mg/kg (adult 5 mg) daily oral; slow release (adult): 35 mg wkly, 75 mg twice a month, 150 mg monthly. Paget's: 0.5 mg/kg (adult 30 mg) daily oral.

Risperidone   0.02 mg/kg (adult 1 mg) 12 H, incr if reqd to 0.15 mg/kg (adult 2–4 mg, max 8 mg) 12 H oral.

Rituximab   Leukaemia: 260–370 mg/m^2 by IV infsn wkly x4. Rheumatoid arthritis (adult, NOT/kg): 1 g IV twice, 2 wk apart.

Rivastigmine   Adult (NOT/kg): initially 1.5 mg 12 H, incr every 2 wk to max 6 mg 12 H oral. Patch: apply 4.6 mg (5 cm^2) daily for 4 wk, then 9.5 mg (10 cm^2) daily.

Rizatriptan   Adult (NOT/kg): 10 mg oral, may repeat x1 in 2 hr.

Rocuronium   0.6–1.2 mg/kg IV stat, then 0.1–0.2 mg/kg boluses or 5–15 mcg/kg/min.

Romiplostim   1–10 mcg/kg wkly SC.

Ropivacaine   2–3 mg/kg (adult max 200–250 mg). Intrathecal: 1 mg/kg (0.1 mL/kg of 1%). Postop infusion 0.2–0.4 mg/kg/hr (0.1–0.2 mL/kg/hr of 0.2%).

Rosiglitazone   Adult (NOT/kg): 4 mg daily oral, incr after 6–8 wk to 4 mg 12 H if reqd. See also glimepiride + rosiglitazone and metformin + rosiglitazone.

Rosuvastatin   10 mg daily oral, incr if reqd to 20 mg then 40 mg at 4 wk intervals.

Roxithromycin   2.5–4 mg/kg (adult 150 mg) 12 H oral.

Rufinamide   10 mg/kg (adult 400 mg) daily oral, incr over 1–2 wk to 45 mg/kg (adult 3200 mg). Lower dose if on valproate.

Sacrosidase   ≤15 kg 1 mL or 1 full scoop (8500 u), >15 kg 2 mL or 2 full scoops (17,000 U) oral with each meal or snack.

Salbutamol (and levalbuterol)   0.1–0.15 mg/kg (adult 2–4 mg) 6 H oral. Inhaltn: mild resp soltn (5 mg/mL, 0.5%) 0.5 mL diluted to 4 mL, or nebule 2.5 mg/2.5 mL (0.1%) 3–6 H; moderate 0.5% soltn 1 mL diluted to 4 mL, or nebule 5 mg/2.5 mL (0.2%) 1–2 H; severe (in ICU) 0.5% soltn undiluted continuous. Aerosol 100 mcg/puff: 1–2 puff 4–6 H. Rotahaler: 200–400 mcg 6–8 H. IM or SC: 10–20 mcg/kg (adult 500 mcg) 3–6 H. IV in child: amp 1 mg/mL at 0.3–0.6 mL/kg/hr (5–10 mcg/kg/min) for 1 hr, then 0.06–0.12 mL/kg/hr

(1–2 mcg/kg/min). Preterm labour: (adult, NOT/kg): 200 mcg/mL in 5%D at 3 mL/hr (10 mcg/min), incr until contractions cease (usually at 3–15 mL/hr), then halve dose every 6 hr; max duration usually 48 hr. IV infsn incompatible with aminophylline, ketamine and magnesium.

Salicylic acid   Cradle cap: 6% soltn (Egocappol) 12 H 3–5 days. Plantar warts: 15% soltn x1–2/day, 40% medicated disc 24–48 H. See also benzoic acid + salicylic acid.

Salicylsalicylic acid   See salsalate.

Salmeterol   Aerosol, diskhaler (NOT/kg): 50–100 mcg 12 H. See also fluticasone + salmeterol.

Sargramostim (GM-CSF, Leucomax)   3–5 mcg/kg daily SC, or IV over 6 hr. Keep WCC 5000–10,000/mm^3.

Scopolamine   See hyoscine hydrobromide.

Secretin   1 cu = 4 chr units. 1–2 cu/kg slow IV.

Selegiline   Adult (NOT/kg): 10 mg daily, oral. Transdermal patch: 6 mg daily; incr to max 9–12 mg daily if reqd.

Selenium sulphide   2.5% shampoo x2/wk for 2 wk.

Senna, Sennoside   Tab 7.5 mg, granules 15 mg/5 mL. Daily (NOT/kg): 6 mo to 2 yr 7.5 mg, 3–10 yr 7.5–15 mg, >10 yr 1–30 mg.

Sermorelin (GHRH)   1 mcg/kg fasting in morning IV.

Sertraline   0.5 mg/kg (adult 25 mg) daily oral, incr if reqd to 1–2 mg/kg (adult 50–100 mg) daily; may give 3–4 mg/kg (adult 150–200 mg) daily for up to 8 wk.

Sevelamer   20–40 mg/kg (adult 800–1600 mg) 8 H oral, titrated to serum phosphorus.

Sevoflurane   7% (child) 5% (adult) induction, then 0.5–3%.

Sildenafil   Adult sexual dysfunction: 25–100 mg (NOT/kg) oral 1 hr before sexual activity (max once/day). Pul hypertensn: oral 0.3 mg/kg 3–6 H incr until effective or systemic hypotension (usual max 2–3 mg/kg/dose); adult (NOT/kg) usually 20 mg 8 H. 1 hr before stop NO: 0.4 mg/kg oral once. IV infsn: 0.4 mg/kg over 3 hr, then 1.6 mg/kg/day.

Silver nitrate, stick   Apply daily to affected area only.

Silver sulfadiazine 1% + chlorhexidine 0.2%   Cream: apply in 3–5 mm layer.

Simethicone   See aluminium hydroxide compound.

Simvastatin   Adult (NOT/kg): 10 mg daily oral, incr 4 wkly if reqd to max 80 mg daily – max 10 mg/day with amiodarone, diltiazem or verapamil; 20 mg/day with amlodipine or ranolazine. See also ezetimibe + simvastatin.

Simvastatin + Sitagliptin (10/50, 20/50, 40/50, 10/100, 20/100, 40 mg/100 mg) tabs   See simvastatin doses.

Sirolimus   3 mg/m^2 (adult 6 mg) stat, then 1 mg/m^2 (adult 2 mg) daily oral.

Sitagliptin   2 mg/kg (adult 100 mg) daily oral. See also metformin + sitagliptin, and simvastatin + sitagliptin.

Sodium   Deficit (mL saline) = Wt (kg) × 4 × (140 − [Na])/% saline. To incr serum Na by 0.5 mmol/L/hr (max safe rate), infusn rate (mL/hr) = 2 × Wt (kg)/(% saline infused); hours of infusion = 2 × (140 − serum Na). 4 mL/kg of X% saline raises serum Na by X mmol/L. Need 2–6 mmol/kg/day. NaCl MW = 58.45, 1 g NaCl = 17.1 mmol Na, NaCl 20% = 3.4 mmol/mL.

Sodium alginate   See alginic acid.

Sodium aurothiomalate   0.25 mg/kg wkly IM, incr to 1 mg/kg (max 50 mg) wkly for 10 wk, then every 2–6 wk.

Sodium benzoate   Neonate: 250 mg/kg over 2 hr stat, then 10–20 mg/kg/hr IV.

Sodium bicarbonate   See bicarbonate.

Sodium calcium edetate (EDTA)   25–40 mg/kg 12 H IM or IV over 1 hr for 5 days; repeat after 3 days if reqd. With dimercaprol: 12.5 mg/kg 4 H for 3–7 days.

Sodium chloride   See sodium.

Sodium citrate   Constipation (adult, NOT/kg): usually 450 mg in 5 mL as enema, often with sodium lauryl sulphoacetate, glycerol, sorbitol or sorbic acid.

Sodium citrotartrate   40–80 mg/kg (adult 2–4 g) in 50 mL water 8–12 H oral.

Sodium cromoglycate   Inhalation (Intal): 1 cap (20 mg) 6–8 H, 2 mL soltn (20 mg) 6–8 H, aerosol 1–10 mg 6–8 H. Eye drops 2%: 1 drop/eye 4–6 H oral. Oral: 5–10 mg/kg (max 200 mg) 6 H oral. Nasal 2% or 4%: 1 dose to each nostril 3–12 H.

Sodium feredetate   See ferrous salts.

Sodium ferric gluconate Fe 12.5 mg/mL. 0.05 mL/kg (adult 2 mL) test dose IV over 1 hr, then 0.25 mL/kg (adult 10 mL) IV over 1 hr with each dialysis (usually for 8 doses).

Sodium fluoride NOT/kg: <2 yr 0.55 mg oral daily, 2–4 yr 1.1 mg, >4 yr 2.2 mg. Osteoporosis, Paget's, bone secondaries in adult (NOT/kg): 20–40 mg 8–12 H.

Sodium fusidate Tablets: 10–15 mg/kg (adult 250–500 mg) 8 H oral. IV over 2–8 hr: 10 mg/kg (adult 500 mg) 8 H; severe inftn 15 mg/kg (adult 750 mg). Peak level 30–200 µmol/L (x0.52 = mcg/mL). For suspension, see fusidic acid.

Sodium hyaluronate Adult (NOT/kg). Cystitis 800 mcg/mL: 50 mL into bladder wkly x4, then 4 wkly. Ophthalmic: 10–15 mg/mL (1–1.5%) 0.2–0.6 mL into anterior chamber; 0.18% drops 1/eye as reqd. Osteoarthritis 10–15 mg/mL: 2–2.5 mL intra-articular wkly x3–5.

Sodium nitrite 3%: 0.2 mL/kg (max 10 mL) IV over 5 min.

Sodium nitroprusside <30 kg: 3 mg/kg in 50 mL 5%D at 0.5–4 mL/hr (0.5–4 mcg/kg/min) IV. >30 kg: 3 mg/kg made to 100 mL in 5%D at 1–8 mL/hr (0.5–4 mcg/kg/min). If used for >24 hr, max rate 4 mcg/kg/min. Max total 70 mg/kg with normal renal function (or sodium thiocyanate <1725 µmol/L, x0.058 = mg/L). Protect from light.

Sodium phenylbutyrate 10–13 g/m²/day divided into equal amounts with each feed or meal, oral.

Sodium phosphate See phosphate, sodium.

Sodium picosulphate 2.5 mg (1–4 yr), 2.5–5 mg (4–10 yr), 5–10 mg (>10 yr) at night oral.

Sodium polystyrene sulphonate (Resonium) 0.3–1 g/kg (adult 15–30 g) 6 H NG (give lactulose) or PR.

Sodium salicylate 1 g = 1.1 g aspirin.

Sodium valproate 5 mg/kg (adult 200 mg) 8–12 H oral or IV, incr if reqd to max 20 mg/kg (adult 1 g) 8–12 H. Slow release 15–60 mg/kg (adult 1000–3000 mg) daily. Level 2 hr after dose 350–900 µmol/L (x0.14 = mg/L).

Somatostatin See octreotide.

Somatropin 1 mg = 3 iu. Usually 0.5–1 mg/m² on 5–7 days a wk SC, or 1–2 mg/m² on 3 days a wk IM. Short bowel: 0.1 mg/kg (max 8 mg) daily SC.

Sorbitol 70% 0.2–0.5 mL/kg (adult 20–30 mL) 8–24 H oral. With activated charcoal: 1 g/kg (1.4 mL/kg) NG, x1–2.

Sorbolene cream; pure, with 10% glycerin, or with 5% or 10% olive oil or peanut oil Skin moisturiser: apply p.r.n.

Sotalol IV: 0.5–2 mg/kg (adult 25–120 mg) over 10 min 6 H. Oral: 1–4 mg/kg (adult 50–160 mg) 8–12 H.

Spironolactone Oral (NOT/kg): 0–10 kg 6.25 mg 12 H, 11–20 kg 12.5 mg 12 H, 21–40 kg 25 mg 12 H, over 40 kg 25 mg 8 H. Female hirsutism 50 mg 8 H. IV: see potassium canrenoate.

Stanolone 2.5% gel. Male: apply 5–10 g daily to a large area of skin and allow 5 min to dry. Female (lichen sclerosus): apply 2.5 g to vulva on alternate days.

Streptokinase (SK) Short term (myocardial infarction): 30,000 U/kg (max 1,500,000 U) IV over 1 hr, repeat if occlusion recurs <5 days. Long term (DVT, pul emb, art thrombosis): 2000 U/kg (max 100,000 U) IV over 10 min, then 1000 U/kg/hr (max 100,000 U/hr); stop heparin and aspirin, if PTT <x2 normal at 4 hr give extra 10,000 U/kg (max 500,000 U) IV over 30 min, stop SK if PTT >x5 normal then give 1000 U/kg/hr. Local infsn: 50 U/kg/hr (continue heparin 10–15 U/kg/hr). Blocked IV cannula: 5000 U/kg in 2 mL in cannula for 2 hr then remove, may repeat x2.

Streptomycin 20–30 mg/kg (max 1 g) IM daily.

Succimer 350 mg/m² 8 H for 5 days, then 12 H x14 days oral.

Succinylcholine See suxamethonium.

Sucralfate 1 g tab (NOT/kg): 0–2 yr quarter tab 6 H, 3–12 yr half tab 6 H, >12 yr 1 tab 6 H oral.

Sucrose Analgesia in infants: 0.17 g/kg (0.5 mL/kg of 33% soltn) 2 min before procedure.

Sufentanil 2–50 mcg/kg slow IV; may then infuse so that total dose is 1 mcg/kg/hr of expected surgical time.

Sulbactam See ampicillin + sulbactam.

Sulfadiazine 50 mg/kg (max 2 g) 6 H slow IV.

Sulfadoxine See pyrimethamine + sulphadoxine.

Sulfamethoxazole + trimethoprim See cotrimoxazole.

Sulfasalazine See sulphasalazine.

Sulindac 4 mg/kg (adult 200 mg) 12 H oral.

Sulphacetamide   100 mg/mL 1 drop/eye 2–3 H during the day.

Sulphadoxine   See pyrimethamine + sulphadoxine.

Sulphamethoxazole + trimethoprim   See cotrimoxazole.

Sulphasalazine   Active colitis: 20 mg/kg 6–12 H (max 4 g/day) oral; remission 7.5 mg/kg (max 0.5 g) 6–8 H, suppos (NOT/kg) adult 0.5–1 g 12 H. Arthritis: 5 mg/kg 12 H, incr if reqd to 10 mg/kg 8–12 H (max 2 g/day).

Sumatriptan   Oral: 1–2 mg/kg (adult 50–100 mg) stat, may repeat twice. SC or needle-free: 0.12 mg/kg (max 6 mg) stat, may repeat once after 1 hr. Nasal: 10–20 mg, may repeat x1 after 2 hr. See also naproxen.

Surfactant   See beractant (Survanta), calfactant (Infasurf), colfosceril palmitate (Exosurf), poractant alfa (Curosurf), pumactant (ALEC).

Suxamethonium   IV: neonate 3 mg/kg, child 2 mg/kg, adult 1 mg/kg. IM: double IV dose.

Tacrolimus   IV infusion: 2 mg/m^2/day. Oral: 3 mg/m^2 12 H. Trough level: whole blood 10–15 ng/mL (sent to Austin daily at 1000 from RCH).

Tacrolimus ointment   2–16 yr: apply 0.03% sparingly 12 H for max 3 wk, then daily. >16 yr: apply 0.1% sparingly 12 H for max 3 wk, then 0.03% 12 H.

Tamoxifen   Adult (NOT/kg): 20 mg daily, incr to 40 mg daily if no response after 1 mo.

Tar   See coal tar.

Tazobactam   See piperacillin + tazobactam.

Teicoplanin   250 mg/m^2 IV over 30 min stat, then 125 mg/m^2 IV or IM daily. Severe inftn: 250 mg/m^2 12 H x3 doses, then 250 mg/m^2 IV or IM daily.

Telmisartan   1 mg/kg (adult 40 mg) daily, incr if reqd to 2 mg/kg (adult 80 mg) daily oral. See also hydrochlorothiazide + telmisartan.

Temazepam   0.3 mg/kg (adult 20–40 mg) oral.

Temocillin   25–50 mg/kg (adult 1–2 g) 12 H IV or IM.

Temozolomide   200 mg/m^2 daily oral for 5 days per 28-day cycle (150 mg/m^2 for first cycle if previous chemotherapy).

Temsirolimus   Adult (NOT/kg): 25 mg IV over 1 hr wkly.

Tenecteplase   1 mg = 200 U. Myocardial infarction (adult): 100 U/kg (max 10,000 U) IV over 10 sec once; also give aspirin 150–325 mg/day, and heparin to maintain APTT 50–75 sec.

Tenoxicam   0.2–0.4 mg/kg (adult 10–20 mg) daily oral.

Terbinafine   62.5 mg (<20 kg), 125 mg (20–40 kg), 250 mg (adult) daily oral. 1% cream, gel: apply 12–24 H to dry skin.

Terbutaline   Oral: 0.05–0.1 mg/kg (adult 2.5–5 mg) 6 H. SC: 5–10 mcg/kg (adult 0.25–0.5 mg). IV: child 3–6 mcg/kg/min for 1 hr, then 0.4–1 mcg/kg/min; adult 0.25 mg stat over 10 min, then 1–10 mcg/kg/hr. Inhaltn: mild resp soltn (1%, 10 mg/mL) 0.25 mL diluted to 4 mL 3–6 H; moderate 0.5 mL of 1% diluted to 4 mL, or respule 5 mg/2 mL 1–2 H; severe (in ICU) undiluted continuous. Aerosol 250 mcg/puff: 1–2 puffs 4–6 H.

Terfenadine   30 mg (6–12 yr), 60 mg (adult) 12 H oral.

Terlipressin   0.04 mg/kg (adult 2 mg) IV, then 0.02–0.04 mg/kg (adult 1–2 mg) 4–6 H for max 72 hr. Slow onset, long action: continuous infsn may cause necrosis.

Testolactone   5–10 mg/kg (max 250 mg) 6 H oral.

Testosterone   NOT/kg. Esters: 100–500 mg IM every 2–4 wk. Implant: 8 mg/kg (to nearest 100 mg) every 16–24 wk. Undecanoate: 40 mg daily oral, incr to 80–120 mg daily; depot 750 mg IM, after 4 wk, then every 10 wk. 1% gel: 5 g tube (50 mg testosterone) to skin daily. Transdermal patch: 2.5–5 mg daily; gel 40–50 mg. Metered dose pump: 40–60 mg daily. 30 mg buccal tab: applied just above incisor 12 H. Post-menopausal breast cancer: 100 mg x2–3/wk IV or IM. Testosterone level: <16 yr 5–10 nmol/L, >16 yr 10–30 nmol/L.

Tetracaine   See amethocaine.

Tetracosactrin zinc injection (Synacthen Depot)   600 mcg/m^2 (max 1 mg) IM every 1–7 days.

Tetracycline   >8 yr (NOT/kg): 250–500 mg 6 H oral. Acne (NOT/kg): 500 mg 12 H, reducing to 250 mg 12 H. Eye: apply 2–8 H. See also rolitetracycline.

Theophylline   80 mg theophylline = 100 mg aminophylline). Loading dose: 8 mg/kg (max 500 mg) oral. Maintenance: 1st wk life 2 mg/kg 12 H; 2nd wk 3 mg/kg 12 H; 3 wk to 12 mo ((0.1 × age in wk) + 2.7) mg/kg 8 H; 1–9 yr 4 mg/kg 4–6 H, or 10 mg/kg slow release 12 H; 10–16 yr or adult smoker 3 mg/kg

4–6 H, or 7 mg/kg 12 H slow release; adult non-smoker 3 mg/kg 6–8 H; elderly 2 mg/kg 6–8 H. Serum level: neonate 60–80 μmol/L, asthma 60–110 (x0.18 = mcg/mL).

Thiabendazole   25 mg/kg (max 1.5 g) 12 H oral 3 days.

Thiamine   Beriberi: 1–2 mg/kg IV, IM or oral daily. Metabolic dis (NOT/kg): 100 mg 8 H IV, IM, SC, oral.

Thiopental   See thiopentone.

Thiopentone   2–5 mg/kg slowly stat (beware hypotension). IV infsn: amp 25 mg/mL at 0.04–0.2 mL/kg/hr (1–5 mg/kg/hr). Level 150–200 μmol/L (x0.24 = mcg/mL).

Thiosulphate   See sodium thiosulphate.

Thrombin glue   10,000 U thrombin in 9 mL mixed with 1 mL 10% calcium chloride in syringe 1, 10 mL cryoprecipitate in syringe 2: apply to bleeding sites together. Do not inject.

Thrombin, topical   100–2000 U/mL onto bleeding surface.

Thymidine   75 g/m^2 every 4–6 wk IV over 24 hr.

Thyroxine   50 mcg tab. 100 mcg/m^2 rounded to nearest quarter tab (adult 100–200 mcg) daily oral. IV: 50 mcg/m^2 daily.

Tiagabine   0.1 mg/kg (adult 5 mg) 12 H oral, incr wkly to 0.1–0.2 mg/kg (adult 5–10 mg) 8 H; 0.2–0.3 mg/kg (adult 10–15 mg) 8 H if on carbamazepine, phenobarb, phenytoin, primidone.

Ticarcillin   50 mg/kg (adult 3 g) IV 6–8 H (1st wk life), 4–6 H or constant infsn (2+ wk). Cystic fib: 100 mg/kg (max 6 g) 8 H IV.

Ticarcillin + clavulanic acid   Dose as for ticarcillin.

Tigecycline   2 mg/kg (adult 100 mg) IV over 1 hr stat, then 1 mg/kg (adult 50 mg) IV over 30 min 12 H.

Tilactase   200 U/drop: 5–15 drops/L added to milk 24 hr before use. 3300 U/tab: 1–3 tabs with meals oral.

Tiludronate   Adult 400 mg daily for 12 wk oral.

Tiludronic acid   See tiludronate disodium.

Timolol   0.1 mg/kg (adult 5 mg) 8–12 H, incr to max 0.3 mg/kg (adult 15 mg) 8 H. Eye drops (0.25%, 0.5%): 1 drop/eye 12–24 H; see also bimatoprost + timolol, latanoprost + timolol.

Timolol 5 mg/mL + travoprost 40 mcg/mL   1 drop/eye daily.

Tinidazole   Giardia, trichomonas: 50 mg/kg (adult 2 g) daily for 2 days oral, or 25 mg/kg (adult 1 g) daily x5 days. Amoebiasis: 50 mg/kg (adult 2 g) daily for 3–5 days, usually followed by diloxanide furoate 10 mg/kg (adult 500 mg) 8 H × 10 days.

Tinzaparin   1 mg = 75 anti-Xa IU. Prophylaxis: 50 U/kg SC 2 hr before surgery, then daily for 7–10 days. Treatment: 175 U/kg SC daily for at least 6 days.

Tiotropium   NOT/kg: 18 mcg cap daily by inhaler.

Tissue plasminogen activator   See alteplase.

Tobramycin   IV or IM. 1 wk to 10 yr: 8 mg/kg day 1, then 6 mg/kg daily. >10 yr: 7 mg/kg day 1, then 5 mg/kg (max 240–360 mg) daily. Neonate, 5 mg/kg dose: <1.2 kg 48 H (0–7 days of life), 36 H (8–30 days), 24 H (>30 days); 1.2–2.5 kg 36 H (0–7 days of life), 24 H (>7 days); term 24 H (0–7 days of life), then as for 1 wk to 10 yr. Trough level <1.0 mg/L. Inhaltn: 80 mg in 4 mL 12 H; 28 mg cap 12 H or TOBI 300 mg 12 H alternate months. Eye: 1 drop or 1 cm cream 4 H. See also dexamethasone.

Tocopherol   See alpha-tocopheryl acetate, and vitamin E.

Tolazamide   2–5 mg/kg (adult 100–250 mg) 6–24 H oral.

Tolazoline   Newborn: 1–2 mg/kg slowly stat (beware hypotension), then 2–6 mcg/kg/min (0.12–0.36 mg/kg/hr) IV. Note: 1–2 mg/kg/hr too much (Pediatrics 1986;77:307).

Tolbutamide   Adult (NOT/kg): initially 1 g 12 H oral, often reducing to 0.5–1 g daily.

Tolfenamic acid   4 mg/kg (adult 200 mg) oral, may repeat once after 2 hr.

Topiramate   1 mg/kg (adult 50 mg) 12–24 H oral, incr if reqd to 4–10 mg/kg (adult 100–500 mg) 12 H. Slow release: same total dose given once a day oral. See also phentermine.

Torasemide   0.1–1 mg/kg (adult 5–50 mg) daily oral or IV. Rarely up to 4 mg/kg (adult 200 mg) daily in renal failure.

Tramadol   2–3 mg/kg (adult 50–100 mg) stat, then 1–2 mg/kg (adult 50–100 mg) 4–6 H (usual max 400 mg/day, up to 600 mg/day) oral or IV over 3 min. Slow release (adult, NOT/kg): 100–300 mg daily oral. IV infusion 2–8 mcg/kg/min.

Tramazoline   Nasal: 82 mcg each nostril x3–6/day. See also dexamethasone + tramazoline.

Trametinib   Adult (NOT/kg): 2 mg daily oral with dabrafenib.

Trandolapril   0.01–0.1 mg/kg (adult 0.5–4 mg) daily oral.
Tranexamic acid   Oral: 15–25 mg/kg (adult 1–1.5 g) 8 H for ≤5 days. IV: 10–15 mg/kg (adult 0.5–1 g) 8 H;
   surgery for cyanotic congenital heart disease 100 mg/kg load, then 10 mg/kg/hr.
Travoprost   40 mcg/mL (0.004%): 1 drop/eye in evening. See also timolol + travoprost.
Trazodone   1–4 mg/kg (adult 50–200 mg) 8 H oral. Slow release (adult, NOT/kg): 75–150 mg each evening
   oral, incr by 75 mg every 3 days to 375–600 mg daily.
Tretinoin   22.5 mg/m^2 12 H oral. Cream or lotion 0.05%, gel 0.01%: apply daily for 3–4 mo, then x1–3/wk.
Triamcinolone   Joint, tendon (NOT/kg): 2.5–15 mg stat. IM: 0.05–0.2 mg/kg every 1–7 days. Cream or
   ointment 0.02%, 0.05%: apply sparingly 6–8 H. Triamcinolone has no mineralcorticoid action, 1 mg = 5 mg
   hydrocortisone in glucocorticoid action. See also gramicidin + neomycin + nystatin + triamcinolone cream
   and ointment.
Triamterene   2 mg/kg (adult 100 mg) 8–24 H oral. See also benzthiazide + triamterene.
Triazolam   0.005–0.01 mg/kg (adult 0.125–0.5 mg) at night oral. 30 min preop: 0.01–0.03 mg/kg (adult
   0.5 mg) oral.
Triclosan   0.5–5% lotion: 2 mL to wet skin for 30 sec, rinse and repeat. Bath oil: 20 mL in 20 cm bath, soak
   15 min.
Triethylenethiophosphoramide   See thiotepa.
Trifluoperazine   0.02–0.4 mg/kg (adult 1–10 mg, occasionally 20 mg) 12 H oral. Capsule: adult 15 mg daily.
Trifluridine   1% soltn: 1 drop/eye 2 H (max 9 drops/day) until epithelialised, then 4 H (max 5 drops/day) for
   7 days.
Trihexyphenidyl   See benzhexol.
Triiodothyronine (T3)   See liothyronine.
Trilostane   0.5–4 mg/kg (adult 30–240 mg) 6 H oral.
Trimethoprim   4 mg/kg (adult 75–150 mg) 12 H, or 6–8 mg/kg (usual max 300 mg) daily oral or IV. Urine
   prophylaxis: 2 mg/kg (adult 150 mg) at night oral.
Trimethoprim + sulphamethoxazole   See cotrimoxazole.
Tropicamide   0.5%, 1%: 1 drop/eye, repeat after 5 min.
Uracil   See tegafur + uracil.
Urea   10% cream: apply 8–12 H.
Urofollitrophin   See follicle stimulating hormone.
Urokinase   4000 U/kg IV over 10 min, then 4000 U/kg/hr for 12 hr (start heparin 3–4 hr later). Blocked
   cannula: instill 5000—25,000 U (NOT/kg) in 2–3 mL saline for 2–4 hr. Empyema: 2 mL/kg of 1500 U/mL in
   saline, position head up/down and right side up/down 30 min each, then drain. Pericard eff: 10,000 U/mL,
   1 mL/kg (max 20 mL), clamp 1 hr, drain.
Ursodeoxycholic acid   5–10 mg/kg (adult 200–400 mg) 12 H oral.
Ursodiol   See ursodeoxycholic acid.
Valaciclovir   20 mg/kg (adult 1 g) 8 H oral. Genital herpes (NOT/kg): treatment 500 mg 12 H, prevention
   500 mg daily (<10 episodes/yr) 1 g daily (>9 episodes/yr). Orolabial: 40 mg/kg (adult 2 g) 12 H for 2 doses.
Valganciclovir   15 mg/kg (max 900 mg) 12 H (treatment) daily (prophylaxis) oral with food.
Valproic acid, valproate   See sodium valproate.
Valrubicin   Adult (NOT/kg): 800 mg wkly x6 intravesical.
Valsartan   0.8–3 mg/kg (adult 40–160 mg) daily oral. See also amlodipine + valsartan, hydrochlorothiazide
   + valsartan.
Vancomycin   Infuse IV over 90 min. Usually 25 mg/kg IV, then 15–20 mg/kg 8–12 H; trough 10–15 mg/L.
   Severe inftn: 30 mg/kg IV, then 15–20 mg/kg 8–12 H; trough 15–20 mg/L, MIC <1 mg/L, AUC/MIC 400. C.
   difficile: 10 mg/kg (adult 500 mg) 6 H oral. Intraventric (NOT/kg): 10 mg 48 H.
Vasopressin, aqueous   IM, SC: 2.5–10 U 6–12 H. IV: put 2–5 U in 1 L fluid, and replace urine output +
   10% each hour. Hypotension (brain death, sepsis, post-bypass): 1 U/kg in 50 mL at 1–3 mL/hr (0.02–0.06
   U/kg/hr) + adrenaline 0.1–0.2 mcg/kg/min. GI hge: 6 U/kg in 50 mL at 1–5 mL/hr IV, 1 mL/hr local IA. See
   desmopressin, lypressin.
Vasopressin, oily   2.5–5 U (NOT/kg) IM every 2–4 days.
Vecuronium   ICU: 0.1 mg/kg p.r.n. IV. Theatre: 0.1 mg/kg stat, then 0.5–2 mcg/kg/min; up to 10 mcg/kg/min
   occasionally.

Venlafaxine   Adult (NOT/kg): 37.5 mg 12 H oral, incr if reqd to max 150 mg 12 H. Slow release: 75 mg daily oral, incr if reqd to max 225 mg daily.

Verapamil   IV: 0.1–0.2 mg/kg (adult 5–10 mg) over 10 min, then 5 mcg/kg/min. Oral: 1–3 mg/kg (adult 80–120 mg) 8–12 H.

Vidarabine   Eye ointment: x5/day until epithelialised, then 12 H 7 days. IV infsn: 10 mg/kg/day 5–10 days (varicella-zoster), 15 mg/kg/day 10 days (herpes encephalitis).

Vigabatrin   25 mg/kg (adult 500 mg) 12 H oral, incr if reqd to max 75 mg/kg (adult 1.5 g) 12 H.

Vitamin A   High risk (NOT/kg): 100,000 i.u. (<8 kg), 200,000 i.u. (>8 kg) oral or IM every 4–6 mo. Severe measles: 400,000 i.u. (NOT/kg) once. Cystic fib: 1500 U daily (<3 yr) 5000 U daily (3–10 yr) 10,000 U daily (>10 yr) oral. >10,000 i.u. daily or >25,000 U per wk may be teratogenic.

Vitamin A, B, C, D compound (Pentavite, infant)   <3 yr (NOT/kg): 0.15 mL daily, incr by 0.15 mL/day to 0.45 mL/day.

Vitamin A, B, C, D compound (Pentavite, child)   <3 yr (NOT/kg): 2.5 mL daily. >3 yr (NOT/kg): 5 mL daily.

Vitamin B group   Amp: IV over 30 min. Tab: 1–2/day.

Vitamin B1   See thiamine.

Vitamin B2   Metabolic disease: 50–150 mg 12–24 H oral.

Vitamin B6   See pyridoxine.

Vitamin B12   See hydroxocobalamin.

Vitamin C   See ascorbic acid.

Vitamin D2   See ergocalciferol.

Vitamin D3   See cholecalciferol.

Vitamin E   1 U = 1 mg. Preterm babies, Coperol E (NOT/kg): 40 U (2 drops) daily oral. CF, malabs: 50–100 U (<3 yr) 200–400 U (>3 yr) daily oral. Cholestasis: 50 U/kg daily oral, incr if reqd in 50 U/kg increments. A-beta-lipoproteinaemia: 35–70 U/kg 8 H oral. HUS: 0.25 g/m^2 6 H oral. See alpha-tocopheryl.

Vitamin K1   See phytomenadione.

Vitamin K3   See menapthone sodium bisulphite.

Vitamins, parenteral   MVI-12 (for adult): 5 mL in 1 L IV fluid. MVI Paediatric, added to IV fluid: 65% of a vial (<3 kg), 1 vial (3 kg to 11 yr).

Vitaprem (RCH: Pentavite, folate, B12, C)   1 mL daily oral.

Von Willebrand factor/Factor VII concentrate (Wilate)   Minor hge: 20–40 IU/kg then 20–30 IU/kg 12–14 H. Surgery: 35–50 IU/kg, then 30–40 IU/kg 12–24 H.

Voriconazole   Oral, IV over 2 hr: child 8 mg/kg load then 7 mg/kg 12 H; adult 6 mg/kg repeated after 12 hr, then 4 mg/kg 12 H. Incr maintenance by 50% if reqd. Trough 1–5 mg/L.

Warfarin   Usually 0.2 mg/kg (adult 5 mg) stat, 0.2 mg/kg (adult 5 mg) next day if INR <1.3, then 0.05–0.2 mg/kg (adult 2–5 mg) daily oral. Usual INR 2–2.5 for prophylaxis, 2–3 for treatment, 3–4 mechanical valve. Beware drug interactions. Severe hge: reverse with either coagulation factor (Prothrombinex) 25 U/kg (adult 500 U) or factor 7a (rFVIIa) 20 mcg/kg, and phytomenadione 0.3 mg/kg (adult 10 mg), and fresh frozen plasma 10 mL/kg; repeat according to INR.

Whole blood   6 mL/kg raises Hb 1 g%. 1 bag = 400 mL approx.

Xylometazoline   <6 yr: 0.05% 1 drop or spray 8–12 H. 6–12 yr: 0.05% 2–3 drops or sprays 8–12 H. >12 yr: 0.1% 2–3 drops or sprays 6–12 H.

Zanamivir   Adult (NOT/kg): 10 mg 12 H for 5 days inhaled. Prophylaxis: 10 mg daily inhaled.

Zileuton   Adult (NOT/kg): 600 mg 6 H oral.

Zinc chloride   5.3 mg/mL = 2.5 mg/mL Zn = 38 μmol/mL Zn. 2–4 μmol/kg/day (<1 yr), 1 μmol/kg/day (child), 40–60 μmol/day (adult). Serum zinc 11–22 μmol/L.

Zinc sulphate   (220 mg cap = 50 mg Zn = 765 μmol Zn). Deficiency, acroderm enteropath: initially 3 mg/kg (adult 220 mg) 8–12 H oral, adjusted to achieve serum zinc 11–22 μmol/L (0.7–1.4 mg/L). Diarrhoea child (NOT/kg): 10–20 mg daily oral.

Zoledronate   0.025–0.05 mg/kg (adult 4 mg) IV over 15 min; usually repeated every 4 wk. Post-menopausal osteoporosis (adult, NOT/kg): 5 mg IV every 1–2 yr.

Zoledronic acid   See zoledronate.

Zolmitriptan   Adult (NOT/kg): 2.5–5 mg oral, repeat in 2 hr if reqd; max 15 mg in 24 hr. Nasal: 5 mg spray in each nostril, repeat in 2 hr if reqd; max twice in 24 hr.

Zolpidem   0.1–0.4 mg/kg (adult 5–20 mg) nocte oral; lower dose for women. Sublingual: 5–10 mg nocte; *Intermezzo* 1.75 mg (women) 3.5 mg (men). Oral spray 5 mg: 1–2 sprays nocte.

Zonisamide   2 mg/kg (adult 100 mg) daily oral, incr if reqd after 2 wk to 12 H, then 3 mg/kg (adult 150 mg) 12 H, then 4 mg/kg (adult 200 mg) 12 H; rarely up to 6 mg/kg (adult 300 mg) 12 H. Level 10–20 mg/L.

Zopiclone   0.1–0.3 mg/kg (adult 5–15 mg) at bedtime oral.

Antimicrobial guidelines

Nigel Curtis
Mike Starr

Paediatric Handbook, Ninth Edition. Edited by Amanda Gwee, Romi Rimer and Michael Marks.

Infection	Likely organisms	Initial antimicrobials[1] 0 = maximum dose	Duration of treatment[2] and other comments
CENTRAL NERVOUS SYSTEM/EYE			
Brain abscess	S. milleri and other streptococci Anaerobes Gram-negatives S. aureus	Flucloxacillin 50 mg/kg (2 g) iv 6 H *and* Third generation cephalosporin[3] *and* Metronidazole 15 mg/kg (1 g) iv stat, then 7.5 mg/kg (500 mg) iv 8 H	3 weeks minimum Penicillin hypersensitivity: substitute Flucloxacillin with Vancomycin 15 mg/kg (500 mg) iv 6 H
Post-neurosurgery	As above plus S. epidermidis	As above but substitute Flucloxacillin with Vancomycin 15 mg/kg (500 mg) iv 6 H	
Encephalitis	Herpes simplex virus Enteroviruses Arboviruses M. pneumoniae	Aciclovir 20 mg/kg iv 8 H (age <3 months) 500 mg/m[2] iv 8 H (age 3 months to 12 years) 10 mg/kg iv 8 H (age >12 years)	3 weeks minimum Consider adding Azithromycin if M. pneumoniae suspected
Meningitis Over 2 months of age	S. pneumoniae[4] N. meningitidis H. influenzae type b[5]	Third generation cephalosporin[3]	S. pneumoniae 10 days N. meningitidis 5–7 days H. influenzae type b 7–10 days Consider addition of Dexamethasone
Over 2 months of age and possibility of penicillin-resistant pneumococci[4] (www.snipurl .com/vanco)	As above	Third generation cephalosporin[3] *and* Vancomycin 15 mg/kg (500 mg) iv 6 H	
Under 2 months of age	As above plus Group B streptococci E. coli and other Gram-negative coliforms L. monocytogenes	Benzylpenicillin 60 mg/kg iv 12 H (1st week of life) 6 H (1–4 weeks of age) 4 H (>4 weeks of age) *and* Third generation cephalosporin[3]	Gram-negative 3 weeks GBS/Listeria 2–3 weeks Substitute Benzylpenicillin with Vancomycin if possibility of penicillin-resistant pneumococci[4]
With shunt infection, post-neurosurgery, head trauma or CSF leak	As for over 2 months of age plus S. epidermidis S. aureus Gram-negative coliforms incl. P. aeruginosa	Vancomycin 15 mg/kg (500 mg) iv 6 H *and* Ceftazidime 50 mg/kg (2 g) iv 8 H	10 days minimum
Contact prophylaxis	N. meningitidis	Rifampicin 10 mg/kg (600 mg) po 12 H	2 days (alternatives: see Table 18.2)
Contact prophylaxis	H. influenzae type b	Rifampicin 20 mg/kg (600 mg) po 24 H	4 days (alternatives: see Table 18.2)

Postseptal (orbital) cellulitis *S. aureus* *H. influenzae* spp. *S. pneumoniae* *M. catarrhalis* Gram-negatives Anaerobes	Flucloxacillin 50 mg/kg (2 g) iv 6 H **and** Third generation cephalosporin[3]	10 days minimum Rule out meningitis Consider adding Metronidazole if not responding
Preseptal (periorbital) cellulitis Mild Group A streptococci *S. aureus* *H. influenzae* spp.	Amoxycillin/clavulanate [400/57 mg per 5 mL] 22.5 mg/kg (875 mg) (Amoxycillin component) = 0.3 mL/kg (11 mL) po 12 H	7–10 days Consider non-infective cause in trivial cases
Severe, or not responding, or under 5 years of age and non-Hib immunised As above plus *H. influenzae* type b[5]	Flucloxacillin 50 mg/kg (2 g) iv 6 H **and** Third generation cephalosporin[3]	
CARDIOVASCULAR		
Endocarditis Native valve or homograft Viridans streptococci Other streptococci *Enterococcus* spp. *S. aureus*	Benzylpenicillin 60 mg/kg (2 g) iv 6 H **and** Flucloxacillin 50 mg/kg (2 g) iv 6 H **and** Gentamicin 7.5 mg/kg (360 mg) iv daily (<10 years) 6 mg/kg (360 mg) iv daily (≥10 years)	4–6 weeks Gentamicin 1 mg/kg (80 mg) iv 8 H for 1–2 weeks when used only for synergy (Gentamicin monitoring is generally not required with low dose in this setting)
Artificial valve or post surgery As above plus *S. epidermidis*	Vancomycin 15 mg/kg (500 mg) iv 6 H **and** Flucloxacillin 50 mg/kg (2 g) iv 6 H **and** Gentamicin 7.5 mg/kg (360 mg) iv daily (<10 years) 6 mg/kg (360 mg) iv daily (≥10 years)	
Endocarditis prophylaxis For dental procedures only Viridans streptococci *S. aureus* *S. pneumoniae* Other Gram-positive cocci *Enterococcus* spp.	Amoxycillin 50 mg/kg (2 g) Local anaesthetic: give po 1 hour before procedure General anaesthetic: give iv with induction	Penicillin hypersensitivity: substitute Amoxycillin with Clindamycin 20 mg/kg (600 mg) po or iv

Infection	Likely organisms	Initial antimicrobials[1] () = maximum dose	Duration of treatment[2] and other comments
GASTROINTESTINAL			
Diarrhoea *Salmonella* spp. isolated in infant under 3 months of age or in immunocompromised	*Salmonella* spp.	Third generation cephalosporin[3]	5–7 days Antibiotic treatment is generally unnecessary for most other organisms
Antibiotic associated	*C. difficile*	Metronidazole 7.5 mg/kg (400 mg) po 8 H	7–10 days
Giardiasis	*G. lamblia*	Metronidazole 30 mg/kg (2 g) po daily *or* Tinidazole 50 mg/kg (2 g) po stat	3 days Single dose
Peritonitis or ascending cholangitis	Gram-negative coliforms Anaerobes *Enterococcus* spp.	Ampicillin or Amoxycillin 50 mg/kg (2 g) iv 6 H *and* Gentamicin 7.5 mg/kg (360 mg) iv daily (<10 years) 6 mg/kg (360 mg) iv daily (≥10 years) *and* Metronidazole 15 mg/kg (1 g) iv stat, then 7.5 mg/kg (500 mg) iv 8 H	Up to 14 days See footnote 6 re Gentamicin dosing/monitoring
Threadworm (Pinworm)	*Enterobius vermicularis*	Mebendazole 50 mg po (<10 kg) 100 mg po (≥10 kg) *or* Pyrantel 10 mg/kg (1 g) po daily	Single dose; may need to repeat after 14 days 3 days Treat whole family
GENITOURINARY			
Urinary tract infection Over 6 months of age and not sick	*E. coli* *P. mirabilis* *K. oxytoca* Other Gram-negatives	Trimethoprim 4 mg/kg (150 mg) po 12 H *or* Co-trimoxazole (Trimethoprim/Sulphamethoxazole 8/40 mg/mL) 0.5 mL/kg (20 mL) po 12 H	5 days
Under 6 months of age or sick or acute pyelonephritis	As above plus *Enterococcus* spp.	Benzylpenicillin 60 mg/kg (2 g) iv 6 H *and* Gentamicin 7.5 mg/kg (360 mg) iv daily (<10 years) 6 mg/kg (360 mg) iv daily (≥10 years) 5 mg/kg (360 mg) iv daily (1st week of life)	5–7 days for UTI 10–14 days for pyelonephritis See footnote 6 re Gentamicin dosing/monitoring
Prophylaxis	As above	Trimethoprim 2 mg/kg (150 mg) po daily *or* Co-trimoxazole (Trimethoprim/Sulphamethoxazole 8/40 mg/mL) 0.25 mL/kg (20 mL) po daily	Routine prophylaxis is no longer recommended

RESPIRATORY

Epiglottitis	*H. influenzae* type b[5]	Ceftriaxone 50 mg/kg (1 g) iv daily	5 days Consider addition of Dexamethasone
Gingivostomatitis In immunocompromised	Herpes simplex virus	Aciclovir 500 mg/m^2 iv 8 H (age 3 months to 12 years) 10 mg/kg iv 8 H (age >12 years)	7 days Treatment is only recommended in the immunocompromised
Otitis externa Acute diffuse	*S. aureus* *S. epidermidis* *P. aeruginosa* *Proteus* spp. *Klebsiella* spp.	Topical steroid/antibiotic drops	7 days Clean ear canal (± insertion of wick soaked in drops if ear canal oedematous)
Acute localised (furuncle) ± cellulitis	*S. aureus* Group A streptococci	Flucloxacillin 50 mg/kg (2 g) iv 6 H	5 days
Failure of first-line treatment, high fever or severe persistent pain	As above plus *P. aeruginosa*	Ticarcillin/Clavulanate 50 mg/kg (3 g) (Ticarcillin component) iv 6 H	14 days minimum Consider fungal infection
Otitis media	Viruses *S. pneumoniae* *M. catarrhalis* *H. influenzae* spp. Group A streptococci	Consider no antibiotics for 48 hours if over 6 months of age *or* Amoxicillin 15 mg/kg (500 mg) po 8 H	5 days Consider Amoxycillin/Clavulanate after 48 hours if inadequate response to Amoxycillin
Pertussis	*B. pertussis*	Azithromycin 10 mg/kg (500 mg) daily *or* Clarithromycin 7.5 mg/kg (500 mg) po 12 H	5 days 7 days Can be given up to 3 weeks after contact with index case or if symptoms <3 weeks

(continued)

Infection	Likely organisms	Initial antimicrobials[1] () = maximum dose	Duration of treatment[2] and other comments
Pneumonia Mild (outpatient)	Viruses S. pneumoniae H. influenzae spp.	Amoxycillin 25 mg/kg (500 mg) po 8 H	5 days
Moderate (inpatient)	As above	Benzylpenicillin 60 mg/kg (2 g) iv 6 H	
Severe systemic toxicity or pneumatocoele	As above plus S. aureus Group A streptococci Gram-negatives	Flucloxacillin 50 mg/kg (2 g) iv 6 H **and** Third generation cephalosporin[3]	10 days minimum Consider adding Azithromycin 15 mg/kg (500 mg) iv stat, then 5 mg/kg (200 mg) iv daily to cover M. pneumoniae and other atypical pathogens
Tonsillitis	Viruses Group A streptococci	Consider no antibiotics (particularly if <4 years) *or* Phenoxymethylpenicillin (Penicillin V) 250 mg po 12 H (<10 years) 500 mg po 12 H (≥10 years)	10 days
SKIN/SOFT TISSUE/BONE			
Bites (animal/human)	Viridans streptococci S. aureus Group A streptococci Oral anaerobes E. corrodens Pasteurella spp. (cat and dog) C. canimorsus (dog)	Amoxycillin/Clavulanate (400/57 mg/5 mL). 22.5 mg/kg (875 mg) (Amoxycillin component) 0.3 mL/kg (11 mL) po 12 H	5 days for infected bite For otherwise healthy individuals, antibiotic therapy is usually not necessary for bites with a low risk of infection Check tetanus immunisation status
If severe, penetrating injuries, esp. involving joints or tendons	As above	Ticarcillin/Clavulanate 50 mg/kg (3 g) (Ticarcillin component) iv 6 H	14 days
Cellulitis Mild (outpatient)	Group A streptococci S. aureus	Cephalexin 25 mg/kg (500 mg) po 6 H *or* Cephalexin 33 mg/kg (500 mg) po 8 H	5–10 days
Moderate/severe (inpatient)	As above	Flucloxacillin 50 mg/kg (2 g) iv 6 H	

(continued)

Facial cellulitis in child under 5 yr of age and non-Hib immunised	As above plus *S. pneumoniae* *H. influenzae* spp.[5]	Flucloxacillin 50 mg/kg (2 g) iv 6 H *and* Third generation cephalosporin[3]	
Necrotising fasciitis	As above	Vancomycin 15 mg/kg (500 mg) iv 6 H *and* Meropenem 25 mg/kg (1 g) iv 8 H *and* Clindamycin 15 mg/kg (600 mg) iv 8 H	Consider IVIG
Head lice	*Pediculus humanus* var. *capitis*	1% permethrin liquid or cream rinse	Repeat after one week
Impetigo	Group A streptococci *S. aureus*	Mupirocin 2% ointment top 8 H if localised *or* Cephalexin 33 mg/kg (500 mg) po 8 H	5–10 days
Lymphadenitis (cervical) Mild	*S. aureus* Group A streptococci Oral anaerobes	Cephalexin 25 mg/kg (500 mg) po 6 H *or* Cephalexin 33 mg/kg (500 mg) po 8 H	7 days
Severe	As above	Flucloxacillin 50 mg/kg (2 g) iv 6 H	
Osteomyelitis Uncomplicated	*S. aureus* Group A streptococci *S. pneumoniae*	Flucloxacillin 50 mg/kg (2 g) iv 6 H	3 weeks for uncomplicated cases[2]
If under 5 yr of age and non-Hib immunised	As above plus *H. influenzae* type b[5]	Flucloxacillin 50 mg/kg (2 g) iv 6 H *and* Third generation cephalosporin[3]	
In patient with sickle cell anaemia	As above plus *Salmonella* spp.	Flucloxacillin 50 mg/kg (2 g) iv 6 H *and* Third generation cephalosporin[3]	
With penetrating foot injury	As above plus *P. aeruginosa*	Ticarcillin/Clavulanate 50 mg/kg (3 g) (Ticarcillin component) iv 6 H	Surgical intervention important

(continued)

489

Infection	Likely organisms	Initial antimicrobials[1] () = maximum dose	Duration of treatment[2] and other comments
Scabies	Sarcoptes scabiei	Permethrin 5% cream top	One application from neck down; leave on for minimum of 8 H (usually overnight) May need to repeat after 7 days Treat whole family
Septic arthritis	As for osteomyelitis	As for osteomyelitis	3 weeks for uncomplicated cases.[2] Always consider surgical drainage
Shingles In immunocompromised or involving eye	Varicella zoster virus	Aciclovir 500 mg/m[2] iv 8 H (age 3 months to 12 years) and 10 mg/kg iv 8 H (age >12 years) and Aciclovir ointment to eye 5 times per day	7 days Shingles in immunocompetent children does not generally require treatment
SEPTICAEMIA (UNDER 2 MONTHS OF AGE)			
Septicaemia Community-acquired infection	Group B streptococci E. coli and other Gram-negative coliforms L. monocytogenes H. influenzae spp.[5] plus those listed below for 'Septicaemia with unknown CSF'	Benzylpenicillin 60 mg/kg iv 12 H (1st week of life) 6 H (1–4 weeks of age) 4 H (>4 weeks of age) and Third generation cephalosporin[3]	Add Flucloxacillin 50 mg/kg iv 12 H (1st week of life) 8 H (1–4 weeks of age) 6 H (>4 weeks of age) if infection with S. aureus suspected (e.g. umbilical infection) Duration depends on culture results Premature neonates require special dosing consideration
If abdominal source suspected	As above plus Anaerobes	Amoxicillin or Ampicillin 50 mg/kg (2 g) iv 6 H and Gentamicin 5 mg/kg iv 24 H (1st week of life) 7.5 mg/kg iv daily thereafter and Metronidazole 15 mg/kg iv stat, then 7.5 mg/kg iv 8 H	
SEPTICAEMIA (OVER 2 MONTHS OF AGE)			
Septicaemia with unknown CSF	S. pneumoniae[4] N. meningitidis S. aureus Group A streptococci Gram-negatives	Flucloxacillin 50 mg/kg (2 g) iv 6 H and Third generation cephalosporin[3]	Substitute Flucloxacillin with Vancomycin 15 mg/kg (500 mg) iv 6 H if central line in situ or suspected MRSA infection Consider adding IVIG and Clindamycin 15 mg/kg (600 mg) iv 8 H if suspect Gram-positive toxic shock syndrome Duration depends on culture results

(continued)

490

Septicaemia with normal CSF	As above	Flucloxacillin 50 mg/kg (2 g) iv 6 H *and* Gentamicin 7.5 mg/kg (360 mg) iv daily (<10 years) 6 mg/kg (360 mg) iv daily (≥10 years)	
In non-Hib immunised	As above plus *H. influenzae* type b[5]	Flucloxacillin 50 mg/kg (2 g) iv 6 H *and* Third generation cephalosporin[3]	
In neutropenic patient	As above plus *Enterococcus* spp. *P. aeruginosa*	Piperacillin/Tazobactam 100 mg/kg (4 g) (Piperacillin component) iv 6 H (8 H if <6 months) *and* Amikacin 22.5 mg/kg (1.5 g) iv daily (<10 years) 18 mg/kg (1.5 g) iv daily (≥10 years)	Local protocols for fever and neutropenia may differ Target trough (<2 mg/L pre 3rd dose)
In neutropenic patient with potential line infection	As above plus Gram-positive cocci incl. *S. epidermidis*	Piperacillin/Tazobactam as above *and* Amikacin as above *and* consider Vancomycin 15 mg/kg (500 mg) iv 6 H	

Notes to antimicrobial guidelines

- Further information available at www.snipurl.com/RCHantibiotics.
- These guidelines have been developed to assist doctors with their choice of initial empiric treatment.
- Except where specified, they **do not apply to neonates or immunocompromised patients**.
- Always ask about previous hypersensitivity reactions to antibiotic.
- The choice of antimicrobial, dose and frequency of administration for continuing treatment may require adjustment according to the clinical situation.
- The recommendations are not intended to be prescriptive and alternative regimens may also be appropriate.

1 Antimicrobial choice and dose

- Antibiotics should be changed to narrow spectrum agents once sensitivities are known.
- Dose adjustments may be necessary for neonates, and for children with renal or hepatic impairment.
- Alternative antimicrobial regimens may be more appropriate for neonates, immunocompromised patients or others with a special infection risk (e.g. cystic fibrosis, sickle cell anaemia).
- Resistance to antimicrobials is an increasing problem worldwide. Of particular concern is the increasing incidence of penicillin-resistant pneumococci (see footnote 4). It is important to take into account local resistance patterns when using these guidelines.

2 Duration of treatment

Duration of treatment is given as a guide only and may vary with the clinical situation. 'Step down' from intravenous to oral treatment is appropriate in many cases. **Durations given generally refer to the minimum total intravenous and oral treatment.**

3 Third generation cephalosporins

Cefotaxime: 50 mg/kg (2 g) iv 6 H
Ceftriaxone: usual 50 mg/kg (2 g) iv daily;

severe (including meningitis and brain abscess) 100 mg/kg (2 g) iv daily or 50 mg/kg (1 g) iv 12 H.
NB. Ceftriaxone should be avoided in neonates, particularly if <41 weeks gestation, jaundiced or receiving calcium containing solutions, including TPN.

4 Penicillin-resistant pneumococci (www.snipurl.com/vanco)

The prevalence of invasive strains that are highly resistant to Penicillin or cephalosporins in Melbourne remains low. A third generation cephalosporin remains the drug of first choice for the empiric treatment of meningitis. However, Vancomycin should be added if *S. pneumoniae* is suspected (www.snipurl.com/vanco). This should be stopped if sensitivity to a third generation cephalosporin is shown, as will be the case with most isolates. The prevalence of resistant strains is being monitored and this recommendation may change.

Penicillin remains the drug of first choice for the empiric treatment of suspected pneumococcal pneumonia and other non-CNS infections, regardless of susceptibility. High doses of penicillin overcome resistance in this setting and should be used for confirmed non-CNS infection caused by penicillin-resistant pneumococci.

5 Invasive *H. influenzae* type b disease

Since the introduction of *H. influenzae* type b (Hib) immunisation, there has been a dramatic decline in the incidence of invasive disease. However, in children with potential invasive disease, who are not fully immunised against Hib, therapy should include cover against Hib.

6 Gentamicin therapeutic dose monitoring

Once-daily administration of Gentamicin is safe and effective for most patients. Certain patients, such as neonates and those with cystic fibrosis, endocarditis or renal failure, may require special dosing consideration.

The regimen for monitoring Gentamicin levels is different for once-daily and 8, 12 or 18 H dosing, and depends on renal function:

(continued)

Once-daily dosing
- Normal renal function – if the patient is to have more than 3 doses, the trough level (pre-dose) should be checked before the third dose and then every 3 days (target level <1 mg/L).
- Abnormal renal function – trough levels may need to be checked earlier and more frequently (target level <1 mg/L).
- Renal failure – levels should be checked prior to each dose and the results should be discussed with a specialist familiar with therapeutic drug monitoring before the next dose is given.

7 Vancomycin therapeutic drug monitoring
- Target trough level 10–15 mg/L for most infections.
- Severe infections may require higher trough levels.

APPENDIX 4
Formulae

ETT tube size and position (p. 1)
Neonates Table 21.1, p. 333
Tube size (internal diameter) = (age/4) + 4 mm (for patients over 1 year of age)
Depth of insertion is approximately (age/2) + 12 cm from the lower lip

Anion gap (p. 328)
Anion gap = Na − bicarbonate − Cl

Bicarbonate administration (pp. 109, 188)
mmol of HCO_3 required = basic deficit (mmol/L) × weight (kg) × 0.3 (child)
mmol of HCO_3 required = basic deficit (mmol/L) × weight (kg) × 0.5 (newborn)
Infuse half with cardiac monitoring, then reassess

Dose Na replacement (p. 112)
Dose of Na^+ (mmol) = bodyweight × 0.8 × (140 − current serum Na^+)

Additives (p. 109)
Molar potassium chloride (0.75 g in 10 mL) = 1 mmol/mL of K^+ and Cl^-
Sodium chloride (20%) = 3.4 mmol/mL of Na^+ and Cl^-
Molar sodium bicarbonate (8.4%) = 1 mmol/mL of Na^+ and HCO_3^-
Calcium gluconate 10% = 0.22 mmol/mL of Ca^{2+}, which is 8.9 mg/mL of Ca^{2+}
Magnesium chloride for injection (0.48 g anhydrous in 5 mL) = 1 mmol/mL of Mg^{2+}

Conversion factors
Sodium chloride 1 g contains 17 mmol Na and 17 mmol Cl
Potassium chloride 1 g contains 13 mmol K and 13 mmol Cl
Sodium bicarbonate 1 g contains 12 mmol Na and 12 mmol HCO_3

Formulae
Anion gap = Na − (bicarbonate + Cl); normal <12
Number mmol = mEq/valence = mass (mg)/mol. wt
Sodium deficit: mL 20% NaCl = wt × 0.2 × (140 − serum Na)
Water deficit (mL) = 600 × wt (kg) × [1 − (140/Na)] (if body Na normal)
Non-catabolic anuria: urea rises of 3−5 mmol/L per day

kcal (p. 119)

$$kcal = \frac{mJ \times 1000}{4.2}$$

Estimated weight
Weight = (age + 4) × 2

Surface area (p. 437)

$$\text{Surface area (m}^2\text{)} = \sqrt{\frac{\text{height (cm)} \times \text{weight (kg)}}{3600}}$$

Paediatric Handbook, Ninth Edition. Edited by Amanda Gwee, Romi Rimer and Michael Marks.
© 2015 John Wiley & Sons, Ltd. Published 2015 by John Wiley & Sons, Ltd.

BMI (p. 206)

BMI = bodyweight in kg divided by the square of height in metres (kg/m^2); standard growth charts now include BMI centile charts.

- Overweight = BMI between 85th and 95th centile for age and sex
- Obesity = BMI greater than 95th centile for age and sex

Osmolality (p. 186)

Calculated values

Serum osmolality = ($Na^+ \times 2$) + glucose + urea

Adjusted Na^+ = plasma Na^+ + 0.3 × (plasma glucose − 5.5)

Normal (270 − 295 mmol/L)

Transfusion volume (p. 171)

Packed red cells (mL) = weight (kg) × Hb rise required (g/L) × 0.4

Index

Paediatric Handbook, Ninth Edition. Edited by Amanda Gwee, Romi Rimer and Michael Marks.
© 2015 John Wiley & Sons, Ltd. Published 2015 by John Wiley & Sons, Ltd.

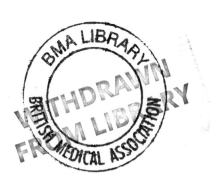